Clinical Voice Pathology

Theory and Management

Fifth Edition

Clinical Voice Pathology

Theory and Management

Fifth Edition

Joseph C. Stemple, PhD, CCC-SLP, ASHAF
Nelson Roy, PhD, CCC-SLP, ASHAF
Bernice K. Klaben, PhD, CCC-SLP, BRS-S

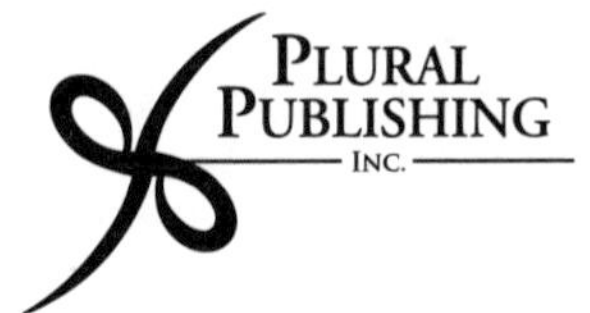

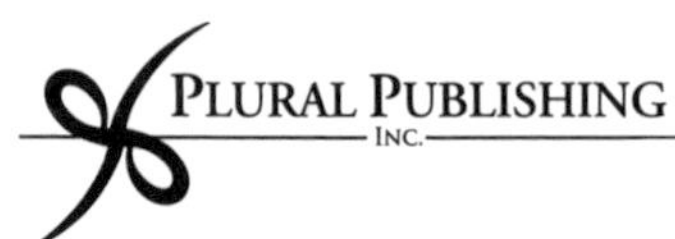

5521 Ruffin Road
San Diego, CA 92123

e-mail: info@pluralpublishing.com
Website: http://www.pluralpublishing.com

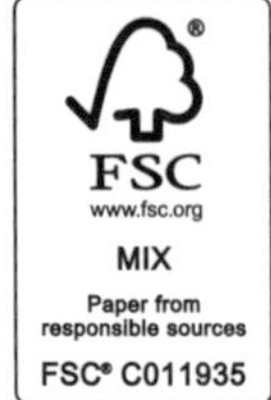

Typeset in 11/13 Garamond by Flanagan's Publishing Service, Inc.
Printed in the United States of America by McNaughton & Gunn, Inc.
17 16 15 14 2 3 4 5

Library of Congress Cataloging-in-Publication Data

Stemple, Joseph C., author.
Clinical voice pathology : theory and management / Joseph C. Stemple, Nelson Roy, Bernice Klaben.—Fifth edition.
p. ; cm.
Includes bibliographical references and index.
ISBN-13: 978-1-59756-556-1 (alk. paper)
ISBN-10: 1-59756-556-3 (alk. paper)
I. Roy, Nelson, author. II. Klaben, Bernice, author. III. Title.
[DNLM: 1. Voice Disorders. WV 500]
RF510
616.2'2—dc23

2013042556

Contents

Preface

This fifth edition of *Clinical Voice Pathology: Theory and Management* marks the 30-year anniversary of this text. As this preface is written, the memories of 1984 are in the forefront of our minds. It was an exciting time for the profession—the beginning of a new age of voice pathology. Desktop computers were new and provided clinicians the opportunity to instrumentally assess voice production. Laryngeal videostroboscopy was introduced as a voice care tool, and the importance of preserving the vocal fold cover was realized. To understand the influence and growth of technology in the field, one need only observe the differences between the Apple IIE computer that was used to prepare the first edition of this text and the iMac being used today for the fifth edition. We have seen remarkable changes in these 30 years.

This edition also introduces the end of one era and the beginning of another. The past 3 editions have included the wonderful contributions of our friend and colleague Dr Leslie Glaze. Her scientific knowledge, masterful writing, and attention to detail have all added to the quality and fabric of this text. Leslie is now enjoying retirement, but her influence upon this text will live through this and future editions of *Clinical Voice Pathology: Theory and Management*.

We are excited to introduce Dr Nelson Roy as a new coauthor for this fifth edition. Dr Roy's research and clinical contributions to the field of voice pathology are nationally and internationally recognized. He is a master clinician and scientist who will continue the tradition of "clinical scientist as author." We are pleased to have Nelson on board and know that his contributions will enhance the quality of the learning experience for our students and professionals alike.

The advances in our field in the past 30 years have been extraordinary. However, when one studies the history of our specialty, it is remarkable how much of our past remains in terms of assessment and treatment. As an example, with all the available technology to aid in voice evaluation, we would submit that the skilled patient interview remains the most important part of the voice assessment. In the same vein, many of the therapy techniques that we currently use have their foundations in skills that were practiced centuries ago to enhance singing and speaking voices. The advances in our knowledge have significantly enhanced the diagnostic process and have helped confirm whether our chosen treatments are truly effective.

The authors of this text have been privileged to serve those with voice disorders for many years. While we have had the opportunity to work in clinical voice centers, side-by-side with our laryngology partners, we fully understand that voice therapy is needed and provided in practically every setting in which speech-language pathologists work. This text is designed to help prepare all clinicians, not only those who specialize in the area of voice, to evaluate and treat voice disorders. This unique and eclectic population of patients encompasses all ages across the life span and represents etiologies arising from medical, environmental, social, psychological, and occupational threats to vocal health. Our patients may be typical voice users, occupational voice users, elite vocal performers, individuals with head and neck cancer, and others who suffer with upper airway symptoms. Each patient provides us with a unique diagnostic dilemma: How do we best return the voice to optimal condition?

This text is organized to systematically build the knowledge base and clinical skills necessary to successfully answer this question. We seek to organize, explain, and illustrate the comprehensive hierarchy of knowledge necessary to manage the many types of voice disorders. **Chapter 1** begins with an entertaining history of voice disorders from ancient foundations to the present. This information clarifies the role of speech-language pathologists in the care of voice-disordered patients and introduces the interdisciplinary background that has permeated our history of successful voice therapy.

A progressive development of essential clinical knowledge areas begins with **Chapter 2**, the anatomy and physiology of voice production. Understanding the structure and function of the laryngeal mechanism is an essential basis for evaluating phonatory function, examining the larynx and vocal folds, recognizing the impact of abnormal changes or adaptations on voice production, and sharing information with our physician partners in care. This fifth edition updates the descriptions of the 3 subsystems of voice production—respiration, phonation, and resonance—and expands the discussion of vocal fold histology and DNA microarray gene expression analysis.

Chapter 3 provides a thorough update on the common etiologies of voice disorders including behavioral, medical, and personality related. Common factors associated with the cause and maintenance of voice disorders are discussed to understand best options for treatment planning.

Chapter 4 presents the pathologies of the laryngeal mechanism, organized according to the *Classification Manual for Voice Disorders-I* developed by Special Interest Division 3 (Voice and Voice Disorders) of the American Speech-Language-Hearing Association (2006). The pathologies are presented in 8 major groups: (1) structural pathologies; (2) inflammatory conditions; (3) trauma or injury; (4) systemic conditions affecting voice; (5) aerodigestive conditions affecting voice; (6) psychiatric or psychological disorders affecting voice; (7) neurologic voice disorders; and (8) other disorders of voice. Many of the pathologies are illustrated with color plates.

Chapters 5 and 6 discuss the objectives and procedures of a systematic diagnostic voice evaluation. Chapter 5 introduces traditional evaluation techniques, including the patient interview, audioperceptual judgments, patient self-assessment, determining the cause(s) and maintaining factor(s) of the voice disorder, and educating the patient about these findings to establish a collaborative management plan based on these clinical data. Chapter 6 provides a state-of-the-art overview of the instrumental measures that comprise a comprehensive voice assessment, including the scientific principles that underlie their development, application, and interpretation. In addition to standard measures of acoustics, aerodynamics, electromyography, and stroboscopy, this edition explains the utility of high-speed digital imaging and videokymography tools. The appendix includes instrumental measurement norms and a helpful glossary of terms.

Knowledge of anatomy and physiology, pathologies, etiologies, and the diagnostic process have prepared the reader for **Chapter 7** that explores an array of voice therapy approaches following the orientations of hygienic, symptomatic, psychogenic, physiologic, and eclectic treatments. Using patient cases to illustrate major insights about voice treatment that we have each gathered from our 30-plus years of clinical experience, we orient the reader to the theories, selection criteria, and clinical methods for specific voice management principles. This treatment framework is appropriate for common, yet diverse voice complaints due to a variety of laryngeal pathologies and vocal dysfunctions. Finally, we highlight the current clinical evidence that either supports or refutes popular treatments used in voice therapy.

Because of the exceptional concerns of voice performers, **Chapter 8** introduces the factors that influence clinical management approaches for this artistic population, such as personalities, temperament, performance routines and schedule, and other special considerations needed for their care and treatment. The chapter defines the roles of the expanded interdisciplinary team and identifies the affiliate organizations that represent and support voice performers. In addition to traditional voice therapy considerations, the chapter discusses nontraditional alternative treatments that are popular with this population.

Chapter 9, Rehabilitation of the Laryngectomized Patient, serves as a stand-alone manual on the management of this special patient population. This chapter reflects the current "best practice" in voice rehabilitation or restoration in head and neck cancer patients. By outlining the complementary roles of the interdisciplinary treatment team, we understand the multiple management goals: cure the disease; select optimal communication methods; ensure safe swallowing; and address any associated physical, social, and emotional changes that affect each patient. The chapter also contains photographs of the latest communication and airway management devices currently on the market.

Over the past four decades, our chosen specialty of clinical voice pathology has expanded greatly within the field of communication disorders. Nonetheless, this fifth edition of our text retains its original purpose: to provide students and clinicians with a strong foundation of basic voice science infused with a deep clinical understanding of the best methods for assessing and treating voice disorders. We hope that you, the reader, will find this text clear, informative, and a worthwhile addition to your professional library.

As always, text development requires a team. We are indebted to Angie Singh, Valerie Johns, Milgem Rabanera, and McKenna Bailey for encouraging and supporting this fifth edition. In addition, we wish to thank our students and colleagues who have suggested ways to improve the text with each new writing. Finally, it is our patients who have taught us so much about what is important in the care of their voices and to them we are greatly indebted.

Joseph C. Stemple,
Nelson Roy, and
Bernice K. Klaben

1

Voice: A Historical Perspective

Voice, articulation, and language are the major elements of human speech production. When a disorder related to any of these elements is present, the ability to communicate may be impaired. Voice is the element of speech that provides the speaker with the vibratory signal upon which speech is carried. Regarded as magical and mystical in ancient times, today the production of voice is viewed as both a powerful communication tool and an artistic medium. It serves as the melody of our speech and provides expression, feeling, intent, and mood to our daily articulated thoughts. As it is expressed artistically through the many varieties of vocal performance, voice provides great expression and joy for both the listener and the performer.

This text is concerned with the study of both normal and disordered voice production. It is meant to introduce the reader to the science of voice production, the causes of voice disorders, and the pathologies of vocal function. You will explore methods of evaluation of voice disorders and delve into the wide array of management techniques; all are designed to return the pathologic voice to an improved state of equilibrium. Treating voice disorders is extremely rewarding. The vast majority of patients with vocal difficulties who follow the prescribed treatment plans significantly improve their voice quality in a relatively short period of time.

A voice disorder exists when a person's quality, pitch, and loudness differ from those of people of similar age, gender, cultural background, and geographic location.[1–4] In other words, when the perceptual properties of voice are so deviant that they draw attention to the speaker, a voice disorder may be present. A voice disorder also may exist when the structure and/or function of the laryngeal mechanism no longer meet the voicing requirements established for the mechanism by the speaker. These requirements include vocal difficulties that others do not readily recognize, such as the negative effects of vocal fatigue or instability in the singing voice, but are reported to be present by the speaker. Successful management of a voice disorder is dependent on the individual recognizing the problem and accepting the need for improvement.

The effects of a voice disorder depend on the voicing needs of the individual. Those with a great need for normal voice production, such as professional voice users, may be unusually concerned with the presence of even minor vocal difficulties. Those with low vocal needs may not be greatly concerned with even more severe vocal problems. Identifying the vocal needs of each patient is extremely important in successfully treating voice disorders.[5]

The speech-language pathologist (SLP) plays a major role in the evaluation and management of voice disorders. This role focuses on three major goals: (1) evaluation of laryngeal function using auditory and visual perceptual tasks, acoustic analysis, and aerodynamic measures of vocal function; (2) identification and modification or elimination of the functional causes that have led to the development of the voice disorder; and (3) development of a therapy plan that will remediate the voice disorder and return the voice to improved function. To accomplish these goals, SLPs must have an extensive understanding and knowledge of the normal anatomy and physiology of the laryngeal mechanism, as well as knowledge of common laryngeal pathologies. They also must understand etiologic factors that lead to the development of voice disorders, as well as appropriate diagnostic techniques and skills for discovering the causes. Finally, based on previous knowledge, SLPs must develop a bank of clinical management approaches for remediating the voice disorder.

Speech-language pathologists have been involved in the evaluation and management of voice disorders since the beginning of our profession in the 1930s.[6,7] The advent of voice therapy was a unique blend of the knowledge that speech correctionists, as speech-language pathologists were then called, gained from training in the areas of public speaking, oral interpretation, and theater arts. This training was combined with understanding in the areas of anatomy, physiology, psychology, and pathologies of the laryngeal mechanism. In more recent history, voice pathologists have been required to also gain knowledge in other areas such as vocal fold histology, biomechanics of laryngeal tissue, voice acoustics, aerodynamics of voice production, and visual imaging and interpretation of vocal function.[8–13] (SLPs who specialize in voice disorders are often called voice pathologists; both terms will be used in this text.) These years during which SLPs have dealt with the remediation of voice disorders represent only a small segment of time when compared with the total history of the evaluation and treatment of voice disorders. We begin by looking to the past as a means of gaining an understanding and appreciation of the current knowledge of clinical voice pathology.

ANCIENT HISTORY

The earliest accounts of voice disorders, as with other medical information, were handed down orally. These accounts were mainly represented by folk remedies for various recognized disorders. Folklore remedies for disorders of the throat included rubbing liniment derived from centipedes on the neck, gargling the juice of crabs, and inhaling the ashes of a burned swallow. Plant remedies included gargles made from cabbage, garlic, nettles, pennyroyal, and sorrel. Wearing beads of various kinds or a black silk cord around the throat was also recommended, as was the excommunication of sore throats in the name of God.[14]

One of the earliest written histories of a voice disorder was presented about 1600 BC in the Edwin Smith Papyrus. One of many Egyptian papyri discovered in burial tombs, the Edwin Smith Papyrus contained early medical writings. It described 50 traumatic surgical cases, beginning with injuries to the head and continuing down the body to the thorax. One of these cases was a detailed description of a crushing injury to the neck, which caused the loss of speech. The Egyptian writings contained a hieroglyph portraying the lungs and trachea (Figure 1–1). The larynx was not pictured because no organ for voice had yet been identified.[15]

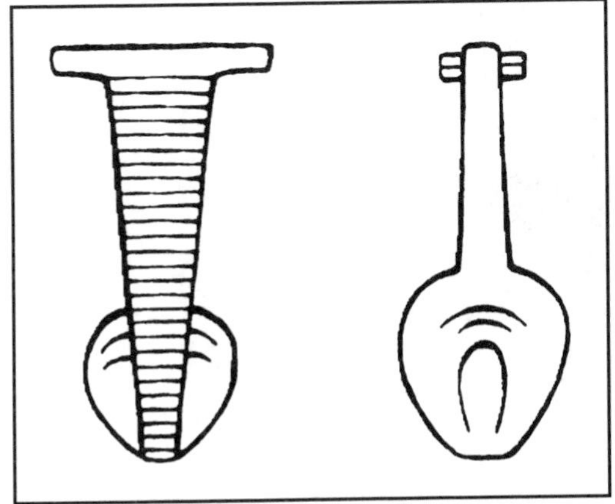

FIGURE 1–1. Egyptian hieroglyph of the trachea and lungs.

The ancient Hindu civilization presented much medical information including mention of diseases of the throat. The most notable information was presented in the Sanskrit-Atharva-Veda (700 BC). Among the Hindus, surgical achievements included tonsillectomy and rhinoplasty. Nose flaps became a necessity in this civilization, for cutting off the nose was the corporal punishment for adultery. Hindu gargles for throat disorders included oils, vinegar, honey, the juices of fruit, and the urine of sacred cows.[16]

In the fifth century BC, Hippocrates, the "Father of Medicine," was responsible for finally separating medicine from magic. One of Hippocrates' greatest contributions to medicine was his insistence on the value of observation. Hippocrates made many observations regarding diseases associated with the throat and voice, although he, too, failed to identify the source of voice. Several of these observations, as translated by Chadwick and Mann,[17] include the following:

- Aphorism 58: Commotion of the brain, from any cause, is inevitably followed by loss of voice.
- Coan Prognosis 240: Aphonia is of the most serious significance if accompanied by weakness.
- Coan Prognosis 243: Aphonia during fever in the manner of that seen in seizure, associated with a quiet delirium, is fatal.
- Coan Prognosis 252: A shrill, whining voice and dimness of the eyes denote a spasm.

These examples demonstrate that Hippocrates studied symptoms more than treatments of diseases. Hippocrates was the first person to write that observation of voice quality, whether it be clear or hoarse, is one means by which a physical diagnosis may be reached.[17]

Observation of voice quality remains a powerful diagnostic tool.

Aristotle was the first writer to refer to the larynx as the organ from which the voice emanates. In his *Historia Animalium*,[18] written in the late fourth century BC, he stated that the neck was the part of the body between the face and the trunk, with the front being the larynx and the back, the gullet. He further stated that phonation and respiration took place through the larynx and the windpipe.[15]

This information lay dormant until five centuries later when the first true anatomist, Claudius Galenus, was born in Asia Minor in 131 AD. Galen (Figure 1–2) derived his knowledge of anatomy from the dissection of animals. He greatly advanced the knowledge of the upper air passages and the larynx and described the warming and filtering functions of the nose. He also distinguished six pairs of intralaryngeal muscles and divided them into abductor and adductor muscles. The thyroid, cricoid, and arytenoid cartilages were described, as was the activity of the recurrent laryngeal nerves.

In experiments with pigs, Galen demonstrated that pigs would always cease squealing when the recurrent laryngeal nerve was severed. This led him to conclude that muscles move certain parts of the body on which breathing and voice depend and that these muscle movements are dependent on nerves from the brain. Galen, therefore, proved that the larynx was the organ of voice, thus disproving that the "voice was sent forth by the heart,"[14] which was still a popular belief.

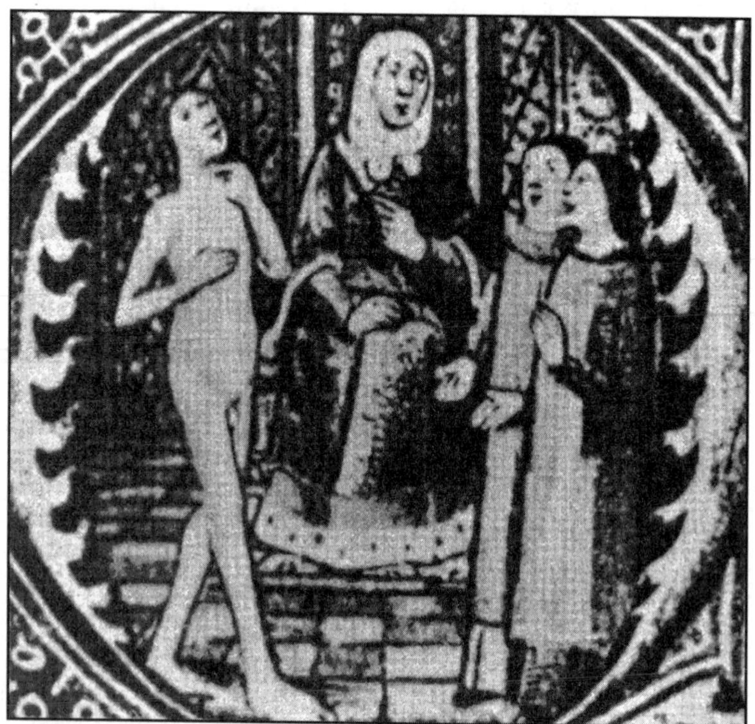

FIGURE 1–2. Claudius Galenus (Galen).

THE RENAISSANCE

Galen did much to further medical progress, but his theories and views, which were by no means totally accurate, were blindly accepted for 1500 years as the world went through the Dark Ages. This historical period of intellectual and artistic stagnation was finally broken in the late 14th and early 15th centuries AD with the invention of the printing press, the astronomic discoveries of Copernicus and Galileo, and the discovery and exploration of the Western Hemisphere. With these and other discoveries, the world began the great growth period known as the Renaissance.

A genius of the Renaissance, the bold artist Leonardo da Vinci (1452–1519) did not hesitate to exchange his painting brush for a dissection scalpel to explore human anatomy. Andreas Vesalius (1514–1564) reformed the knowledge of anatomy (Figure 1–3). In his 1542 publication, *De Humani Corporis Fabrica*,[19] this 29-year-old anatomist and artist corrected many of the age-old errors of Galen. He clarified the laryngeal anatomy and presented the function of the epiglottis. Vesalius' work is considered to be the anatomic classic of all time.[14]

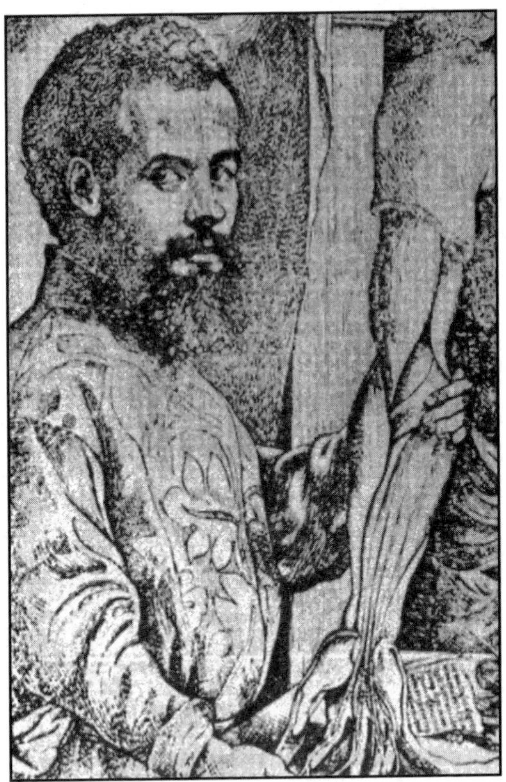

FIGURE 1–3. Andreas Vesalius, 1514–1564.

During this time period, Bartolomeus Eustachius (1520–1574; Figure 1–4) was one of the first anatomists to accurately describe the structure, course, and relations of the eustachian tube. More interesting were his descriptions and carvings of the anatomy of the larynx, which were not discovered until the 18th century in the Vatican Library and are even more detailed and accurate than those of Vesalius. Fabricius, of Padua, authored the first monograph of the larynx (1600) entitled *De Visione Auditu*.[20] In his monograph, Fabricius named the posterior cricoarytenoid muscles and described the action of the other laryngeal muscles.

THE 17TH TO 19TH CENTURIES

The discoveries of anatomy, physiology, and pathology of the laryngeal mechanism continued, highlighted by descriptions of the laryngeal ventricles by the Italian anatomist Giovanni Morgagni (1682–1771); further clarification of the purpose of the epiglottis by Francois Magendie (1783–1855) of Paris; the functions of the laryngeal cartilages and

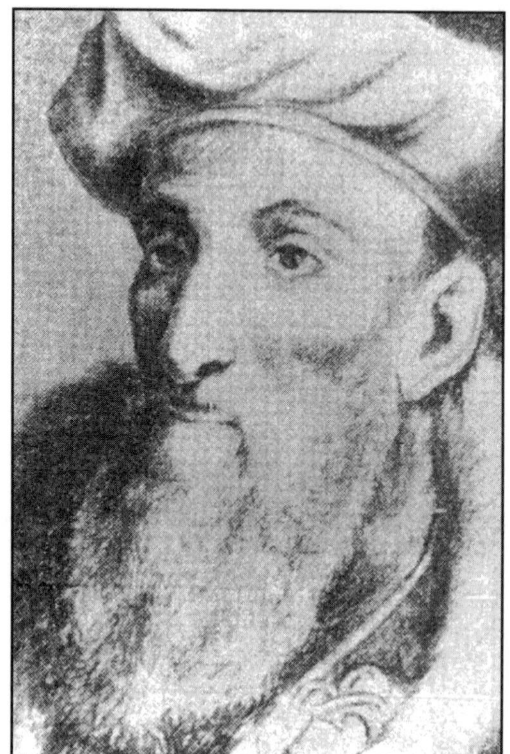

FIGURE 1–4. Bartolomeus Eustachius, 1520–1574.

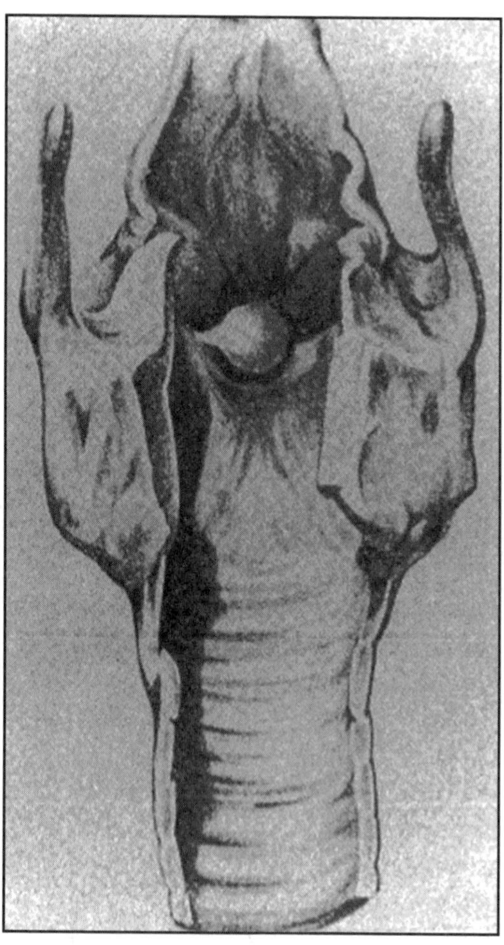

FIGURE 1–5. Polyps of the larynx; from Ryland.[21]

muscles in the production of voice by Robert Willis in Cambridge in 1829; and finally, in Frederick Ryland's (1837) publication called *Treatise on the Disease and Injuries of the Larynx and Trachea*.[21] This important publication clearly described the diseases of the larynx (Figure 1–5) as they were understood before the use of the laryngeal mirror.

THE LARYNGEAL MIRROR

Since the time of Aristotle, many minds had considered the idea of examining the larynx in living humans. It was not until 1854, however, that a Parisian singing teacher named Manuel Garcia (1804–1906; Figure 1–6) made the discovery that ushered in what became known as the modern era of laryngology.

Strolling through the gardens of Palais-Royal on a bright September day, Garcia observed the flashing sun in the windowpanes of the quadrangle buildings:

> Suddenly I saw the two mirrors of the laryngoscope in their respective positions, as if actually present before my eyes. I went straight to Charriere, the surgical instrument maker, and

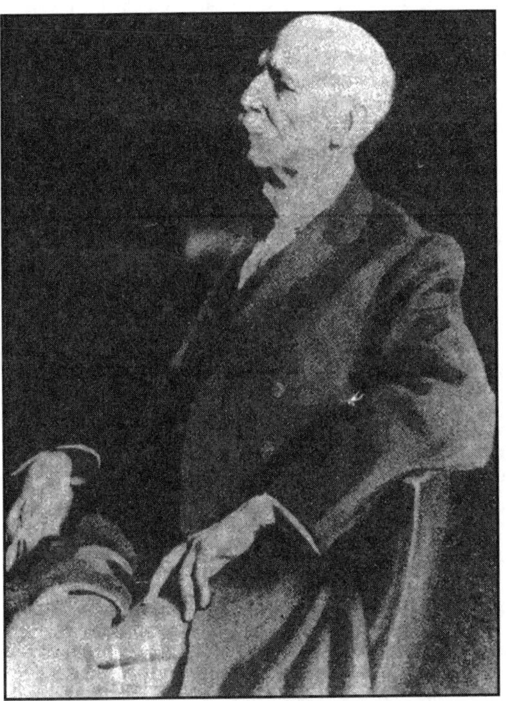

FIGURE 1–6. Manuel Garcia at age 100 years.

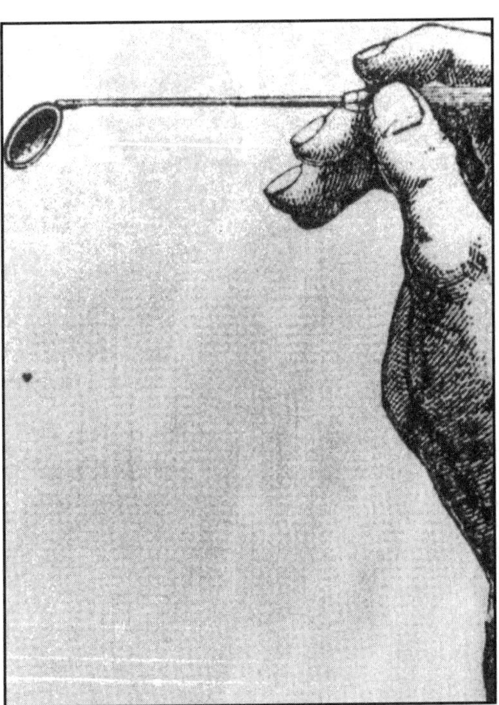

FIGURE 1–7. The position of the hand with the laryngeal mirror.

asking if he happened to possess a small mirror with a long handle, was informed that he had a little dentist's mirror, which had been one of the failures of the London exhibition of 1851. I bought it for six francs. Having also obtained a hand mirror, I returned home at once, very impatient to begin my experiments. I placed against the uvula the little mirror (which I heated in warm water and carefully dried), then flashing upon its surface with the hand mirror a ray of sunshine, I saw at once, to my great joy, the glottis, wide and open before me, and so fully exposed that I could perceive a portion of the trachea. When my excitement had somewhat subsided, I began to examine what was passing before my eyes. The manner in which the glottis silently opened and shut and moved in the act of phonation, filled me with wonder.[22]

FURTHER ADVANCEMENTS

The use of the laryngeal mirror (Figure 1–7) was taken up quickly in the major medical centers of the world, with the major improvement of artificial illumination made in Budapest by Johann Czermak in 1861.[23] The laryngeal mirror was first introduced in the United States in 1858 by Ernst Krakowizer, but credit for the development of laryngology as a specialty in the United States was given to Louis Elsberg of New York and J. Dobs Cohen of Philadelphia. Elsberg taught laryngoscopy in the University Medical School of New York in the 1860s, and Cohen published the first American textbook on diseases of the throat in 1872. Cohen also performed the first total laryngectomy in the United States.

Other laryngeal examination techniques followed including stroboscopy (1878), direct laryngoscopy (1895), and ultrahigh-speed photography developed at the Bell Telephone Laboratories in 1937. These techniques are further described in Chapters 5 and 6 of this text. Medical treatment of laryngeal pathologies has advanced greatly just in the past 30 years. The philosophy of surgical intervention has changed from one of lesion excision to a philosophy of vocal conservation. A subspecialty in otolaryngology was developed known as phonosurgery, which is defined as surgery to improve voice quality.[24] Special microsurgical instruments have been designed specifically for the purpose of permitting laryngologists to excise laryngeal lesions while maintaining the integrity of the vocal fold mucosa and thus voice quality. Phonosurgical techniques have also been applied to problems associated with vocal fold closure such as paralysis and bowing in an effort to improve voice quality. New procedures and techniques are rapidly developing, leading to improved voice production for a variety of voice disorders.

VOICE THERAPY

The evaluation and treatment of voice disorders remained the province of the medical profession until about 1930. At this time, a few laryngologists, as well as singing teachers, instructors in the speech arts, and a fledgling group of speech correctionists became interested in retraining individuals with vocal disorders.[25] Using drills and exercises borrowed from training manuals designed to enhance the normal voice, these specialists attempted to modify the production of the disordered voice. Enterprising teachers created many of these rehabilitation techniques and tailored them to individual students' needs. The techniques, however, were not based on scientific principles of laryngeal, respiratory, and resonatory physiology. Nonetheless, it is particularly interesting how many of these techniques remain with us today, as testimony to the insight and creativity of early speech pathologists.

In the 1930s, the study and practice of voice therapy were greatly advanced with the publication of two books, *The Rehabilitation of Speech* by West, Kennedy, and Carr,[26] and Charles Van Riper's *Speech Correction Principles and Methods*.[27] In their chapter related to voice disorders, West, Kennedy, and Carr concentrated on the organic problems of voice and diseases related to laryngeal dysfunction. These authors understood that when the voice is disordered, there is always a reason, and if properly studied, the reason will be discovered. Causes of the disorder may be neuropathologic, emotional, or the result of improper vocal habits and structural pathology. To rehabilitate voice, the authors suggested techniques including ear training, breathing exercises, relaxation training, articulatory compensations, emotional retraining, and special drills and exercises to be used with cleft palate and velopharyngeal insufficiency.

Van Riper stressed remedial measures to be used specifically by speech correctionists. He was the first author to suggest that voice disorders could be classified under the major headings of disorders of pitch, loudness, and quality. Van Riper advocated that voice therapy should follow a medical examination, to rule out organic pathology, and a detailed evaluation of pitch, loudness, and quality. His description of therapy techniques was the most elaborate of the time and included several therapy approaches:

- Recognition of the problem by the patient
- Production of a new, more appropriate sound
- Stabilization of the new vocal behavior in many contexts
- Habituation of the new voicing behavior in all situations.

These early foundations of voice rehabilitation have evolved into several general voice management orientations. These orientations may be classified as follows:

- Hygienic voice therapy
- Symptomatic voice therapy
- Psychogenic voice therapy
- Physiologic voice therapy
- Eclectic voice therapy

In short, hygienic voice therapy concentrates on discovering the behavioral causes of the voice disorder and focuses on modifying or eliminating these causes. Symptomatic voice therapy modifies the deviant vocal symptoms identified by the voice pathologist, such as breathiness, low pitch, glottal attacks, and so on. The focus of psychogenic voice therapy is on the emotional and psychosocial status of the patient, which led to and maintained the voice disorder. The physiologic orientation of voice therapy relies on direct modification of respiration, phonation, and resonance to improve the balance of laryngeal muscle effort to the supportive airflow, as well as the correct focus of the laryngeal tone. Finally, the eclectic approach to voice therapy is the combination of any and all of the previous voice therapy orientations. None of these philosophical orientations is pure. Much overlap is present, often leading, of course, to the use of eclectic voice therapy.

CLINICAL VOICE PATHOLOGY

The role of the speech-language pathologist has expanded significantly in the evaluation and management of voice disorders. The "voice pathologist" has become an integral part of a team responsible for treating individuals with such disorders. This team is composed primarily of the laryngologist and voice pathologist, with other team members including relevant medical specialists, vocal coaches, and singing instructors. Never before in the history of the treatment of voice disorders have patients had the opportunity for such integrated multidisciplinary care. The physician's medical expertise combined with the voice pathologist's knowledge of speech and voice processes and behavioral management have significantly improved the accuracy of diagnosis and the management care of patients.

This text is designed to introduce and integrate the artistic nature of voice care with the scientific areas of knowledge that are necessary for the development of a "voice pathologist." Voice analysis and treatment is a unique blend of art and science. The artistic nature of voice care involves sensitive human interactions. The vocal mechanism is quite strong and resilient physiologically but sensitive psychologically. The voice pathologist must develop a caring compassion, empathy, and understanding for the patient and the problems the voice disorder creates.

These interaction skills require that a person have the ability to listen not only to the characteristics of the voice quality, but also to what the patient says. In turn, gathering appropriate information related to the voice disorder is dependent on the interview skills of the voice pathologist. Despite many integral parts of a diagnostic voice evaluation, the patient interview remains the most valuable tool in the assessment and remediation of a voice disorder.

Considering the strong relationship between voice production and the emotional state of the patient, the voice pathologist must also develop effective counseling skills. It is common for patients with voice disorders to share personal information regarding their thoughts, feelings, and relationships. Often, this information must be discussed in depth as it relates to the voice problem. The role of the voice pathologist demands that professionals can discuss and consider sensitive issues related to voice. However, the voice pathologist also must be aware of the potential need to refer emotional concerns to other mental health care professionals.

Finally, developing and maintaining patient motivation is the "art" of clinical intervention. Motivational skill is the ability to instill action for change. Although many patients come to the voice pathologist highly motivated to improve voice production, some do not. The voice pathologist must have not only the ability to motivate the somewhat noncompliant patient, but also the creativity and perseverance to maintain motivation in those who proceed through the sometimes arduous tasks of therapy. In our experience, the ability to monitor progress through objective measures and laryngeal imaging procedures has significantly improved patient compliance and motivation.

The scientific nature of voice care involves a broad knowledge base, including the following:

- normal anatomy and physiology
- laryngeal pathologies
- etiologic correlates
- diagnostic methods including
  - perceptual assessment
  - vocal acoustics
  - vocal aerodynamics
  - laryngeal imaging techniques
  - patient self-assessment
- therapy methods

The voice pathologist must be completely familiar with the anatomy and physiology of the normal laryngeal mechanism, respiratory system, and supraglottic structures. Based on the specific physiologic needs of the patient, voice management approaches may be planned and implemented. The voice pathologist must learn to recognize various laryngeal pathologies, including their causes, signs, symptoms, and typical management approaches. Laryngeal pathologies encompass a broad range, from tissue lining changes of the vocal fold cover to neurologically induced, psychologically induced, or functionally induced changes in voice production.

The many causes of laryngeal pathologies also must be well understood by the voice pathologist. These causes include behavioral origins, medical etiologies, or psychologically based onset. The voice pathologist who recognizes the critical etiologic correlates will likely be very successful in discovering specific causes of voice disorders, which is the first step in successful remediation.

The ability to objectively measure many aspects of voice production has added important clinical tools in voice evaluation and management. Along with these tools comes the need to develop additional knowledge bases, including knowledge related to the science of voice acoustics, aerodynamics, and laryngeal imaging. Many commercial instruments are available that provide multitudes of measures related to voice production. It is the responsibility of the voice pathologist to understand the science of the specific measures and to utilize the measures as only one part of the diagnostic voice evaluation. The clinical ear remains the most valuable perceptual assessment tool.

The practice of clinical voice pathology has a deep, rich, and interesting history that continues to rapidly evolve at this writing. By combining the speech-language pathologist's natural artistic abilities related to human interaction skills, expertise in our knowledge of the upper airway, a strong scientific base, and expertise in behavioral management, the voice pathologist has emerged as a specialist in the treatment of voice disorders. Improved patient care is the ultimate result.

Our study of voice production begins in Chapter 2 with the anatomy and physiology of the mechanisms of voice. A complete understanding of this area of knowledge is an essential foundation in the preparation of the clinical voice pathologist.

REFERENCES

1. Aronson A. *Clinical Voice Disorders: An Interdisciplinary Approach.* New York, NY: Brian C. Decker; 1980.
2. Boone D. *The Voice and Voice Therapy.* 2nd ed. Englewood Cliffs, NJ: Prentice-Hall; 1977.
3. Greene M. *The Voice and Its Disorders.* 3rd ed. Philadelphia, PA: JB Lippincott; 1972.
4. Moore P. *Organic Voice Disorders.* Englewood Cliffs, NJ: Prentice-Hall; 1971.
5. Koufman J, Isaccson G. *The Spectrum of Vocal Dysfunction.* Philadelphia, PA: WB Saunders; 1991.
6. Moore GP. Have the major issues in voice disorders been answered by research in speech science? A 50-year retrospective. *J Speech Hear Disord.* 1977;42(2):152–160.
7. Stemple J. *Voice Therapy: Clinical Studies.* San Diego, CA: Singular Thomson Learning; 2000.
8. Hirano M. *Clinical Examination of Voice.* New York, NY: Springer-Verlag; 1981.
9. Hirano M, Bless D. *Videostroboscopic Examination of the Larynx.* San Diego, CA: Singular Publishing Group; 1993.
10. Hixon T. *Respiratory Function in Speech and Song.* Boston, MA: College-Hill Press; 1987.
11. Kent R, Reed C. *The Acoustic Analysis of Speech.* San Diego, CA: Singular Publishing Group; 1992.
12. Sapienza CM, Stathopoulos ET. Respiratory and laryngeal measures of children and women with bilateral vocal fold nodules. *J Speech Hear Res.* 1994;37(6):1229–1243.
13. Titze I. *Principles of Voice Production.* Englewood Cliffs, NJ: Prentice-Hall; 1994.
14. Stevenson S, Guthrie G. *A History of Otolaryngology.* Edinburgh, Scotland: E & S Livingstone; 1949.
15. Fink R. *The Human Larynx: A Functional Study.* New York, NY: Raven Press; 1975.

16. Wright J. *A History of Laryngology and Rhinology*. 2nd ed. Philadelphia, PA: Lea and Febiger; 1941.
17. Chadwick G, Mann W. *The Medical Works of Hippocrates*. Oxford, UK: Blackwell Scientific Publications; 1950.
18. Peck A. *Aristotle: Historia Animalium*. Cambridge, UK: Howard University Press; 1965.
19. Vesalius A. *De Humani Corporis Fabrica*. Basle; 1542.
20. Fabricius. *De Visiona Voce Auditu*. Venice; 1600.
21. Ryland F. *Treatise on the Diseases and Injuries of the Larynx*. London, UK: Longmans; 1837.
22. Garcia M. Paper presented at: Transaction Section of Laryngology. VII International Congress of Medicine; 1881; London, England.
23. Czermak J. *Du laryngoscope et Son Emploi en Physiologie et Nen Medicine*. Paris, France; 1860.
24. Ford CN. G. Paul Moore lecture: lessons in phonosurgery. *J Voice*. 2004;18(4): 534–544.
25. Murphy A. *Functional Voice Disorders*. Englewood Cliffs, NJ: Prentice-Hall; 1964.
26. West R, Kennedy L, Carr A. *The Rehabilitation of Speech*. New York, NY: Harper & Brothers; 1937.
27. Van Riper C. *Speech Correction Principles and Methods*. Englewood Cliffs, NJ: Prentice-Hall; 1939.

2

Anatomy and Physiology

Knowledge of the anatomy and physiology of the laryngeal mechanism is paramount to understanding voice disorders, as a foundation for examining the larynx, evaluating phonatory function, and recognizing the impact of abnormal changes or adaptations on voice production. A solid understanding of the normal structure and function of the larynx is the basis for interpreting evaluative findings and developing appropriate voice treatment plans.

ANATOMY

The larynx is essentially a cartilaginous tube that connects inferiorly to the respiratory system (trachea and lungs) and superiorly to the vocal tract and oral cavity. This orientation in the body is important, because it exploits the interactive relationship between these three subsystems of speech: the pulmonary power supply, the laryngeal valve, and the supraglottic vocal tract resonator. When considering the *vocal mechanism,* it is common to emphasize the complex and intricate structures of the larynx and vocal folds, but this limited perspective is flawed if it fails to include the broader contributions of subglottic breath support and supraglottic vocal tract resonance. Vocal function of the larynx relies heavily on the integration of this three-part system: respiration, phonation, and vocal tract resonance (Figure 2–1).

The lungs function as the power supply by providing aerodynamic (subglottal) tracheal pressure that blows the vocal folds apart and sets them into vibration. This vocal fold oscillation provides the sound source for phonation. As the tissues open and close in repeated cycles, the vocal folds modulate subglottal pressure and transglottal flow as short pulses of sound energy. The vocal tract serves as the resonating cavity, which shapes and filters the

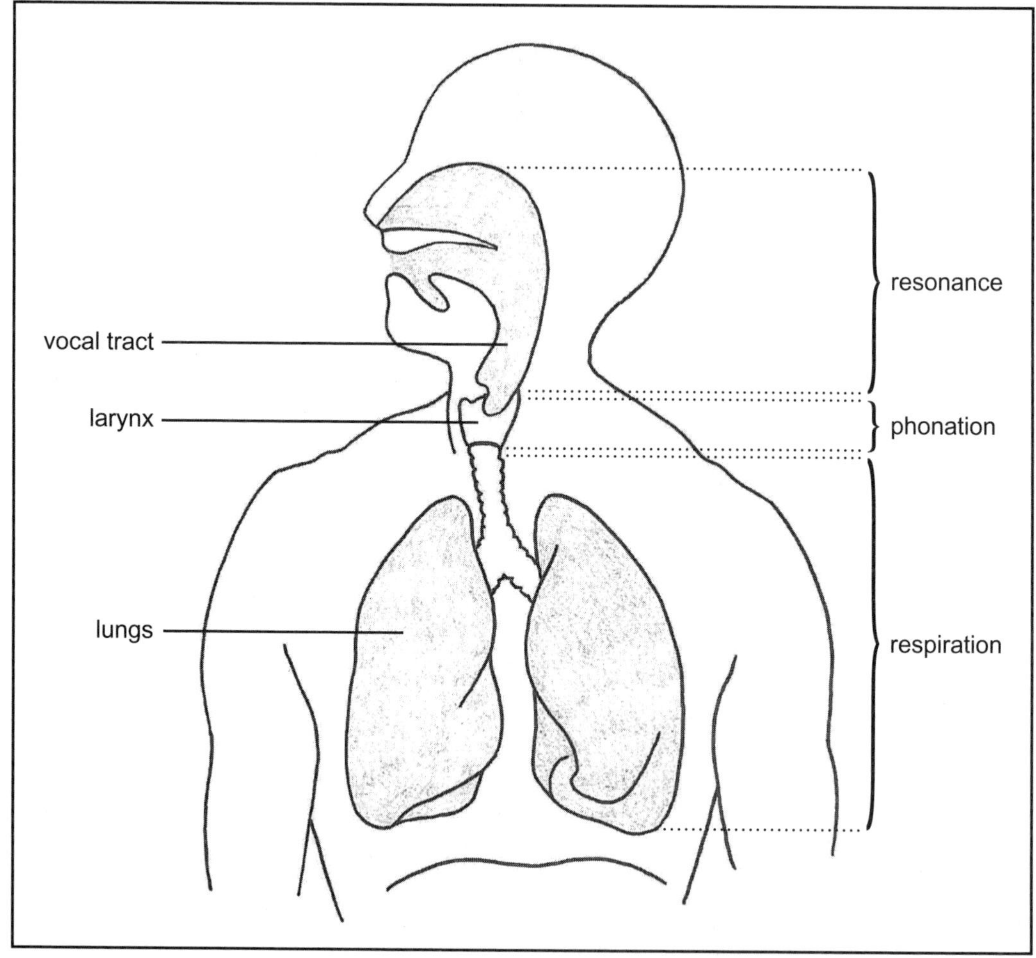

FIGURE 2–1. Orientation of the larynx in the body, at the juncture between the subglottic trachea and lungs and the supraglottic pharyngeal and oral cavities. These structures form the three subsystems of voice: respiration, phonation, and resonance.

acoustic energy to produce the sound we recognize as human voice.[1–7]

Differential diagnosis of voice disorders requires careful assessment of these three components. Obviously, laryngeal health and vocal function will influence the quality of voice production, but respiratory support and supraglottic resonance will also affect the speech product. For example, adequate or insufficient lung pressure can either maximize or limit vocal fold vibration, respectively. A patient with weak or compromised lung capacity may be unable to generate sufficient subglottal pressure required to produce normal vocal loudness or quality. Similarly, altering the shape and size of the vocal tract can either improve or diminish vocal resonance by enhancing or constricting the phonatory sound source generated by the vocal folds. The loss of either of the subglottal or supraglottal contributions could violate the potential for normal voice quality.[6,7] The resulting voice product radiated from the lips is a truly interactive result of these subsystems: respiration, phonation, and resonance.

The Laryngeal Valve

The larynx consists of a complex arrangement of cartilages, muscles, connective tissues, and mucosa that allows wide degrees of variation in position, movement, and tension to support three basic functions: airway preservation (opening) for ventilation, airway protection (closing) to block or repel environmental infiltrates, and phonation (vocal fold vibration) for communication and singing. The laryngeal valve achieves these three functions through three levels of *folds* (from most superior to most inferior):

1. Aryepiglottic folds connect the anterior attachment of the epiglottis cartilage to the arytenoid cartilages to form the superior border of the circular laryngeal column (Figure 2–2). The upper rim of the larynx is formed by the

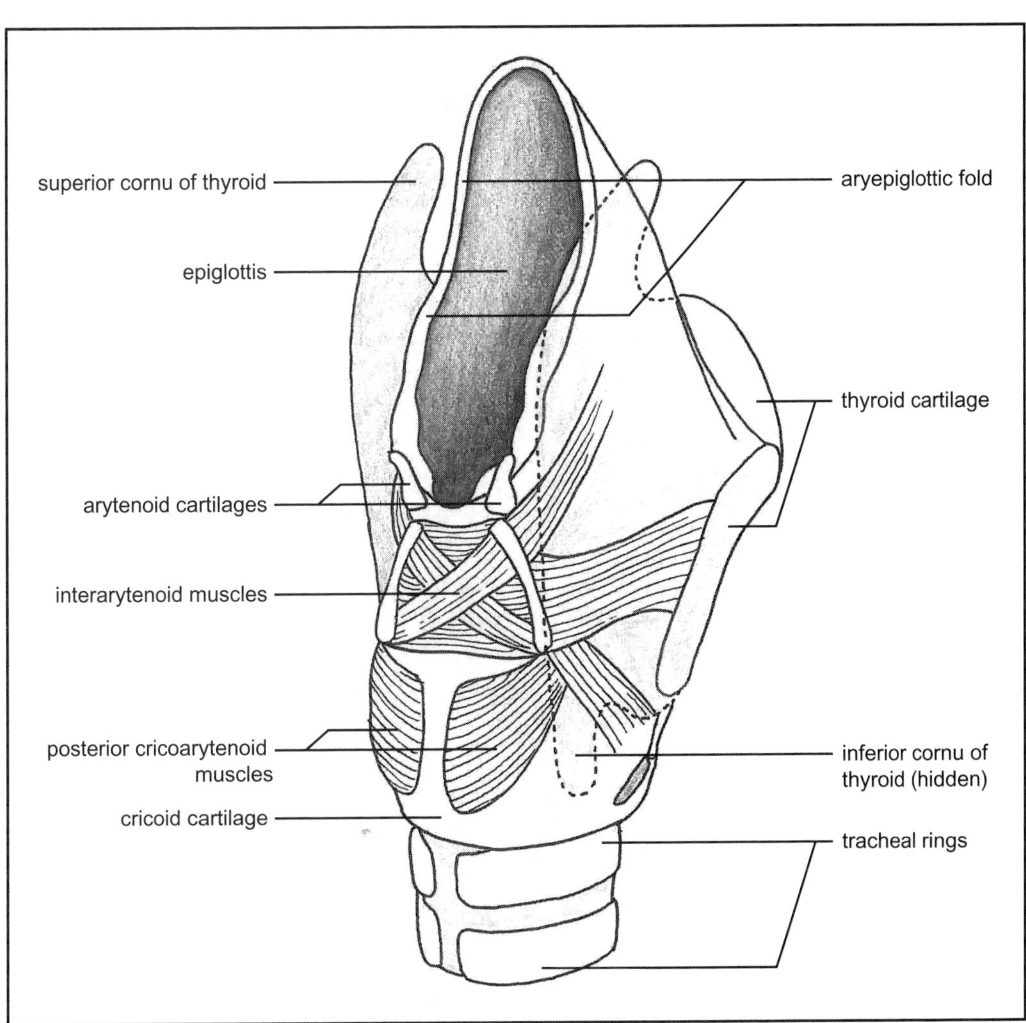

FIGURE 2–2. Oblique view of the larynx.

aryepiglottic folds, strong fibrous membranes that connect the lateral walls of the epiglottis to the left and right arytenoid cartilage complexes. When the epiglottis cartilage folds posteriorly and inferiorly over the laryngeal vestibule, it separates the pharynx from the larynx and offers the first line of defense for preserving the airway.[1,2,8,9]

2. Ventricular (or false) folds lie superior and parallel to the true vocal folds just above the ventricles. The ventricular folds form the second sphincter. They are not normally active during phonation but may become hyperfunctional during effortful speech production or extreme vegetative closure. The ventricular folds are directly superior to the ventricles, which function as variable pockets of space above the true vocal folds. The ventricular folds form a "double layer" of medial closure, if needed. The principle function of this sphincter is to increase intrathoracic pressure by blocking the outflow of air from the lungs. For example, the ventricular folds compress tightly during rapid contraction of the thoracic muscles (eg, coughing or sneezing) or for longer durations when building up subglottic pressure to stabilize the thorax during certain physical tasks (eg, lifting, emesis, childbirth, or defecation). The ventricular folds also assist in airway protection during swallowing.[1,2,8,9]

3. True vocal folds, which open for breathing, close for airway protection, and vibrate to produce sound. The third and final layer of this folding mechanism is the true vocal folds. For speech communication, the vocal folds provide a vibrating source for phonation. They also close tightly for nonspeech and vegetative tasks, such as coughing, throat clearing, and grunting, by functioning as a variable valve, modulating airflow as it passes through the vibrating vocal folds during phonation, closing off the trachea and lungs from foods and liquids during swallowing actions, and providing resistance to increased abdominal pressure during effortful activities. The angles of true vocal fold closure are multidimensional and include the potential for valving in both horizontal and vertical planes, depending on the variable shape, tension, and compression of the medial edge. Communicative maneuvers include narrow and rapid opening and closing gestures to produce momentary phonetic contrasts for voiced and voiceless speech sounds, as well as sustained vocal fold closing to produce vibration for phonation.[1,2,8,9]

All three of these folding structures —the epiglottis, ventricular folds, and true vocal folds—exhibit variable shape, tension, and position to accomplish these communicative and vegetative functions in the body. Together, these three levels of airway preservation and protection perform constant adjustments in the airway aperture (Figure 2–3).

Respiration for Phonation

Vocal fold vibration is the sound source that produces phonation and provides the speech signal. Phonation relies on pulmonary respiratory power, supported by the abdominal and thoracic musculature. The lungs are housed within the ribcage in the thorax and separated from the viscera (digestive organs in the abdomen) by a large, dome-shaped muscle called the diaphragm. The bottoms of the lungs are attached to the top of the diaphragm by a double-walled pleural lining. During inhalation, the diaphragm contracts (flattening downward in the body),

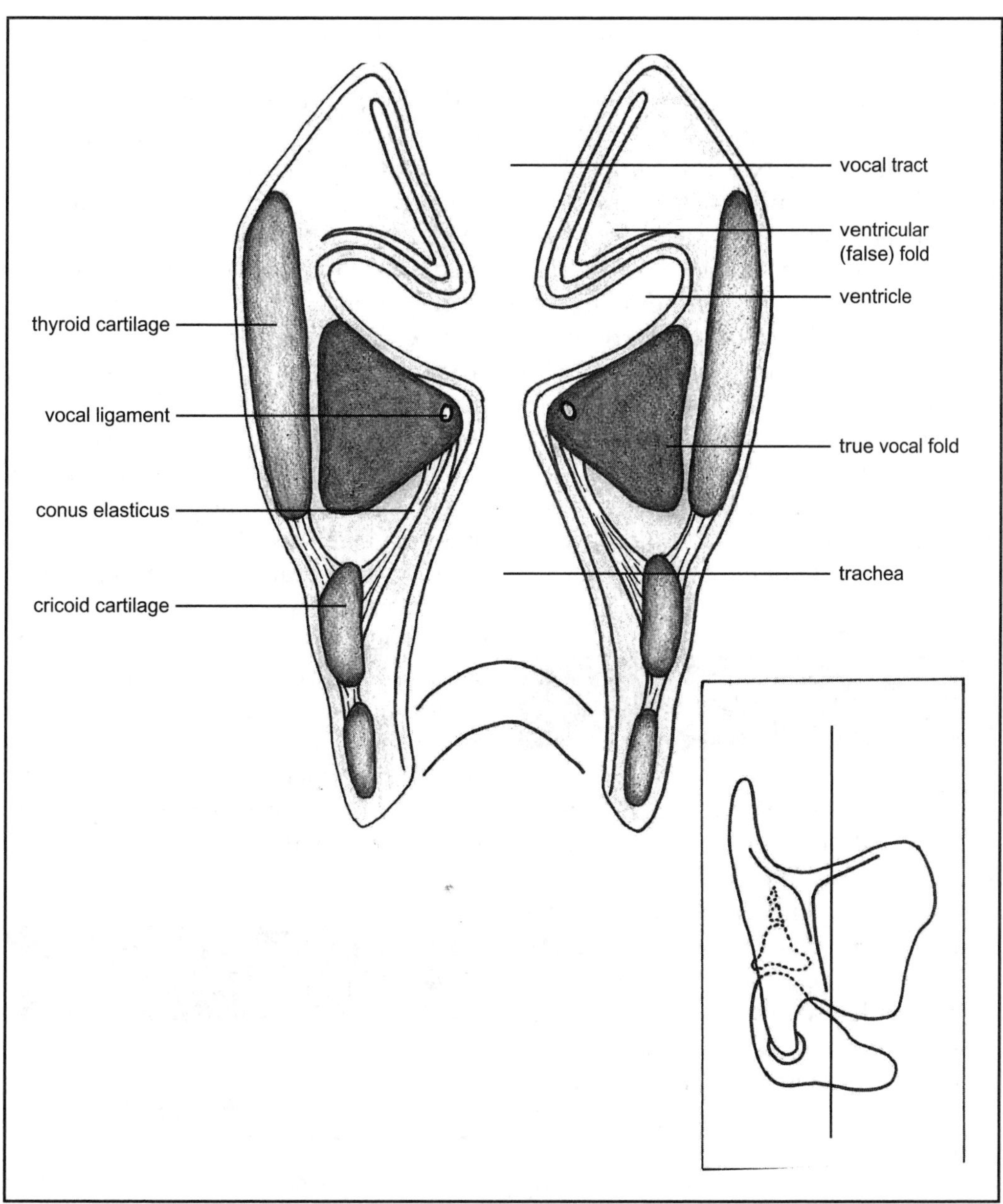

FIGURE 2–3. Coronal view of the ventricular and true vocal folds (insert: Coronal plane of Figure 2–3).

compressing the viscera, and simultaneously pulling the lungs downward, thereby expanding the lung volume. As this lung volume expands, air is drawn passively into the lungs. During exhalation, the diaphragm relaxes and rises back up to its resting position, as passive elastic recoil pushes air out of the lungs and upward through the vocal folds and vocal tract. During quiet exhalation, the vocal folds are abducted (opened) in the paramedian position (approximately

60% of the full glottal aperture), so no sound is generated. To exhale for speech, however, the vocal folds adduct (close) at midline, constricting the airflow stream as it exits the lungs. This aerodynamic breath stream builds up pressure below the vocal folds until they are blown apart and set into oscillation, creating the vibratory sound source of phonation.[10–12] Without this airflow, no sustained phonatory sound source can be achieved. The interactive relationship between the subglottal air pressure buildup and transglottal airflow rate passing through the vibrating vocal fold valve influences the overall pitch, loudness, and quality of phonation.[4,5,10–14]

VOCAL TRACT RESONANCE

As sound waves generated by the vocal folds travel through the supraglottic air column into the pharynx, oral and nasal cavities, and across articulatory structures such as the velum, hard palate, tongue, and teeth, the excitation of air molecules within this space creates a phenomenon called resonance. Resonance occurs when sound is reinforced or prolonged as acoustic waveforms reflect off another structure. The model of acoustic energy (phonation) traveling through a filter (vocal tract) modified in variable shape, size, and constriction characteristics (articulatory gestures) is the basis for Fant's Acoustic Theory of Speech Production.[15] This theory underlies our understanding of the three components of the acoustic speech product: *glottal sound source* provided by the vibrating vocal folds, coupled with the supraglottic contributions of *vocal tract filtering* and *resonant characteristics*.[15,16]

The fluctuating dimensions of vocal tract cross-sectional area, cavity shape, and points of articulatory contact (eg, tongue, teeth, and lips) each directly influence the quality and strength of the acoustic product radiated from the lips and perceived by listeners. The sound of vocal fold vibration without the supraglottic resonating cavity (eg, in intraoperative conditions or in excised larynx studies) reveals a flat, atonal buzz, devoid of any "ring" and completely unrecognizable as human voice. The contribution of this resonating filter is essential to creating the perceptual attributes of voice, including pitch, loudness, nasality, and quality. Manipulating resonance characteristics by changing the vocal tract shape and oral posturing has been the study of vocal pedagogues, actors, and singers for several centuries.[5,7,11,13–16] Modifying resonance has also been applied directly to voice treatment methods for disordered speakers and professional voice users.[17–20]

STRUCTURAL SUPPORT FOR THE LARYNX

Hyoid Bone

The larynx is composed of a complex system of mucosa, connective tissues, muscles, and cartilages, all suspended from a single semicircular bone, the hyoid. The hyoid bone marks the superior border of the laryngeal complex of muscles and cartilage. It articulates with the superior cornu of the thyroid cartilage and attaches to the thyroid through the thyrohyoid membrane. Although the hyoid serves as the muscular attachment for many extrinsic muscles of the larynx, it is notable as the sole bone in the body that does not articulate with any other bone. This has an important benefit clinically, because chronic elevation of the hyoid can reflect excessive tension of the muscular sling that supports the larynx. Speech-language pathologists and vocal pedagogues may palpate the neck to assess hyoid positioning and monitor vocal tension in patients or performers (Figure 2–4).[1,2,9,10]

Laryngeal Cartilages

There are nine laryngeal cartilages that extend from just below the hyoid bone superiorly to the first tracheal ring inferiorly. Together, these cartilages attach to muscles and connective tissues to form the surrounding columnar housing for the vocal folds. The three largest cartilages are (from most superior to inferior) the epiglottis, thyroid, and cricoid. Additionally, there are three smaller pairs of cartilages that form the posterior wall of the laryngeal column; they are (from most inferior to superior) the arytenoid, corniculate, and cuneiform cartilages.

Epiglottis

The epiglottis cartilage is shaped like a long leaf, with its narrow base (petiole) attached to the inner portion of the anterior rim of the thyroid cartilage. This attachment allows the blade of

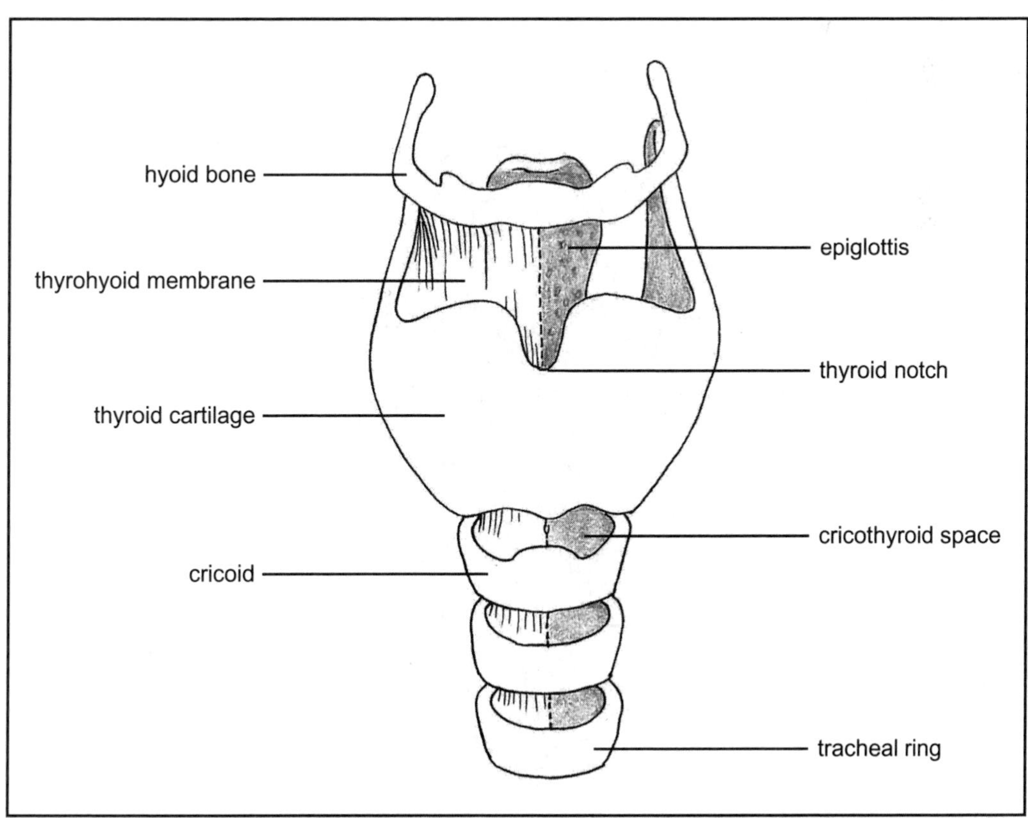

FIGURE 2–4. Anterior view of the hyoid bone and laryngeal cartilages.

the epiglottis cartilage to fold along its midline and move forward and back, closing down inferiorly and posteriorly over the laryngeal vestibule. Although the position of the epiglottis may influence vocal tract resonant properties, the epiglottis normally has no direct role in phonation or communication. Its primary role is airway protection, as it forms the top level of the three tiers of a sphincteric folding mechanism to divert particles of food or liquid away from the glottis during swallowing. Unlike other laryngeal cartilages, the epiglottis is composed of elastic cartilage and therefore does not ossify, or harden, with age. This composition is important because this structure must remain flexible throughout life to allow a pliable free edge to assist in closing the airway (Figures 2–5 and 2–6).[1,2,9,10]

Thyroid

The thyroid cartilage is a three-sided saddle-shaped curve that creates the anterior border of the airway column. The thyroid cartilage attaches the true vocal folds to the internal rim of the anterior curve. Posteriorly are two superior cornu, or "horns," that extend upward to articulate with the hyoid bone, and two inferior cornu that articulate with the cricoid cartilage below it.[1,2,9,10] The thyroid is composed of hyaline cartilage that ossifies and limits flexibility with age.[21] The lateral walls form quadrilateral plates, called laminae, that attach at the anterior midline in a thyroid notch or prominence. In newborns, these laminae form a curve of about 130°, and the angle becomes more acute with age. A fully matured thyroid angle will be

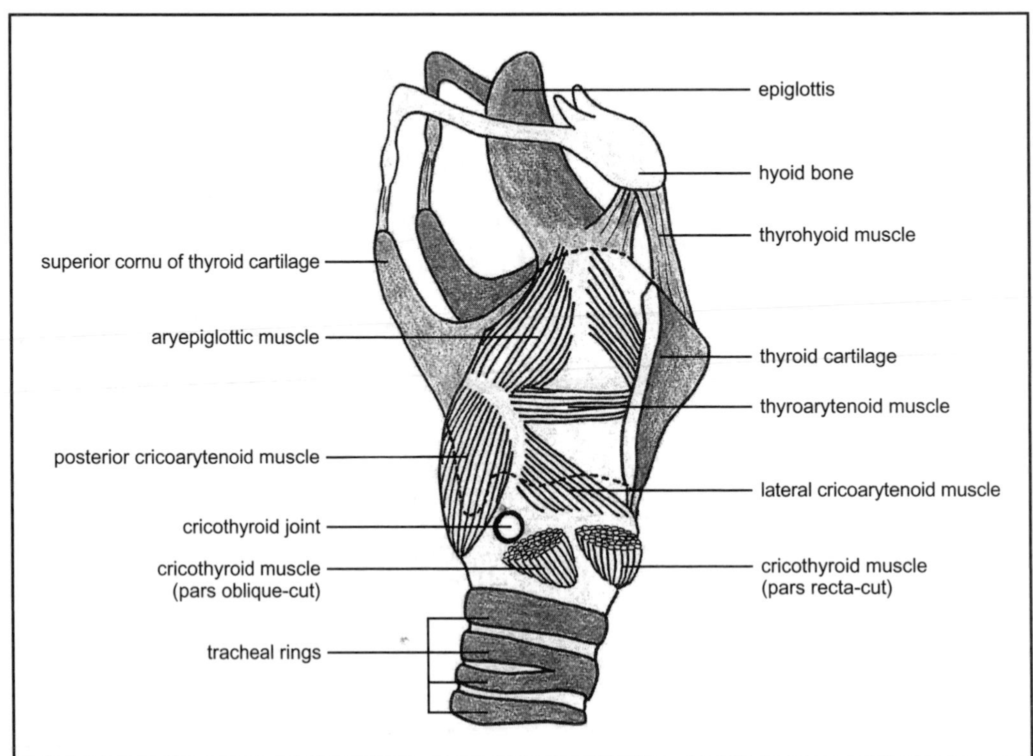

FIGURE 2–5. Lateral view of the larynx.

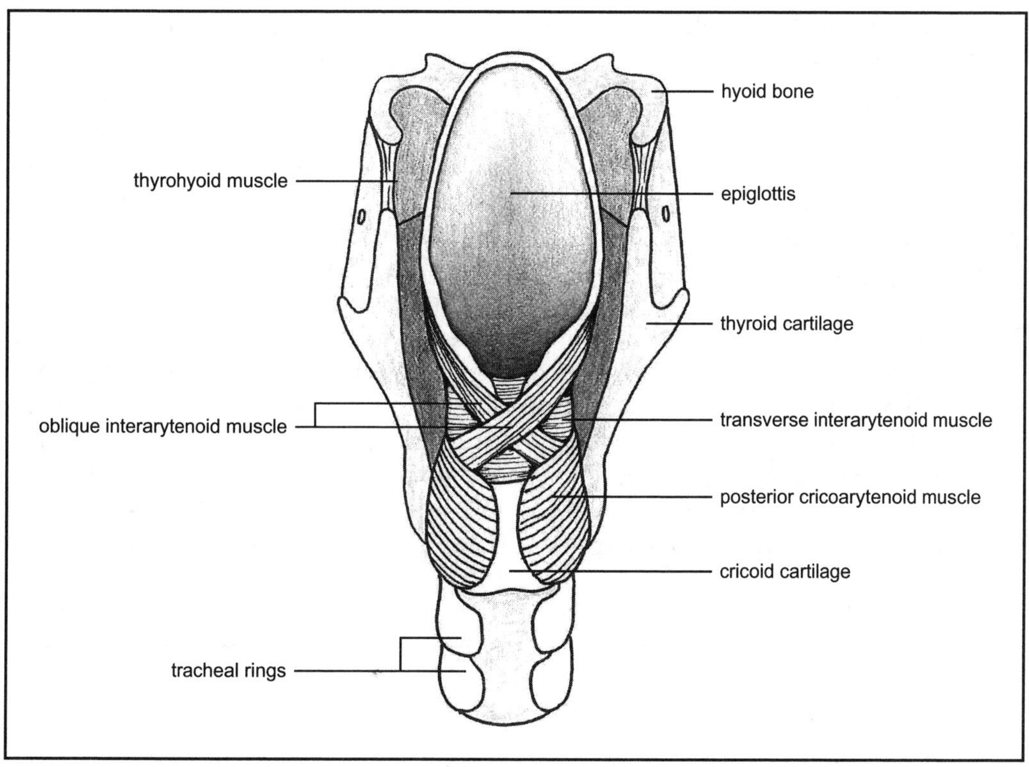

FIGURE 2–6. Posterior view of the larynx.

more acute for adult males (90°) than for adult females (110°).[9] In males, the thyroid notch will become more prominent anteriorly, resulting in the characteristic male "Adam's apple." This thyroid notch can be seen or palpated at the front of the neck. Clinically, malposition or aberrant movement of the thyroid notch can signal extrinsic laryngeal muscle hyperfunction or voice misuse.[18–20]

Cricoid

Below the thyroid cartilage is the cricoid, another hyaline cartilage. It is the only circular cartilage, and its shape is described as a "signet ring," with a narrow anterior curve and broad posterior back.

The cricoid sits above the first tracheal ring and provides a stable round entry to the pulmonary airway. The cricoid has two sets of paired facets, or flat surfaces that articulate with the thyroid and arytenoid cartilages. The cricothyroid joints connect the lateral facets of the cricoid to the inferior cornu of the thyroid cartilage above it, thus allowing the thyroid cartilage to rock forward from its vertical position. The convex facets on top of the posterior cricoid rim are where the concave pyramidal bases of the paired arytenoid cartilages rest to form the cricoarytenoid joint.[1,2,9,10] Both the cricothyroid and cricoarytenoid joints are lined with a synovial membrane that provides a connective tissue cushion supplied with secretions for lubrication, blood supply, adipose cells, and lymph tissue. Both articular joint surfaces and the synovial joint membranes display normal, age-related deterioration, although no gender differences have been noted (Figure 2–7).[21,22]

Arytenoids, Corniculates, and Cuneiforms

The three paired cartilages are the arytenoid, corniculate, and cuneiform cartilages. The arytenoid cartilages are pyramid shaped, with three quasitriangular surfaces: the anterior, lateral, and medial sides. The arytenoids have a pointed apex on top and a concave base. The anterior points of the arytenoid base project farther forward than the lateral and median sides to form the vocal processes. The bilateral vocal processes form the cartilaginous portions of the vocal fold and are the posterior points of attachment for the membranous left and right true vocal folds. The arytenoids are composed of hyaline cartilage, except for these vocal processes, which have elastin cartilage at their tips. The lateral arytenoid angles are called the muscular processes, because two different intrinsic laryngeal muscles attach in separate locations. When these muscles contract, they move the bilateral vocal

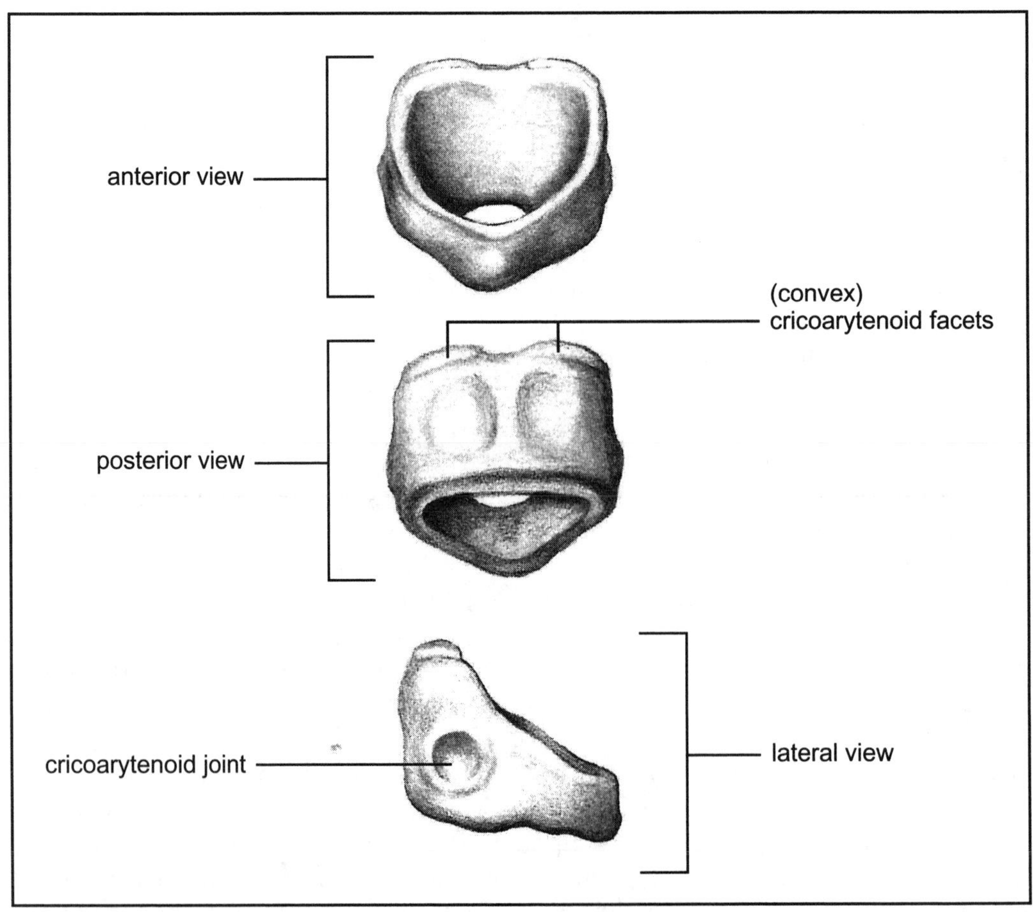

FIGURE 2–7. Cricoid cartilage: anterior, posterior, and lateral views.

processes laterally to open (abduct) or medially to close (adduct) the vocal folds. The medial arytenoid angle faces its arytenoid pair, forming an even surface for midline glottic closure (Figure 2–8).[1,2,9,10]

The base of the arytenoid cartilage is a concave cylinder, allowing it to articulate smoothly with the convex superior surface of the posterior cricoid cartilage. The arytenoid base fits neatly over the posterior cricoid similar to an empty half-cylinder resting over a rounded bar. The movement of the cricoarytenoid joint is complex and has been the subject of discovery and clarification over many years. When the tips of the vocal processes are directed medially (facing each other), normal vocal folds meet at midline and are closed (adducted). When vocal process tips are pointed laterally, the vocal folds are drawn open (abducted). Formerly, these arytenoid movements were thought to rotate on an axis, because a superior view of the vocal process tips (that attach to the membranous vocal folds) confirms that the vocal process tips appear to twist medially and laterally. However, that oversimplified presumption is inaccurate. In fact, these movements are not accomplished by simple rotation, but rather by two separate types of arytenoid motion: rocking and sliding. To understand these degrees of movement, first consider that the concave base (empty half-cylinder) of the arytenoid allows it to rock anteriorly and posteriorly over the superior convex cylindrical cricoid rim (bar). Second, the cricoid rim slopes downward laterally and anteriorly along its circular curve, allowing the arytenoid cartilage

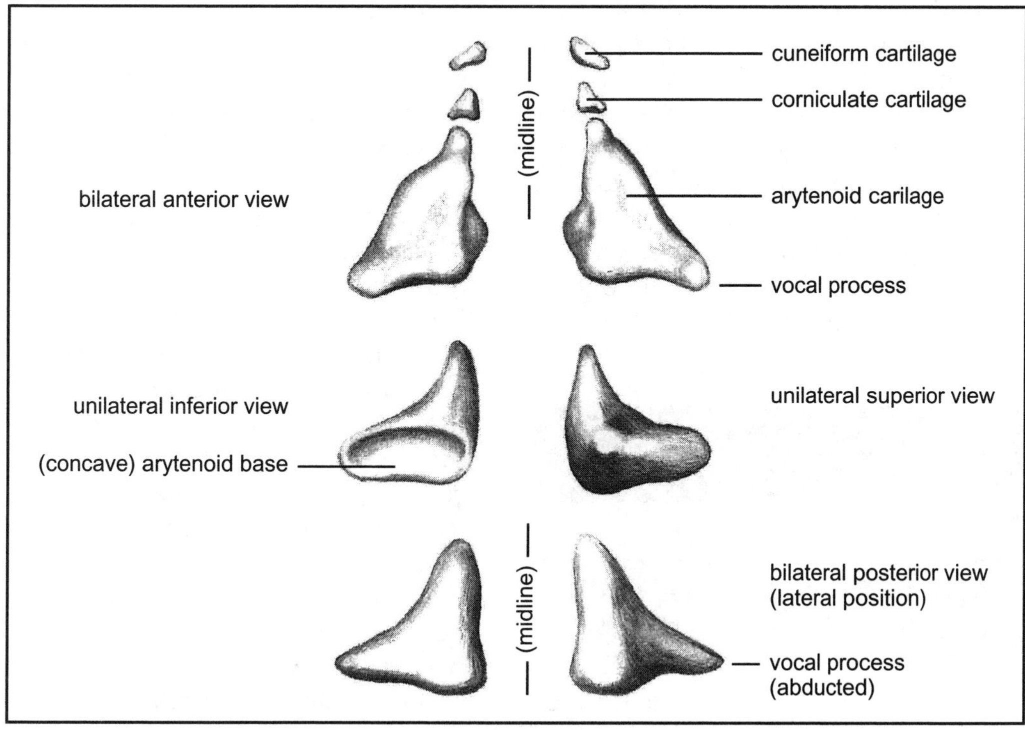

FIGURE 2–8. Arytenoid cartilage complex: arytenoid, corniculate, and cuneiform cartilages.

to slide in the same lateral and anterior direction to produce these rocking and sliding motions.[1,2,9,10,23,24]

Three different muscles attach to the lateral or posterior facets of the arytenoid base. Their discrete contractions adjust the position of the arytenoid base on the cricoid rim and direct the vocal process tips to orient the membranous vocal folds into varying degrees of fully opened (abducted) to fully closed (adducted). During this rocking and sliding, the vocal process tips can achieve both the medial and lateral angle orientations needed to adduct or abduct the membranous vocal folds and, consequently, alter the shape and size of the glottis.[22–24]

The corniculate cartilages (also called the cartilages of Santorini) are attached by a synovial joint to the superior tips of the arytenoids. The cuneiform cartilages (also known as the cartilages of Wrisberg) do not articulate with other cartilages but are embedded in the muscular complex superior to the corniculates. Both of these tiny cartilages consist of hyaline cartilage. They provide no clear function but may add structure and stability to preserve the airway by extending the column of muscular tissue superiorly to form the posterior border of the aryepiglottic fold.[22–24]

MUSCLES

Muscles for Respiration: Inspiration and Exhalation

The muscles of respiration are divided functionally into muscles of inspiration and expiration. These muscles respond differently in quiet breathing versus respiration for phonation. The muscles of inspiration (Figure 2–9) are as follows:

- Diaphragm: a dome-shaped muscle that attaches to the inferior border of the rib cage, active in both quiet and speech breathing. When it contracts, it depresses the abdomen and increases the vertical dimensions of the lungs and thoracic cavity.
- External intercostals: a series of muscles situated between each of the ribs, originating from the inferior surface of one rib and coursing down and medially to attach to the superior surface of the rib below. These muscles are active in both quiet and speech breathing; when they contract, the external intercostals elevate the rib cage and increase the transverse and anteroposterior dimensions of the thoracic cavity.
- Sternocleidomastoid: a major accessory muscle of inspiration that attaches at its upper end to the mastoid process of the skull and at its lower end to the sternum and clavicle, active only during deep breathing. When it contracts, it elevates the sternum and rib cage.
- Scalenes: three muscle pairs that originate at the cervical vertebrae (C2 through C7) and attach to the first and second ribs. They are active during forced inspiration; when they contract, they elevate the rib cage.
- Pectoralis major and pectoralis minor: two accessory muscles of inspiration. Pectoralis major originates in the sternum and attaches to the humerus; pectoralis minor originates in the costal cartilages and attaches to the scapula. They are active only during

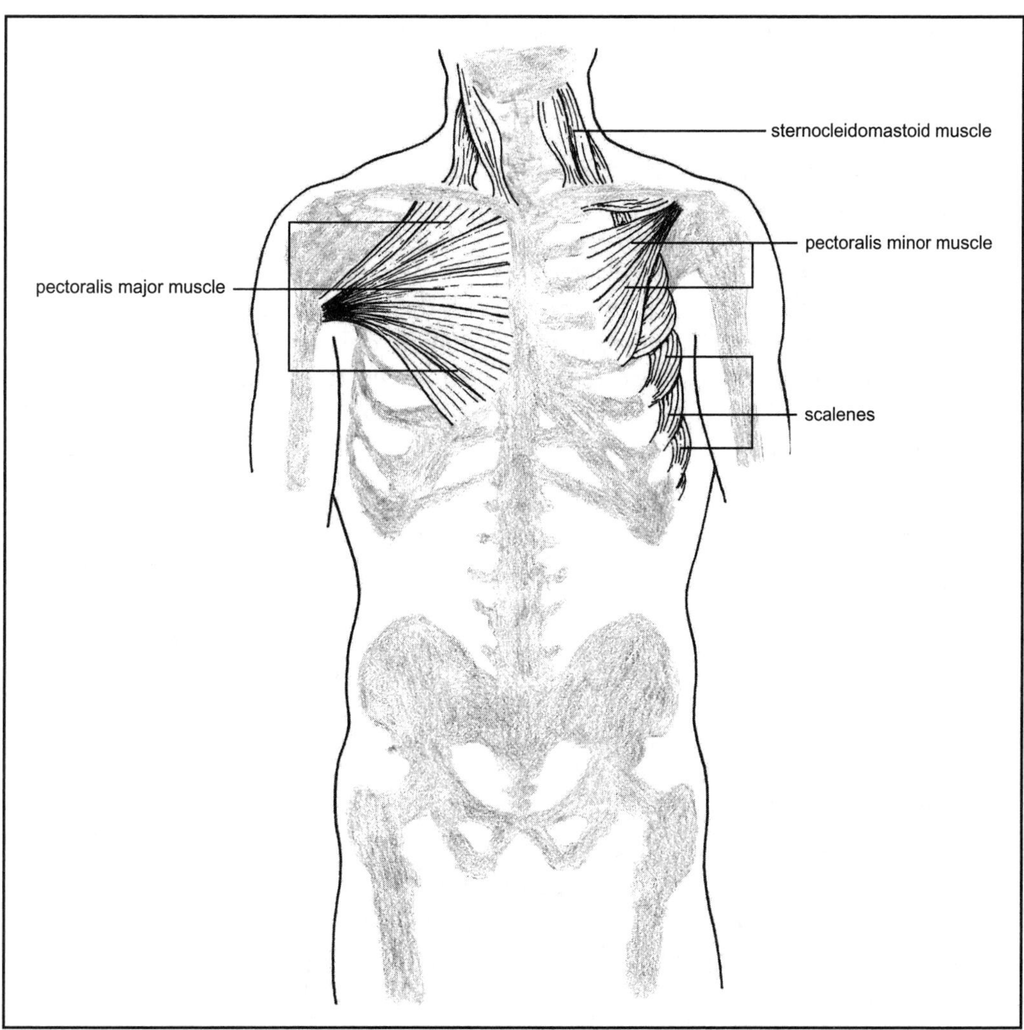

FIGURE 2–9. Muscles of inspiration.

the final phase of maximal inspiration; when they contract, they elevate the rib cage.

The muscles of expiration work in concert with the passive forces of torque, tissue elasticity, and gravity. At the end of a normal inspiratory cycle, the muscles of inspiration relax and passive recoil decreases the thoracic cavity dimensions. This decrease occurs as a result of: (1) gravity pulling downward on the rib cage; (2) tissue elasticity pulling the rib cage downward and inward; (3) the diaphragm moving upward into its normal, relaxed position; and (4) the torque on the twisted ribs causing them to lower. During speech breathing, expiratory muscles assist these passive forces by compressing the abdominal viscera, to force the diaphragm upward and depress the lower ribs, to decrease thoracic cavity size and thereby sustain pulmonary pressure. The muscles that support expiration (Figure 2–10) are as follows:

- Internal intercostals: a series of muscles situated between each of the ribs, originating from the inferior surface of one rib and coursing down and laterally to attach to the superior surface of the rib below. Active only in speech breathing; when they contract, the internal intercostals depress the rib cage to reduce dimensions of the thoracic cavity.
- Rectus abdominis: long, vertical muscle that covers the central abdomen, originating at the pubis and attaching to the sternum and lower ribs. Active only during speech breathing; when it contracts, it compresses the abdomen.
- Transverse abdominis: broad muscle that originates at the posterior vertebral column and fans anteriorly to attach to the abdomen at various points from the diaphragm down to the pubis. Active only during speech

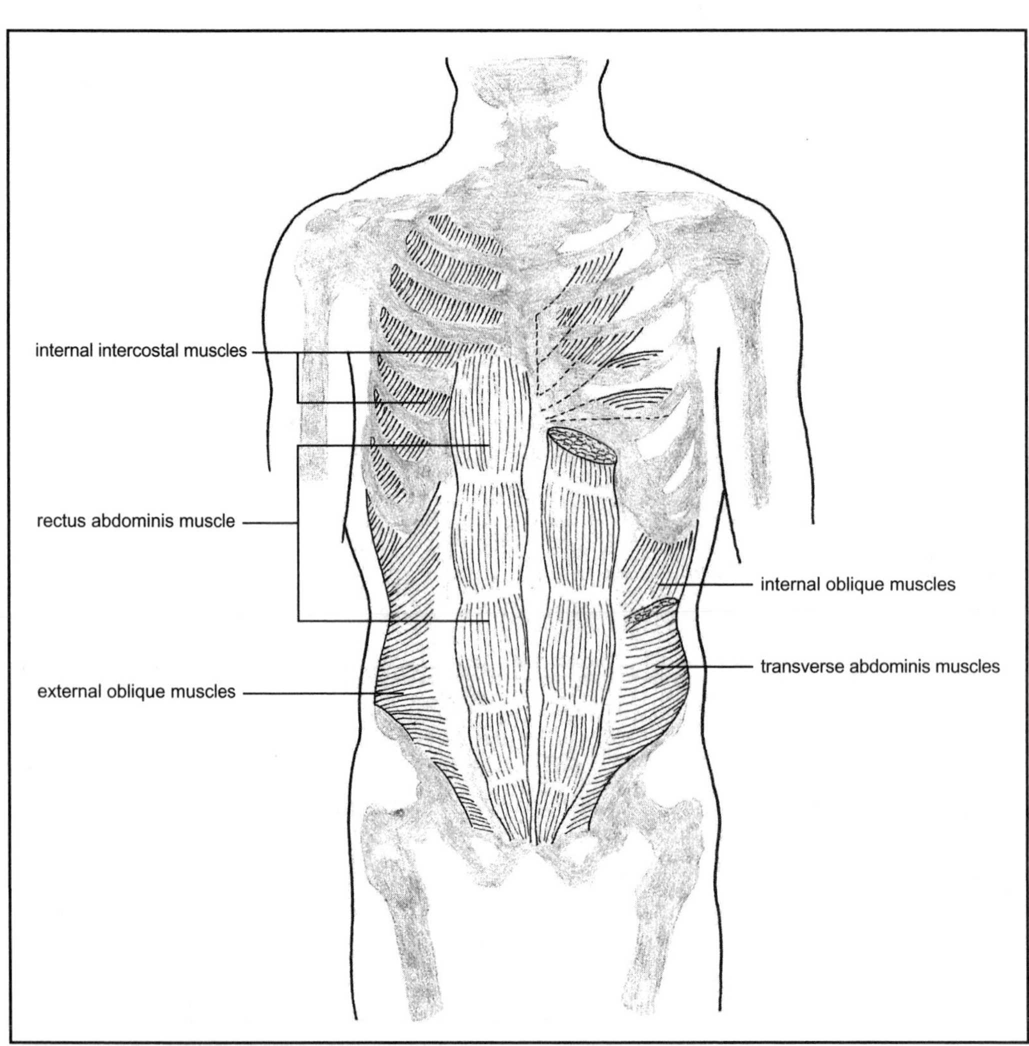

FIGURE 2–10. Muscles of expiration.

breathing; when it contracts, it compresses the abdomen.

- Internal obliques: upward fanlike muscle that originates at the iliac crest and attaches to the cartilage of the lower ribs. Active only during speech breathing; when it contracts, it lowers the rib cage.
- External obliques: downward fanlike muscle that originates at the lower ribs and attaches at abdominal points and the iliac crest. When contracting for speech breathing, it lowers the rib cage and compresses the abdomen.

Laryngeal Muscles

There are two logical groupings of the laryngeal muscles: extrinsic and intrinsic. Extrinsic laryngeal muscles are so named because they attach to both a site in the larynx and to an external point, such as the hyoid bone, sternum, mandible, or skull base. The intrinsic muscles have both ends attached to a laryngeal cartilage. When contracted, all muscles increase tension and shorten, providing a "pull" between the attachments. The primary function of the extrinsic muscles is to influence overall laryngeal height or position in the neck. For example, the larynx moves vertically (superiorly and inferiorly) and horizontally (anteriorly and posteriorly) as a whole for lifting, swallowing, phonating, and many vegetative acts. Extrinsic muscle manipulations also alter the shape and filtering characteristic of the supraglottic vocal tract, which modifies vocal pitch, loudness, and quality. The primary function of the intrinsic laryngeal muscles is to alter the shape and configuration of the glottis, by modifying the position, tension, and edge of the vocal folds. These intrinsic laryngeal manipulations consist of adduction (closing), abduction (opening), and modifications in vocal fold length, tension, and thickness. Both intrinsic and extrinsic muscle groups are necessary to accomplish the many vital and complex movements required for ventilation, airway protection, and communication, and all are integral to maintaining a functioning laryngeal valve.[1,2,9,10,25]

Extrinsic Laryngeal Muscles

The many extrinsic muscles of the larynx (Figure 2–11) can be divided into two regional groupings: suprahyoid above the hyoid bone and infrahyoid below the hyoid bone (Table 2–1). The muscles' locations can usually be identified based on their names that describe the structural attachments. By knowing the attachments, one can predict the effect of individual muscle contraction (shortening) between those sites. For example, the thyrohyoid attaches to the hyoid bone superiorly and the thyroid cartilage inferiorly. When contracted, this muscle draws these structures closer together. The sternocleidomastoid, although not technically an extrinsic laryngeal muscle, forms a broad sheath in the neck that extends from the sternum to the mastoid, without attaching directly to the larynx. Nonetheless, it is an accessory muscle for respiration and contributes to head and neck movements and stability.

Suprahyoid Muscles. The suprahyoid muscles generally raise the larynx by pulling the hyoid bone upward. This action is particularly important during a swallow, when laryngeal elevation can help protect the airway from aspiration. Clinically, laryngeal elevation

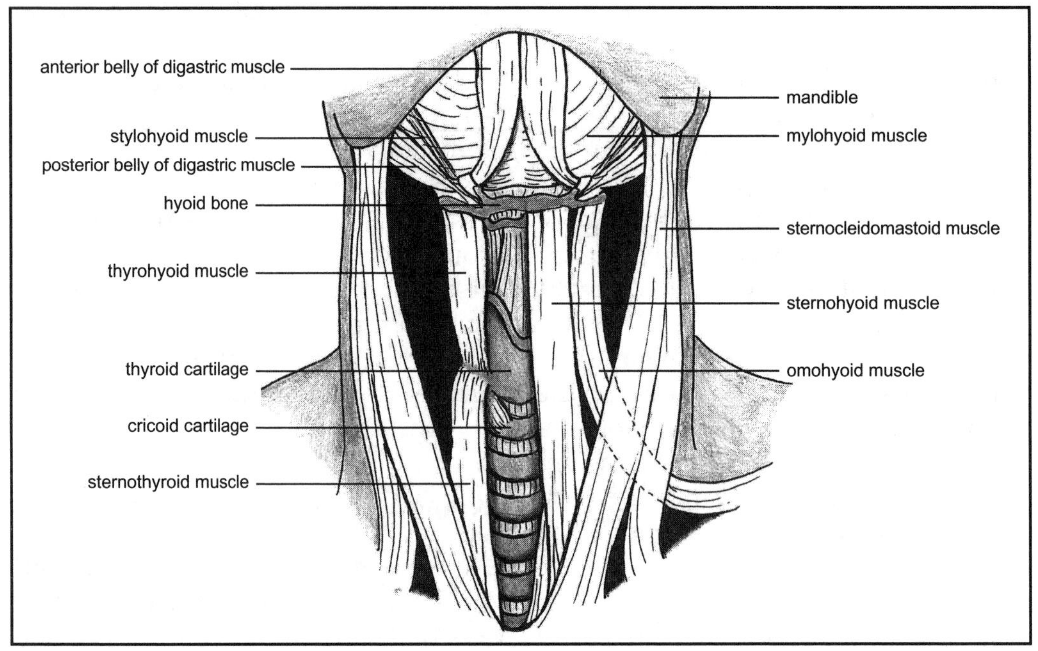

FIGURE 2–11. Extrinsic laryngeal muscles.

Table 2–1. Extrinsic Laryngeal Muscles

Muscle	*Attachments*	*Function*
	Suprahyoid Muscles	
Stylohyoid	Temporal bone (styloid process) to hyoid	Raises hyoid bone posteriorly
Mylohyoid	Mandible to hyoid	Raises hyoid bone anteriorly
Digastric	Two compartments: anterior and posterior	
Anterior	Mandible to hyoid	Raises hyoid bone anteriorly
Posterior	Temporal bone (mastoid process) to hyoid	Raises hyoid bone posteriorly
Geniohyoid	Mandible to hyoid	Raises hyoid bone anteriorly
	Infrahyoid Muscles	
Thyrohyoid	Thyroid to hyoid	Brings thyroid cartilage and hyoid bone closer together
Sternothyroid	Sternum to thyroid	Lowers thyroid cartilage
Sternohyoid	Sternum to hyoid	Lowers hyoid bone
Omohyoid	Scapula to hyoid	Lowers hyoid bone
	Regional	
Sternocleidomastoid	Sternum and clavicle to mastoid process of the temporal bone	Rotates the neck

during phonation may be a sign of excessive extrinsic laryngeal muscle tension and is often an accurate indicator of hyperfunctional voice use.[2,8,9,18,19] The suprahyoid extrinsic laryngeal muscles include the stylohyoid, the mylohyoid, the digastric (anterior and posterior bellies), and the geniohyoid (not seen). All elevate the hyoid bone and larynx in the neck, but the specific repositioning of other structures depends on the muscular attachments. For example, both the posterior diagastric and the stylohyoid muscles move the hyoid posteriorly. The digastric may depress the mandible; the mylohyoid may elevate the tongue.

Infrahyoid Muscles. The infrahyoid muscles include the thyrohyoid, the sternothyroid, the sternohyoid, and the omohyoid. In general, the infrahyoid muscles pull the hyoid bone and larynx to a lower position in the neck. The sternothyroid depresses the thyroid cartilage. The thyrohyoid contracts the distance between the hyoid and the thyroid, as mentioned previously.

Intrinsic Laryngeal Muscles

There are five intrinsic laryngeal muscles (Table 2–2), each of which attaches to cartilages in the larynx to modify the cricothyroid and cricoarytenoid joint relationships, and thereby affect the position, length, and tension of the vocal folds. Specifically, these intrinsic muscles create three critical effects:

1. Change the position of the cartilage framework that houses the vocal folds
2. Alter the length, tension, and shape of the vocal fold edge
3. Change the shape of the glottal opening between the vocal folds.

As with the extrinsic muscles, the intrinsic muscles of the larynx are also identifiable by their names that describe the cartilaginous attachments. Intrinsic laryngeal muscles are skeletal muscles, predominantly Type IIA, which are fast acting and fatigue resistant. Moreover, there are multiple muscle fiber inputs to each motor unit, suggesting high capacity for fine motor control.[9,10]

Cricothyroid. The cricothyroid is a broad, fan-shaped muscle that attaches inferiorly to the anterior arch of the cricoid cartilage and courses superiorly and laterally to the anterior rim of the thyroid cartilage. The cricothyroid is the only intrinsic laryngeal muscle that is not innervated by the recurrent laryngeal nerve; rather, the cricothyroid is innervated by the external branch of the superior laryngeal nerve. When the cricothyroid muscle contracts, it decreases the distance between these two cartilages, simultaneously stretching, lengthening, and creating longitudinal tension that stiffens the entire membranous vocal fold and thins the medial vibrating edge. This vocal fold lengthening is achieved as the thyroid cartilage is pulled inferiorly, as the cricoid is pulled superiorly, or by a combination of these movements. The cricothyroid muscle has been described traditionally as having two distinct compartments: pars rectus (vertical) and pars oblique (angled). However, a third "horizontal" belly has also been recently identified. The exact function of these muscle bellies is not clear, but recent study suggests that pars recta and pars oblique function in variable patterns for different speakers and at different portions of the fundamental frequency range.[26] Regardless, cricothyroid contraction always reduces the vibrating mass of the vocal fold by

Table 2–2. Intrinsic Laryngeal Muscles

Muscle	*Attachments*	*Innervation*
Cricothyroid (CT)	Cricoid to thyroid	External branch of the superior laryngeal nerve
Two compartments:		
Pars recta	Cricoid to inferior border of the thyroid lamina	
Pars oblique	Cricoid to inferior cornu of the thyroid	
Thyroarytenoid (TA)	Thyroid to arytenoid vocal process	Recurrent laryngeal nerve
Two compartments:		
Thyromuscularis	Lateral portion of the TA	
[Thyro]vocalis	Medial portion of the TA	
Lateral cricoarytenoid (LCA)	Lateral cricoid to the arytenoid muscular process	Recurrent laryngeal nerve
Interarytenoid	Joins the left and right muscular processes of the arytenoids	Recurrent laryngeal nerve
Two compartments:		
Transverse	Unpaired muscle sheath attaching to the lateral laminae of the left and right arytenoids; runs horizontally	
Oblique	Paired muscles coursing from the base of one arytenoid upward and across to the apex of the other, forming an X-configuration	
Posterior cricoarytenoid (PCA)	Posterior medial aspect of the cricoid to the lateral arytenoid muscular process	Recurrent laryngeal nerve

separating the vocal folds slightly to prevent tight adduction, increasing overall stiffness, and limiting the vibratory wave to the thinnest portion of the vocal fold, located at the medial edge. Therefore, the cricothyroid serves as the largest contributor to fundamental frequency control, especially in higher tones (Figure 2–12).[1,2,9,10,26]

Thyroarytenoid. The thyroarytenoid is attached anteriorly to the internal angle of the thyroid cartilage and posteriorly to the vocal process of the arytenoid (Figure 2–13). The thyroarytenoid is innervated by the recurrent laryngeal nerve. The thyroarytenoid usually contains two muscle compartments arranged in parallel. The lateral belly is

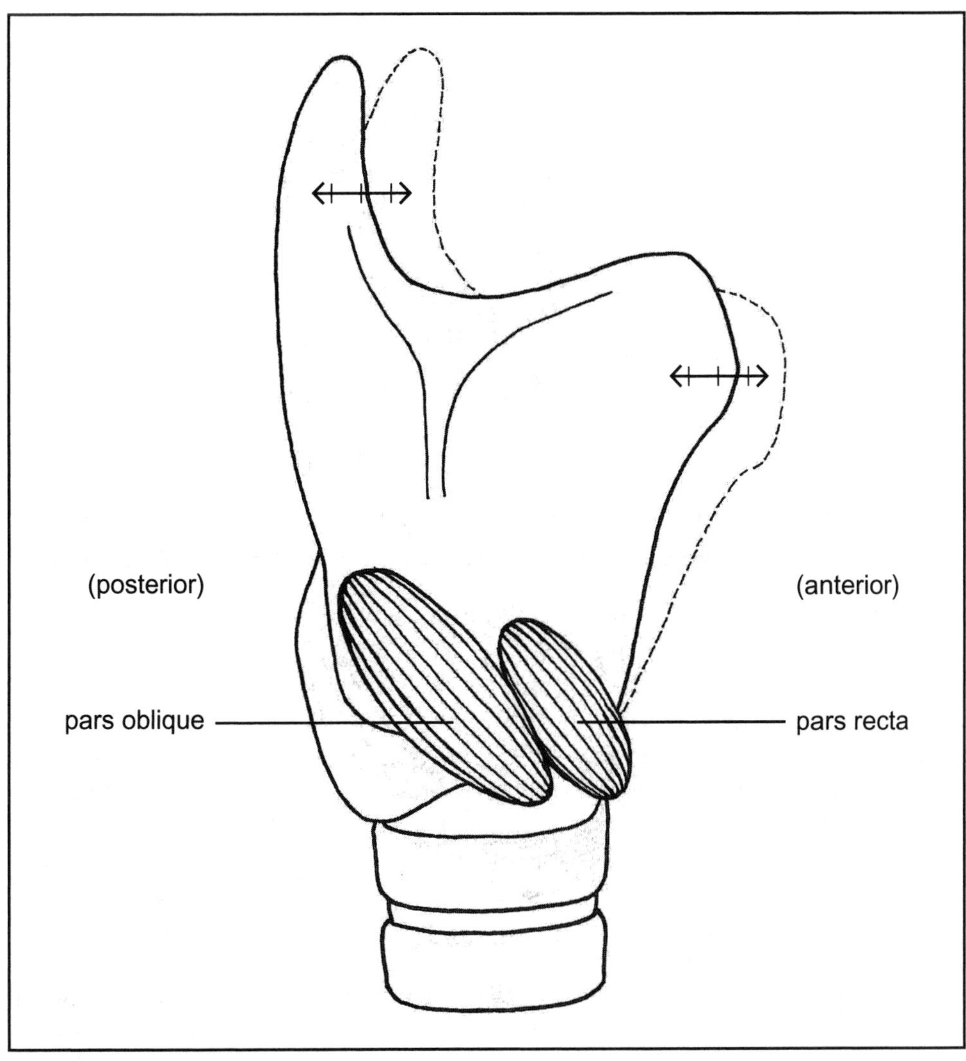

FIGURE 2–12. Lateral view of cricothyroid muscle contraction that pulls the thyroid anteriorly.

called the thyromuscularis; the medial belly is the thyrovocalis, or simply, the vocalis. Often, the general name thyroarytenoid (reflecting both compartments) and vocalis are used interchangeably. The thyroarytenoid muscle is the actual "body" of the vocal fold. When contracted, it shortens the fold length and lowers its vertical level in the larynx by drawing the arytenoid cartilages anteriorly. This muscle also influences the vocal fold shape and glottic closure patterns because thyroarytenoid contraction thickens and rounds the vocal fold by increasing the mass of the vibrating medial edge. As the vocal fold body stiffens, the superficial cover and transition become looser, allowing greater vocal fold closure and larger vibratory amplitude. Thus, the thyroarytenoid

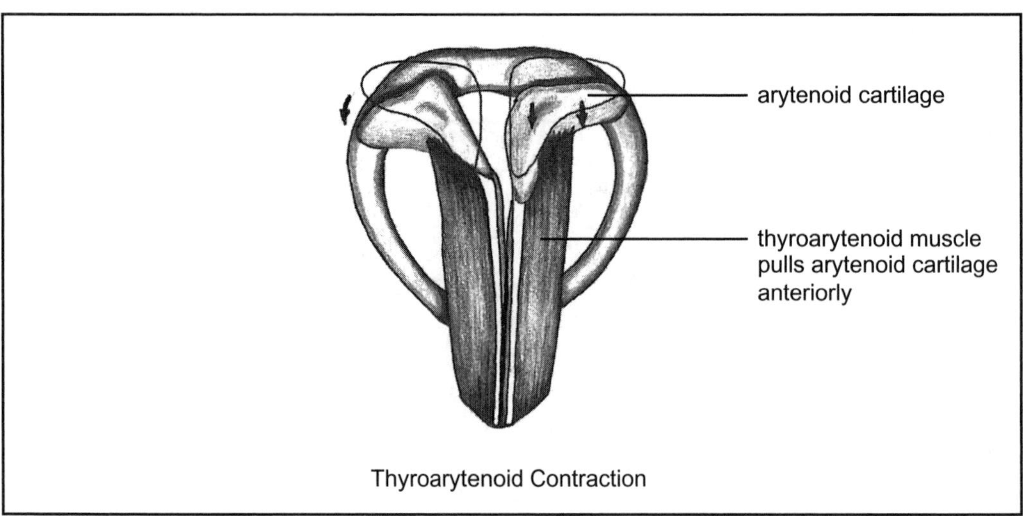

FIGURE 2–13. Superior view of thyroarytenoid muscle contraction that shortens and rounds the vocal folds.

contributes directly to lowering fundamental frequency, increasing loudness, and tightening of the glottic closure.[1,2,9,10,25] Historically, the thyromuscularis (lateral portion) was thought to contribute more to vocal fold adduction, due to its high concentration of fast twitch muscle fibers, whereas the thyrovocalis, which has predominantly slow-twitch fibers, was thought to exert greater control over phonation.[27]

Lateral Cricoarytenoid. The lateral cricoarytenoid is another broad, fan-shaped muscle that attaches to the lateral superior rim of the cricoid and to the lateral arytenoid muscular process (Figure 2–14). The lateral cricoarytenoid is innervated by the recurrent laryngeal nerve. When the lateral cricoarytenoid contracts, it rocks the arytenoids anteriorly and slides the muscular processes laterally. This movement redirects the tips of the vocal processes medially, bringing the membranous vocal folds to midline adduction and lowering the vocal folds. The lateral cricoarytenoid serves as one of the strongest vocal fold adductors (closers) by closing the glottis and creating medial compression for loud voice and strong vegetative closure, as in coughing, grunting, throat clearing, and Valsalva maneuvers.[1,2,9,10]

Interarytenoid. The interarytenoid muscles attach the left and right arytenoid cartilages (Figure 2–15). When they contract, the medial walls of the cartilage are drawn together, contributing to forceful closure of the vocal folds, especially in the posterior glottis. The interarytenoid muscles are composed of two separate compartments, the transverse and the oblique bellies. Both the transverse and oblique bellies of the interarytenoids are innervated by the recurrent laryngeal nerve. The transverse (horizontal) belly is the only unpaired intrinsic laryngeal muscle; it attaches to the posterior plane of each arytenoid and brings the medial facets of the arytenoids together. The oblique (crossed) bellies attach at a 45°

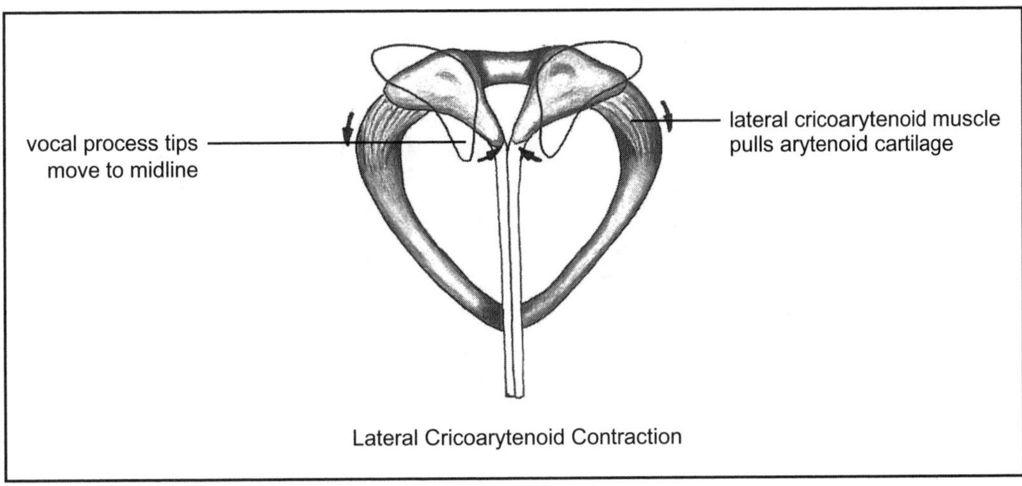

FIGURE 2–14. Superior view of lateral cricoarytenoid muscle contraction that moves the vocal processes to midline and adducts the vocal folds.

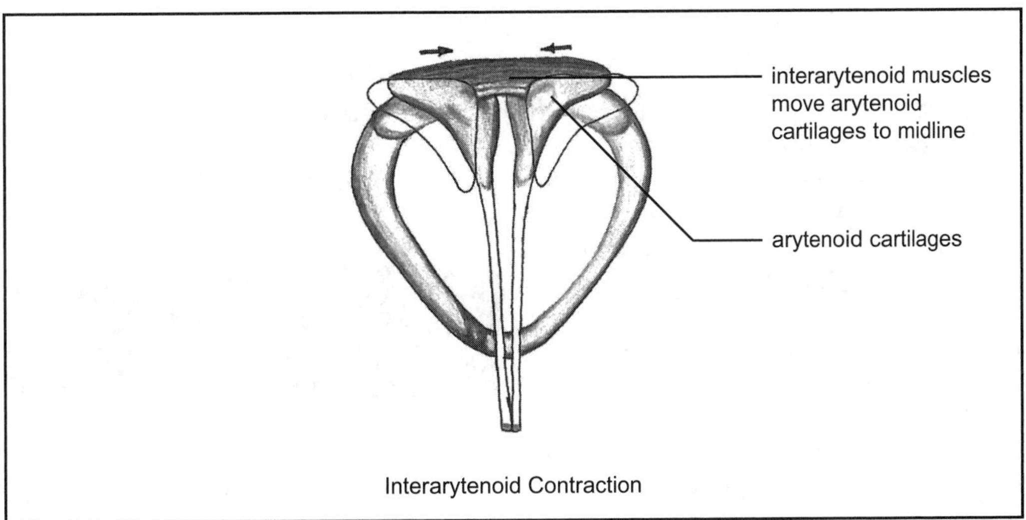

FIGURE 2–15. Superior view of interarytenoid muscle contraction that moves the arytenoids to midline and adducts the vocal folds.

angle from the inferior border of one arytenoid to the superior border of its contralateral pair. When the bellies contract, the space between the corniculate and cuneiform cartilages decreases, pulling the apices of the arytenoids medially, and decreasing the aperture in the vertical column above the true vocal folds.[1,2,9,10]

Posterior Cricoarytenoid. The posterior cricoarytenoid is the sole abductor of the vocal folds (Figure 2–16). Its attachments are the posterior lamina of the cricoid and the muscular (lateral) arytenoid cartilage. The posterior cricoarytenoid is innervated by the recurrent laryngeal nerve. When the posterior

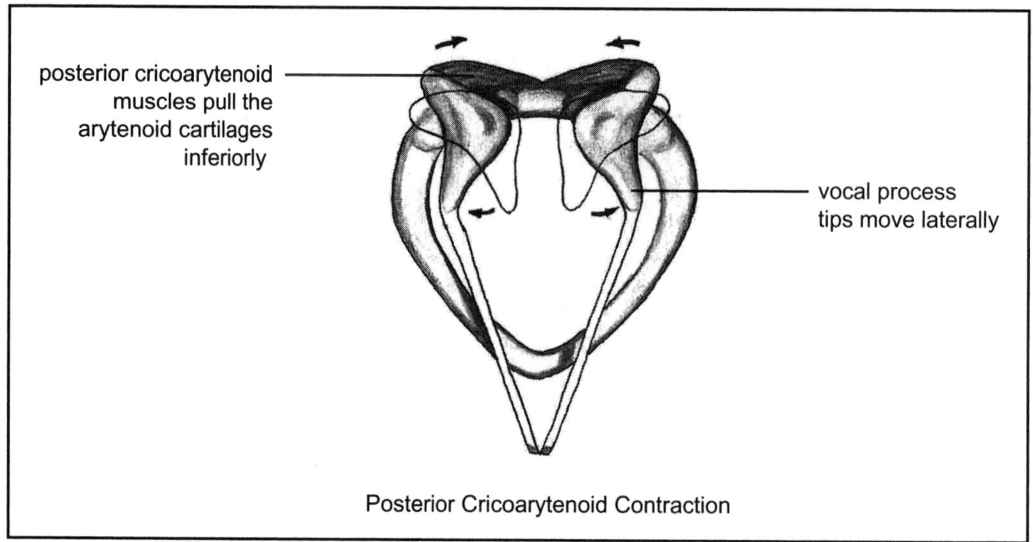
posterior cricoarytenoid muscles pull the arytenoid cartilages inferiorly
vocal process tips move laterally
Posterior Cricoarytenoid Contraction

FIGURE 2–16. Superior view of posterior cricoarytenoid muscle contraction that moves the vocal processes laterally and abducts the vocal folds.

cricoarytenoid contracts, it rocks the arytenoid apices posteriorly to widen the laryngeal vestibule and redirects the vocal processes laterally to separate the membranous portions of the vocal folds, thus widening the glottal aperture by elevating and abducting the vocal folds. The posterior cricoarytenoid abducts fully for respiration and only partially during quick glottal opening gestures to produce unvoiced sounds.[1,2,9,10]

The importance of the intrinsic laryngeal muscles is their remarkable variability to modify the tone, posture, length, and shape of the vocal folds in a wide range of functions, from forceful closure to complex phonation to quiet respiration. Table 2–3 lists each specific muscle function, including its effect on abduction and adduction, vocal fold length, tension, and medial edge. It is worth noting that in clinical circles the intrinsic laryngeal muscles are often discussed using their abbreviations. For instance, the cricothyroid muscle is referred to as the *CT*, thryoartenoid as the *TA*, lateral cricoarytenoid as the *LCA*, interarytenoid as the *IA*, and the posterior cricoarytenoid as the *PCA*.

TRUE FOLDS, VENTRICULAR (FALSE) FOLDS, AND VENTRICLE

Recall from Figure 2–3 that immediately superior to the true vocal folds are another set of folds, called the ventricular (false) folds. Unlike the true vocal folds, the ventricular folds do not vibrate during normal phonation and do not share the same intricate histologic layer structure, nor do they perform discrete adjustments in movement range or position. Perhaps the most important role of the ventricular vocal folds is to create strong adduction for vegetative maneuvers that require very forceful midline closure, such as cough-

Table 2–3. Intrinsic Laryngeal Muscle Functions

Parameters	
Function	Abduction or adduction of the vocal fold
Length	Shortening or lengthening of the vocal fold
Thickness	Thickening or thinning of the vocal fold body
Edge	Sharpening or rounding of the vocal fold free edge
Tension	Increasing or decreasing stiffness of the vocal fold

Muscle Actions					
	CT	***TA***	***LCA***	***IA***	***PCA***
Function	Tensor	Adductor	Adductor	Adductor	Abductor
Length	Longer	Shorter	Shorter		
Thickness	Thinner	Thicker	Thicker		
Edge	Sharper	Rounder	Rounder		
Tension	Stiffer body and cover	Stiffer body; looser cover			

Abbreviations: *CT*, cricothyroid; *TA*, thyroarytenoid; *LCA*, lateral cricoarytenoid; *IA*, interarytenoid; *PCA*, posterior cricoarytenoid.

ing or grunting, or during swallowing. Between the ventricular and true vocal folds is a longitudinal furrow, or space, known as the ventricle. The shape and size of this space vary with the tension and vertical dimensions of the vocal tract, thus influencing vocal resonant quality for professional vocal performers. These three structures mark vertical anatomic regions of the laryngeal vestibule. The supraglottic region is defined as the space above the true vocal folds and between the ventricles and ventricular folds; the intraglottic region (or glottis) is the space between the true vocal folds; and finally, the subglottic region is the space extending from the inferior surface of the true vocal folds down to the cricoid cartilage.

VOCAL FOLD MICROSTRUCTURE

The membranous portions of the vocal folds oscillate (vibrate) to create sound in the larynx. The integrity of the vibrating pattern for phonation relies on a pliable, elastic structure. To achieve this, the fully developed adult vocal folds contain five discrete histologic layers that vary in composition and mechanical properties to provide variable amounts of flexibility and stability. From most superior to deep, the five layers are arranged from a thin, pliable superficial epithelium to progressively stiffer strata of the superficial, intermediate, and deep layers of the lamina propria, to the densest tissue, the vocalis muscle. The epithelium and lamina propria are passive layers that contribute most to vocal fold vibration. Any compromise to these loose, gelatinous structures will impair phonatory quality. Consequently, there is an important microcellular transition zone between the epithelium and the superior layer of the lamina propria which helps preserve vocal fold tissue health or assist in recovery from traumatic injury.[1,2,9,10,28,29]

Epithelium

The free edge of the vocal fold is covered by the epithelium, a mucosal layer of stratified squamous cells that wraps over the internal contents of the vocal folds. The epithelium is the thinnest of the five layers, consisting of only six to eight cell layers, and has been described as a pliable capsule. The deep epithelial cell layer forms a border membrane to divide it from the lamina propria below it. The epithelium offers no mass and is totally compliant but needs a thin layer of slippery mucous lubrication to oscillate best. This lubrication is managed by microstructures that promote water adherence, distribution, and fluid transport along the epithelial surface. First, a mucociliary blanket, divided into mucinous and serous layers, covers the surface. The outermost layer is mucinous; its molecules create a viscous protective cover that prevents dehydration of the underlying serous layer. The serous layer is more watery and contains cilia, which actively beat to and fro to propel water and irritants to the posterior glottis and eventually to the digestive tract. This activity also serves to continually rehydrate and replenish chemical balance in the epithelium.[30,31]

Because the epithelium is the outermost layer of the vocal fold, its delicate cells are the first to be exposed to environmental influences such as humidity, dehydration, pollution, reflux secretions, and other factors that may affect laryngeal health. Besides the mucociliary blanket, microvilli and microridges protect the epithelial surface by distributing fluids and secretions across the epithelial surface. Another internal regulatory system of active fluid and chemical balance has been identified in the vocal fold epithelium. Mucosal chemical receptors can detect and rapidly respond to osmotic changes in the vocal fold environment due to dehydration or other irritant stimuli, by altering the chemical ion balance of sodium, potassium, and other enzymes (eg, adenosine triphosphate, or ATPase). Bidirectional water fluxes transport chemical ions in and out of the mucosa, as needed, to regulate surface fluid, adjust tissue fluid absorption, and restore homeostasis to the vocal fold epithelium.[32,33]

Basement Membrane Zone

The basement membrane zone (BMZ) is a well-defined microcellular transition region that lies between the epithelium, the first layer of the vocal fold, and the next layer, the superficial layer of the lamina propria. Its unique histochemical composition provides a structural juncture between the epithelial cells and the rather loose matrix of proteins present in the superior layer of the lamina propria, where great mechanic shearing forces occur during vocal fold vibration. Accordingly, the BMZ consists of a complex organization of anchoring filaments and collagen fibers organized in horizontal layers to allow tissue in the vocal fold mucosa to shift and glide. These anchoring fibers tether the epithelial mucosa to the underlying lamina propria and appear to provide a small margin of protection from mechanical stress posed by vocal fold vibration. The protein composition and the number and density of anchoring fibers in BMZ have been reported to be genetically influenced. Although normal fiber density is 80 to 120 anchoring fibers per unit area, some specimens display lower or even absent concentrations, which may increase the susceptibility to mechanical injury of the vocal fold. Because BMZ proteins are active in helping repair the epithelial layer when mucosal damage is present, this genetic influence on anchoring fiber density raises questions for future study about genetic predisposition to vocal fold injury (Figure 2–17).[34]

Lamina Propria

The next three layers of the vocal fold form the lamina propria, divided into superficial, middle, and deep layers. Each layer is composed of distinct concentrations of two important fibrous proteins, elastin and collagen, which provide separate contributions to the vibratory properties of the vocal fold cover. Elastin fibers are very thin and have a large dynamic range, allowing tissue to deform (stretch), yet return to its original shape. In contrast, collagen does not stretch easily but can tolerate stress and offers tensile strength and resilience to the extracellular matrix. Both fibers are found in linear arrangements parallel to the vocal fold edge. Accordingly, elastin fibers predominate

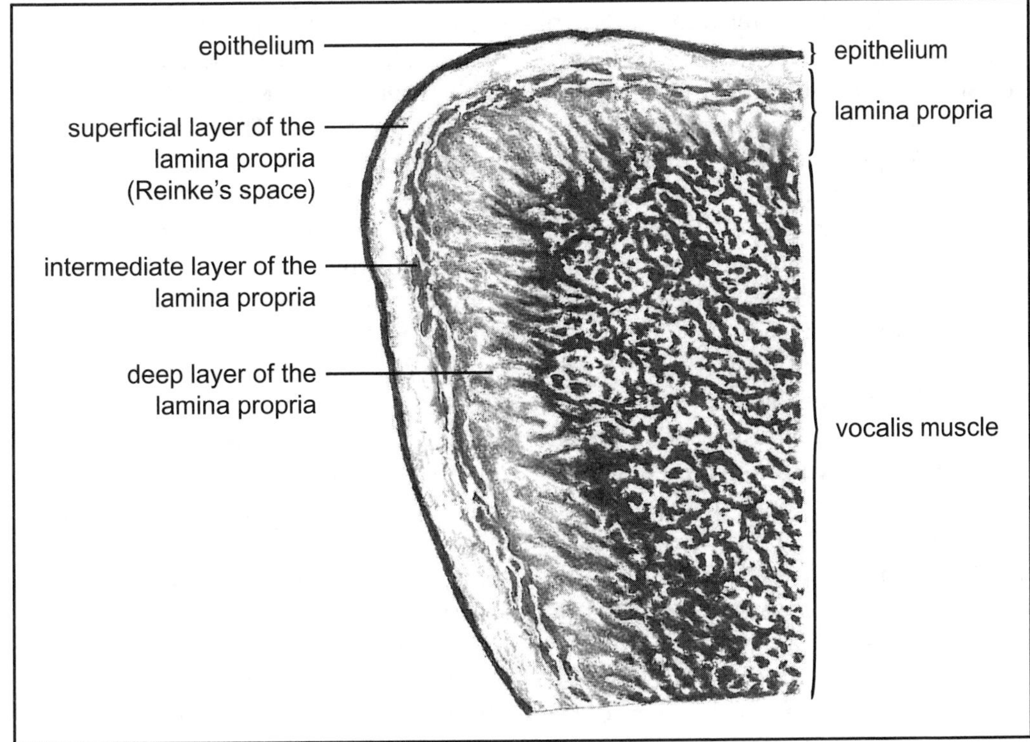

FIGURE 2–17. Vocal fold histologic layer microstructure.

in the superficial and intermediate layers of the lamina propria, where the need for flexible vibratory excursion is greatest, whereas collagen fibers are concentrated in the intermediate and especially the deep layer, where these denser tissues provide cushioning and stability. Elastin fibers develop within the first year in newborn vocal folds and continue to increase in concentration with age, with the largest concentration present in geriatric vocal folds.[9,10,35] Four different types of collagen are present in the basement membrane zone of the vocal fold, but two specific types, collagen Types I and III, were found most commonly in the lamina propria. Collagen Type I fibers, which are thinner and provide tensile strength, were found in both the superficial and deep layers, whereas collagen Type III, which forms larger, wavy fiber bundles, was present throughout all layers, with high concentrations in the superficial and intermediate layers of the lamina propria (I).[9,10,36] All forms of collagen contribute to the flexibility and elasticity of the vocal fold cover.

The superficial layer of the lamina propria is also known as Reinke's space. It is thicker and slightly more dense than the epithelium, although still loose and flexible. This superficial layer is composed of a loose matrix of a few elastin and collagen fibers to provide flexibility and elasticity. It has the appearance of and functions as a soft, slippery, gelatinlike substance, which allows it to vibrate significantly during phonation. When the pliability or health of this layer is violated by vocal fold pathology, the vibratory waveform and resulting voice quality will be significantly impaired. There is a clear border between the superficial layer and the next deeper histologic layer, the intermediate layer of the lamina propria.[9,10,37]

The intermediate layer of the lamina propria is composed principally of elastin fibers, which can stretch to approximately twice their original length, as well as a few collagen fibers to offer tensile strength. Although this layer offers slightly more mass, it also vibrates during phonation. The fourth histologic layer is called the deep layer of the lamina propria. This layer is denser still and composed principally of collagen fibers, and fewer elastin fibers. The tissues of the intermediate and deep layers of the lamina propria (third and fourth layers) together are known as the vocal ligament.[9,10,37,38] These layers are not present in newborn vocal folds, and appear first between the ages of 1 and 4 years. The vocal ligament continues to develop throughout childhood until the larynx reaches full maturity at puberty. Unlike the rather linear cellular divisions between the superficial, intermediate, and deep layers of the lamina propria, the transition between the deep layer fibers and the underlying vocalis muscle is irregular. The deep layer fibers are interspersed with muscle fibers to join these layers firmly together. This architectural fiber organization lends stability at the juncture of the vibrating lamina propria and the stiffer muscle below.[37,39–41]

Other cells present in the lamina propria include fibroblasts, myofibroblasts, and macrophages. Fibroblasts are special cells that produce the fibrous proteins, collagen and elastin. They are present in various concentrations throughout the lamina propria, where they produce enzymes that regulate the tissue environment by destroying old cells and replenishing proteins and other cells. Myofibroblasts, which are differentiated cells designed to repair minor tissue damage, are most concentrated in the superior layer of the lamina propria, where vocal fold injuries from mechanical shearing are common. Macrophages are yet another type of specialized cell that inhibits inflammation; it is most concentrated in the subepithelial juncture between the basement membrane zone and the superior layer of the lamina propria, where infectious agents or environmental irritants may be present.[37,42,43]

The Extracellular Matrix

In addition to the cellular composition described above, all three layers of the lamina propria contain an intricate extracellular (or noncellular) matrix (ECM), designed to provide structural scaffolding and support to the vibrating vocal fold. The ECM is composed of fibrous proteins, interstitial proteins, carbohydrates, and lipids. Recall that the fibrous protein elastin allows tissue to deform flexibly for elasticity during vocal fold vibration, whereas the fibrous protein collagen provides tensile strength to support tissues during mechanical stress and strain.

The interstitial proteins of the lamina propria consist of proteoglycans and glycoproteins that fill the space between the fibrous proteins to control tissue viscosity, layer thickness, and internal fluid content. Tissue viscosity can be thought of as its resistance to flow, or thickness. Tissue with low viscosity is loose, pliable, and vibrates easily; tissue with high viscosity resists easy vibration due to increased thickness, stiffness, or mass. Viscosity is an important variable in vocal fold vibration, and one proteoglycan, hyaluronic acid (HA), appears to influence this factor positively. HA is present throughout the lamina propria but has a larger concentration in the intermediate layer, where it attracts water to form large, space-filling molecules that create a flexible gel. Thus, HA concentrations seem to decrease tissue viscosity while acting as a cushion by resisting compressive and shearing mechanical forces during vocal fold vibration. HA and other proteoglycans in the lamina propria also protect cells from deterioration and assist in tissue repair and clotting.[30,31,35,38] Initially, HA concentration in male vocal folds was reported to exceed that in females by a 3:1 ratio. This gender difference corresponds to there being a thicker intermediate layer of vocal fold lamina propria in males than in females.[35] However, a more recent report using different staining techniques found very large concentrations of HA in female vocal folds, exceeding amounts observed in men, and suggesting that HA concentrations may be variable.[43]

Glycoproteins, lipids, and carbohydrates are also present in the lamina propria. Although less is known about their functional role in the ECM, one glycoprotein, called fibronectin, has been seen extensively in the ECM, in both normal and injured vocal folds. Recent work has identified a large presence of fibronectin in the ECM of embryonic vocal folds and injured folds, including those with benign lesions, such as nodules, polyps, edema, and scar. These histologic findings and work from genetic analyses suggest that this protein is activated when there is a need for tissue regeneration and wound healing.[31,44]

Connective Tissues

Two special connective tissue structures support the vocal folds at points of greatest mechanical stress. First are the anterior and posterior macula flava, which are small oval bundles of elastic and collagen fibers and fibroblasts, connected anteriorly and posteriorly to the membranous lamina propria at the level of the vocal ligament. These connective tissue bundles help to anchor the pliable membranous vocal fold to the cartilage on either end and add elasticity to the cartilaginous membranous attachment. The anterior macula flavae are at the juncture of the vocal folds and the collagenous fibers of the thyroid cartilage, whereas the posterior macula flavae are positioned between the vocal folds and each vocal process tip of the arytenoid cartilage. The cell density of the macula flavae is greater than that seen in the lamina propria, reflecting its function as a stabilizing cushion at the end points of the membranous vocal folds.[1,2,9,10]

The second connective tissue is the conus elasticus, a fibrous membrane that serves as a supportive "shelf" that underlies the vocal fold layers. The conus elasticus arises from the subglottic tracheal wall, coursing superiorly and medially, and inserting into the inferior border of vocal ligament, where it presumably supports the superficial vocal fold tissue vibration.[1,2,9,10]

Vocal Muscle

The fifth and final histologic layer is the vocalis muscle, which has been described previously. The vocalis forms the main body of the vocal fold and provides tonicity, stability, and mass. Although the muscle tissue is far denser than the lamina propria layers above, it still oscillates during vocal fold vibration. Furthermore, because of its nervous innervation, this muscle is the only true "active" tissue, capable of contracting and relaxing to modify vocal fold tone and tension. The lamina propria and epithelium layers vibrate passively in response to the aerodynamic breath stream, but the vocalis muscle is the only portion of the true vocal fold that can contract and relax in response to neurologic control. Therefore, vibration of the vocalis is both active and passive.

BLOOD SUPPLY AND SECRETIONS

The internal fluid balance of the larynx is controlled by the blood supply, whereas external secretions control the external "hydration" of the vocal folds. The blood supply arises from the superior thyroid, superior laryngeal, and inferior laryngeal arteries. These arteries branch from the external carotid artery in the neck. Venous return is transmitted through the jugular vein.[1,2,9] The predominant blood supply is found in the intermediate and deep layers of the lamina propria and the vocalis muscle. Those small blood vessels, arterioles, and capillaries that lie closest to the free vibrating edge run parallel to the vocal fold. In general, the blood supply to the vocal fold is arranged similarly to the histologic layer organization, in that larger arterial supply is found in the deeper layers, whereas smaller capillaries are seen in the lamina propria. There is limited blood supply to the superficial layers and epithelium of the vocal fold, which likely offers some protection from injury to the superficial surface of the vocal fold. When hemorrhage does occur, it creates an extra mass that inhibits its vibration, due to the stiffness formed by the subepithelial clot (varix).[1,2,9,10]

Serous and mucous glands are located in the tissues lateral, superior (in the ventricle), and inferior to the vocal folds, again avoiding the medial edge.[45,46] Mucus propagation along the margin of the fold is assisted by the texture of the epithelial layer, which has microscopic irregularities (microvilli and microridges). These microstructures serve two purposes: increasing the surface tension of the outer membrane to adhere fluids to the vocal fold surface and channeling them to distribute a thin film of liquid along the vocal fold.[32,33,46] This thin, watery, and healthy mucus contributes the characteristic "shine" seen on normal vocal folds. However, in dehydrated or pathologic conditions, the vocal folds may appear dry and dull, and thick clumps of white tacky mucus can appear, especially over lesion sites.

NEUROLOGIC SUPPLY

Central Nervous System Control

Central nervous system (CNS) mechanisms relay afferent (sensory) information from the larynx to the brain and send efferent (motor) commands from the brain to the body. In the larynx, these CNS relays and commands are not entirely understood, because of the difficulty in studying relevant respiratory and phonatory function in vivo and the complex range of vegetative and communicative laryngeal activities required for respiration, phonation, and deglutition. Consider that respiration alone involves very carefully timed acts both of glottal opening for respiration and airway preservation, and glottal closing for swallowing and thoracic stabilization (eg, grunting) as well as coughing, throat clearing, and other airway protective gestures. Similarly, CNS control of phonation requires modulation of many vocalizations, from vegetative sounds produced in nonspeech sounds (eg, laughter, crying) to complex communicative demands of speech and voice, as well as skilled vocalizations for acting and singing performance.

The sensory receptors in laryngeal mucosa and respiratory passages send information from the larynx to the CNS, transmitted along the afferent pathway by the internal branch of the superior laryngeal nerve, through the vagus, to terminate in a region of the medulla called the nucleus tractus solitarius (NTS). This region contains areas that are involved in the control of respiration, laryngeal maneuvers, and swallowing. In anesthetized animal studies, NTS fiber activity has been shown to occur in phase with the timing of evoked swallowing or respiratory events. Other sensory fibers do not terminate in NTS but continue to another section of the midbrain called the periaqueductal gray area (PAG).[47,48] There is also some limited evidence of sensory projection from the larynx to even higher order centers (above the midbrain) in the cortex, including projections to the thalamus (a major sensory relay center), superiorly through the corona radiata, and finally to the postcentral gyrus of the cortex.[49–51]

Efferent (motor) commands for voice production originate in the precentral gyrus of the cerebral cortex, which communicates with motor nuclei in the brainstem and spinal cord, before transmitting commands to the peripheral nervous system to trigger muscle contractions. Both pyramidal and extrapyramidal motor pathways are involved in laryngeal control for phonation. Conclusions from experimental work suggest the PAG is a crucial center for voluntary control over vocalizations, by projecting motor commands through the nucleus retroambiguus (NRA) located in the medulla, which in turn projects to the motor nucleus ambiguus, located in the reticular formation. It has been suggested that this PAG-NRA projection may serve as a final common pathway for vocalization.[47,48] The nucleus ambiguus contains the central origins of the laryngeal motoneurons for all of the intrinsic laryngeal muscles. The localized site of cricothyroid motoneurons is more distinct than the motoneuron groupings of the other intrinsic muscles, which appear to converge in a general area. Motoneurons for esophageal and respiratory control are also located in the nucleus ambiguus. Studies that examine laryngeal motoneuron activity have found that units may be task-specific for vocalization, inspiration, or a combination of expiration and vocalization.[47,48] Thus, the interaction between phonation, deglutition, and respiration is inherent to understanding the central pathways of laryngeal control, reflexive activity, and voluntary laryngeal maneuvers for nonspeech gestures and speech production.[2,9,10,47,48]

Peripheral Innervation

The 10th cranial nerve (X), the vagus, innervates the larynx peripherally (Figure 2–18). Vagus means "wandering," and the name appropriately describes its circuitous and far-reaching route through the body to innervate sites from the skull to the abdomen. The vagus innervates the larynx via two important branches, the recurrent and superior laryngeal nerves, which contain all the sensory and motor fibers that supply the larynx. The first portion is the superior laryngeal nerve (SLN), which branches off the vagus near the nodose ganglia in the neck. After coursing alongside the carotid artery, the SLN forms internal and external branches. The internal branch inserts through the thyrohyoid membrane, superior to the vocal folds, and provides most of the sensory information to the larynx. The external branch is primarily a motor nerve that has been regarded historically as innervating the cricothyroid muscle only.[1,2,9,10] However, recent studies have suggested that the external branch of the SLN can also innervate the ipsilateral thyroarytenoid muscle, inferior pharyngeal constrictor (and upper esophageal sphincter), as well as connect with the recurrent laryngeal nerve in some cases.[52]

The second branch off the vagus is the recurrent laryngeal nerve (RLN), which extends to the thorax, where it forms long loops through the heart before coursing superiorly back up under the thyroid gland and on to the larynx. The pattern of recurrence is different on the right and left sides of the body. The right RLN courses under the subclavian artery; the left RLN courses under the aortic arch before it reaches the larynx.[1,2,9,10] Consequently, these nerves (especially on the left) are susceptible to injury, and a patient with an unexplained idiopathic vocal fold paralysis should always be evaluated to rule out possible cardiac, lung, or thyroid compromise.

The RLN supplies all sensory information below the vocal folds and all

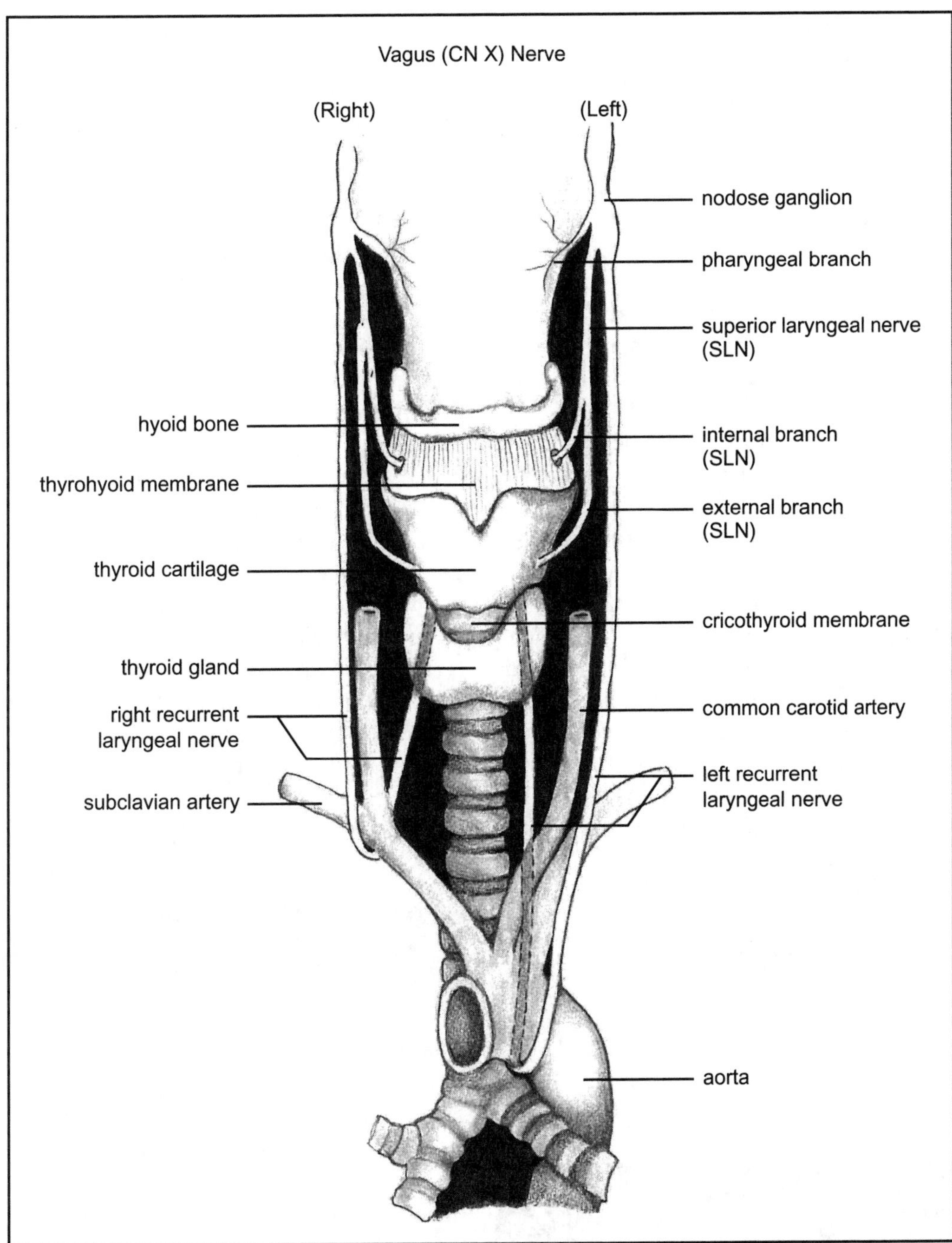

FIGURE 2–18. Vagus (cranial nerve X) innervation of the larynx.

motor innervation to the posterior crico-arytenoid, thyroarytenoid, lateral crico-arytenoid, and interarytenoid muscles. Two characteristics of the SLN and RLN ensure the ability of the intrinsic laryngeal muscles to move quickly and with fine motor control. First, the laryngeal nerves have a high conduction velocity (second only to the eye), which allows rapid contractions. Second, the innervation ratio is low, meaning that many cells (estimated at 100 to 200) are innervating a single motor unit, allowing very specific motor control and tuning.[47,48]

Peripheral muscle receptors are present in all intrinsic laryngeal muscles, to control vocal fold tone and movement. Part of this specialized control arises from the discrete nerve innervation to separate muscle compartments in three of the muscles: the posterior cricoarytenoid, the cricothyroid, and the thyroarytenoid (thryomuscularis and thyrovocalis). Muscle spindles are special proprioceptive receptors common in skeletal muscles that must control dynamic changes in muscle length to adjust for fluctuating structural posture, weight bearing, or position, by creating graduated changes in muscle length under variable stimuli. These receptors occasionally have been identified in the intrinsic laryngeal muscles, most prominently in the thyromuscularis compartment of the thyroarytenoid.[27] However, a later investigation failed to identify the presence of any muscle spindles in the thyroarytenoid muscle, which reinforces the need for additional study confirming the presence and function of muscle spindles in the larynx.[51]

LARYNGEAL REFLEXES

A complex system of laryngeal reflexes preserves the airway through a series of sensory receptors located in mucosal tissue, articular joints, and muscle. These receptors have the ability to elicit tight sphincteric closure, also known as a laryngeal adductor response, to close off the trachea and lungs to protect the airway from foreign materials or aspiration. Mucosal tissue receptors respond to touch, vibration, changes in air pressure, and liquid stimuli; mechanoreceptors respond to stimuli in articular joints and muscles.[53] These life-protecting reflexes occur rapidly, and some have been shown to respond normally (neither interrupted nor delayed) even during speech or respiratory tasks, such as quiet inspiration, humming, forced exhalation, and vowel prolongation, which demonstrates their ability to preserve the airway, regardless of laryngeal activity.[54] Stimulants that irritate the vocal fold mucosa may also incite an extreme glottic closure reflex, called laryngospasm. In an awake individual, laryngospasm usually lasts under a minute, but in aggravated cases (eg, under anesthesia), this prolonged vocal fold adduction can pose a threat to ventilation.[9,10]

DEVELOPMENTAL CHANGES

In newborns, the larynx is situated high in the neck, with the cricoid positioned at the approximate level of C3 to C4 in the cervical column. As babies grow in the first year, the larynx begins its descent in the neck, while the pharynx lengthens and widens. By puberty, the larynx has descended to the level of C6 or C7, accompanied by significant skeletal facial growth to create a much larger vocal tract length and area. This increase in supraglottic dimensions contributes importantly to the precipitous drop in vocal fundamental frequency and development of resonant speech characteristics that develop from childhood to physical maturation.

The intrinsic larynx also undergoes dramatic changes from birth through puberty. Hirano, Kurita, and Nakashima have examined the size and structure of the vocal folds across age ranges (Table 2–4).[39] The vocal fold length of boys and girls appears to be similar until about age 10 years. After that point, there is gradual but consistent gender-specific development that increases the overall length of the vocal folds and changes the covarying ratio between the membranous to cartilaginous portions of vocal folds, in different dimensions for males and females. By adulthood, the female overall vocal fold length is 11 to 15 mm, whereas the male length is 17 to 21 mm. The greater ratio of cartilage-to-membrane length in newborns recedes with development, so that at maturity, the ratio of membranous to cartilage portions is 4:1 in adult females and 5.5:1 in adult males.[39] This growth correlates with other standard indicators of physical maturation, including height, weight, and onset of puberty. For example, in males, the rise in testosterone at puberty stimulates the anterior growth of the thyroid notch and wide growth of the pharynx.

In newborn infants, the total vocal fold length ranges from 1.25 to 3 mm, and the ratio from membranous to cartilage portions is approximately 1.5:1. The macula flava connective tissues at the juncture of the membranous and cartilaginous attachments are already present at birth.[39] Stellate cells and cell surface receptors for hyaluronic acid (prominent in the ECM of the lamina propria) are present in the newborn macula flava, even though the newborn membranous vocal fold has no identifiable layer structure at this time.[1,3] By the age of 2 to 5 months, cells begin to differentiate into 2 layers, progressing to 3 different layers of cell density by about 11 months. These cell differentiations will ultimately develop throughout childhood into discrete transition layers with different cellular concentrations of elastin and collagen. Although clear changes in cellular layer composition are observable from the first year through age 12 or 13, the final 5-layer structure of the lamina propria, including the vocal ligament, is not completely developed until puberty.[41]

Table 2–4. Laryngeal Growth and Development

	Newborns	*Adult Females*	*Adult Males*
Total vocal fold length	2.5–3 mm	11–15 mm	17–21 mm
Membranous portion	1.3–2 mm	8.5–12 mm	14.5–18 mm
Cartilaginous portion	1–3 mm	2–3 mm	2–3 mm
Membranous to cartilaginous ratio	1.5:1	4.0:1	5.3:1
Thyroid cartilage angle	130°	110°	90°
Cricoid level in the neck	C2–C3	C6	C7

GERIATRIC VOCAL FOLDS

Changes in vocal fold anatomy with aging have received increasing attention over the last 2 decades. Clinicians have long been aware of the deterioration in voice quality, pitch and loudness range, and vocal endurance among geriatric speakers. Laryngeal imaging techniques have provided information about the common appearance of thinned (bowed) vocal folds in elderly patients, especially those who have no other apparent contributing pathology except advanced chronological age.[55,56] The clinical observation of these geriatric changes in voice quality and laryngeal appearance has been termed *presbylaryngeus*, or aging larynx.

Histologic evidence of age-based changes in laryngeal anatomy has demonstrated that the intermediate layer of the lamina propria in geriatric vocal folds becomes looser and thinner, which could contribute to a loss of tissue bulk, resulting in the characteristic bowed appearance of glottic closure patterns seen clinically in patients with presbyphonia. Histologically, there is evidence of morphologic disorganization and breakdown of the collagen and elastin fibers in aging vocal folds as well as changes in the composition and concentrations of fibrous and interstitial proteins. With age, fibroblast cellular regulation declines, and fibrous proteins do not regenerate as quickly. Elastin fibers proliferate with age but may become broken or cross-linked with other cells, which adds stiffness and decreases overall tissue elasticity. The delicate layer structure that characterized the young adult lamina propria deconstructs as elastin fibers become denser and less pliable, and broken fibers are replaced by more fibrous collagen throughout the lamina propria.[57]

In the past decade, investigators have also examined aging intrinsic laryngeal muscle to detect changes due to muscle fiber injury or atrophy, which is anticipated with advanced age. Immunohistologic analyses have revealed two important processes present in the aging thyroarytenoid muscle. First, there is a proliferation of myonuclei and associated satellite cells that accompany a specialized process called *apoptosis*, or planned cell death (suicide). This apoptosis results in selective, age-related loss of type 1 muscle fibers in the vocal fold.[58] Second, aging thyroarytenoid muscle tissues exhibit proportional increases in the developmental myosin isoform, which is only present in adults when muscle fibers are regenerating. This finding suggests that despite the inevitable age-related decline of muscle function due to fiber injury or cell death, human vocal fold muscle fibers retain the ability to partially compensate for these tissue changes by spontaneously regenerating with age.[59] However, newly regenerated muscle fibers require motoneuron innervation to function; without sufficient nerve supply, muscle fibers will continue to denervate and atrophy, and contribute to the characteristic loss of muscle tone and bulk (ie, bowing) seen clinically in the aging vocal folds.[55,56] Laryngeal motoneurons also demonstrate variable age-related motor unit remodeling, through cycles of denervation, followed by nerve collateral sprouting, and finally reinnervation. This process results in longer motor unit durations, especially after age 60.[60] Other signs of neurologic decline include fewer motor units, less efficient nerve connections, and larger muscle territory supplied by each motor unit.

DNA MICROARRAY GENE EXPRESSION ANALYSIS

The most recent advance in our knowledge of laryngeal tissue anatomy and physiology emerges from the field of molecular biology, where rapid DNA microarray analysis techniques have been applied to examine patterns of gene expression in vocal fold tissue. DNA contains our gene code, which contains all of the information needed to regulate the cell biology of living tissue. When specific cellular functions are required, a DNA response will trigger a molecular message, through a process called *transcription*, making a special molecule, mRNA (called *mRNA* to reflect the "message" function) with instructions to execute a specific task, such as sending information to build the proper protein to repair tissue injury. The genetic expression of any given tissue will reflect the type and number of mRNA present. This information provides important clues not only about the cellular environment, but also the gene's recent exposure to toxins or disease, as well as its history of mechanical strain or injury. Thus, gene expression provides information about the biological state of current health and the tissue's response to ongoing cellular activities and exposures.[61]

Microarray analysis allows rapid and simultaneous analysis of mRNA by thousands of genes. By using known information about DNA and statistical analyses that factor the presence of mRNA in various samples, it is possible to identify whether a specific gene expression is typical, overexpressed (or upregulated), or underexpressed (downregulated) as compared to findings from control tissues. From that information, researchers can determine what mRNA are present, which are deficient, and how they are altering the tissue environment. The timing of microarray analyses is also important. Whereas DNA lasts for the lifetime of the cell, mRNA is present only long enough to execute the messenger command. Therefore, DNA can be studied at any time in the life of the cell, but mRNA genetic expression reflects only the current status of a cell. This timing has great implications for measuring gene expression in healthy versus pathologic vocal folds because it provides a current profile of the coordinated regulatory processes underway at a given point in time. For example, DNA microarray analyses of vocal fold polyp and granuloma tissues have identified the proliferation of select genes that were not present in microarray analyses of healthy control tissue. Specifically, upregulated epithelial and epidermal genes were present in the vocal fold polyp. In contrast, the granuloma exhibited overexpression of inflammatory, wound healing, and extracellular matrix remodeling genes.[62] More recently, microarray analysis was used to compare tissue samples from Reinke's edema and polyps. Gene transcription profiles exhibited the presence of distinct molecular and cellular DNA processes in these two lesions; 65 genes differentiated Reinke's edema and polyps.[63] To further test the model, the transcription profiles for Reinke's edema and polyps were used to classify two lesions that were previously determined to be "unknown" by five voice specialists. Using a predictor analysis, genetic profiles successfully classified both unknown lesions with a minimum of 13 genes.[63] Although much further study is needed, this important finding confirms the feasibility of using genetic microarray analysis to verify differential diagnoses of laryngeal tissue abnormalities. In the future, mRNA information about cellular homeostasis and protein production in the tissues will assist in developing translational treatment protocols for vocal fold pathologies, including genetic tissue engineering or protein therapies.[61,62]

PHYSIOLOGY OF PHONATION

Theories of Vibration

Van den Berg's Aerodynamic-Myoelastic Theory

Vocal fold vibration is achieved based on the physical process of flow-induced oscillation, where a consistent stream of air flows past the tissues, creating a repeated pattern of opening and closing. In van den Berg's aerodynamic-myoelastic theory, both airflow (aerodynamic) and muscular (myoelastic) properties account for the passive convergent and divergent motions of the vocal folds during phonation. This classical theory emphasizes the reciprocal role of subglottal pressure and transglottal flow as they interact with vocal fold tissue resistance and elasticity. At the onset of phonation, subglottal pressure rises below the adducted vocal folds.[1,9,64–67] When pressure rises to overcome this resistance, the folds are blown apart and subglottal pressure diminishes, accelerating the flow rate through the glottis. Because pressure and flow are inversely proportional, when flow increases, a momentary pressure drop occurs between the vocal folds, which also draws the vocal folds back together, according to the Bernoulli principle. Elastic tissue recoil also pulls the vocal folds back toward midline, completing a full cycle of vibration. With the vocal folds reapproximated, subglottal pressure builds again to repeat the process. Oscillation is a function of two contributions: covarying pressure and flow and the mechanical properties of tissue deformation and collision. Van den Berg's aerodynamic myoelastic theory provided an early understanding of vocal fold vibration, but later discoveries of the histologic tissue composition and vibratory mucosal waveforms have generated more advanced theories about vocal fold vibration.[1,9,64–67]

Hirano's Body-Cover Theory

Hirano's body-cover theory recognizes the important role of the passive (nonmuscular) superficial layers (epithelium and lamina propria) to vocal fold vibration.[1,3,4,10,65–67] Each of the five histologic layers, from epithelium to three-layered lamina propria to muscle tissue, present different properties of vibratory mass and compliance. The epithelial layer is the most elastic component; subsequent layers form a complex transition to stiffer muscle tissue. The functional layer differences are not as discrete; often they are regrouped into three vibratory divisions: cover (epithelium and superficial layer of the lamina propria), transition (intermediate and deep layers of the lamina propria), and body (vocalis muscle). The theory of vocal fold vibration is based on these functional divisions. The vibrating cover forms the compliant, fluid oscillation seen in vocal fold vibratory patterns, whereas the body provides the stiffer, underlying stability of vocal fold mass and tonus. The transition serves as the coupling between the superficial mucosa and the deep muscle tissue of the vocal fold during vibration. Thus, the body-cover theory of vibration accounts for the mass and stability provided by the vocalis muscle and deep layer of the lamina propria over which the compliant and flexible layers of the lamina propria and epithelium oscillate.[1,3,4,10,65–67]

This "undulation" or oscillation of the superficial vocal fold layers creates an infinitely variable ripple of tissue deformation and recoil. Vocal fold vibration is a complex waveform that challenges advanced vibration theory and modeling techniques. Some investigators have explored applications of chaos theory (fractal analysis) to vocal fold vibration in an attempt to account for both the complexity and redundancy of vibratory patterns.[37,68] Clinically, it is useful to consider at least three vibratory phases of wave motion that can be seen from a superior view during endoscopy:

- Horizontal (medial to lateral movements), as seen during the opening and closing patterns of vibration
- Longitudinal (anterior to posterior "zipperlike" wave), as seen in a front-to-back traveling wave
- Vertical phase (inferior to superior opening and closing of the vocal folds), seen as an upper versus lower lip difference in some views of vocal fold vibration.[5,28,37]

Reports of mucosal wave amplitudes estimate that the horizontal excursion (medial to lateral motion) during normal vocal fold vibration ranges from 1 to 2 mm. The vertical-phase change appears to be much larger, however, in the realm of 3 to 5 mm.[39] Clinically, only horizontal and longitudinal changes can be seen readily during most imaging techniques (ie, supraglottic view), although some close images of vocal folds will display vertical phase differences. This is an unfortunate limit, because experimental evidence suggests that this (mostly) unseen vertical-phase change in mucosal wave probably affects the overall vibratory waveform significantly (Plate 1).[5,12,28,37,66]

Titze's Self-Oscillation Theory

Most recently, Titze has expanded on these theories to describe the vocal folds as a flow-induced self-oscillating system, sustained across time by the aerodynamic forces of pressure and flow. Scherer, Titze, Jiang, and others have described a sequence of vocal fold oscillation that explains the interchange between these aerodynamic events and associated mechanical tissue response.[5,12,28,37,66] Recall that pressure and flow are reciprocal in this context; when flow is high, pressure is low, and vice versa. In this model, respiration is the driving force that sets the vocal folds in motion (oscillation), and the interchange between pressure and flow at three critical sites keeps the vocal folds vibrating, as follows:

1. Subglottal region: At the area directly beneath the vocal folds, the "leading edges" of the folds are blown apart and set into motion by subglottal air pressure. As the vocal folds are

blown open, translaryngeal (glottal) flow is positive. When the folds recoil to midline, flow is negative.

2. Intraglottal space: In the small space directly between the paired vocal folds, intraglottal pressure keeps the vocal folds oscillating as the convergent and divergent shaping of vocal folds in a back-and-forth motion creates the alternating exchange of airflow and pressure peaks. When the vocal folds are open, intraglottal pressure is positive but dropping as flow increases. When the vocal folds close, intraglottal pressure is negative but rising with the narrowing glottis. As soon as the subglottal pressure blows vocal folds apart, tissue elastic recoil draws them back together at midline closure, which then begins the cycle of subglottal pressure buildup all over again.
3. Supraglottal air column: At the outlet of the glottis, immediately above the vocal folds, the air molecules in the vocal tract are alternately compressed or rarified in a delayed response to the alternate subglottal pressure and transglottal flow puffs created by the vibrating vocal folds. Before vibration begins, the molecules in the vocal tract air column just above the vocal folds are at rest. Once vibration begins, air pressure emitted from the oscillating vocal folds alternatively pushes upward and momentarily releases the vocal tract molecules in a slightly delayed response to the sound energy pulses. This vocal tract air column thus assists in sustaining vocal fold oscillation by serving as a "top-down" driving force, transferring energy from the fluid (air pressure) down to the tissue (upper lip of the vocal folds).[5,12,28,37,66]

Fundamental Frequency Control

Fundamental frequency is the rate of vocal fold vibration, usually expressed in cycles per second, or hertz. The acoustic perceptual correlate of fundamental frequency is pitch. The factors that determine fundamental frequency control are vocal fold length and tension, including passive tension on the vocal fold cover and active stiffness of the vocal fold body. To achieve higher pitch, cricothyroid muscle contraction causes the vocal folds to lengthen, as the cover layers become stretched, tensed, and thin, particularly at the medial vibrating edge. To lower pitch, the thyroarytenoid muscle contracts to shorten vocal fold length, thus decreasing tension on the cover and rounding the medial edge for greater amplitude of vibration. Two other parameters appear to covary with fundamental frequency in predictable ways in modal vocal fold vibration. First, subglottal pressure tends to increase proportionally with increased fundamental frequency in the midrange. Second, vibratory amplitude motion is inversely proportional to the rate of vocal fold vibration. The higher the pitch, the smaller is the vibratory amplitude; amplitude increases as pitch decreases.[1,2,4,5,12]

Intensity Control

Vocal intensity is the sound pressure level of the acoustic output, and its perceptual correlate is loudness. Several factors influence vocal intensity, including subglottal pressure, vocal fold vibratory phase closure, transglottal flow, and supraglottic vocal tract tuning. Healthy voice users have a wide dynamic (loudness) range available to produce sounds that are very quiet or very loud across a range of low and high pitches, especially when vocal folds can achieve complete closure and vibrate flexibly (without stiffness or tension). In general, the intensity of the glottal sound source increases proportionally with increased subglottal pressure and is achieved mechanically because of longer vibratory phase closure pattern and a larger amplitude of vibration. Intensity also tends to covary proportionally with the increased subglottal pressure required to raise fundamental frequency. For example, voice range profiles display the characteristic increase in intensity with increased fundamental frequency. Finally, the vocal tract tuning or filtering characteristic can influence the loudness of the glottal source, as increased supraglottic resonance can increase the acoustic radiation of sound energy. This phenomenon is used widely by trained vocalists, who learn to open the mouth and widen the vocal tract area to project loud speech or singing notes for performance needs.[1,2,4,5,12]

Phonation Modes and Voice Quality Control

Audioperceptual judgments of voice quality are highly subjective, but generally, phonatory quality is affected by the integrity of vocal fold vibration, as defined by regularity, symmetry, phase shape of tissue deformation, and the slope of the glottal flow waveform. Deviations in the cycle-to-cycle slope and shape of the waveform characteristics will impair the resulting acoustic signal. The filtering characteristic of the supraglottic vocal tract will also enhance or detract from the perceived voice quality of the signal. Thus, the quality of voice relies on multiple factors, including compliant and symmetric biomechanic properties of the vocal folds, an adequate and consistent subglottic pressure and flow source, and appropriate vocal tract tuning characteristics.[1,2,4,5,12]

Falsetto (loft), modal (chest) voice, and glottal fry (pulse) are three special phonation modes, or registers. They are identifiable perceptually and can be discriminated by their signature variations in subglottal pressure, flow, and vibratory patterns. Falsetto voice occurs predominantly at high fundamental frequencies and is characterized by strong cricothyroid contraction, resulting in thin and high-pitched voice quality due to slightly abducted vocal folds with vibration only at the medial edges, little to no closed phase, and high flow and subglottal pressure. Modal voice occurs at mid-frequency ranges, when the thyroarytenoid is contracted, shortening the effective length of the vocalis and relaxing the passive cover layers to produce rounded vocal fold edges and allow complete glottic closure with large vibratory amplitude and mucosal wave. Glottal fry occurs at the lowest end of the fundamental frequency range and is characterized by pulsed and irregular vocal fold vibration with a prolonged closed phase, low subglottal pressure, and very limited transglottal flow.[1,2,4,5,12]

SUMMARY

The larynx is an immensely complex organ that serves many functions for both vegetative and communicative purposes. Research continues to define laryngeal anatomic, morphologic, and histologic microstructure, its central and peripheral neural control mechanisms, physiologic function, and most recently, genetic properties in normal and pathologic conditions. This scientific knowledge is critical to understanding the relationship between voice disorders and their consequential effects on voice production, and to discovering optimal rehabilitative approaches. Additional chapters in this text describe measurement tools that clarify our understanding of vocal function and its relationship to voice production.

REFERENCES

1. Hirano M. *Clinical Examination of Voice.* New York, NY: Springer-Verlag; 1981.
2. Kirchner JA. *Physiology of the Larynx.* Washington, DC: The American Academy of Otolaryngology-Head and Neck Surgery Foundation Inc; 1984.
3. Hirano M. Phonosurgical anatomy of the larynx. In: Ford CN, Bless DM, eds. *Phonosurgery.* New York, NY: Raven Press; 1991:25–42.
4. Scherer RC. Physiology of phonation: a review of basic mechanics. In: Ford CN, Bless DM, eds. *Phonosurgery.* New York, NY: Raven Press; 1991:77–94.
5. Scherer R. Laryngeal function during phonation. In: Rubin JS, Sataloff RT, Korovin GS, eds. *Diagnosis and Treatment of Voice Disorders.* 2nd ed. Clifton Park, NY: Thomson Delmar Learning; 2003: 87–106.
6. Acker BF. Vocal tract adjustments for the projected voice. *J Voice.* 1987;1:77–82.
7. Lessac A. *The Use and Training of the Human Voice.* New York, NY: Drama Book Publishers; 1967.
8. Fink BR, Demarest RJ. *Laryngeal Biomechanics.* Cambridge, MA: Harvard University Press; 1978.
9. Tucker HM. *The Larynx.* New York, NY: Thieme Medical Publishers Inc; 1987.
10. Noordzij JP, Ossoff RH. Anatomy and physiology of the larynx. *Otolaryngol Clin North Am.* 2006;39(1):1–10.
11. Hixon T. *Respiratory Function in Speech and Song.* Boston, MA: College-Hill Press; 1987.
12. Titze IR. *Principles of Voice Production.* Englewood Cliffs, NJ: Prentice-Hall; 1994.
13. Gauffin J, Sundberg J. Spectral correlates of glottal voice source waveform characteristics. *J Speech Hearing Res.* 1989;32:556–565.
14. Davis PJ, Bartlett D Jr, Luschei ES. Coordination of the respiratory and laryngeal systems in breathing and vocalization. In: Titze IR, ed. *Vocal Fold Physiology.* San Diego, CA: Singular Publishing Group; 1993:89–226.
15. Fant G. The voice source: theory and acoustic modeling. In: Titze IR, Scherer RC, eds. *Vocal Fold Physiology.* Denver, CO: Denver Center for the Performing Arts; 1983:453–464.
16. Kent RD, Read C. *The Acoustic Analysis of Speech.* San Diego, CA: Singular Publishing Group; 1992.
17. Verdolini-Marston K, Burke MK, Lessac A, Glaze L, Caldwell E. Preliminary study of two methods of treatment for laryngeal nodules. *J Voice.* 1995;9(1): 74–85.
18. Erickson D, Baer T, Harris KS. The role of strap muscles in pitch lowering. In: Bless DM, Abbs J, eds. *Vocal Fold Physiology.* San Diego, CA: College-Hill Press; 1983:279–285.
19. Morrison M, Angsuwarangsee T. Extrinsic laryngeal muscular tension in patients with voice disorders. *J Voice.* 2002;16(3):333–343.
20. Verdolini K, Druker DG, Palmer PM, Samawi H. Laryngeal adduction in resonant voice. *J Voice.* 1998;12(3): 325–327.

21. Kahane JC. Connective tissue changes in the larynx and their effects on voice. *J Voice.* 1987;1:27–30.
22. Kahane JC. Age-related changes in the human cricoarytenoid joint. In: Fujimura O, ed. *Vocal Fold Physiology.* Vol 2. New York, NY: Raven Press; 1988: 145–158.
23. Hirano M, Yoshida T, Kurita S, Kiyokawa K, Sato K, Tateishi O. Anatomy and behavior of the vocal process. In: Baer C, Sasaki S, Harris K, eds. *Laryngeal Function in Phonation and Respiration.* Boston, MA: Little, Brown and Company; 1987:3–13.
24. Von Leden H, Moore P. The mechanics of the cricoarytenoid joint. *Arch Otolaryngol.* 1961;73:541–555.
25. Hirano M, Kiyokawa K, Kurita S. Laryngeal muscles and glottic shaping. In: Fujimura O, ed. *Vocal Fold Physiology.* Vol 2. New York, NY: Raven Press; 1988: 49–66.
26. McHenry M, Kuna S, Minton J, Vanoye C, Calhoun, K. Differential activity of the pars recta and pars oblique in fundamental frequency control. *J Voice.* 1997: 11:48–58.
27. Saunders I, Han Y, Wang J, Biller H. Muscle spindles are concentrated in the superior vocalis subcompartment of the human thyroarytenoid muscle. *J Voice.* 1999;12:7–16.
28. Hirano M. Structure and behavior of the vibratory vocal folds. In: Sawashima T, Cooper D, eds. *Dynamic Aspects of Speech Production.* Tokyo, Japan: University of Tokyo Press; 1966:13–23.
29. Hirano M, Matsuo K, Kakita Y, Kawasaki H, Kurita S. Vibratory behavior versus the structure of the vocal fold. In: Titze IR, Scherer, RM, eds. *Vocal Fold Physiology.* Denver, CO: Denver Center for the Performing Arts; 1983:26–40.
30. Gray SD, Hirano M, Sato K. Molecular and cellular structure of vocal fold tissue. In: Titze IR, ed. *Vocal Fold Physiology.* San Diego, CA: Singular Publishing Group; 1993:1–35.
31. Gray SD. Cellular physiology of the vocal folds. *Otolaryngol Clin North Am.* 2000;33(4):679–697.
32. Fisher K, Telser A, Phillips J, Yeates D. Regulation of vocal fold transepithelial water fluxes. *J Appl Physiol.* 2001;91: 1401–1411.
33. Sivasankar M, Fisher K. Vocal folds detect ionic perturbations on the luminal surface: an in vitro investigation. *J Voice.* 2008;22(4):408–419.
34. Gray S. Basement membrane zone injury in vocal nodules. In: Gauffin J, Hammarberg B, eds. *Vocal Fold Physiology.* San Diego, CA: Singular Publishing Group; 1991:21–28.
35. Hammond T, Gray S, Butler J, Zhou R, Hammond E. Age- and gender-related elastin distribution changes in human vocal folds. *Otolaryngol Head Neck Surg.* 1998;119(4):314–321.
36. Tateya T, Tateya I, Bless DM. Collagen subtypes in human vocal folds. *Ann Otol Rhinol Laryngol.* 2006;115(6):469–476.
37. Jiang J, Lin E, Hanson DG. Vocal fold physiology. *Otolaryngol Clin North Am.* 2000;33(4):699–718.
38. Hammond T, Zhou R, Hammond E, Pawlak A, Gray S. The intermediate layer: a morphologic study of the elastin and hyaluronic acid contents of normal human vocal folds. *J Voice.* 1997;11:59–66.
39. Hirano M, Kurita S, Nakashima T. Growth, development, and aging of human vocal folds. In: Bless DM, Abbs J, eds. *Vocal Fold Physiology.* San Diego, CA: College-Hill Press; 1983:22–43.
40. Gray SD, Smith M, Schneider H. Voice disorders in children. *Pediatr Clin North Am.* 1996;43(6):1357–1384.
41. Hartnick CJ, Rehbar R, Prasad V. Development and maturation of the pediatric human vocal fold lamina propria. *Laryngoscope.* 2005:115(1):4–15.
42. Sato K, Sakamoto K, Nakashima T. Expression and distribution of CD44 and hyaluronic acid in human vocal fold mucosa. *Ann Otol Rhinol Laryngol.* 2006;115(10):741–748.

43. Lebl MDA, Martins JRM, Nader HB, Simones MJ, De Biase N. Concentration and distribution of hyaluronic acid in human vocal folds. *Laryngoscope.* 2007;117(4):595–599.
44. Hirschi SD, Gray SD, Thibeault S. Fibronectin: an interesting vocal fold protein. *J Voice.* 2002;16(3):310–316.
45. Gracco C, Kahane JC. Age-related changes in the vestibular folds of the human larynx: a histomorphometric study. *J Voice.* 1989;3:204–212.
46. Fukuda H, Kawaida M, Tatehara T, et al. A new concept of lubricating mechanisms of the larynx. In: Fujimura O, ed. *Vocal Fold Physiology.* Vol 2. New York, NY: Raven Press; 1988:83–92.
47. Larson CR, Wilson KE, Luschei ES. Preliminary observations on cortical and brainstem mechanisms of laryngeal control. In: Bless DM, Abbs J, eds. *Vocal Fold Physiology.* San Diego, CA: College-Hill Press; 1983:82–95.
48. Garrett JD, Larson CR. Neurology of the laryngeal system. In: Ford CN, Bless DM, eds. *Phonosurgery.* New York, NY: Raven Press; 1991:43–76.
49. Udaka J, Kanetake H, Kihara H, Koike Y. Human laryngeal responses induced by sensory nerve stimuli. In: Fujimura O, ed. *Vocal Fold Physiology.* Vol 2. New York, NY: Raven Press; 1988:67–74.
50. Davis P, Zhang SP, Bandler R. Midbrain and medullary regulation of vocalization. In: Davis P, Fletcher N, eds. *Vocal Fold Physiology.* San Diego, CA: Singular Publishing Group; 1996:121–136.
51. Brandon CA, Rosen C, Georgelis G, Horton MJ, Mooney MP, Sciote JJ. Staining of human thyroarytenoid muscle with myosin antibodies reveals some unique extrafusal fibers, but no muscle spindles. *J Voice.* 2003;17(2):245–254.
52. Mu L, Sanders I. The human cricothyroid muscle: three muscle bellies and their innervation patterns. *J Voice* 2009; 23:21–28.
53. Suzuki M. Laryngeal reflexes. In: Hirano M, Kirchner JA, Bless DM, eds, *Neurolaryngology: Recent Advances.* Boston, MA: Little, Brown, and Company; 1987: 142–155.
54. Henriquez VM, Schulz GM, Bielamowicz S, Ludlow CL. Laryngeal reflex responses are not modulated during human voice and respiratory tasks. *J Physiol.* 2007; 585(3):779–789.
55. Biever DM, Bless DM. Vibratory characteristics of the vocal folds in young adult and geriatric women. *J Voice.* 1987; 3:120–131.
56. Linville SE. Glottal gap configurations in two age groups of women. *J Speech Hear Res.* 1992;35:1209–1215.
57. Hirano S, Bless DM, de Rio AM, Connor N, Ford CN. Therapeutic potential of growth factors for aging voice. *Laryngoscope.* 2004;114(12):2161–2167.
58. Malmgren LT, Lovice DB, Kaufman MR. Age-related changes in muscle fiber regeneration in the human thyroarytenoid muscle. *Arch Otolaryngol Head Neck Surg.* 2000;126(7):851–856.
59. Malmgren LT, Jones CE, Bookman LM. Muscle fiber and satellite cell apoptosis in the aging human thyroarytenoid muscle: a stereological study with confocal laser scanning microscopy. *Otolaryngol Head Neck Surg.* 2001;125(1):34–39.
60. Takeda N, Thomas G, Ludlow CL. Aging effects on motor units in the human thyroarytenoid muscle. *Laryngoscope.* 2000; 110(6):1018–1025.
61. Gray SD, Thibeault SL. Diversity in voice characteristics—interaction between genes and environment, use of microarray analysis. *J Comm Disord.* 2002;35:347–354.
62. Thibeault SL, Hirschi SD, Gray SD. DNA microarray gene expression analysis of a vocal fold polyp and granuloma. *J Speech Lang Hear Res.* 2003;46:491–502.
63. Duflo SM, Thibeault SL, Li W, Smith ME, Schade G, Hess MM. Differential gene expression profiling of vocal fold polyps and Reinke's edema by complementary DNA microarray. *Ann Otol Rhinol Laryngol.* 2006;115(9):703–714.

64. Van den Berg J. Myoelastic-aerodynamic theory of voice production. *J Speech Hear Res.* 1958;1:227–244.
65. Hirano M, Yoshida T, Tanaka S. Vibratory behavior of human vocal folds viewed from below. In: Gauffin J, Hammarberg, B, eds, *Vocal Fold Physiology.* San Diego, CA: Singular Publishing Group; 1994:1–6.
66. Titze IR. Mechanisms of sustained oscillations of the vocal folds. In: Titze IR, Scherer RC, eds. *Vocal Fold Physiology.* Denver, CO: Denver Center for the Performing Arts; 1983:349–357.
67. Berke G, Great B. Laryngeal biomechanics: an overview of mucosal wave mechanics. *J Voice.* 1993;7:123–128.
68. Baken R. Irregularity of vocal period and amplitude: a first approach to the fractal analysis of voice. *J Voice.* 1990;4:185–197.

3

Some Etiologic Correlates

Since West, Kennedy, and Carr[1] commented that there is always a reason for a voice disorder, voice pathologists have sought to identify those reasons with each new patient. Sometimes the causes are easily identified, such as in cases of vocal nodules in shouting children. At other times, finding the contributing causes of the disorder requires the skill of a highly experienced diagnostician. To enhance the successful outcome of the search, it is advantageous for those seeking the answers to be familiar with as many etiologic points of reference as possible. This chapter seeks to provide these reference points by discussing some of the more common etiologic factors associated with the development and maintenance of voice disorders. These factors include the following major categories:

- vocal misuse
- medically related etiologies
- primary disorder etiologies
- personality-related etiologies

ETIOLOGIES OF VOCAL MISUSE

Vocal misuse (Table 3–1) refers to functional voicing behaviors that contribute to the development of voice disorders. These include voice behaviors that cause trauma to the vocal folds (phonotrauma) that sometimes leads to benign

Table 3–1. Etiologies of Vocal Misuse

Vocally Abusive Behaviors	*Inappropriate Vocal Components*
1. Shouting	1. Respiration
2. Loud talking	2. Phonation
3. Screaming	3. Resonance
4. Vocal noises	4. Pitch
5. Coughing	5. Loudness
6. Throat clearing	6. Rate

mucosal pathology as well as the use of inappropriate vocal components, such as pitch, loudness, breathing strategies, phonation habits, and speech rate.

Phonotrauma

Phonotrauma may occur whenever the vocal folds are forced to adduct too vigorously causing mechanical trauma to the laryngeal mucosa. This trauma, when repeated or habituated, may contribute to vocal fold mucosal tissue change and maladaptive behavior of the laryngeal musculature.[2,3] Sheer force, in the form of sudden and violent adduction of the vocal folds or a more persistent use of a vocally traumatic behavior, is one of the main elements in the development of many voice disorders.[4] Forceful behaviors associated with vocal hyperfunction include excessive shouting and loud talking, such as children shouting on a playground or a factory worker talking loudly over machine noise. Phonotrauma also occurs during screaming and in the production of vocal noises. Vocal noises refer to those nonspeech laryngeal sounds that children make while playing. Common vocal noises may include the imitation of a car, truck, or motorcycle engine; the piercing scream of sirens; the vocalizations of action figures; and various growls, barks, and howls of animals.

One of the most prevalent forms of phonotrauma is incessant, habitual, nonproductive throat clearing.[5,6] In one study of 206 patients who were referred for voice therapy due to muscle tension dysphonia (MTD), 141 (or 68%) presented with this traumatic throat clearing behavior.[7] Vigorous, aperiodic adduction of the vocal folds, which occurs during even mild throat clearing, was observed through the classic, high-speed motion films of vocal fold vibration that Timcke, Von Leden, and Moore produced as far back as 1959.[8]

Throat clearing may be either a primary or a secondary etiologic factor. As a primary factor, it may appear following a cold or respiratory infection, as described in the following example.

Mrs. M's voice evaluation revealed that she had never experienced vocal difficulties prior to contracting a cold 6 weeks earlier. Accompanying the cold had been excessive coughing and throat clearing. The cold symptoms and the cough subsided after 10 to 12 days, but Mrs. M unknowingly continued to harshly clear her throat. The resultant mucosal trauma caused a mild, persistent dysphonia. Indirect laryngoscopy performed during the sixth week revealed mild bilateral vocal fold edema. The subsequent voice evaluation identified continual throat clearing as the primary etiologic factor associated with the persistent hoarseness. Habitual throat clearing was extinguished using a "forceful swallow" modification approach (see Chapter 7), and the vocal folds returned to their normal structure and function allowing normal voice.

Throat clearing is often identified as a secondary abusive factor for patients who present with various laryngeal pathologies. Individuals frequently develop this behavior as a response to perceived laryngeal sensations. These laryngeal sensations may be caused by the presence of the pathology. Common sensations reported by patients include dryness, tickling, burning, aching, lump in the throat, or a "thickness" sensation. Patients often become hypersensitive to the laryngeal area as the result of the pathology. When this is the case, even normal sensations, such as those associated with mucus drainage, become magnified, and a common response is habitual throat clearing. In more recent years, chronic throat clearing has also been identified as a symptom of laryngopharyngeal reflux (LPR).[9] LPR occurs when acidic stomach contents are refluxed into the posterior laryngeal area causing significant tissue irritation that sometimes affects voice quality. LPR is discussed in detail in Chapters 4 and 7 of this text. In both behavioral and reflux-related cases, throat clearing serves both as a symptom of the pathology and as a maintaining contributor to the disorder.

Coughing is also a vocally abusive behavior. Coughing may be the symptom of many different types of respiratory diseases, such as asthma, chronic obstructive pulmonary disease, or malignant lung lesions.[10] Coughing may also be a symptom of laryngopharyngeal reflux.[11] When associated with a disease process, a physician treats coughing. Chronic cough, as with throat clearing, may be developed as a response to laryngeal pathology and is not always associated with disease processes. When this is the case, the voice pathologist often is called upon to extinguish this behavior as part of a behavioral management protocol.[12]

Inappropriate Vocal Components

Voice production is dependent on the interrelationship of many different vocal components. These voicing components include respiration, phonation, and resonance, as well as the psychophysical components of pitch, loudness, and rate. It is expected that the presence of laryngeal pathology would modify any one or all of these components. Conversely, the functional misuse of any component or combination of components may cause a laryngeal pathology.

Respiration

In Chapter 2, we learned that vibration of the vocal folds is activated by the respiratory airstream overcoming the resistance of the approximated vocal folds, thus blowing the folds apart. The exchanges of pressure and flow interact with tissue compliance to draw the vocal folds back together, completing one vibratory cycle. The subglottic air pressure necessary to initiate phonation for normal conversational voice is between 3 and 7 cm of H_2O.[14] Hirano demonstrated that the normal airflow rate for voice production ranges from 50 to 200 mL H_2O/s.[14] When mass lesion, poor muscular control or incoordination, neural problems, or normal aging influences on the mucosal covering and muscles of the vocal folds compromise glottis closure, airflow rates may increase, and subglottic air pressure may be increased or decreased depending on the individual's compensation strategy.

Normal control of inspiration and expiration is necessary to support normal phonation. Aronson[15] suggested that the vast majority of voice patients use anatomically and physiologically normal respiration to support voice production. Nonetheless, certain functional respiratory habits and behaviors may lead directly to the development of a voice disorder. For example, a patient may habitually use a shallow, thoracic (chest) breathing pattern that does not support normal phonation. Low intensity and breathiness may characterize the resultant voice quality. Another functional breathing behavior that may contribute to the development of a voice disorder is the habit of speaking at the end of normal expiration. This behavior occurs when a person continues to speak when the normal tidal expiration has been completed. Speaking at the end of expiratory volume increases respiratory and laryngeal muscle tension and may contribute to vocal dysfunction.

Phonation

Traumatic hyperadduction of the vocal folds has previously been discussed. Patients who utilize harsh glottal attacks or persistent glottal fry phonation may also demonstrate inappropriate phonation as a functional etiology. Harsh or hard glottal attack, or glottal coup, describes one of three means by which phonation may be initiated. The hard attack is accomplished by complete and rapid adduction of the vocal folds, buildup of subglottic air pressure, and then explosion of the folds while initiating phonation. Habitual use of a hard glottal attack usually causes an increase in laryngeal area muscle tension, as well as an increased and unnecessary impact on the vocal fold mucosa. The increased muscle tension requires a greater buildup of subglottic air pressure, all of which contribute to vocal hyperfunction.

The opposite of the hard glottal attack is the breathy or aspirate attack. When this mode of attack is used to initiate phonation, the vocal folds are abducted as exhalation for phonation begins and then only adduct after phonation has been initiated, creating a moment of breathiness that is heard at the initiation of the vowel. Because of poor glottic closure, the aspirate attack is also a voice misuse that may contribute to vocal dysfunction. The third mode of vocal attack is the even or static attack. This is the most efficient means of initiating voice onset. With the static attack, the vocal folds are nearly approximated as exhalation begins, permitting the onset of phonation to be smooth and effortless.

Glottal fry or pulse register is one of three vocal registers described by Hollien,[16] with the other two being modal and loft registers. Glottal fry is the lowest range of phonation along the frequency continuum and the least flexible. Production of glottal fry is characterized by tightly approximated vocal folds whose free edges appear flaccid.[17] The closed phase of the vibration cycle is long when compared with the total vibration cycle during glottal fry phonation. The tighter closure requires a greater increase in subglottic air pressure, contributing to laryngeal tension. Persistent use of glottal fry, which has been described as sounding like a poorly tuned motorboat engine, will often cause vocal fatigue, laryngeal tension, and a "lump in the throat" feeling.

Opposite the pulse register is the loft register, which includes the higher range of vocal frequencies including the falsetto. Persistent use of the loft register or falsetto voice is a maladaption of the normal voice physiology and may be identified as functional falsetto or juvenile voice. Finally, the range of frequencies normally used in speaking and singing comprise the modal register.

Resonance

Once sound is generated at the level of the vocal folds (the sound source), it then passes through a series of filters (the vocal tract) that dampen and enhance the sound and make each voice unique and distinctive to the owner of the voice. There is a wide range of acceptable voice resonance patterns, although the level of acceptability is often determined by geographic location, such as the Southern "twang." Certain resonance problems may have an organic basis, such as those resulting from velopharyngeal incompetence or a submucous cleft, whereas others are caused by functional disturbances. Functional resonance disturbances may be caused by the improper coupling of the pharyngeal, oral, and nasal cavities or the improper placement of the tongue and larynx.

Hypernasality or rhinolalia aperta occurs when vowels and voiced consonants are excessively resonated in the nasal cavity. This behavior occurs when the velopharyngeal port remains open during production of the phonemes other than the nasal consonants /m/, /n/, and /ng/. The increase in nasal resonance may or may not be accompanied by excessive nasal air emission, which is heard as a friction noise that accompanies the phonemes produced.

Denasality or rhinolalia clausa occurs when normal nasal resonance is not present on the phonemes /m/, /n/, and /ng/. The physical basis is an overclosure of the velopharyngeal port or an obstruction of the nasal cavity. The acoustic result sounds as if the speaker has a head cold.

Assimilative nasality occurs when the phonemes adjacent to the three nasal consonants are nasalized along with these sounds. The cause is presumed to be the premature opening of the port prior to the nasal consonant and a lingering opening of the port following the nasal consonant. This form of nasal resonance is often heard for a brief period following removal of large tonsils and adenoids.

Cul-de-sac nasality is a closed nasality in which all the vowels, semivowels, and nasals are produced with a hollow-sounding or dead-end resonance. This form of nasality is thought to be caused by obstruction in the anterior nasal cavity.

Retracted tongue and elevated larynx are anatomical postures that often accompany each other and contribute to altered resonance and laryngeal tension. When the larynx is elevated, the vocal tract will be shortened, thus raising all the formant frequencies. The increased extrinsic and intrinsic laryngeal muscle tension also tends to raise the fundamental frequency. The combination of these effects yields a perceived higher pitched voice with a pinched resonance quality. Patients who exhibit these behaviors often complain of laryngeal aching and fatigue caused by the increased muscular activity.

Pitch

Pitch is the perceptual correlate of the fundamental frequency of voice. Misuse refers to pitch levels that are too high, too low, or lacking in variability. Habitual use of an inappropriate pitch may create laryngeal tension and strain. Patients we have treated who required direct pitch modification have included young men with pseudoauthoritative voices, speakers who frequently talk and lecture either in noisy locations or to large groups in less-than-adequate acoustical conditions, patients with other illnesses and emotional conditions, patients who have undergone vocal fold surgery who have not automatically made the appropriate pitch adjustments, male patients with functional falsetto, female patients with juvenile voice, and, transsexual patients wishing to develop a more gender-appropriate voice.

Change in pitch is a common symptom of voice disorders, especially those associated with mass lesion or other vocal fold cover changes. Therefore, it seldom is appropriate from a therapeutic point of view to be concerned with direct pitch modification. As the vocal fold mucosa improves, so too would the inappropriate pitch. To try to ascertain an "optimum" pitch from the pathologic voice would be frustrating. The various methods suggested to accomplish this task are flawed due to the presence of the pathology. Therefore, direct pitch modification is reserved for selected cases in which the use of an inappropriate pitch has been isolated as the primary etiologic factor associated with the development of the voice disorder.

Loudness

Loudness is the perceptual term that relates to vocal intensity. The inappropriate use of loudness is demonstrated in voices that are habitually too soft, too loud, or lack loudness variability. The phonotraumatic behaviors of shouting and loud talking have been previously discussed. It is important to note that habitual use of an inadequate loudness level may also lead to vocal dysfunction. Vocal intensity is determined by the lateral excursion of the vocal folds and the speed with which they return to approximate as dictated by the subglottic air pressure and the resultant airflow. When a person speaks very softly, the balance between the airflow and the muscular activity may be disturbed. The decreased airflow causes more demands to be placed on the intrinsic muscle system, thus leading to possible vocal muscle strain and fatigue. Talking softly may be phonotraumatic if not well supported by the airstream.

Rate

As an etiologic factor, rate may contribute to laryngeal pathologies when speech is produced too rapidly. Faulty use of the laryngeal mechanism related to vocal hyperfunction is evident when speakers produce speech in too rapid a manner.[6] The patient who talks too fast typically does not use proper breath support, often talking on insufficient breath support. Increased rate may lead to laryngeal muscle tension.

Rarely will a voice pathologist be presented with a voice disorder in which a single vocal component is isolated as the primary etiology. If inappropriate components are found to be the cause, a combination of components usually will be identified, with misuse of one being the predominant factor contributing to the voice disorder. Inappropriate components may also be the result of laryngeal pathologies that were caused by other etiologic factors. When this is the case, the components are recognized as the symptoms of the disorder (such as low pitch, glottal fry, breathiness, etc).

Vocal misuse represents the most common etiologic factor identified in patients with voice disorders.[4,18,19] Voice therapy is particularly effective in the remediation of voice disorders caused by vocal misuse.

MEDICALLY RELATED ETIOLOGIES

This category of etiologic correlates refers to medical or surgical interventions that directly cause voice disorders and medical or health conditions and treatments that may indirectly contribute to the development of vocal dysfunction (Table 3–2). Voice pathologists' base of knowledge regarding these etiologic factors will aid them during the diagnostic process, especially when discussing the patient's medical history.

Direct Surgery

Direct surgical procedures are those that cause an insult to the anatomical structures responsible for phonation and resonance. These surgeries would include total laryngectomy, hemilaryngectomy, supraglottic laryngectomy, glossectomy, mandibulectomy, palatal surgery, and other head and neck excisions such as radical neck dissection and pharyngeal surgeries. Most of these surgeries are conservation procedures designed to eradicate disease regardless of the effects on phonation. Vocal rehabilitation is essential following these surgeries and is described in Chapter 9.

Indirect Surgery

Surgery for other medical problems may indirectly contribute to the development of voice disorders. Because of the anatomic relationships of the thyroid, heart, lungs, cervical spine, and carotid arteries to the recurrent laryngeal nerves, the superior laryngeal nerves, and the vagus nerve, surgical procedures involving these structures may involve some trauma to the nervous supply of the larynx. Possible consequences may be a vocal fold paresis or paralysis and a loss of sensory innervation to the mucosal lining of the larynx.[20]

Women who have undergone a complete hysterectomy, including the

Table 3–2. Medically Related Etiologies

Trauma	*Chronic Illnesses and Disorders*
Direct surgery • Laryngectomy (total, hemi, supraglottic) • Glossectomy • Mandibulectomy • Palatal • Other head and neck	Sinusitis Respiratory illnesses Allergies Medications Gastrointestinal disorders
Indirect surgery • Thyroid • Cardiac • Carotid • Lung • Cervical • Hysterectomy	Nervous disorder Endocrine disorder Cardiac disease Lung disease Arthritis
Intubation Mechanical trauma Burns	Alcohol/drug abuse Smoking

uterus and both ovaries, may also experience vocal difficulties. A temporary or permanent lowering of the vocal pitch may be caused by hormonal changes. Some patients, in an attempt to maintain the "normal" higher pitch, place increased muscle strain on the laryngeal mechanism, thus setting the stage for the development of vocal dysfunction.[21]

Finally, any surgery that requires general anesthesia and the placement of an endotracheal tube has the potential for causing a voice problem.[22–24] Friedmann[25] suggested two different types of laryngeal injuries caused by intubation: (1) trauma to the mucosa over the vocal processes of the arytenoid cartilages in the posterior larynx and (2) trauma caused by constant pressure of the tube on the vocal process resulting in tissue necrosis. The result in either case is injury to the mucosa that covers the cartilage, with concomitant injury to the perichondrium. In an attempt to repair the damaged area, granulomatous tissue may develop.[26] Other potential problems caused by intubation may be arytenoid cartilage subluxation (especially during an emergent intubation), interarytenoid tissue scarring (causing arytenoid movement problems), and possible paresis/paralysis caused by nerve compression by the tube.[27–29] Treatment for voice disorders caused by intubation injuries often will involve a combination of medical and voice therapy treatments.

Chronic Illnesses and Disorders

Many chronic illnesses and disorders and their treatments may contribute to the development of vocal dysfunction. Because of the importance of these etiologic factors, Chapters 4 and 7 of this text deal with issues related to changes in vocal function associated with each of these disorders and illnesses in much greater detail. As outlined in Table 3–2, voice disorders may develop secondary to other systemic, cardiac, respiratory, immunologic, gastrointestinal, endocrine, inflammatory, and pharmacologic influences.

For example, chronic sinusitis and other upper respiratory infections, although often limited to the supraglottic structures, may contribute to the development of hoarseness. Because the sinus drainage does not touch the vocal folds, it cannot be blamed for the hoarseness, although the patient may perceive it as the cause. Nonetheless, coughing and throat clearing, which often accompany these illnesses, are implicated in phonotrauma and may be the direct cause of the voice problem. Medications used to treat these illnesses and their symptoms may also be implicated as a cause. Antihistamines are commonly used to dry the secretions but will also cause a reduction in the secretions of the salivary and mucous glands, thus contributing to potential dehydration of the vocal folds. Anticough medications, such as codeine and dextromethorphan, are also mucosal drying agents.[30]

Other, more chronic respiratory illnesses, such as asthma, chronic obstructive pulmonary disease, and lung cancer may directly or indirectly contribute to voice disorders. The increased responsiveness and hyperactivity of the trachea and bronchi in individuals with asthma may lead to transitory or prolonged episodes of wheezing, coughing, and dyspnea. Hoarseness may, therefore, result from vocal fold tissue lining abuse, poor respiratory support, and the dehydrating medications used to treat the condition. Bronchodilators, such as albuterol (Proventil and Ventolin), may have the side effects of tremor and nervousness. Corticosteroid inhalants may contribute to vocal fold bowing and an elevation of fundamental frequency.[31,32]

Chronic obstructive pulmonary disease (COPD) is a clinical term used to describe a group of diseases characterized by persistent slowing of airflow during exhalation. The most common of these diseases are emphysema and chronic bronchitis, both of which may cause the vocally abusive wheezing, coughing, dyspnea, and sputum expectoration. Again, medications used to treat these diseases may have a negative effect on the mucous membrane and the fluid secretion to the vocal folds.

Lung cancer may have a more direct effect on the functioning of the vocal folds. A symptom of lung cancer is left vocal fold paralysis caused by damage to the vagus nerve. Radiation treatments, chemotherapy, and direct lung surgery may also violate the nervous supply to the vocal fold, as well as mucous secretion and internal hydration.

About 1 in every 5 persons in the United States has an allergy caused by something inhaled, ingested, touched, or injected.[33] Severity may range from very mild to very severe to fatal. When an airborne allergen (a substance that elicits the allergic response) enters the body, it reacts with an antibody that is fixed to the surface of mast cells found in the nose, lungs, and skin. The allergen-antibody binding triggers the release of histamines, which are responsible for the allergic symptoms. The histamine causes contraction of smooth muscles, dilation of blood vessels, and stimulation of mucous glands to produce increased quantities of mucus.[33] Allergies may cause congestion and edema of the vocal folds, thus negatively affecting voice production. Treatments for allergies may include medicines such as antihistamines and topical steroids, with the side effects as previously described. Decongestants may also be utilized to decrease the edema of the mucous membrane. Long-term use of a vasoconstrictor, however, may show a diminished drug effect with the return of edema and congestion being greater than was previously present.[34] Persistent allergies may be treated through injections of the allergen designed to desensitize the patient to that allergen.

Gastrointestinal disorders may also negatively affect voice production. Though the prevalence is controversial, one disorder in this category is laryngopharyngeal reflux (LPR).[35,36] Reflux of the acidic stomach contents to the posterior larynx has been implicated in the symptoms of chronic hoarseness, voice fatigue, cough, chronic throat clearing, globus sensation (lump in the throat), and a sensation of choking.[37] The burning of the posterior larynx may cause edema, ulceration, and granulation of the laryngeal mucosa as well as pseudosulcus and interarytenoid changes.[38] In two studies, signs and symptoms of LPR have been shown to be present in as many as 50% of individuals seeking treatment for voice disorders.[18,39] A complete treatment regimen is described in Chapter 7.

The presence of lower intestinal disorders, such as spastic colon, irritable bowel syndrome, and diarrhea, may also be implicated in the development of voice disorders. Antispasmodic medications used for these disorders, such as atropine, scopolamine, and diphenoxylate hydrochloride, reduce glandular secretions and are drying agents.[30]

Patients with emotional disorders, such as emotional tension, depression, and anxiety, may also experience voice disorders for a number of reasons, including simple laryngeal area tension, poor respiratory support, and whole-body fatigue from poor sleep habits, to name a few. Psychotropic medications prescribed for nervous tension, depression, psychotic disorders, and sleep disorders may have a negative effect on voice production because of drying and sedation. Some of these common drugs include Elavil, Pamelor, Prozac, and Paxil (antidepressants); Thorazine and Haldol (antipsychotics); and antihistamines that are often used for sleep disorders.[40–43]

Endocrine dysfunction, such as hypothyroidism, hyperthyroidism, hyperpituitarism, amyloidosis, virilization, and minor hormonal changes associated with menstruation, has also been implicated as a cause of voice disorders. Hoarseness, vocal fatigue, pitch changes, loss of range, breathiness, reduced loudness, and pitch breaks have all been observed in individuals with endocrine disorders.[44–46]

Cardiac and circulatory problems may also contribute to the development of voice disorders. We previously discussed the potential negative effects of cardiac surgery on the recurrent laryngeal nerve. Medications used to control high blood pressure, such as methyldopa, reserpine, and captopril, are drying agents, and their diuretic effect could potentially result in dryness and irritation of the mucous membrane of the vocal folds.[41]

Arthritis, an inflammatory disease of the body's synovial joints, has also been implicated in the development of voice disorders. The symptoms of cricoarytenoid joint arthritis are hoarseness, a laryngeal fullness feeling, and pain associated with inflammation of the joint. In more severe cases, the joint may be fixed (cricoarytenoid ankylosis) and imitate the appearance of a vocal fold paralysis. The severity of the symptoms is dependent on the severity of the arthritis.[47–49]

Finally, the negative effects of smoking, alcohol abuse, and illicit drug use on the vocal mechanism cannot be denied. Minimally, the heat and chemicals from tobacco smoke cause erythema, edema, and generalized inflammation of the vocal tract. Even more threatening is the contribution tobacco smoke makes to the development of laryngeal carcinoma. Other conditions that smoking can cause include polypoid mucosal changes and the precancerous conditions of leukoplakia and hyperkeratosis (see Chapter 4).[50–54] Sataloff[55] reported that marijuana smoke is particularly irritating, causing considerable vocal fold mucosal response. He also noted that cocaine could be extremely irritating to the nasal mucosa, causing increased vasoconstriction and altering mucosal sensation, resulting in decreased voice control and a tendency toward vocal abuse. Alcohol is a vasodilator and thus may cause drying of the mucous membrane of the vocal folds. In addition, it is a central nervous system depressant that, when abused, results in symptoms of incoordination, dysarthria, and impaired judgment. Alcohol use also may aggravate LPR. Caffeine is also a drug. It is a central nervous system stimulant, which has the potential to cause hyperactivity and tremor. In addition, it decreases laryngeal secretions causing laryngeal dehydration. As with alcohol, caffeine has a relaxation effect on the upper esophageal sphincter, and it can promote LPR. Smoking and drug and alcohol abuse may directly cause laryngeal pathologies. These chronic external and internal irritants are extremely abusive to the vocal mechanism and have been implicated as causes of many pathologies, from chronic laryngitis to laryngeal neoplasm. In addition to the direct abuse of inhaled chemicals, many smokers also have a "smoker's cough," which adds additional phonotrauma to compound the problem.

When dealing with medically related etiologies, the appropriate physician specialist must identify and treat the primary medical condition. The voice pathologist often proves helpful in identifying for the physician behaviors that may or may not be associated with the medical condition, thus adding to the diagnostic process. Improvement of the medical condition does not automatically improve the concomitant voice disorder. Voice evaluation and therapy prove to be a valuable asset to many patients exhibiting other surgical or medical conditions.

PRIMARY DISORDER ETIOLOGIES

This major etiologic category includes embryologic, physiologic, neurologic, and anatomical disorders (Table 3–3) that have vocal changes as secondary symptoms of the primary disorder. Included in this category are cleft palate and organic velopharyngeal insufficiency, with their characteristic hypernasal vocal components. An inappropriate high pitch and a pharyngeal resonatory focus frequently characterize the vocal components of people with profound hearing loss. Boone[56] found that 17- and 18-year-old male subjects with deafness had a mean fundamental frequency 54 Hz higher than the same measure for males of the same age with normal hearing. Individuals with a severe-profound sensorineural hearing loss often speak with the tongue retracted toward the pharyngeal wall, creating a disturbance in normal voice resonance.

Table 3–3. Primary Disorder Etiologies

Cleft palate
Velopharyngeal insufficiency
Hearing impairment
Cerebral palsy
Other neurogenic disorders
Trauma

The voices of individuals with cerebral palsy will vary widely because the neurologic damage is not related to one form of neurologic lesion.[57] Individuals presenting with cerebral palsy often speak with a labored, monotonous, and strained phonation with a limited frequency range. Control of intensity, caused by body positioning and respiratory support limitations, may also be problematic. These symptoms are also similar to the unpredictable effects of traumatic brain injuries (TBIs).

Many voice symptoms are present in a wide range of neurologic disorders. In his exceptional review of dysphonias associated with neurological disease, Aronson reported that technically, neurologic voice disorders are dysarthrias and are most often embedded "in a complex of respiratory, resonatory, and articulatory dysarthric signs."[58(p77)] The neurologic disorders with associated voice symptoms are discussed in detail in Chapter 4.

Accidental trauma is the final cause of a voice disorder listed in the category of Primary Disorder etiologies. Blunt or penetrating injuries to the larynx often cause edema, fractured laryngeal cartilages, joint dislocations, and lacerations. These injuries may be caused by automobile accidents and sports-related injuries, stabbing and gunshot wounds, strangulation, and, on rare occasions, traumatic intubation injuries. Inhalation of flames, gasses, and fumes and swallowing of caustic substances also may cause serious traumatic injury to the laryngeal mucosa. The primary concern related to severe trauma of the larynx is the establishment and maintenance of an adequate airway. Voice therapy will follow recovery from the acute stage of the injury.

As primary disorders, these conditions require appropriate medical, surgical, educational, and rehabilitative interventions. The voice pathologist will most often serve as part of a team attempting to modify the voice, swallowing, articulation, and language components of these various disorders.

PERSONALITY-RELATED ETIOLOGIES

The relationship between personality, psychological factors, and voice disorders is not well understood. Roy, Bless, and Heisey[59,60] reported that personality may act as a persistent risk factor for voice pathology. One category of voice disorders studied by these authors included functional dysphonia. Functional dysphonia refers to a voice disorder in the absence of identifiable neurologic or structural pathology.[61] In the past, the term *functional dysphonia* has been used to describe a host of medically unexplained voice disorders including hysterical dysphonia/aphonia, conversion dysphonia/aphonia, psychogenic or psychosomatic dysphonia/aphonia, and hyperkinetic or hyperfunctional dysphonia, with muscle tension dysphonia (MTD) as a current popular term.[62] Roy, Bless, and Heisey contend that functional dysphonia may be related to anxiety, inhibitory laryngeal motor behavior, and elevated tension states. The personality traits consistent with this vocal state are elevated neuroticism and low extraversion. The production of these functionally dysphonic voices is likely caused by maladaptive posturing of the laryngeal muscles, both extrinsic and intrinsic, causing an unusual voice quality or aphonia. Functional falsetto or puberphonia and juvenile voice are also likely the result of maladaptive laryngeal posturing and laryngeal muscle disregulation.

Voice is a sensitive indicator of emotions, attitudes, and role assumptions.[62] The quality of voice often directly suggests the way a person feels physically and emotionally. The resulting vocal symptoms may simply reflect a whole-body tension that causes a more specific hypertonicity of the intrinsic and extrinsic laryngeal muscles and, ultimately, a MTD. It has been suggested, but remains unclear, that the symptoms may be a sign of a much more serious underlying psychological disorientation.[63] In either case, the tensions and stresses of everyday life may contribute directly to the abnormal functioning of the sensitive vocal instrument, more so in certain personality types (Table 3–4).

Table 3–4. Personality-Related Etiologies

Environmental stress
Identity conflict

Environmental Stress

Environmental stress represents the many occurrences in human life that can cause emotional and physical stresses, provoking vocal disorders in some individuals. Consider, for example, the following: Mrs. S, an attractive 60-year-old woman, was referred by the laryngologist with the diagnosis of mild bilateral vocal fold edema. She complained of a chronic "hoarseness" and "tiredness" in her voice after only minimal use. Her general voice quality was described as mildly dysphonic, characterized by habitual use of low pitch, breathiness, and intermittent glottal fry phonation. During the voice evaluation, no vocally abusive behaviors, medically related causes, or primary disorders were identified. Without further interview, we may have surmised that the cause of this disorder was use of the inappropriate vocal components of pitch and respiration.

The social history, however, revealed that Mrs. S's husband had died just 2 months prior to the evaluation. She was in the process of trying to close his affairs and sell the house they had shared for 36 years. As you would now expect, this patient was experiencing what may be called a primary muscle tension dysphonia due to the depression and stress she was experiencing. The laryngeal muscle tension caused by her generalized hypertonicity led to the use of inappropriate vocal components, which physically contributed to the development of vocal fold edema. Nonetheless, the major cause of this disorder was the environmental stress.

At times, environmental stress may cause even more severe vocal symptoms: Mrs. P was a 36-year-old homemaker and mother of 2 sons, ages 14 and 16 years. She was referred by the laryngologist with the diagnosis of normal appearing vocal folds. Her voice quality, which she had experienced for 6 weeks, was aphonic with intermittent periods of phonation in the form of a high-pitched squeak. The social history, gathered during the evaluation, revealed that Mrs. P's 16-year-old son recently had been arrested for theft. Until this unfortunate occurrence, he had been a model youth making good grades in school and had participated in sports, drama, and other positive social activities. Mrs. P's vocal difficulties began about the time of his arrest. The maladaptive vocal function was her reaction to this intolerable, stressful situation. Voice therapy was successful in returning the patient's voice to normal within the first session (see Chapter 7).

Identity Conflict

Aronson[64] stated that psychosexual conflicts are neither signs of environmental stress nor psychological reactions to stressful life problems. Identity problems are embedded in the fabric of the personality. Persons who experience difficulties in establishing their own personalities may present with voice problems as a result. These may include maintaining a high-pitched falsetto in the postadolescent male; or a weak, thin, juvenile-sounding voice in an adult female; or the desire of the male-to-female transsexual to raise the pitch of her voice. We would strongly caution the reader that although some individuals with these vocal disorders may present with psychological conflicts, the majority do not. The voice problem may simply be a learned response or the conscious desire to project a particular image. (The pathologies associated with the etiology of identity conflict are discussed in Chapter 4.)

Voice disorders that are the result of personality-related etiologies are particularly amenable to voice therapy. However, it should be noted that the personality types associated with functional dysphonia may have a history of previous voice disorders, and a majority may experience some level of relapse.[65] At times, psychological referral and family counseling may be necessary and appropriate. The voice pathologist must realize the limitations of direct voice therapy and make referrals to mental health professionals as necessary. It must be remembered that treatment of any voice disorder involves treatment of the whole person.

SUMMARY

This chapter has presented some of the etiologic correlates of voice disorders in a categorical manner. It should be understood, however, that most voice disorders have more than one contributing etiologic factor. One of the rewards of working with patients who have voice disorders is the challenge of discovering the pertinent parts of the etiologic puzzle. The perceptual symptoms of many voice pathologies are similar, but the causes for those symptoms are many. The voice pathologist achieves success by finding the causes and then modifying or eliminating them, thus resolving the pathology and improving the voice. Chapter 4 discusses the various laryngeal pathologies that develop as a result of these etiologic factors, and Chapters 5 and 6 present ways of discovering these etiologic correlates.

REFERENCES

1. West R, Kennedy L, Carr A. *The Rehabilitation of Speech*. New York, NY: Harper & Brothers; 1937.
2. Johns M. Update on the etiology, diagnosis, and treatment of vocal fold nodules, polyps, and cysts. *Curr Opin Otolaryngol Head Neck Surg*. 2003;11(6):456–461.
3. Stemple JC, Stanley J, Lee L. Objective measures of voice production in normal subjects following prolonged voice use. *J Voice*. 1995;9(2):127–133.
4. Brodnitz F. *Vocal Rehabilitation*. 4th ed. Rochester, NY: American Academy of Ophthalmology and Otolaryngology; 1971.
5. Greene M. *The Voice and Its Disorders*. 3rd ed. Philadelphia, PA: JB Lippincott; 1972.
6. Wilson D. *Voice Problems of Children*. Baltimore, MD: Williams & Wilkins; 1979.
7. Stemple J, Lehmann, D. Throat clearing: The unconscious habit of vocal hyperfunction. Platform presentation, American Speech-Language-Hearing Association National Convention. Detroit, MI; 1980.
8. Timcke R, Von Leden H, Moore P. Laryngeal vibrations: measurements of the glottic wave, Part 2: physiologic variations. *Arch Otolaryngol*.1959;69:438–444.
9. Belafsky PC, Postma GN, Koufman JA. Validity and reliability of the reflux symptom index (RSI). *J Voice*. 2002;16(2): 274–277.
10. Nagala S, Wilson JA. Chronic cough. *Clin Otolaryngol*. 2008;33(2):94–96.
11. Vaezi MF. Laryngeal manifestations of gastroesophageal reflux disease. *Curr Gastroenterol Rep*. 2008;10(3):271–277.
12. Blager FB, Gay ML, Wood RP. Voice therapy techniques adapted to treatment of habit cough: a pilot study. *J Commun Disord*. 1988;21(5):393–400.
13. Shipp T, McGlone RE. Laryngeal dynamics associated with voice frequency change. *J Speech Hear Res*. 1971;14(4):761–768.

14. Hirano M. *Clinical Examination of Voice.* New York, NY: Springer-Verlag; 1981.
15. Aronson AE. *Clinical Voice Disorders.* 3rd ed. New York, NY: Thieme; 1990.
16. Hollien H. On vocal registers. *J Phonetics.* 1974;2:125–143.
17. Zemlin W. *Speech and Hearing Science: Anatomy and Physiology.* 4th ed. Englewood Cliffs, NJ: Prentice-Hall; 1997.
18. Coyle SM, Weinrich BD, Stemple JC. Shifts in relative prevalence of laryngeal pathology in a treatment-seeking population. *J Voice.* 2001;15(3):424–440.
19. Herrington-Hall BL, Lee L, Stemple JC, Niemi KR, McHone MM. Description of laryngeal pathologies by age, sex, and occupation in a treatment-seeking sample. *J Speech Hear Disord.* 1988;53(1):57–64.
20. Rubin AD, Sataloff RT. Vocal fold paresis and paralysis. *Otolaryngol Clin North Am.* 2007;40(5):1109–1131, viii–ix.
21. Amir O, Biron-Shental T. The impact of hormonal fluctuations on female vocal folds. *Curr Opin Otolaryngol Head Neck Surg.* 2004;12(3):180–184.
22. Balestrieri F, Watson CB. Intubation granuloma. *Otolaryngol Clin North Am.* 1982;15(3):567–579.
23. Peppard SB, Dickens JH. Laryngeal injury following short-term intubation. *Ann Otol Rhinol Laryngol.* 1983;92(4, pt 1):327–330.
24. Whited RE. Laryngeal dysfunction following prolonged intubation. *Ann Otol Rhinol Laryngol.* 1979;88(4, pt 1):474–478.
25. Friedmann I. Granulomas of the larynx. In: Paparella M, Shumrick, D, eds. *Otolaryngology: Head and Neck.* Vol 3. 2nd ed. Philadelphia, PA: WB Saunders; 1980.
26. Doyle P, Martin G. Paradoxical glottal closure mechanism associated with postintubation granuloma. *J Voice.* 1991;5:247–251.
27. Rubin AD, Hawkshaw MJ, Moyer CA, Dean CM, Sataloff RT. Arytenoid cartilage dislocation: a 20-year experience. *J Voice.* 2005;19(4):687–701.
28. Kitahara S, Masuda Y, Kitagawa Y. Vocal fold injury following endotracheal intubation. *J Laryngol Otol.* 2005;119(10):825–827.
29. Bastian RW, Richardson BE. Postintubation phonatory insufficiency: an elusive diagnosis. *Otolaryngol Head Neck Surg.* 2001;124(6):625–633.
30. Martin F. Tutorial: drugs and vocal function. *J Voice.* 1988;2:338–344.
31. Watkin KL, Ewanowski SJ. The effects of triamcinolone acetonide on the voice. *J Speech Hear Res.* 1979;22(3):446–455.
32. Williams AJ, Baghat MS, Stableforth DE, Cayton RM, Shenoi PM, Skinner C. Dysphonia caused by inhaled steroids: recognition of a characteristic laryngeal abnormality. *Thorax.* 1983;38(11):813–821.
33. Spiegel J, Hawkshaw M, Sataloff R. Allergy. In: Sataloff R, ed. *Professional Voice: The Science and Art of Clinical Care.* New York, NY: Raven Press, 1991; 153–157.
34. Colton R, Casper J. *Understanding Voice Problems: A Physiological Perspective for Diagnosis and Treatment.* Baltimore, MD: Williams & Wilkins, 1996.
35. Garrett CG, Cohen SM. Otolaryngological perspective on patients with throat symptoms and laryngeal irritation. *Curr Gastroenterol Rep.* 2008;10(3):195–199.
36. Belafsky PC, Rees CJ. Laryngopharyngeal reflux: the value of otolaryngology examination. *Curr Gastroenterol Rep.* 2008;10(3):278–282.
37. Belafsky PC, Postma GN, Amin MR, Koufman JA. Symptoms and findings of laryngopharyngeal reflux. *Ear Nose Throat J.* 2002; 81(9)(suppl 2):10–13.
38. Belafsky PC, Postma GN, Koufman JA. The validity and reliability of the reflux finding score (RFS). *Laryngoscope.* 2001;111(8):1313–1317.
39. Koufman J. Gastroesophageal reflux and voice disorders. In: Rubin J, ed. *Diagnosis and Treatment of Voice Disorders.* New York, NY: Igaku-Shoin, 1995;161–175.
40. Abaza MM, Levy S, Hawkshaw MJ, Sataloff RT. Effects of medications on the voice. *Otolaryngol Clin North Am.* 2007; 40(5):1081–1090, viii.
41. National Center for Voice and Speech (NCVS). Prescribed medications and

their effects on voice and speech. Retrieved September 23, 2013, from http://www.ncvs.org/rx.html.

42. Damste PH. Voice change in adult women caused by virilizing agents. *J Speech Hear Disord.* 1967;32(2):126–132.
43. Sataloff R. Endocrine dysfunction. In: Sataloff R, ed. *Professional Voice: The Science and Art of Clinical Care.* New York, NY: Raven Press, 1991;201–205.
44. Derman RJ. Effects of sex steroids on women's health: implications for practitioners. *Am J Med.* 1995;98(1A):137S–143S.
45. Habermann G. [Singer and actor under medical attention of the laryngologist]. *Laryngol Rhinol Otol (Stuttg).* 1976; 55(6):433–446.
46. Evans S, Neave N, Wakelin D, Hamilton C. The relationship between testosterone and vocal frequencies in human males. *Physiol Behav.* 2008;93(4–5):783–788.
47. Speyer R, Speyer I, Heijnen MA. Prevalence and relative risk of dysphonia in rheumatoid arthritis. *J Voice.* 2008;22(2): 232–237.
48. Kolman J, Morris I. Cricoarytenoid arthritis: a cause of acute upper airway obstruction in rheumatoid arthritis. *Can J Anaesth.* 2002;49(7):729–732.
49. Vrabec JT, Driscoll BP, Chaljub G. Cricoarytenoid joint effusion secondary to rheumatoid arthritis. *Ann Otol Rhinol Laryngol.* 1997;106(11):976–978.
50. Guimaraes I, Abberton E. Health and voice quality in smokers: an exploratory investigation. *Logoped Phoniatr Vocol.* 2005;30(3–4):185–191.
51. Georgalas C. Interobserver perceptual analysis of smokers voice. *Clin Otolaryngol.* 2005;30(1):74–75.
52. Gonzalez J, Carpi A. Early effects of smoking on the voice: a multidimensional study. *Med Sci Monit.* 2004;10(12): CR649–CR656.
53. Zeitels SM, Hillman RE, Bunting GW, Vaughn T. Reinke's edema: phonatory mechanisms and management strategies. *Ann Otol Rhinol Laryngol.* 1997; 106 (7, pt 1): 533–543.
54. Wynder E, Stellmann, S. Comparative epidemiology of tobacco-related cancers. *Cancer Res.* 1977;37:4608–4622.
55. Sataloff R. Patient history. In: Sataloff R, ed. *Professional Voice: The Science and Art of Clinical Care.* New York, NY: Raven Press; 1991:69–83.
56. Boone D. Modification of the voices of deaf children. *Volta Rev.* 1966;68:686–692.
57. Greene M, Mathieson L. *The Voice and Its Disorders.* 5th ed. London, UK: Whurr Publishers; 1989.
58. Aronson A. *Clinical Voice Disorders: An Interdisciplinary Approach.* New York, NY: Brian C. Decker; 1980.
59. Roy N, Bless DM, Heisey D. Personality and voice disorders: a multitrait-multidisorder analysis. *J Voice.* 2000; 14(4):521–548.
60. Roy N, Bless DM, Heisey D. Personality and voice disorders: a superfactor trait analysis. *J Speech Lang Hear Res.* 2000; 43(3):749–768.
61. Koufman J, Isaccson G. *The Spectrum of Vocal Dysfunction.* In: Koufman J, ed. *The Otolaryngologic Clinics of North America.* Philadelphia, PA: WB Saunders; 1991:985–988.
62. Morrison M, Rammage L. *The Management of Voice Disorders.* San Diego, CA: Singular Publishing Group; 1994.
63. Kinzl J, Bierl W, Rauchegger H. Functional aphonia. A conversion symptom as a defensive mechanism against anxiety. *Psychother Psychosom.* 1988;49:31–36.
64. Aronson A. *Clinical Voice Disorders: An Interdisciplinary Approach.* 2nd ed. New York, NY: Brian C. Decker; 1985.
65. Roy N, Bless DM, Heisey D, Ford CN. Manual circumlaryngeal therapy for functional dysphonia: an evaluation of short- and long-term treatment outcomes. *J Voice.* 1997;11(3):321–331.

4

Pathologies of the Laryngeal Mechanism

Voice disorders arise when an individual's quality, pitch, or loudness differs from voice characteristics typical of speakers of similar age, gender, cultural background, and geographic location. Etiologies arise from many possible factors, including structural, medical, and neurologic alterations of the respiratory, laryngeal, and vocal tract mechanisms. Other pathologies develop following maladaptive or inappropriate voice use. Other voice disorders originate in direct response to psychogenic factors. The complementary relationship among these various physical, voice use, and psychological influences ensures that many voice disorders and laryngeal pathologies will have contributions from more than one etiologic factor, and that there may be considerable overlap among these three groupings.[1–3] For example, inappropriate vocal behaviors or excessive vocal demands may incite structural changes in the vocal fold mucosa that create an organic pathology (eg, polyps or nodules). Psychological trauma or excessive emotional stress may accompany the onset of spasmodic dysphonia. Muscle tension dysphonia that emerges during an upper respiratory infection may persist long after the cold has resolved, presumably because of the effortful phonation and other maladaptive vocal behaviors adopted during the cold. These typical scenarios highlight the overlapping influences of multiple primary factors and secondary components that maintain the voice disturbance. Consequently, the rehabilitative plan must address both the predisposing condition that incited the pathology, as well as any persistent barriers to recovery. Treatment alternatives can be eclectic, including medical or surgical intervention, voice therapy, psychological counseling, or a combination approach. This chapter presents general descriptions and differential diagnostic signs of the most common voice disorders and the underlying contributions from medical, surgical, behavioral, rehabilitative, and psychosocial components.

PREVALENCE OF VOICE DISORDERS

The prevalence of voice disorders is difficult to establish because figures vary with age, gender, and occupation, but estimates range from 3% to 10% in the general population.[3] Twenty years ago, a study of 428 otolaryngology patients, aged 18 to 82 years, found that 7.2% of the males and 5% of the females had some form of laryngeal pathology.[4] Ten years later, 1158 new patient records from the same otolaryngology practice were reviewed to replicate those findings.[5] The most frequent voice pathologies for those treatment-seeking patients were benign vocal fold lesions (such as nodules, granuloma, and edema) and functional voice disorders (including diagnoses of symptoms of vocal fatigue and hoarseness), plus a new, prominent diagnostic category: reflux laryngitis (laryngopharyngeal reflux). Diagnoses of vocal fold paralysis, carcinoma, and vocal fold bowing were frequent but occurred more often in elderly speakers. The largest group of patients ranged in age from 45 to 64 years. Females sought treatment for voice disorders more frequently than did males. The most common pathology seen in females was nodules; in males, the most common diagnoses were papilloma, granuloma, and cancer. Prevalence of specific laryngeal pathologies also varied with the speaker age and sex. Some pathologies were more common in males, including nodules in boys, and cancer, leukoplakia, and hyperkeratosis in adult men. Psychogenic dysphonia was more common in females than males. The most common pathologies from that treatment-seeking age group are presented in Table 4–1.[5]

Sampling voice disorders from an otolaryngology patient roster is helpful to illustrate a comprehensive range of disorders common in that population, but two large, random adult samples were studied in recent years to yield a true prevalence for voice disorders.

Table 4–1. Most Common Laryngeal Pathologies in Adults

Age	*Male*	*Female*	*All*
Young adults (22–44 years)	Edema	Edema Polyps Nodules	Nodules Edema
Middle age (45–64 years)	Polyps	Edema Polyps Nodules	Polyps Edema Cancer
Older adults (>64 years)	Vocal fold paralysis		Vocal fold paralysis Cancer

Telephone interviews with 1326 adults between the ages of 21 and 66 in the states of Utah and Iowa revealed that nearly 30% reported a lifetime prevalence of a voice disorder, and approximately 7% reported a current voice problem.[6] Chronic voice problems were more common in women, in middle adult ages (40–59 years), and in individuals who reported heavy voice demands, reflux symptoms, chemical exposures, and frequent upper respiratory infections.[6]

Another random sampling of 117 elderly individuals between the ages of 65 and 94 in the states of Utah and Kentucky revealed a larger lifetime prevalence of a voice disorder, at 47%, with 29% of participants reporting a current voice problem.[7] Contributors to voice problems in this elderly group included reflux symptoms, history of a neck or back injury, and reports of chronic pain conditions. Moreover, seniors were more likely to report a negative impact of voice disorders on their quality of life, due to the frustration of not being heard, having to repeat oneself, and requiring increased physical effort to speak. These discouraging voice experiences coupled with the sharp increase in the lifetime prevalence and current incidence of voice disorders in elderly speakers may help explain why that group was the largest treatment-seeking cohort in the otolaryngology patient studies conducted previously.[5,6]

Occupations also affect the prevalence of voice disorders.[8] In a study of schoolteachers, 32% self-identified as having had a voice disorder, compared with only 1% of other occupations sampled.[9] Overridingly, occupations that place persons at risk for voice disorders require heavy vocal demands, such as professional voice use (acting, singing, and other vocal performances), telemarketing, and reception service. Threats increase when individuals must talk over loud ambient noise, as in the case of teachers, factory workers, stock traders, aerobic instructors, and restaurant servers.

Estimates of voice disorders for children are also variable but tend to exceed estimates for adult speakers. Typical prevalence rates range from as low as 6% to as high as 23%[10,11] In a major children's medical center, the most common medical diagnoses were subglottic stenosis, vocal nodules, laryngomalacia, dysphonia without visible organic pathology, and vocal fold paralysis.[12] However, that specialist practice may tend to overestimate the type and number of extreme medical conditions in children's voice disorders.

PATHOLOGY CLASSIFICATIONS

To organize the broad and ever-increasing range of laryngeal pathologies and voice disorders, Special Interest Division 3 (Voice and Voice Disorders) of the American Speech-Language-Hearing Association published a collaborative work in 2006 to promote a consistent framework and common terminology for classifying pathologies and conditions that affect voice. This volume, entitled the *Classification Manual for Voice Disorders-I*, emerged after a decade of literature review and discussion by voice pathologists and otolaryngology colleagues.[13] The goal was to produce a systematic overview of clinical descriptions and classification criteria for over 120 different conditions affecting voice. The resource includes medical and voice classification criteria for 30 structural pathologies, 25 neurologic disorders, 20 aerodigestive conditions, 13 psychological disturbances, 15 systemic diseases, 4 inflammatory processes, 4 traumatic conditions, and 5 other miscellaneous voice disorders. Modeled after other interdisciplinary diagnostic classification schemes, each description includes essential and associated features, vocal impairment, clinical history and demographic profile, course and complications, medical and voice differential diagnosis, and severity criteria.

This chapter presents the most common clinical pathologies of the laryngeal mechanism, organized similarly to the *Classification Manual for Voice Disorders I* into eight major groups:

1. Structural pathologies
2. Inflammatory conditions
3. Trauma or injury
4. Systemic conditions affecting voice
5. Aerodigestive conditions affecting voice
6. Psychiatric or psychological disorders affecting voice
7. Neurologic voice disorders
8. Other disorders of voice[13]

A complete listing of the pathologies presented in this chapter is contained in Table 4–2, and a comprehensive description of the treatments used with these voice disorders is presented in Chapter 7.

Structural Pathologies of the Vocal Fold

Pathologies of the vocal fold include those that cause any alteration in its histological structure. Only physicians may make medical diagnoses of laryngeal pathology. However, as interdisciplinary collaborators, voice professionals must be familiar with and able to recognize normal appearing structures (Plate 2) to discriminate from abnormal findings. Changes in the mucosal layers or in the vocal fold muscle body will affect the mass, size, stiffness, flexibility, and tension of the vibrating mechanism and may alter the glottal closure pattern during phonation.[1,2,13] Any one of these vocal fold changes has the potential to alter vocal quality, pitch, and loudness. Differential diagnosis of the voice disorder etiology usually is made through careful visual examination of the lesion, but the history of voice use, disorder onset, course, and remission will also contribute important information critical to understanding the source of the problem and the indications for treatment.

The audioperceptual quality of voice in patients with any lesion varies tremendously as a function of lesion severity, the patient's habitual voice use pattern, and any compensatory strategies he or she may adopt. These adjustments include both productive and maladaptive changes. Productive changes might include improved breath support, enhanced vocal tract tuning, or appropriate loudness and pitch changes. Maladaptive compensations include effortful phonation, poor tone focus, or inappropriate pitch and loudness. These perceptual attributes are common in many types of vocal fold lesions; rarely will distinctive audioperceptual features differentially discriminate the vocal pathology. Part of the difficulty in associating perceptual attributes to select pathologies is that vague and inconsistent terms are used to describe voice quality. For example, the generic term *dysphonia* can encompass breathiness, roughness, increased strain or effort with phonation, intermittent voice breaks or aphonia, loss of pitch and loudness range, and vocal fatigue.

Table 4–2. Classification of Pathologies and Disorders

- I. Structural Pathologies of the Vocal Fold
  - A. Malignant Epithelial Dysplasia of the Larynx
  - B. Benign Epithelial and Lamina Propria Abnormalities of the Vocal Fold
    1. Vocal Nodules
    2. Vocal Fold Polyps
    3. Vocal Fold Cysts
    4. Reactive Vocal Fold Lesion
    5. Reinke's Edema and Polypoid Degeneration
    6. Vocal Fold Scarring
       - a. Vocal Fold Sulcus/Sulcus vocalis
    7. Vocal Fold Granuloma and Contact Ulcer
    8. Keratosis, Leukoplakia, and Erythroplasia
    9. Recurrent Respiratory Papilloma (RRP)
    10. Subglottic and Laryngeal/Glottic Stenosis; Acquired Anterior Glottic Web
    11. Vascular Lesions: Vocal Fold Hemorrhage, Hematoma, Varix, and Ectasia
  - C. Congenital and Maturational Changes Affecting Voice
    1. Congenital Webs (Synechia)
    2. Laryngomalacia
    3. Puberphonia: Mutational Falsetto and Juvenile Voice
    4. Presbyphonia or Presbylaryngeus
- II. Inflammatory Conditions of the Larynx
  - A. Cricoarytenoid and Cricothyroid Arthritis
  - B. Acute Laryngitis
  - C. Laryngopharyngeal Reflux
  - D. Chemical Sensitivity/Irritable Larynx Syndrome
- III. Trauma or Injury of the Larynx
  - A. Internal Laryngeal Trauma
    1. Thermal and Chemical Exposure
    2. Intubation/Extubation Injury
  - B. External Trauma and Arytenoid Dislocation
- IV. Systemic Conditions Affecting Voice
  - A. Endocrine Disorders
    1. Hypothyroidism and Hyperthyroidism
    2. Sexual Hormonal Imbalances
    3. Growth Hormone Abnormalities (Hyperpituitarism)
  - B. Immunologic Disorders
    1. Allergies

continues

Table 4–2. *continued*

- V. Nonlaryngeal Aerodigestive Disorders Affecting Voice
  - A. Respiratory Diseases
    - 1. Asthma and Chronic Obstructive Pulmonary Disease
  - B. Gastroesophageal Reflux Disease (GERD)
  - C. Infectious Diseases of the Aerodigestive Tract
    - 1. Laryngotracheobronchitis (Croup)
    - 2. Mycotic (Fungal) Infections: Candida
- VI. Psychiatric and Psychological Disorders Affecting Voice
  - A. Psychogenic Conversion Aphonia and Dysphonia
  - B. Factitious Disorders or Malingering
  - C. Gender Dysphoria or Gender Reassignment
- VII. Neurologic Disorders Affecting Voice
  - A. Peripheral Nervous System Pathology
    - 1. Superior Laryngeal Nerve Paralysis: Unilateral or Bilateral
    - 2. Recurrent Laryngeal Nerve Paralysis: Unilateral
    - 3. Recurrent Laryngeal Nerve Paralysis: Bilateral
    - 4. Superior Laryngeal Nerve and Recurrent Laryngeal Nerve Paresis
    - 5. Myasthenia Gravis
  - B. Movement Disorders Affecting the Larynx
    - 1. Spasmodic Dysphonia
      - a. Adductor Spasmodic Dysphonia (ADSD)
      - b. Abductor Spasmodic Dysphonia (ABSD)
      - c. Mixed Adductor and Abductor Spasmodic Dysphonia
    - 2. Essential Vocal Tremor
  - C. Central Neurologic Disorders Affecting Voice
    - 1. Amyotrophic Lateral Sclerosis
    - 2. Parkinson's Disease
    - 3. Multiple Sclerosis
    - 4. Huntington's Chorea
- VIII. Other Disorders of Voice Use
  - A. Vocal Abuse, Misuse, and Phonotrauma
  - B. Vocal Fatigue
  - C. Muscle Tension Dysphonia (Primary and Secondary)
  - D. Ventricular Phonation (Plica Ventricularis)
  - E. Paradoxical Vocal Fold Motion (Vocal Fold Dysfunction) or Episodic Dyspnea

Malignant Epithelial Dysplasia of the Larynx

Cancer of the larynx (Plate 3) is among the most devastating of all laryngeal pathologies because of the life-threatening implications of the disease and its effect on vocal communication. Most laryngeal carcinomas are of the squamous cell type and originate from the epithelium. If the lesion develops further, it will invade the deeper layers of the vocal fold including the vocalis muscle, which will affect the mass and stiffness of all affected mechanical layers.[1,3] The most common symptom of this pathology is persistent hoarseness or difficulty breathing. Vocal symptoms will vary from a very mild to severe dysphonia depending on the location and the extent of the tumor. Rarely, sensations of laryngeal pain or referred pain to the ear may be present in later stages of the disease. In advanced cases, the extent of the tumor may create an airway compromise, swallowing problems, or both.

Laryngeal carcinoma is most often caused by chronic irritation of the laryngeal epithelium and mucosa by such agents as tobacco smoke and alcohol, but rarely there may be other etiologies. Carcinoma can also occur in other sites of the larynx external to the true vocal folds. When a suspicious lesion is identified, a surgical biopsy is conducted to excise a tissue sample for histopathologic analysis and a definitive diagnosis. Once the presence of malignancy is confirmed, treatment options include radiation therapy, surgical excision, chemotherapy, or a combination approach. Surgical management options vary widely, based on the size, extent, and type of the malignancy. The procedure to remove malignant tissue may range from a soft tissue excision to a partial resection of the laryngeal cartilage and soft tissue to a total laryngectomy, which removes the entire larynx from the hyoid bone to the first trachea rings. Obviously, the total laryngectomy has the most severe impact on communication. Increasingly, head and neck surgeons are assessing tumor size and, if possible, using laryngeal preservation surgeries for appropriate candidates, so that the tumor can be excised without sacrificing one or both vocal folds.[14,15] These techniques preserve the laryngeal vibratory sound, produced from the reconstructed tissue. Regardless of the management approach, the voice pathologist plays an important role in preparing the patient and the family for the consequences of the various forms of surgery and in the subsequent delivery of appropriate laryngeal or alaryngeal voice rehabilitation. A complete review of laryngeal cancer diagnosis, treatment, and rehabilitation options is presented in Chapter 9.

Benign Epithelial and Lamina Propria Abnormalities of the Vocal Fold

Benign lesions of the superficial layers of the vocal fold are the most prevalent pathology group. Historically, it has been difficult to achieve consensus on the precise clinical and diagnostic features that discriminate various lesions, such as polyps, nodules, and cysts, as well as newer terms such as *pseudocyst*, *fibrous masses*, and *reactive lesions*. Laryngeal imaging techniques that present a magnified image of the lesion during vibration have augmented our ability to recognize consistent visual features and typical lesion location.[16] All laryngeal pathologies involve some disruption of the extracellular matrix of the lamina propria, but in the future, the histological composition and genetic profiles of lesions will help resolve clinical diagnostic uncertainties.

Vocal Nodules. Vocal nodules (Plates 4 and 5) are one of the most common benign vocal fold lesions. Nodules represent an inflammatory degeneration of the superficial layer of the lamina propria with associated fibrosis and edema.[1,3] These lesions usually are bilateral and symmetric and vary in size from as small as a pinhead to as large as a pea. They tend to arise on the medial edge between the anterior one-third and posterior two-thirds of the true vocal fold, or at the point of greatest amplitude of vocal fold vibration. At least 2 types of nodules have been described: acute and chronic. Acute nodules arise from traumatic or hyperfunctional voice use and appear rather gelatinous and floppy, as the overlying squamous epithelium is normal. Chronic nodules appear harder and more fixed to the underlying mass of the mucosa because of increased fibrosis and a thickened epithelium. During vibration, the mass and stiffness of the vocal fold cover are increased, but the mechanical properties of the transition and body may not be affected.[13,16,17]

Nodules can occur at any age but occur most frequently in both male and female children and in female adults.[18–20] Nodules are rarely present in adult males. The resulting effects on voice can be variable, depending on the extent of the lesions, the length of time since onset, and any accompanying laryngeal inflammation. The symptoms of vocal nodules include mild to moderate dysphonia characterized by roughness, breathiness (caused by glottal gaps anterior and posterior to the bilateral nodules), and increased laryngeal muscle tension. Nodules occur commonly in untrained singers, especially in those using inappropriate vocal technique or in talkative, socially aggressive, and tense individuals. The first line of management for vocal nodules is voice therapy. When nodules are removed surgically without the benefit of voice rehabilitation therapy, they may quickly recur. Even chronic nodules may resolve when the patient follows the appropriate management program. When nodules do not respond to therapy in the patient who has been compliant with voice therapy, surgical management may be required, followed by postsurgical voice rehabilitation.

Vocal Fold Polyps. A vocal fold polyp (Plate 6) is a fluid-filled lesion composed of gelatinous material that develops in the superficial layer of the lamina propria, usually in the middle one-third of the membranous vocal fold. Most polyps are exophytic (rising above the tissue surface) and have an active blood supply, which may account for their sudden onset and rapid increase in size. Although polyps most often occur unilaterally, they also may appear bilaterally. Polyps may present in sessile (blisterlike) or pedunculated (attached to a stalk) forms.[1,3,13,16,17] As with nodules, the cause of vocal fold polyps is thought to be acute vocal trauma or some form of voice abuse. However, most polyps occur in adults, and these lesions are seen rarely in children. Vocal symptoms will vary significantly from mild to severe dysphonia depending on the type and location of the polyp and its interference with glottic closure and vocal fold vibration. For example, a pedunculated polyp may not affect phonatory quality if the lesion lies above or below the vibrating edge of the vocal folds. Large vocal fold polyps also can obstruct the glottis and create audible inspiration. A polyp will cause the mass and stiffness of the vocal fold cover to increase, especially when a hemorrhagic blood vessel is "feeding the lesion." Occasionally, a proliferation of collagen fibers or cyst development will accompany polyps. Unlike nodules, larger polyps may require surgery, especially if rapid improvement is not seen following stringent voice conservation. The combination of phonosurgery and voice rehabilitation therapy is optimal in those patients who require a rapid definitive approach.

Vocal Fold Cysts. Cysts are fluid-filled, sessile growths (Plates 7 and 8) that can be present congenitally or be acquired later in life. There are no clear etiologic factors, although mucous gland blockage and vocal abuse have both been proposed as possible contributors. These epithelial sacs are located most frequently on the cephalic surface or the medial edge of the vocal fold but may occur anywhere in the membranous portion of the true vocal fold, in the laryngeal ventricle, or in the ventricular folds. Vocal fold cysts are embedded in the superficial layer of the lamina propria, sometimes with extension into the intermediate and deep layers of the vocal ligament.[1,3,13,21] They appear as a whitish oval form, sometimes transparent below the epithelium. Although cysts usually occur unilaterally, bilateral cysts may be present. Because cysts often arise in the medial edge of a fold, contralateral reactive tissue thickening may occur, creating the erroneous appearance of bilateral lesions (eg, nodules). However, unlike nodules, cysts create a stiff adynamic segment due to reduced mucosal wave and amplitude of the vocal fold cover at the lesion site. Therefore, vibratory imaging is often helpful to differentiate cysts from nodules.[16,22] As with other mass lesions, cyst size and severity will influence the extent of voice quality changes, from mild to moderate dysphonia to near aphonia in the case of large cysts. Because of the predominant stiffness characteristics posed by these lesions, even a small cyst may have a significant negative effect on the singing voice. Cysts do not respond to behavioral voice therapy, and the definitive treatment is surgical excision, usually from a superior and lateral approach to avoid scarring of the medial edge of the vocal fold.

Reactive Vocal Fold Lesion. A reactive vocal fold lesion is a generic term given to describe new tissue changes due to the known impact stress and mechanical irritation of a primary lesion (eg, polyp, cyst, or other mass) contralateral to the site.[13] The lesion may appear to be thickened, rough, or as a concave depression to accommodate the convex bulge of the primary lesion (ie, "cup and saucer" effect). Usually, these tissue abnormalities add minimal disruptions to voice quality and resolve quickly following successful surgical or behavioral treatment for the primary lesion. However, naïve observers may mistake reactive vocal fold tissue for primary, bilateral lesions.

Reinke's Edema and Polypoid Degeneration. Reinke's edema (Plates 9 and 10) occurs when the superficial layer of the lamina propria becomes filled with viscous fluid because of long-standing trauma. In its most severe form, the entire membranous portions of the vocal folds become infiltrated with thick, gelatinous fluid, giving them the appearance of enlarged, fluid-filled bags or balloons. This extreme form is called polypoid degeneration.[1,3,13,23] Both Reinke's edema and polypoid degeneration are caused by chronic vocal abuse and smoking. Because this excessive swelling affects the entire length of the vocal folds, glottic closure usually is complete. The increased mass and stiffness of the vocal fold cover reduce the superficial mucosal wave and amplitude during vocal fold vibration. Unlike many other laryngeal pathologies, Reinke's edema and polypoid degeneration tend to result in a consistent signature change in voice quality, including mild to moderate dysphonia, characterized by dramatically lower pitch and a husky hoarseness. This voice quality has traditionally been described as a "whiskey" or "smoker's" voice.

Surgical treatment for polypoid degeneration and Reinke's edema is common, using a lateral incision to extract the superfluous contents while protecting the medial edge of the vocal fold.[3] Voice therapy is valuable both preoperatively in identifying the causes of the pathology and postoperatively for reestablishing good vocal hygiene and improved voice production. Most patients have become accustomed to the low-pitched vocal roughness, so preoperative consultation should inform them of the pitch increase and quality change that will occur following surgery. In postoperative therapy, clinicians can assist the patient in using his or her "new" voice correctly.

Vocal Fold Scarring. Scar is the general term given to permanent tissue changes in the cellular structure of the lamina propria following any number of etiologic factors, including lesion presence, chronic tissue irritation from vocal abuse, and iatrogenic (postsurgical) changes. Scar tissue increases the stiffness and reduces mucosal wave during vocal fold vibration. In severe cases, a nonvibrating scar may limit the glottic closure pattern.[24,25] Voice quality changes associated with scarring include roughness, strain and loss of vocal flexibility in pitch, loudness, and endurance. Treatment usually includes behavioral compensations, but dysphonia due to scarring is notoriously persistent.

Vocal Fold Sulcus/Sulcus Vocalis. A vocal fold sulcus (Plate 11) is a special form of vocal fold scarring that forms a ridge or furrow that runs along the superficial layer of the lamina propria, causing the vocal fold edge to appear bowed and resulting in a characteristic spindle-shaped gap. Sulci may occur unilaterally or bilaterally and can extend from a small pit or divot to a furrow running the entire length of the medial surface of the membranous portion of the vocal fold, to create a bowed appearance. The sulcus significantly decreases the mucosal wave of the vibrating cover, though the deeper vocal fold structures are unaffected.[1,3,13,25,26] There is no clear etiology for sulcus vocalis. One proposed theory is that vocal fold sulci develop following abnormal embryologic maturation of the vocal fold cover, resulting in a furrowed appearance of the membranous vocal fold edge. Apparent acquired onset of sulcus vocalis is also possible, especially because of laser surgery or changes with age. Sulcus vocalis can be difficult to identify reliably because the furrow is often overlooked without vibratory imaging to reveal the medial edge of the fold.[16] Even with that imaging, the sulcus may be difficult to detect if the overlying cover obscures the view of a midline furrow. Voice quality changes with a vocal fold sulcus may range from mild to severe dysphonia, depending on the extent of the defect into the lamina propria. Often, sulcus increases vocal fold stiffness, reduces vibratory mucosal wave and amplitude, and creates a characteristic spindle-shaped glottal gap. As for all forms of vocal fold scarring, behavioral and phonosurgical treatments have had mixed success.

Vocal Fold Granuloma and Contact Ulcer. Granulomas (Plates 12 and 13) are vascular exophytic and inflammatory lesions that develop following tissue irritation in the posterior larynx, usually on the medial surface of the arytenoid cartilage.[1,3,13,27–29] A contact ulcer is an ulcerated lesion that occurs in the same site, often perceived as an aggravated consequence of granuloma. In some cases, a cup and saucer effect occurs when a granuloma on one arytenoid meets a concave ulcerated area on the contralateral side. Both lesions are unique among vocal fold pathologies because they can be painful, and initial signs may include complaints of a sore throat or referred pain to the ear, with or without voice disturbance. Two principal etiologies are associated with the mechanical or chemical tissue irritants that produce a granuloma or contact ulceration. First, these lesions may form following laryngeal intubation due to surgery or the need for long-term airway ventilation, presumably due to the endotracheal tube pressure on the superficial mucosa of the arytenoid cartilages. Second, these lesions form in patients with laryngopharyngeal reflux, likely due to the chemical irritation from gastric acids present in the posterior glottis. Another factor associated with granuloma and contact ulcer is persistent voice misuse, especially for speakers with pressed, low-pitched voice, due to the extra tension needed to maintain that quality.[29]

Unless the lesion is large or accompanied by localized edema or erythema of the membranous vocal fold, the presence of a granuloma does not necessarily affect vocal fold vibration. Nonetheless, besides throat pain, patients may complain of restricted pitch range and vocal endurance. Treatment may be medical, surgical, behavioral, or a combination, depending on the size and etiology of the lesions. A medical antireflux regimen is a common first approach, followed by surgery, if needed. Behavioral voice treatment will seek to eliminate vocal strain and pressed voice, elevate pitch, if needed, and reduce hard glottal onsets or other forms of excessive medial compression. However, granulomas and contact ulcers arise in areas of constant movement and mechanical pressure, so these lesions are notoriously recalcitrant and frequently recur.[27–29]

Keratosis, Leukoplakia, and Erythroplasia. Keratosis, leukoplakia, and erythroplasia are three pathologies that are sometimes termed more generally as *epithelial hyperplasia*, meaning "abnormal mucosal changes."[1,3,13,30] Although the three conditions are related, they present as three visibly distinct tissue changes. Leukoplakia (Plate 14) means "white plaque," which accurately describes this condition, marked by a thick white substance that covers the vocal folds in diffuse patches, usually on the superior surface of the vocal fold as opposed to midline margins. The pathology of leukoplakia is variable and may include both benign and malignant lesions.[1,13]

Hyperkeratosis (Plate 15) means "excessive keratin," which reflects the buildup of keratinized (horny) cell tissue, distinctive for its leaflike appearance and irregular, rough vocal fold margins.[1,13] Erythroplasia refers to thickened and abnormal tissue that is red. These changes usually occur in response to combinations of hyperfunctional voice use and chemical irritants, especially alcohol and tobacco use. Although the pathologies are benign, hyperkeratosis and leukoplakia are hyperplastic epithelial changes, which may enter and involve the superficial, intermediate, and even deep layers of the lamina propria. The lesions usually are bilateral but can occur unilaterally. They increase the mass and stiffness of the cover of the fold while leaving the transition and the body unaffected. Patients are instructed to avoid future exposure to tobacco smoke, chemical inhalants, and other irritants. Usually, phonosurgery will be conducted to confirm the diagnosis with a small biopsy and to remove the hyperplasia from the vocal fold mucosa. If the tissue around the lesion is abnormal (called *atypia*), these lesions may signal early carcinoma.[30] Voice therapy often can help restore voice quality and ensure that the patient modifies any behaviors that contributed to the epithelial changes.

Recurrent Respiratory Papilloma (RRP). Papillomas (Plate 16) are wartlike growths that develop in the epithelium and invade deeper into the lamina propria and vocalis muscle. They can grow rapidly and in large clusters. If they proliferate in the upper aerodigestive airway, this excessive growth can compromise the airway. Papillomas have a cellular composition of highly vascular, stratified squamous epithelium with connective tissue cores.[1,3,13] The lesions are caused by the human papilloma virus (HPV) infection, and although the presence of HPV in the birth canal may predispose the baby to childhood papilloma, the incidence is inconsistent. Papillomas occur in 4.3 out of 100,000 children, found equally in boys and girls and usually appearing between 2 and 4 years. Often, papilloma growth decreases with age and may disappear altogether during puberty. Adult-onset papillomas are rising but are still less common, with only 1.8 out of 100,000 and a male-to-female predominance of 2:1.[13]

Papillomas affect the mass and stiffness of the cover, transition, and body of the vocal fold, resulting in severe dysphonia. Because of the diffuse locations and rapid spread of the papilloma, medical treatments are aggressive and have included interferon therapy, injections, and laser excision.[3] Multiple surgeries are often required to control these tumors, and these repeat procedures can create vocal fold scarring, thus producing a secondary voice disorder.[31]

Most worrisome, however, is the fact that papillomas are known to spread within the upper airway, involving the larynx, trachea, and bronchus, potentially leading to compromised respiration and occasionally death. Because of the diffuse locations of these growths and the speed at which they tend to proliferate, tracheostomy is sometimes required to guarantee the patient a functional airway. The role of voice therapy in treatment of papilloma is twofold. First, patients can learn to reduce hyperfunctional voice use to lessen excessive vocal fold medial compression. Second, treatment may assist patients in recovering appropriate or optimal voice quality postsurgery, especially when vocal folds are scarred by multiple procedures. The resulting voice quality may range from mild dysphonia to complete aphonia, depending on the extent of the disease and the aggressiveness of the required treatment(s).

Subglottic and Laryngeal/Glottic Stenosis and Acquired Anterior Glottic Web. Stenosis (Plate 17) is a fibrous tissue overgrowth that narrows the airway, either in the subglottis just below the vocal folds or in the laryngeal plane. Glottic stenosis or anterior glottic webbing is an acquired scar that connects the medial edges of the vocal folds, beginning in the anterior commissure and extending posteriorly. In severe cases, the stenosis at either vertical level can compromise the airway, resulting in stridor. Stenosis arises from multiple sources, including congenital maldevelopment of the cricoid cartilage or the conus elasticus or postintubation scarring, any of which might produce a narrowing of the larynx below the glottis. Stenosis can create an airway obstruction with associated inhalatory stridor, even from birth. In some cases, as the cricoid cartilage grows in infancy or early childhood, the problem is alleviated. In more severe cases, surgical repair of the subglottic region is required, including tracheostomy in extreme cases.[32,33]

Other small acquired microwebs may develop in the anterior commissure in the postoperative period following vocal fold surgeries that involve the anterior membranous portion of the folds or following vocal trauma. These microwebs occur when irritation of the anterior commissure reheals as a small fibrotic web.[1,3,13] The effect of this microweb on voice quality can be variable, and surgical management is occasionally warranted, especially in elite performers.

Vascular Lesions: Vocal Fold Hemorrhage, Hematoma, Varix, and Ectasia. Vascular vocal fold lesions, including hemorrhage, hematoma, varix, and ectasia (Plate 18) occur because of some traumatic (usually acute) injury to the small blood vessels of the vocal fold, such as excessive coughing, crying, or screaming. Vascular lesions are thought to occur more frequently among premenstrual women using aspirin products.[1,3,13] Often, a hemorrhage occurs abruptly when a small capillary on the superior surface of the vocal fold ruptures, causing a bleed into the superficial layer of the lamina propria (Reinke's space). A hematoma is the accumulation of blood that has leaked from the vessel. A varix is a mass of blood capillaries that appears as a small, long-standing "blood blister" that has hardened over time, creating an adynamic segment in vocal fold vibration and contributing to loss of pitch and loudness range. It may also appear as a blunt end of a varicose vein, seen on the surface of the vocal fold after the hemorrhage has resolved. The term *ectasia* refers to a larger collection of varices. All of these vascular injuries can present with focal or diffuse discoloration of the vocal fold surface, ranging from bright red to brownish yellow, depending on the time since initial bleeding.[1,3,13] These injuries have the potential to increase mucosal stiffness and, in more severe cases, create localized scarring of the vocal fold cover. Voice quality changes can be severe at the time of the bleed, and dysphonia may continue in the period after the injury. When other laryngeal inflammation or edema accompanies vocal fold hemorrhage and hematoma, the submucosal vocal fold space may also combine with the vascular trauma to create a secondary mass lesion. Small varices or ectasias may not cause noticeable voice change, despite observable loss of vibratory amplitude and mucosal wave. However, even these slight disruptions may be significant for professional voice users. Aggressive voice conservation and rest may resolve acute hemorrhage or hematoma. When vascular injuries persist, medical and surgical treatments include steroids, cauterization to stop the bleed, or, in the case of a persistent varix, microexcision of the lesion.

Congenital and Maturational Changes Affecting Voice

Congenital Webs (Synechia)

Webs of the vocal folds occur when there is a tissue bridge between the two vocal folds at the anterior commissure. Congenital webs (Plate 19) arise when the vocal folds fail to separate during the 10th week of embryonic development. Webbing may occur anywhere from the anterior to the posterior glottis. If the web is complete at birth, airway compromise is a threat. More commonly, webbing of the anterior glottis causes various degrees of dyspnea and stridor, depending on the extent of the web.[1,3,13] Phonosurgery is conducted to separate the web, using a keel to maintain separation of the raw edges of the folds and to avoid reformation of the web caused by postoperative scarring. The keel is removed after several weeks. During the healing period, the airway is maintained via tracheostomy. The voice qualities of children with congenital webs will range from normal voice to a severe dysphonia, depending on the length and thickness of the web. In some cases, virtually no effects are noted in either breathing or voice quality. Occasionally, a congenital web may go undetected in males until puberty, when the vocal pitch fails to lower because of the reduced vibratory length of the folds.

Laryngomalacia

Laryngomalacia is a congenital pediatric laryngeal abnormality that is not necessarily a voice disorder. Rather, the condition creates an airway threat due to a soft, flexible omega-shaped epiglottis.[3,13] As the child inhales, the floppy epiglottis is drawn into the airway, causing audible stridor. Unless severe airway obstruction or feeding problems ensue, no treatment is required for this condition, as the epiglottis will continue to develop, and the condition will spontaneously clear by age 3 with normal maturation.

Puberphonia: Mutational Falsetto and Juvenile Voice

The laryngeal mechanism undergoes dramatic change in both males and females during puberty. The male voice lowers about 1 octave, and the female voice lowers 2 to 3 semitones. When this acoustic change does not take place despite normal laryngeal maturation, puberphonia occurs. Males with puberphonia may speak in falsetto voice or near the top of their modal frequency range, hence the clinical term *mutational falsetto*. Females with similar speech and voice distortions are said to have a *juvenile resonance disorder* or *childlike voice*, due to a higher pitch accompanied by anterior tongue posturing during speech production. Some proposed causes of mutational falsetto in males include resistance to puberty, feminine self-identification, the desire to maintain a competent childhood soprano singing voice, and embarrassment when the voice lowers dramatically, perhaps earlier than those of one's peers. The juvenile voice of the postadolescent female is recognized less commonly than mutational falsetto because the vocal symptoms of this disorder are less socially aberrant. Women who demonstrate a juvenile voice may have resisted the transition into adulthood or may have habituated this altered laryngeal and vocal tract posture.

The voice qualities associated with these disorders are typically mild dysphonias characterized by high pitch, low intensity, cul-de-sac nasality, and breathiness. Physiologically, this is caused by persistent hyperfunction of the cricothyroid muscles, a high-postured tongue, and pronounced laryngeal elevation. Patients with puberphonia cannot build appropriate subglottic air pressure to increase intensity; common complaints are vocal fatigue and the inability to shout or compete with background noise. Young males may also demonstrate raspy voice quality if they attempt to lower pitch level despite an elevated larynx positioned for falsetto register. Mutational falsetto and juvenile voice most often are identified during the first few postadolescent years, with the social consequences being more negative for the male. In both disorders, it is critical that the clinical examination has ruled out underlying structural or movement anomalies. For example, an occult vocal fold paralysis in a postadolescent male or female may present as a high-pitched, breathy voice. Falsetto may also result from primary muscular incoordination or dysfunction that could affect speech articulation as well. Occasionally these pathologies are not identified until the adult years, when it often is more difficult to achieve normal voice. Nonetheless, behavioral voice therapy has been consistently successful in triggering appropriate pitch and resonance, often in the very first session, but consistent follow-up is needed to familiarize and stabilize the "new" voice.

Presbyphonia or Presbylaryngeus

"Presby" means "aging," and presbyphonia or presbylaryngeus is a term used to describe a voice disorder that develops during normal processes of laryngeal aging, without other contributing etiology.[34,35] The laryngeal changes presumed to underlie this disorder include reduced respiratory efficiency, loss of elasticity of the vocal fold mucosa, and possibly deterioration of the tone of the vocal fold body.[36] Also, ossification of the hyaline laryngeal cartilages may contribute to a slight decline in range and speed of intrinsic laryngeal adjustments. The perceptual effects of these aging changes are consistent with older sounding voice: "thin" or muffled voice quality, decreased loudness, increased breathiness, pitch instability, and lack of vocal endurance and flexibility. Presbyphonia begins typically after age 65, but individuals who are in excellent physical condition or speakers who have professional voice training and have remained active vocal users may be more resistant to age-related deterioration.[34–38] The classic appearance of the vocal folds in presbylaryngeus is a slightly bowed glottal gap during vibration due to thinned vocal folds, presumably because of loss of vocal fold cover elasticity and vocal fold body tonus.[38] Voice rehabilitative therapy, especially vocal function exercises, may improve voice quality dramatically in patients with presbyphonia.

Inflammatory Conditions of the Larynx

Cricoarytenoid and Cricothyroid Arthritis

Rheumatoid arthritis is a chronic immunologic and inflammatory disorder that disrupts the normal structure and function of synovial joints, including the cricoarytenoid and cricothyroid joints in approximately 25% of patients with the disease. (Note that rheumatoid arthritis is distinct from osteoarthritis, which is a mechanical deterioration of connective tissues that does not involve laryngeal joints.) Vocal fold inflammation and edema may accompany arytenoid mucosal erythema. During symptomatic periods, laryngeal function for both respiration and voice production may be compromised by pain, swelling, and, in the most severe form, mechanical fixation or ankylosis (fusion) of the cricoarytenoid joints. Mechanical fixation or ankylosis cannot be determined visually, due to possible confounds with paralysis; rather, diagnosis is made by direct palpation. The fixation may occur unilaterally or bilaterally and at any point along the cricoid rim, from midline to laterally abducted positions. Thus, resulting airway and voice complications could include aspiration risk and breathy aphonic voice quality in cases of unilateral or bilateral lateral fixation. In rare cases of bilateral arytenoid midline fixation, the airway obstruction requires a tracheotomy or unilateral arytenoidectomy to reestablish adequate ventilation. Unilateral arytenoid fixation at midline creates stridor and dysphonia that can usually be managed with anti-inflammatory and corticosteroid medications, to relieve the exacerbation.[39–41]

Acute Laryngitis

The nonspecific term *laryngitis* is used to describe an inflammation of the vocal fold mucosa, causing mild to severe dysphonia with lowered pitch and intermittent phonation breaks.[42] The cause of acute laryngitis is unknown, but it is usually associated with upper respiratory inflammation due to bacterial, viral, or fungal infections, or behavioral trauma (eg, vocal abuse). Vocal folds usually appear edematous and erythematic. The most effective treatments for acute laryngitis include external and internal hydration, antibiotics, if prescribed, and rest. Occasionally, a cough suppressant may be prescribed to limit additional damage to the vocal folds. Many patients will not feel pain with repeated coughing and may unknowingly aggravate the vocal injury if they are unaware of the deleterious effects of severe or prolonged coughing. Usually, acute laryngitis resolves spontaneously as other upper respiratory symptoms recede, often within a few weeks to a month. Persistent laryngitis for weeks or months after other recovery is complete always warrants a closer look by the voice pathology team, to rule out other inflammatory laryngeal etiologies.

Laryngopharyngeal Reflux

Laryngopharyngeal reflux (LPR) (Plate 20) occurs when gastric fluids from the upper esophageal sphincter leak into the pharynx and larynx, irritating and inflaming the mucosa. Symptoms are diverse, including possible dysphonia, excessive mucus, coughing, throat pain, swallowing difficulties, and globus (sensation of a lump in the throat).[43–45]

Often, patients with one or more of these symptoms deny any history of heartburn, indigestion, or "hot burps." Voice problems associated with LPR are similarly variable, ranging from none to severe dysphonia, often fluctuating with other symptoms. Because of this known inconsistency in signs and symptoms, Belafsky, Postma, and Koufman have proposed a Reflux Finding Score (RFS) to help standardize medical observations made on a laryngeal examination. The RFS rates common visual signs of tissue inflammation in LPR: subglottic edema, ventricular obliteration, erythema/hyperemia, vocal fold edema, diffuse laryngeal edema, posterior commissure hypertrophy, granuloma/granulation, and thick endolaryngeal mucus.[46] The Reflux Symptom Index (RSI) is a patient self-rating on the severity of select factors associated with LPR over the past month on a scale of 1 (not at all) to 5 (severe). These factors are hoarseness, throat clearing, mucus or postnasal drip, dysphagia, coughing, breathing difficulties, throat sensations or tickle, and heartburn symptoms. A score of 13 or above is thought to reflect the presence of LPR.[47] Because LPR is a medical diagnosis, pharmaceutical management with over-the-counter or prescription medication is a common treatment approach. Behavioral changes may also reduce LPR symptoms, including dietary changes, losing excess weight, eliminating caffeine, alcohol, and other substances that can aggravate or inhibit digestion, wearing loose clothing that does not bind the midriff, elevating the head of the bed at night, and avoiding unnecessary bending in activities such as bowling or gardening. Surgery is usually reserved for chronic and unremitting cases that fail to respond to conservative therapies.

Chemical Sensitivity/Irritable Larynx Syndrome

Some individuals appear to develop consistent and repeated sensitivity to airborne chemical exposures that trigger abnormal airway and voice changes, including dysphonia, weak voice quality, and vocal fatigue. These responses are highly individualized and impossible to predict on the basis of patient or chemical features. Nonetheless, these patients typically report symptom onset following a known exposure to some airborne chemical, such as toxic gases, fumes, carpet or fabric treatments, smoke, aerosols, pollution, perfumes or scents, and other stimulants in the environment.[48–52] Irritable larynx syndrome (ILS) is the term given to the cluster of symptoms reported commonly in these patients, including one or more of the following: dysphonia following exposure, airway distress or episodic laryngospasm, globus, chronic cough, throat pain or dryness, and reflux.[53] Differential diagnosis of ILS is difficult unless the symptoms are consistently acute and time locked with a known chemical exposure as a trigger. Symptoms may exacerbate, plateau, or recede, some lasting only brief periods of time, whereas others persist for years. Treatment typically includes antireflux medications and reasonable precautions against repeated exposure to chemical stimulants, if known.

Trauma or Injury of the Larynx

Trauma to the larynx and vocal folds may injure the cartilaginous framework, the soft tissues, or both. Consequently, airway threats as well as voice disorders may arise from laryngeal trauma. Some common sources of laryngeal injuries are external factors, such as a blunt force trauma, or internal factors, such as chemical or heat inhalation, ingestion of toxic or corrosive fluids, or intubation/extubation trauma. The type and severity of the trauma will determine the nature and extent of the associated airway disruption or voice disorder.

Internal Laryngeal Trauma: Thermal and Chemical Exposure; Intubation/Extubation Injury

Airway exposure to toxic chemicals or heat may result in a thermal injury to the laryngeal mucosa. Short-term laryngeal changes may include inflammatory edema and erythema, coughing, hypersensitivity to airborne irritants, dysphagia, and throat pain or irritation. In the long term, tissue scarring and glottic stenosis may form if the mucosal tissues suffer burns. Another common form of internal laryngeal injury is trauma due to endotracheal tube intubation or extubation.[54] These injuries are rare complications of surgery and occur most frequently if the tracheal tube was inserted emergently or if the airway was either very small (eg, premature infants) or abnormal due to head and neck misalignment. Intubation and extubation injuries are also more common following prolonged intubation periods for mechanical ventilation, because the inflatable cuff places additional pressure on the laryngeal tissues. Short-term laryngeal changes may include pain, localized inflammation, ulceration of the posterior laryngeal mucosa, and granuloma. Long-term complication may include scar or glottic web formation, subglottic stenosis, and arytenoid dislocation.

External Trauma and Arytenoid Dislocation

External laryngeal trauma occurs acutely whenever blunt force or penetrating wounds injure the laryngeal cartilages or soft tissues. Examples include strangulation, injuries due to car or snowmobile accidents, stabbing, and numerous other possibilities. The location, type, and severity of the physical trauma will determine the nature and extent of any subsequent voice disorder, which obviously is a secondary concern to the biological need for airway preservation and protection. Like external trauma, arytenoid dislocation also can occur following external mechanical injury to the neck or throat or from difficult intubation or extubation for surgery.[55] When dislocated, the vocal process of the arytenoid cartilage may not move normally and may rest at a different vertical level than its contralateral pair. Vocal fold adduction and abduction will be asymmetric, and incomplete glottic closure is likely, resulting in dysphonia, breathiness, weakness, and strain. If acute onset follows a traumatic injury, it is easy to rule out paralysis or mechanical fixation. Depending on the injury, pain may be present during voicing.

Systemic Conditions Affecting Voice

Systemic or "whole-body" influences such as endocrine function, allergies, and immunologic responses may also affect the larynx, so it is important for the voice pathologist to recognize these medical disorders that may influence voice production.[1,3,13,56] To understand the relationship between body systems that affect the larynx, some researchers have examined normal and pathologic physiology and measured vocal function as a dependent variable. For example, voice performance may fluctuate with changing female hormonal levels, both within a menstrual cycle and across pregnancy trimesters.[3,57–60] This research supports a long-standing clinical impression among elite professional singers that vocal range, quality, stability, and endurance are affected by the hormonal cycle. Other researchers have used vocal function measures to mark the time-locked association between certain disease processes and associated effects on voice quality, related to sex hormones, thyroid function, allergies, and endocrine disorders.[58–64]

Medical pathologies affecting voice rely predominantly on pharmacologic agents for treatment, although phonosurgery and behavioral voice rehabilitation may be appropriate as second-order approaches. For all voice disorders arising from a systemic condition, pharmacologic treatment is managed by the appropriate medical specialist. The voice pathologist plays a supportive role by assisting in the correct diagnosis and monitoring the changes in vocal function through the treatment course. Although the effects of medications on voice quality and function have not been explored exhaustively, some general predictions are possible, based on known drug actions and reactions.[65,66] Most commonly, drugs used to treat systemic diseases that affect voice produce one of the following four effects on body systems:

- Increasing airflow through bronchodilators, which expand the diameter of pulmonary bronchioles to increase oxygen and carbon dioxide exchange when treating allergies, asthma, and other upper respiratory diseases[3,13,65,66]
- Reducing fluid level in tissues through diuretics, corticosteroids, and decongestants, which each act separately to reduce edema due to inflammation[3,13,65–68]
- Reducing upper respiratory secretions through antihistamines, antitussives (cough suppressants), and antireflux medications, used to treat upper respiratory infections and gastrointestinal disease[3,13,42,65,66]
- Modifying vocal fold structure through long-term use of hormonal therapies, especially estrogen or testosterone, used to treat sexual hormone imbalance.[3,13,57,61,65,66]

Endocrine Disorders

Hypothyroidism and Hyperthyroidism. Thyroid function controls many chemical processes in the body, influencing organs, secretions, tissue health, and emotions. Although thyroid disorders affect voice production, their impact is inconsistent across individuals and difficult to predict.[3,13,69] Like other systemic conditions that may affect voice quality, thyroid etiologies may often be identified retroactively, once treatment has resolved the associated voice disorder. Hypothyroidism, or reduced thyroid hormone production, causes loss of tissue fluids throughout the body, influencing hair, skin, and organ health. Some patients experience a persistent, unexplained dry cough. The vocal fold lamina propria may lose fluids, while the vocal fold body increases mass due to edema in deeper tissues. These changes result in lower pitch, roughness, loss of range and endurance, and vocal fatigue due to a thickened vocal fold body and decreased flexibility of the cover.[3,13,69] Treatment usually includes thyroid replacement medication. Hyperthyroidism results from excessive secretions of the thyroid hormone, and physical symptoms include prominent eyeballs, goiter, tremor, tachycardia, and weight loss. Voice quality changes associated with hyperthyroidism include slight vocal instabilities including "shaky" voice, breathy quality, and reduced loudness. Hashimoto's thyroiditis involves initial hyperthyroidism followed by hypothyroidism.[13] Although thyroid levels can be altered pharmacologically, they do not change rapidly, so vocal and physical symptoms may persist for weeks or months before appropriate hormone levels are achieved and stabilized.

Sexual Hormonal Imbalances. As a general rule, hormonal imbalances arise whenever levels are excessive or diminished, often without apparent cause. Most commonly these disorders are identified at or near puberty, when absent or abnormal reproductive maturation is apparent in either males or females. The greatest and most consistent effect on voice quality is change in habitual pitch and pitch range. *Virilization* is the term given to abnormal secretion of androgenic hormones in females, resulting in male gender characteristics. The vocal effects are low pitch, hoarseness, and occasionally voice breaks.[3,13,57,61] Other specific hormone therapies, including estrogen, androgen, and testosterone replacement and oral contraceptives, may alter voice quality. Behavioral voice therapy can be used to augment the "feminine" quality of voice and speech. Treatment with estrogen or other hormonal therapy may improve voice quality, but pitch changes usually are permanent. Sensitivity to hormonal changes is more common in females than it is in males, perhaps due to the known sexual hormone cycles associated with menstruation, oral contraceptive use, pregnancy, and menopause. In elite female vocal performers, variations in vocal range and stability correspond to changes in these hormonal cycles. During menstruation, for example, the resulting edema may result in dysphonia, reduced pitch and loudness range, and loss of phonatory stability.[58,59] Postmenopause, structural changes in the female vocal fold may lower fundamental frequency and affect vocal endurance.

Growth Hormone Abnormalities (Hyperpituitarism). Endocrine glands secrete hormones that control body growth and development, so growth hormone disorders can alter or limit vocal fold development. Hyperpituitarism results in excessive growth due to oversecretion of the growth hormone, somatotrophin.[13] In this condition, many body structures grow rapidly and disproportionally, including the larynx and vocal folds. This abnormal growth may first become apparent at puberty, when anticipated changes in body growth and voice quality are most prominent. Changes in the oral, nasal, and pharyngeal structures including soft tissue, cartilages, and bones may cause vocal, articulatory, and resonatory distortions, including low pitch, rough voice, and dysarthria.

Immunologic Disorders

Voice disorders seem to occur in persons with immunologic disease but without other obvious contributing etiologies.[3,13,70] Although there are few published reports of the impact of immunologic disorders on laryngeal health and voice quality, some patients with these disorders complain of voice change and deterioration with advancing symptoms. Certainly, not every patient with these diagnoses will exhibit voice problems. In general, these patients report throat pain during talking, dysphonia, vocal fatigue, and loss of vocal flexibility and range. Following is a brief description of some of these disorders most commonly seen in voice disorders clinics. Systemic lupus erythematosus (SLE) is a rheumatologic disease that deposits fibrotic lesions in various organs. Laryngeal involvement may result in ulcerations, scarring, and cyst formation. Sjögren's syndrome is an autoimmune disorder that creates xerostomia (dry mouth) and dry eyes. In the larynx, symptoms include dry (sometimes crusty) epithelial mucosa, thick and tacky secretions, persistent dry cough, dysphagia, rough voice quality, and throat pain. Scleroderma creates fibrotic changes throughout the body due to excessive collagen formation. Typical sequella that may affect voice include gastroesophageal reflux, shortness of breath, and xerostomia. Fibromyalgia is a connective tissue syndrome that creates chronic fatigue and pain; if either of these complaints are localized in the larynx, voice problems may result.[3,13,70] For all of these and other inflammatory disorders, associated voice quality changes are inconsistent and unpredictable.

Allergies

Allergies are perhaps the most common group of inflammatory disorders that affect voice production because of the localized secretions and irritation in the pharyngeal, laryngeal, and nasal mucosa. Increased mucus consistency, nasal drainage or congestion, and edema of the vocal folds and other respiratory mucosa will alter vocal tract resonance and may inhibit phonation, especially when excessive secretions settle on the vocal folds.[3,13,62–64] It is common for patients who have allergies to experience symptoms of sneezing, chronic cough, throat clearing, inflamed nasal and pharyngeal tissues, and other respiratory ailments that may further aggravate the allergic inflammation and edema in the vocal folds and upper airway. Often, symptoms vary with the severity of the allergic response and may cycle with seasons, pollen counts, and specific exposures. Although medications may treat allergic symptoms effectively, they may have a detrimental effect on voice quality, creating a secondary problem for the patient with allergy-related dysphonia. For example, antihistamine medications prescribed to treat allergies may negatively influence voice because of their dehydrating effects.[65,66] Also, some patients experience increased dysphonia after prolonged use of steroid inhalers, which are used to counteract edema and inflammation from allergies.[67,68]

Nonlaryngeal Aerodigestive Disorders Affecting Voice

Respiratory Diseases

Respiratory disease, including asthma, chronic obstructive pulmonary disease, and croup (acute laryngotracheobronchitis) all result in acute or chronic symptoms of dyspnea, with audible inhalatory stridor and expiratory wheeze.[3,13] In children, laryngeal edema associated with asthma or croup may threaten the airway because of its smaller dimension. Although voice quality is clearly a secondary concern relative to ventilatory needs and airway preservation, any chronic compromise of respiratory support for vocal fold vibration may impair voice quality. Treatment for these respiratory disorders usually involves bronchodilators and inhaled steroids to suppress the symptoms of dyspnea and laryngeal edema, if present.[65,66] As with other medical conditions, voice quality changes due to respiratory disease are usually commensurate with symptom severity and treatment success.

Asthma and Chronic Obstructive Pulmonary Disease. Asthma is a respiratory disease that arises from various sources, including allergic responses, infectious processes, or a combination.[3,13,71] When asthma is active, the tracheal and bronchial lining are hypersensitive to external or internal stimuli, resulting in airway constriction, dyspnea, coughing, inhalatory stridor, and expiratory wheeze. Voice quality is not necessarily affected by asthma, but inhaled steroids and bronchodilators that are used to treat the condition may impair voice production. Chronic obstructive pulmonary disease (COPD) is a term given to any pulmonary condition that continually irritates or destroys healthy lung tissue, thereby obstructing airflow and reducing inhalatory and exhalatory gas exchange. Two examples are emphysema, which reduces the alveolar wall elasticity, and chronic bronchitis, which inflames the bronchi. Voice quality may not be affected by these respiratory diseases, but decreased breath support can limit vocal loudness, endurance, flexibility, and range. Similar to asthma, medications that treat COPD may also impair voice quality.[65,66]

Gastroesophageal Reflux Disease (GERD)

Gastroesophageal reflux is an aerodigestive condition that occurs when gastric fluids from the stomach leak from the lower esophageal sphincter into the esophagus. Because GERD involvement is confined to the lower esophagus, the disorder is distinct from laryngopharyngeal reflux (LPR), which affects the posterior laryngeal mucosa and can result in moderate to severe dysphonia. Nonetheless, the terms GERD and LPR are often used interchangeably. Formal assessment for GERD involves a double-probe transnasal pH monitor to assess the rise of gastric acids in the upper and lower esophagus over a 24-hour period.[3,13,43–45] GERD treatment is similar to that for LPR, including over-the-counter or prescription antacids or other medications, coupled with a behavioral antireflux protocol, as described previously.

Infectious Diseases of the Aerodigestive Tract

Certain infectious diseases, whether viral, bacterial, or fungal in origin, can also contribute to chronic laryngitis.[72] Examples include upper respiratory infections, pneumonia, sinusitis, tuberculosis, pertussis (whooping cough), and others.[3,13,72–78] Their impact on voice quality is inconsistent but certainly may be aggravated by severe and prolonged symptoms of chronic cough, sore (or tickling) throat sensations, chest congestion, increased or thickened phlegm, mucus drainage and postnasal drip, and other irritations of the larynx, pharynx, and lungs. The associated dysphonia generally resolves following appropriate medical treatment of the microorganism, when possible.

Some cases may develop a secondary chronic laryngitis (Plate 21) that persists even after the infection has resolved, due to long-standing laryngeal mucosal inflammation, viscous mucus, and epithelial thickening. Voice quality may be mildly to severely dysphonic depending on the severity of the epithelial changes and the voice production habits that may have developed, such as nonproductive coughing and throat clearing. Vocal fatigue is common, but local pain is seldom present. Chronic laryngitis may be aggravated further by occasional exposures and behaviors that would be otherwise tolerated in a healthy larynx, such as vocal misuse and abuse, smoking, poor laryngeal hydration, airborne pollutants or allergens, dehydrating medications, and laryngopharyngeal reflux. The typical treatment for chronic laryngitis is to identify and eliminate potential causative factors and devise compensatory strategies to modify these harmful elements.

Laryngotracheobronchitis (Croup). Croup is a viral infection that affects babies and preschool children. The mucosal lining of the subglottis and trachea become inflamed and edematous, resulting in a dramatic narrowing of the airway.[3,13] Symptoms can be frightening for parents: a harsh, barking cough, inspiratory stridor, shortness of breath, and in severe cases, neck extension and chest wall retraction associated with overt airway distress. Croup attacks last a variable period from 30 minutes to an hour or more, and repeated attacks are common. The treatment priority is understandably airway preservation, but rough, strained, and low-pitched voice quality can be present during croup episodes.

Mycotic (Fungal) Infections: Candida. Some patients with infectious disease are prone to overgrowth of oral and pharyngeal fungus. Candida, or yeast, is a common fungal infection that affects the aerodigestive system, including the larynx and vocal folds (Plate 22). Normal yeast is present in the larynx, pharynx, and trachea. This infectious overgrowth is most common in infants, the elderly, and individuals with decreased immune response, such as with human immunodeficiency virus (HIV/AIDS), status postchemotherapy, and bone marrow or organ transplantation. The candida infection deposits thick white yeast patches on the larynx and vocal folds, which are inflamed with edema and erythema. Laryngeal symptoms of candida include throat and tongue pain, cough, dry mouth, thick and tacky white oral strands, and rough or strained voice quality.[3,13,76–78] Treatment is conducted using antifungal medications but can be particularly difficult to manage in patients who are immunocompromised. Despite a long treatment course, recurrence is common.

Psychiatric and Psychological Disorders Affecting Voice

Functional Dysphonia

The human voice is acutely responsive to changes in emotional state, and the larynx plays a prominent role as the instrument for the expression of intense emotions like fear, anger, grief, and joy. Consequently, many regard the voice as a sensitive "barometer of emotions," and the larynx is considered the control valve that regulates the release of these emotions.[79] Furthermore, the voice is one of the most unique and characteristic expressions of the individual—a "mirror of personality." Thus, when the voice becomes disordered, it is not uncommon for clinicians to offer personality traits, psychological factors, or emotional or inhibitory processes as primary causal mechanisms. This is especially true in the case of "functional dysphonia or aphonia," where no visible structural or neurological laryngeal pathology exists to explain the partial or complete loss of voice. Some ambiguity surrounds the term *functional dysphonia* (FD), and confusion exists because FD is often used as the general descriptive term for a host of medically unexplained voice disorders. FD is sometimes broadly synonymous with "hysterical," "psychogenic," "conversion," "psychosomatic," "hyperkinetic," "hyperfunctional," "muscle misuse," or "muscle tension" dysphonia. Although each diagnostic label implies some degree of etiologic heterogeneity, whether these disorders are qualitatively different and etiologically distinct remains unclear. When applied clinically, these various diagnostic labels often reflect clinician supposition, bias, or preference. However, at the purely phenomenological level, there may be few empirically tractable differences that reliably distinguish these voice disorders.

To improve nosological precision, some clinicians prefer the term *psychogenic voice disorder* to put emphasis on the presumed psychological origins of the disorder. According to Aronson,[79] a psychogenic voice disorder is synonymous with a functional one but has the advantage of stating confidently, after an exploration of its causes, that the voice disorder is a manifestation of one or more forms of psychological disequilibrium. It is essential to recognize, however, that in clinical practice, "psychogenic voice disorder" should not be a default diagnosis for a voice problem of undetermined etiology. Rather, Sapir advises that at least 3 criteria should be met before such a diagnosis is offered: symptom psychogenicity, symptom incongruity, and symptom reversibility.[80] Symptom psychogenicity refers to the finding that the voice disorder is logically linked in time of onset, course, and severity to an identifiable psychological antecedent, such as a stressful life event, or interpersonal conflict. Such information is acquired through a complete case history and psychosocial interview. Symptom incongruity refers to the observation that vocal symptoms are physiologically incompatible with existing or suspected disease, are internally inconsistent, and are incongruent with other speech and language characteristics. An often-cited example of symptom incongruity is complete aphonia (whispered speech) in a patient who demonstrates a normal throat clear, cough, laugh, or hum, whereby the presence of such normal nonspeech vocalization is at odds with assumptions regarding neural integrity and function of the laryngeal system. Finally, symptom reversibility refers to the complete, sustained amelioration of the voice disorder with short-term voice therapy (usually 1 or 2 sessions) and/or through psychological abreaction. Furthermore, maintenance of voice improvement requires no compensatory effort on the part of the patient. In general, psychogenic dysphonia should be suspected when strong evidence exists for symptom incongruity and symptom psychogenicity, but confirmed only when there is unmistakable evidence of symptom reversibility.[80]

Although a wide array of psychopathological processes contributing to voice symptom formation in FD has been proposed, the dominant psychological explanation for dysphonia unaccounted for by pathological findings is the concept of conversion disorder. Conversion disorder involves unexplained symptoms or deficits affecting voluntary motor or sensory function which suggest a neurological or other general medical condition.[81] The conversion symptom represents an unconscious simulation of illness that ostensibly prevents conscious awareness of emotional conflict or stress, thereby displacing the mental conflict and reducing anxiety. When the laryngeal system is involved, it is referred to as conversion dysphonia or aphonia. In aphonia, patients lose their voice suddenly and completely and articulate in a whisper. The whisper may be pure, harsh, or sharp, with occasional high-pitched squeaklike traces of phonation. In dysphonia, phonation is preserved but disturbed in quality, pitch, and/or loudness. Myriad dysphonia types are encountered including hoarseness (with or without strain), breathiness, high-pitched falsetto, as well as voice and pitch breaks that vary in consistency and severity. Vegetative vocal tasks, such as coughing, throat clearing, laughing, sighing, grunting, and humming are usually intact.[3,13,82,83] The majority of conversion voice disorders occur in women, but men and children of all ages are susceptible.[1,5,6]

In conversion voice disorders, psychological factors are judged to be associated with the voice symptoms because conflicts or other stressors precede the onset or exacerbation of the dysphonia. In short, patients convert intrapsychic distress into a voice symptom. Onset is normally sudden, typically in response to some real or imagined stress, tension, or trauma that induces a psychological conversion reaction. This reaction response is a direct attempt to draw attention away from the real problem. It permits the individual to focus on the voice instead of the true source of the stress or emotional conflict. These voicing behaviors are unconscious methods of avoiding the strong interpersonal conflicts that cause the stress, depression, or anxiety. The voice loss, whether partial or complete, is also often interpreted to have symbolic meaning. Primary or secondary gains are thought to play an important role in maintaining and reinforcing the conversion disorder. Primary gain refers to anxiety alleviation accomplished by preventing the psychological conflict from entering conscious awareness. Secondary gain refers to the avoidance of an undesirable activity/responsibility and the extra attention or support conferred to the patient.

Butcher and colleagues[84–86] argued that there is little research evidence that conversion disorder is the most common cause of functional voice loss. Butcher advised that the conversion label should be reserved for cases of aphonia where lack of concern and motivation to improve the voice coexist with clear evidence of a temporally linked psychosocial stressor. In the place of conversion, Butcher[84] offered two alternative models to account for psychogenic voice loss. Both models minimized the role of primary and secondary gain in maintaining the voice disorder. The first was a slightly reformulated psychoanalytic model that stated: "if predisposed by social and cultural bias as well as early learning experiences, and then exposed to interpersonal difficulties that stimulate internal conflict, particularly in situations involving conflict over self-expression or voicing feelings, intrapsychic conflict or stress becomes channeled into musculoskeletal tension, which physically inhibits voice production."[84(p472)] The second model, based on cognitive-behavioral principles, stated: "life stresses and interpersonal problems in an individual predisposed to having difficulties expressing feelings or views would produce involuntary anxiety symptoms and musculoskeletal tension, which would center on and inhibit voice production."[84(p473)] Both models clearly emphasized the inhibitory effects of excess laryngeal muscle tension on voice production, although via slightly different causal mechanisms.

Recently, Roy and Bless proposed a theory to link specific personality traits to the development of FD.[87,88] The "Trait Theory of FD" shared Butcher's theme of inhibitory laryngeal behavior but attributed this muscularly inhibited voice production to specific personality typologies. In brief, the authors speculated that the combination of personality traits, such as introversion and neuroticism (trait anxiety), contributes to predictable and conditioned laryngeal inhibitory responses to certain environmental signals/cues. For instance, when undesirable punishing or frustrating outcomes have been paired with previous attempts to speak out, Roy and Bless postulated that this might lead to muscularly inhibited voice production in individuals predisposed by specific personality characteristics. The theory asserts that this conflict between laryngeal inhibition and activation (that has its origins in personality and nervous system functioning) results in elevated laryngeal tension states and can give rise to incomplete or disordered vocalization in a structurally and neurologically intact larynx.

In research designed to test the theory and to assess the role of personality in common voice disorders, Roy and colleagues[89–90] compared a vocally normal control group and 4 groups with voice disorders—functional dysphonia (FD), vocal nodules (VNs), spasmodic dysphonia (SD), and unilateral vocal fold paralysis (UVFP)—using Eysenck's Personality Questionnaire (EPQ). The EPQ—a popular personality assessment tool—provides scores for personality superfactors: extraversion (E) and neuroticism (N). Extraversion involves the willingness to engage and confront the environment, including the social environment. Extraverts (high E) tend to be dominant, sociable, and active, whereas introverts (low E) tend to be quiet, unsociable, passive, and careful. Neuroticism, the second personality dimension, can be likened to emotionality and is related to anxious, depressed, tense, and emotional characteristics. High N individuals tend to be emotionally unstable, worried, and highly reactive to environmental stimuli.[89] The results showed that distinct personality characteristics were present within the FD and VN groups and were conspicuously absent in the other groups. Group comparisons revealed that the majority of FD and VN subjects were classified as introverts and extraverts, respectively. As compared to the other groups, the FD group scored significantly higher on the Neuroticism dimension, thereby providing evidence to support the role of elevated N in FD development. Comparisons involving the SD, UVFP, and control subjects did not identify any consistent personality differences. On the whole, these differences in personality were compatible with the predictions of the Trait Theory of the dispositional bases of FD. In contrast, the disability hypothesis, which suggests that personality features and emotional maladjustment are solely a negative consequence of vocal disability, was not supported. The investigators concluded that the results largely support the contention that individuals with certain personality traits may be susceptible to developing FD.[89–90]

Despite considerable controversy surrounding causal mechanisms, the clinical voice literature is replete with evidence that symptomatic voice therapy for psychogenic disorders can often result in rapid and dramatic voice improvement.[91] The long-term effectiveness of direct voice therapy for these disorders has not been rigorously evaluated, however. It should be acknowledged that following behavioral voice therapy, only the voice symptom has been removed, not the underlying cause of the disturbance itself. Therefore, the nature of precipitating and perpetuating factors, including possible psychological dysfunction, needs to be better understood. If the situational, emotional, and/or personality features that contributed to the development of the voice disorder remain unchanged following behavioral treatment, it would be logical to expect that such persistent factors would increase the probability/risk of future recurrences.

In conclusion, the larynx can be a site of neuromuscular tension arising from stress, emotional inhibition, fear/threat, communication breakdown, and certain personality typologies. This tension can produce severely disordered voice in the context of a structurally normal larynx. While the precise mechanism(s) underlying and maintaining psychogenic voice problems remains unclear, the voice disorder is a powerful and tangible reminder of the intimate relationship between mind and body.

Factitious Disorders or Malingering

Factitious psychiatric disorders occur when a patient purposefully feigns illness or injury for psychological gain, also known as malingering.[13] Such patients are uncommon in voice disorders clinics, but typical profiles include patients seeking legal compensation, disability certification, or work relief due to the vocal illness or injury. For those with vocally demanding occupations (eg, receptionist, telemarketer, teacher, etc), it is very difficult to discriminate between bona fide threats to dysphonia and psychological overlay. Sometimes, patients will visit multiple health care professionals in an attempt to find a practitioner willing to confirm the factitious disorder. Typical voice symptoms include inconsistent or vague complaints of throat pain, vocal fatigue, dysphonia or aphonia (especially when performing work activities), roughness, breathiness, and strain. During the clinical examination, voice quality may fluctuate between normal and dysphonic, depending on the task and patient awareness. It may be helpful to observe the patient's speech in natural contexts (eg, talking on a cell phone) and to probe vegetative or singing tasks, which may be normal. Sometimes, the patient's responses to case history questions will give clues to the nature of the disorder, especially when signs and symptoms are conflicting (ie, too ill to teach, yet coaching a soccer team) or if the patient acknowledges the secondary gain potential.

Gender Dysphoria or Gender Reassignment

Patients whose biological sexuality conflicts with desired gender may assume the role of the opposite sex either full or part time, with or without undergoing gender reassignment surgery.[3,13,92] These individuals do not have voice disorders but do need consultation to achieve new, gender-appropriate speech and voice quality. These patients can benefit from hormonal therapies, behavioral therapy, and occasionally from phonosurgery to alter voice production.[93] Regardless of whether the transition is from male to female or female to male, voice goals are to modify vocal pitch to an ambiguous or desired range, stabilize voice quality and endurance, and alter speech articulation and prosody to create and maintain a communication style consistent with the desired gender.

Neurologic Disorders Affecting Voice

Neurologic voice pathologies are those voice disorders directly caused by an interruption of the nervous innervation supplied to the larynx, including both central and peripheral insults. Some of these disorders are confined to voice and laryngeal manifestations, such as vocal fold paralysis, whereas broader progressive neurologic diseases may cause deterioration of many central and peripheral motor control systems, including impairment of respiration, resonance, swallowing, and other functions beyond the head and neck.

Peripheral Nervous System Pathology

The peripheral nervous system consists of nerves and their branches after they leave the spinal cord. Peripheral nerve pathology affecting the larynx and vocal folds consists of paresis or paralysis of the superior or recurrent laryngeal nerves. Vocal fold paralysis is the most common neurologic voice disorder and typically is caused by peripheral involvement of the recurrent laryngeal nerve and less commonly of the superior laryngeal nerve. The location of the lesion along the nerve pathway will determine the type of paralysis and the resulting voice quality. More proximal involvement of the vagus (cranial nerve X) would affect both the recurrent and superior laryngeal nerves; more distal injury may affect just one nerve. There are many possible etiologies of vocal fold paralysis including surgical trauma, cardiovascular disease, neurologic diseases, and accidental trauma.[3,13,94–96] Historically, estimates of idiopathic unilateral vocal fold paralysis have been as high as 30% to 35%,[94] but two more recent reports of 117 and 159 patients each reported that idiopathic (unknown) etiologies were identified in unilateral vocal fold paralysis 16.3%[87] and 23%[96] of the time. Rather, chest disease and surgery, such as nonlaryngeal malignancies, anterior cervical fusion, and thyroid surgery contributed in greater proportions. Moreover, improved diagnostic techniques, such as imaging studies and laryngeal electromyography, may account for the smaller number of patients for whom onset appeared truly "idiopathic."[97,98] In cases of idiopathic onset of paralysis, patients frequently report that hoarseness began following a viral infection.

Superior Laryngeal Nerve Paralysis: Unilateral or Bilateral. The external branch of the superior laryngeal nerve (ESLN) innervates the cricothyroid (CT) muscle, which arises from the lateral arch of the cricoid cartilage and inserts into the thyroid cartilage. By lengthening and tensing the vocal folds, contraction of the CT muscle contributes to control of vocal fundamental frequency, and its perceptual correlate "vocal pitch." But, its effects on voice seem to extend beyond just vocal fundamental frequency. For example, in the clinical domain, unilateral CT dysfunction purportedly produces a wide array of phonatory and laryngeal effects, leading some authorities to conclude that dysphonia secondary to unilateral ESLN paralysis is an easily overlooked and often missed clinical entity.[99,100] At present, however, there is no uniform set of laryngoscopic features that are considered definitive of ESLN denervation.

Over the years, numerous descriptions have been offered regarding the laryngeal behaviors associated with unilateral partial or complete ESLN denervation. However, the exact nature and degree, as well as the tasks that provoke these laryngeal signs, are not well documented or understood. The earliest descriptions of ESLN dysfunction seem to reflect assumptions regarding how asymmetric CT tension should intuitively affect laryngeal appearance and function during phonation.[101,102] Regrettably, more recent reports describing laryngeal signs of ESLN denervation have been neither universal nor consistent. For instance, often-cited manifestations of unilateral ESLN dysfunction include, but are not limited to the following: (1) axial rotation of the anterior larynx creating an oblique glottis; (2) decreased longitudinal tension and length of the ipsilateral vocal fold with glottic insufficiency secondary to mild bowing; (3) sluggish abduction or adduction (hypomobility) of the ipsilateral fold during repetitive phonatory tasks; (4) asymmetrical, irregular, or aperiodic vocal fold vibration; and (5) reduced vocal fold amplitude, and mucosal wave in some cases.[103] In an attempt to shed light on this controversy, Roy and colleagues selectively blocked the ESLN using lidocaine, in order to identify the salient laryngeal features associated with acute, unilateral cricothyroid (CT) muscle dysfunction.[104] Flexible videolaryngostroboscopic (FVLS) recordings of participants performing a wide variety of vocal tasks were acquired before and during the block. Contrary to clinical reports, the investigators reported no evidence of hypomobility/sluggishness of the ipsilateral vocal fold, or a consistent pattern of axial rotation of the larynx. Instead, the analysis revealed deviation of the petiole of the epiglottis to the side of CT weakness in 60% of participants during a glissando up maneuver produced at normal volume. This finding had not been reported previously as a manifestation of unilateral CT paralysis. High-pitch voice tasks were found to most reliably reveal laryngeal dysfunction associated with unilateral ESLN paralysis. The same authors recently published a series of clinical cases with LEMG confirmed, longstanding ESLN denervation, who also showed epiglottic petiole deviation to the side of muscle weakness during high-pitched phonation, thus supporting this sign as a possible diagnostic marker of unilateral ESLN paralysis.[105]

In summary, although numerous laryngeal features have been ascribed to unilateral ESLN denervation, regrettably no consensus has emerged as to which laryngeal features, if any, should be considered pathognomonic. Differential diagnosis remains one of the greatest challenges. Deviation of the petiole of the epiglottis to the side of CT muscle weakness during extreme high-pitch voice represents a promising diagnostic sign of both acute and chronic unilateral ESLN denervation. However, further research is necessary to determine the factors that influence the expression and detection of this potential diagnostic sign, as well as its diagnostic precision.

Although much of the literature describing the effects of ESLN denervation has focused on laryngeal correlates, precise descriptions of the auditory-perceptual, aerodynamic, and acoustic consequences of ESLN damage are almost nonexistent. Little is known regarding how the voice sounds or functions following ESLN injury. Only cursory, vague, and unvalidated descriptions exist of the perceptual correlates of ESLN denervation. The speaking voice has been described as weak, breathy, raspy, monotonous, low pitched, and characterized by a loss of the upper pitch range. Regrettably, these vocal signs occur frequently in an array of voice disorders, and by themselves are not particularly unique to unilateral cricothyroid muscle paralysis (UCTP). Although numerous reports assert that UCTP can be disastrous for patients who are singers or professional voice users such as teachers, lawyers, politicians, or broadcasters, most reports have not objectively quantified the degree of impairment or surveyed a variety of voice tasks to reveal specific UCTP-related dysfunction (ie, extended loud talking, singing versus speaking, soft or loud voice production). Additionally, there are few patient-based assessments of the degree of voice-related handicap encountered by the individual who lives with the disorder. Only 2 clinical studies exist that have attempted to formally evaluate the phonatory effects of UCTP. Eckley and colleagues[106] reported on a group of adults (singers and nonsingers) diagnosed with unilateral or bilateral SLN paresis or paralysis (based upon laryngeal EMG findings). Common symptoms among the patients included vocal fatigue, breathiness, hoarseness and volume disturbance during loud phonation, and loss of the upper portion of the pitch range. Only one study exists that has described aerodynamic and acoustic correlates of chronic SLN paresis.[107] Thirty-five nonsingers with unilateral SLN paresis displayed higher than normal laryngeal airflow rates and reduced maximum phonation times. Acoustic correlates reportedly included decreased phonatory frequency range and elevated measures of aperiodicity. It is unclear, however, whether the observed voice effects reflected pure CT dysfunction or compensatory adaptations to chronic, incomplete denervation.

In an attempt to better understand the adverse phonatory effects of acute UCTP, Roy and colleagues[108] also collected multiple measures of phonatory function as part of their lidocaine simulation study described previously. The authors reported that during the unilateral ESLN block, phonatory frequency range (PFR-Hz) was significantly reduced with compression of both upper and lowermost regions of the pitch range. Mean speaking fundamental frequency (SFF) increased significantly during oral reading. Acoustic analysis, aerodynamic assessment, and auditory-perceptual evaluation revealed modest increases in phonatory instability, increased laryngeal airway resistance with no objective evidence of glottic insufficiency, and mild deterioration in voice quality most evident during high-pitched voice productions, respectively. Participants uniformly rated their speaking and singing voices as worse during the block with vocal weakness and effort that they described as a "mild" level of impairment. These results point to fairly modest changes to the speaking voice which extend beyond reductions in pitch range only. As expected, the most consistent adverse effect of UCTP was compression of PFR for all voice tasks. In addition to a reduction in the uppermost region of the pitch range, an unexpected finding was the apparent reduced access to lower parts of the pitch range, and changes in the mean SFF of the voice. That is, the lowest frequency attained was often higher during the block as compared to baseline, suggesting that PFR was not only compressed by lowering the upper range, but also by raising the bottom part of the frequency range. Furthermore, there was also a general pattern of increased fundamental frequency for all voice tasks which targeted normal-pitch or low-pitch productions. This general pattern of pitch elevation was an unexpected finding that was seemingly at odds with previous descriptions associating UCTP with lowered habitual pitch. The authors suggested that this tendency toward pitch elevation could reflect immediate attempts to compensate for loss of CT-induced longitudinal tension, by recruiting other vocal fold tensors such as the ipsilateral or contralateral thyrovocalis belly of the thyroarytenoid (TA) muscle. Hyperfunctioning of the TA may also help to explain why there was no evidence of glottic insufficiency on the aerodynamic measures. The aerodynamic results were not indicative of frank glottic insufficiency as reported by others, but they confirm the laryngoscopic findings described earlier from the same simulation study, which showed no laryngoscopic evidence of glottic insufficiency (ie, bowing or incomplete glottic closure) during acute UCTP. Despite the lack of objective evidence to support glottic insufficiency, the participants viewed their speaking voices as noticeably weaker with increased physical effort expended to produce voice. These participant-based data perhaps provide valuable insight regarding the impetus to compensate for perceived vocal weakness, and the increased muscular effort required to produce such compensations. This may shed valuable light on "compensatory" or "secondary" muscle tension dysphonias, as reactive muscular adjustments to perceived weakness in the voice.

Differential diagnosis of UCTP remains a significant challenge. At present, there is no uniform set of laryngoscopic features that can be considered definitive of unilateral ESLN paralysis. As such, it is impossible to establish the true prevalence, impact, and treatment of UCTP. Recent in vivo simulations combined with clinical case studies suggest that epiglottic petiole deviation to the side of CT muscle weakness during high-pitch voice production deserves further study as a potentially valuable diagnostic sign. Further research is necessary to distinguish acute laryngeal and phonatory effects of UCTP from short- and long-term compensatory muscular adjustments related to chronic denervation.

Recurrent Laryngeal Nerve Paralysis: Unilateral. The RLN innervates the thyroarytenoid, lateral cricoarytenoid, posterior cricoarytenoid, and interarytenoid laryngeal muscles. Patients with unilateral RLN paralysis (Plates 23 and 24) present with varied vocal symptoms, ranging from mild to severe dysphonia. The characteristic perceptual symptoms of paralysis are breathiness, low intensity, low pitch, and intermittent diplophonia. These vocal impairments result from irregular and incomplete vocal fold valving during phonation. Two physical dimensions account for this loss of vocal power and quality:

- Inadequate vocal fold closure, due to the altered resting position of the paralyzed fold
- Loss of vocal fold muscle tone in the paralyzed fold, resulting in flaccidity, weakness, and bowing.

Both factors contribute to the asymmetric, aperiodic, and incomplete vibratory closure during phonation seen in patients with unilateral vocal fold paralysis.[109,110] Because the RLN serves both adductor and abductor functions of the vocal folds, the location of the paralyzed fold, which can vary from full abduction to paramedian position to midline, will influence the nature and severity of the associated voice impairment. The paralyzed fold may rest at midline, fully abducted, or in between, in the paramedian position. If the condition is unilateral, the contralateral fold continues to adduct and abduct normally. Therefore, with a paralyzed fold in the midline position, quasinormal voice quality may still be preserved, as long as the contralateral fold can adduct to meet the paralyzed fold to vibrate. But, the loss of medial compression and a possible difference in vertical height will still disrupt voice production, due to vocal instability, weakness, and loss of endurance.[109,110] Voice quality for contextual speech can approach near normal; however, the patient may experience difficulty in building the necessary subglottic pressure for increased vocal loudness because of the laxness of the paralyzed fold. The midline position of the paralyzed fold may also pose a breathing problem during strenuous activities such as sports or heavy labor, due to inhalatory stridor and reduced airway. Overall, this form of unilateral vocal fold paralysis does not severely compromise the patient's voice or respiratory status.

The most common outcome of unilateral RLN paralysis is a paralyzed fold in a paramedian (partially abducted) position, approximately 1 to 2 mm from midline. This resting lateral position and altered vertical level of the paralyzed fold will determine the size of the resulting glottal gap and the effect on phonation. Voice quality is usually characterized by breathiness and diplophonia. The ability to build subglottic air pressure is also impaired resulting in decreased vocal intensity and the inability to be heard in even low levels of background noise. Patients with this pathology often complain of physical fatigue resulting from the increased effort to produce voice and the breathlessness associated with phonation. When unilateral RLN paralysis results in a fully abducted (cadaveric) position, approximately 3 to 4 mm from midline, voice quality will consistently be severely breathy and aphonic. Without tight glottic closure, it will be difficult to build subglottic pressure for vegetative maneuvers such as coughing, grunting, lifting, and defecating. The airway is well preserved for ventilation, but aspiration risks increase due to lack of glottic closure during swallowing. Treatment approaches for unilateral vocal fold paralysis include a large range of behavioral, surgical, and combination approaches, all of which are described in Chapter 7.

Recurrent Laryngeal Nerve Paralysis: Bilateral. The most serious form of vocal fold paralysis is a bilateral impairment. Usually the etiology is a higher vagal injury or progressive neuropathy. When vocal folds are paralyzed in the adducted position (at midline), they cannot open (abduct) to create sufficient airway for respiration. This critical condition is called bilateral abductor paralysis and requires a surgical procedure to reestablish adequate airway, often through a tracheostomy. Surgical manipulation of one arytenoid cartilage also will create sufficient airway by either removing the arytenoid entirely or suturing it laterally.[110–112] If an arytenoid lateralization is performed, voice quality will be permanently weakened and aphonic. When bilateral paralysis occurs with vocal folds positioned in a paramedian or laterally abducted position, ventilation is no longer a concern, but airway protection becomes a much larger threat because of failure of the vocal folds to close to avoid aspiration. This condition is termed *bilateral adductor paralysis*, and in this configuration, neither voice production nor airway protection can be achieved satisfactorily. Patients with this form of paralysis often require gastrostomy tube feedings because of insufficient airway protection. They may also need augmentative communication aids to compensate for the complete aphonia. Both speech amplifiers and electrolarynx devices have been used to augment the "whispered" voice. In 6 to 9 months following the onset, vocal fold contracture and fibrosis may occur, drawing the folds to midline and permitting a harsh, breathy phonation. This development also improves airway protection during swallowing.

Superior Laryngeal Nerve (SLN) or Recurrent Laryngeal Nerve (RLN) Paresis. Vocal fold paresis occurs when there is partial injury to one or both of the SLN or RLN branches. RLN paresis is presumed by the appearance of reduced vocal fold movement or tone, including a loss in the speed and range of adduction and abduction, especially when unilateral asymmetry is evident. As discussed previously, however, some experts have asserted that hypomobility of one vocal fold may also be a sign of unilateral SLN paresis. It appears then that neither RLN nor SLN paresis can be ascertained empirically.[113,114] Rather, LEMG has been used to define the presence of peripheral nerve paresis and improve clinical prognostication.[98,99,113,114] Paresis has variable effects on voice quality, which may include typical mild deficits, such as dysphonia, breathiness, and decreased pitch range, loudness, and endurance. Often paresis will recover spontaneously within 6 to 12 months, reversing these impairments. There are no medical or surgical treatments for vocal fold paresis, but behavioral voice therapy may help speakers compensate for the voice disorder.

Myasthenia Gravis. Myasthenia gravis is a lower motor neuron impairment of the neuromuscular junction that results in rapid muscle fatigue. Persons with myasthenia gravis may have symptoms confined to the larynx (myasthenia laryngis), but more commonly, they experience broad-based decline across many skeletal muscles. In speech and voice, prolonged speech tasks or concentrated repetitions will result in rapid quality deterioration due to vocal weakness, breathiness, limited pitch and loudness range, and flaccid dysarthria.[3,13,115–119] Although symptoms improve temporarily following rest, the condition is chronic. Medical treatment may help manage and reduce the symptoms of myasthenia gravis. The focus of voice therapy is to maintain and conserve voice efficiency, often through augmentative amplification.

Movement Disorders Affecting the Larynx

Spasmodic Dysphonia

Spasmodic dysphonia is the diagnostic term that describes an unusual voice disorder, marked by consistent and unremitting perceptual symptoms of phonatory spasms without evidence of any other motor speech disorder or laryngeal pathology.[3,13,114–118,120–123] The National Spasmodic Dysphonia Association (NSDA) estimates that approximately 15,000 people are affected by this disorder.[13] Its cause has been debated for many years, and early descriptions linked the condition to psychoneurosis.[3,13,120,124] Currently, we understand that spasmodic dysphonia is a focal, action-induced dystonia, occurring only when the individual speaks. Spasms affect laryngeal movements during voicing, resulting in abnormal and involuntary cocontraction of the laryngeal muscles. There is no evidence of spasm during nonspeech vegetative laryngeal gestures, such as laughing, crying, swallowing, or coughing. Spasmodic dysphonia is considered to be similar to other focal dystonias (eg, blepharospasm, writer's cramp, torticollis, and Meige's oral-facial dystonia) that are similarly affected by abnormal involuntary contractions that are action induced, task specific, and wholly unrelated to other pathology or etiology.[13,123]

The onset of spasmodic dysphonia usually occurs in the middle adult years, but it has been identified in both children and elderly speakers. Because spasmodic dysphonia represents a complex of symptoms rather than a specific diagnosis, the disorder can be difficult to identify empirically.[123] Symptoms may begin gradually, progress over a period of a few months to a few years, and then plateau. Often, patients delay evaluation and diagnosis because initial symptoms are intermittent and fluctuating, or because of the misperception (sometimes on the part of the health care provider, as well as the patient) that these voice changes are sequelae from a prior upper respiratory infection. Perceptual attributes of spasmodic dysphonia may also be confused with other organic, behavioral, or psychogenic voice disorders, especially because many voice symptoms develop following prolonged or extreme vocal demands or following a period of unusual stress or trauma. Thus, decisions about the presence and management of spasmodic dysphonia require careful examination of the individual's speech and voice symptoms across time, attending to the severity and, most importantly, the continued presence of spasms during speech.

There are three types of spasmodic dysphonia: adductor type, abductor type, and mixed. Each type has well-defined perceptual features: the adductor type is characterized by strained-strangled voice stoppages, the abductor type by involuntary breathy bursts, and the mixed containing both features. These speech symptoms coexist with apparently undisrupted nonspeech laryngeal maneuvers, including singing, laughing, coughing, throat clearing, and humming. Symptoms may worsen with stress or heavy speech demands, but they persist regardless of the patient's emotional state or voice use patterns. Overall, severity seems to peak within the first year following the onset of the disorder; however, recent reports suggest that a subset of patients may experience further deterioration over time.[125]

Many patients with spasmodic dysphonia have experienced long and discouraging searches for an accurate diagnosis and for a treatment to cure or reduce the symptoms. Many have seen otolaryngologists, neurologists, psychologists, and speech pathologists. They may have received voice therapy, psychotherapy, stress reduction interventions, drug therapies, EMG and thermal biofeedback, relaxation training, acupuncture, hypnosis, and faith healing. Unfortunately, none of these approaches can relieve vocal symptoms; in fact resistance to any traditional medical or behavioral voice treatments is a hallmark of diagnostic certainty in spasmodic dysphonia. In the past 3 decades, chemodenervation via percutaneous injections of botulinum toxin (BOTOX) into the intrinsic laryngeal muscles have provided temporary reprieve from symptoms of spasmodic dysphonia. A full discussion of this treatment approach is presented in Chapter 7.

Adductor Spasmodic Dysphonia (ADSD). There are two principle types of spasmodic dysphonia: adductor and abductor. Adductor spasmodic dysphonia (ADSD) is the more common and results in a severely hyperfunctional voice, including a classic strained-strangled quality due to the hyperadduction of the vocal folds during spasm. Other perceptual features of the spasms include pitch or voice breaks and occasional voicing "blocks" of tension or effort that interrupt the continuity of phonation. Struggle is often a salient feature of voice onset patterns. The laryngeal behavior is characterized by an intermittent, tight adduction of the vocal folds creating spontaneous and irregular strained voice stoppages, often with momentary pitch changes. ADSD spasms occur more frequently in voiced contexts than in voiceless. Under flexible laryngoscopy, the vocal folds appear normal in structure and function, but visible spasms are obvious during connected speech. Brief periods of normal phonation may occur during speech production, and some patients are able to reduce the frequency and severity of the spasms when talking at a pitch level that is slightly higher than normal, singing in falsetto, or whispering. Many patients with ADSD complain of physical fatigue, tightness of the neck, back, and shoulder muscles, and shortness of breath caused by their efforts to phonate through the closed glottis. Symptom severity varies within and among individuals. Some patients experience only a mild interruption in normal phonation, whereas others may be rendered voiceless by the severity of the spasms. Approximately 25% to 30% of individuals with ADSD also have concomitant vocal tremor, which is a separate disorder.[126–128] In the more severe cases, patients may compensate by whispering or phonating on inspired air. Secondary behaviors similar to those observed in stutterers, such as head jerking, eye blinking, and vocalized starters, may also develop.

Abductor Spasmodic Dysphonia (ABSD). Abductor spasmodic dysphonia (ABSD) is a virtual "mirror image" of the adductor type. Instead of hyperadduction, spasms interrupt phonation with a sudden, involuntary period of aphonia, which is accompanied by a burst of air, as the vocal folds involuntarily abduct. The vocal fold spasms occur primarily during unvoiced consonants in all word positions, on whole words, and on several words in succession. Voice quality consists of involuntary breaks and intermittent aphonia, with uncontrolled, prolonged bursts of breathy phonation. Voice onset may be normal, and then spasms begin with continued speaking. The pattern of involuntary vocal fold abduction is visible on connected speech during flexible endoscopy. Patients often report that their voices improve when they are angry, using a louder voice, or using an elevated pitch and worsen when they are anxious or fatigued. However, patients with ABSD report that speech is effortful due to the spasmodic air escape, and some individuals limit their communication to reduce that fatigue.

Mixed Adductor and Abductor Spasmodic Dysphonia. Some patients present with a combination of ADSD and ABSD symptoms: intermittent, involuntary spasms of vocal fold hyperadduction, and sudden, breathy bursts of involuntary abduction. This sequence of both voice stoppage and breathy aphonia is inconsistent and otherwise similar in onset and patient profile as other clinical descriptions of ADSD and ABSD. Patients with mixed ADSD and ABSD often describe communication as frustrating and tiresome, especially because the combined perceptual features of strained-strangled voice and breathy bursts during phonation are irksome for the speaker, negatively distracting to the listener, and can limit speech intelligibility.

Essential Vocal Tremor. Essential tremor is a movement disorder characterized by rhythmic tremors that may involve the head, arms, neck, tongue, palate, face, and larynx, either in isolation or in combination. In some patients, the tremor may only be observed when the affected body part is being used (intentional tremor), whereas other patients will exhibit the tremor behavior even at rest. The onset of essential tremor is usually gradual and begins most commonly in the fifth or sixth decade of life. The disorder occurs more frequently in females, is often hereditary, and may accompany other neurological signs.[3,13,126,127]

Laryngeal tremor is most noticeable during prolonged vowels, due to the regular wavering of pitch and intensity at a consistent range from 4 to 7 hertz. The tremor will affect connected speech as well and, in severe cases, may include voice breaks or complete stoppages similar to spasmodic dysphonia. Spasmodic dysphonia and essential vocal tremor may exist concurrently in some patients. The perceptual difference between the conditions is evident during sustained vowels: spasmodic dysphonia will sound nearly normal during vowel prolongations, except for brief intermittent spasms; essential vocal tremor will produce consistent rhythmic modulations.[128] In addition to the persistent perceptual features, the laryngeal tremor is visible during sustained phonation during the laryngeal examination. This disorder is different from tremor in other neurologic processes, such as Parkinson's and cerebellar disease. There is no uniformly successful treatment for essential vocal tremor. For example, patients with coexisting ABSD or ADSD and essential vocal tremor who receive BOTOX commonly report relief from the focal dystonia, without any dramatic change in tremor activity.

Central Neurologic Disorders Affecting Voice

Neurologic disorders that affect the larynx do not occur in isolation, and as such, voice impairments will accompany other disordered motor speech functions, including changes in respiration, articulation, resonance, and prosody. The range and type of neurologic voice problems are as varied as the underlying dysarthrias, encompassing both laryngeal and supralaryngeal factors.[3,13,115–118] The classic audioperceptual clusters of speech and voice patterns in neurologic disease may be diagnostic when used in combination with findings from the neurologic examination. These perceptual features include vocal fold hypoadduction, hyperadduction, phonatory instability, and incoordination of both prosody and voiced-voiceless contrasts. Therapy for neurologic disorders that affect voice production is compensatory and will not reverse the underlying etiology but may help maximize the patient's communicative skills, by addressing either select vocal behaviors (eg, increasing loudness or reducing effort) or global speech targets (eg, increasing respiratory support or articulatory precision). Table 4–3 displays the specific voice characteristics associated with different types of dysarthria. The

Table 4–3. Voice Deviations Associated with Dysarthrias

Type	*Audioperceptual Symptoms*	*Examples*
Flaccid	Vocal fold hypoadduction resulting in weak, breathy phonation; reduced loudness; diplophonia; hypernasality; nasal air emission	Myasthenia gravis
Spastic	Vocal fold hyperadduction resulting in low pitch; strained-strangled, effortful, and rough phonation; slow speech rate	Dystonia
Ataxic	Irregular, random variations in pitch, loudness, prosody, and speech rate, including excess and equal stress	Cerebellar disorders
Hyperkinetic	Vocal dystonia; respiratory irregularities resulting in random and sudden changes in pitch and loudness; tremor; myoclonus; intermittent aphonia	Huntington's chorea
Hypokinetic	Monopitch and monoloudness; hypernasality; imprecise articulations and weak phonation; limited vocal endurance; rapid speech rate	Parkinson's disease
Mixed	Symptoms of both spastic and flaccid dysarthria characteristics	Amyotrophic lateral sclerosis

following section describes voice characteristics for some of the most common neurologic disorders that are referred to the voice pathologist.

Amyotrophic Lateral Sclerosis

Amyotrophic lateral sclerosis (ALS) is a degenerative neurological disorder that affects adults between the ages of 30 and 60 years.[115–118,129–131] The primary pathology affects both upper and lower motoneurons, including spread to the motoneurons of the spinal cord, brainstem, and cortex. The resulting dysarthria is a mixed spastic-flaccid type. Muscle weakness, fasciculation, and atrophy provide evidence of lower motor neuron involvement, whereas spasticity, strain, and effortful speech represent upper motor neuron impairment. The severity and sequence of symptom onset and expression are varied. Approximately 75% of patients experience early "limb onset" symptoms, and for these individuals, speech and voice may be unaffected in the early stages. The other 25% present with "bulbar onset" symptoms, including slurred speech, dysphagia, and spastic and flaccid dysarthria.[13] The bulbar presentation of the disease progresses more rapidly than limb presentation in this terminal disease. Features of spastic dysarthria include slow speech rate, strained-strangled voice, and reduced stress and prosody. Features of flaccid dysarthria include hoarse, breathy voice, consonant distortions, and short phrases. Hypernasality may be a feature of both spastic and flaccid dysarthria. The voice of patients with ALS has sometimes been described as "wet" or "gurgly" or having a tremor or flutter on vowel prolongation.[115–118] Because ALS symptoms always progress, inevitably, longitudinal assessment is most helpful to verify the diagnosis and discriminate perceptual features of ALS from other stable disorders, such as ADSD.[129–131] Although voice therapy may address compensatory strategies, there is no successful medical or rehabilitative treatment identified for ALS.

Parkinson's Disease

Parkinson's disease is an extrapyramidal disorder that arises from loss of dopamine in the basal ganglia of the motor cortex, resulting in bradykinesia (slowing of movements), hypokinesia (decreasing range of movements), rigidity, and resting tremor.[3,13,115–118] The disease affects individuals at a mean age of 60 years, with more men affected than women. Speech and voice impairments are consistent with hypokinetic dysarthria. Phonation is characterized by monopitch and monoloudness, with weak, breathy voice and occasional vocal tremor. Speech intelligibility is reduced in advanced stages of the disease and may be aggravated by lack of facial expression and the patient's inability to perceive the dramatic loss of articulatory movement and range and associated speech imprecision.[115–118,132,133] Both medical and surgical treatments have had some success in stabilizing parkinsonian symptoms. A behavioral voice program, the Lee Silverman Voice Therapy, has a long record of positive, peer-reviewed treatment outcomes in improving the loudness and intelligibility of speech in patients with idiopathic Parkinson's disease.[132,133] The central targets of this program are loud productions of steady-state phonation conducted in a rigorous exercise routine, including multiple trials daily. Despite the focus on respiration and phonatory loudness, treatment effects have generalized to increased articulatory strength, precision, and intelligibility, as well as improved vocal loudness and quality.

Multiple Sclerosis

Multiple sclerosis is an example of hyperkinetic dysarthria that affects young adults from late teens through age 40, with higher predominance in women than men. The disorder is a progressive inflammatory demyelinating disease that results in both sensory and motor impairments of many functions, including gait, mobility, and coordination, vision, and cognition.[3,13,115–118,134,135] Similar sensory and motor deficits can spread to include the vocal tract and other head and neck musculature. Speech and voice characteristics, if present, are typical of spastic-ataxic dysarthria, due to effortful bursts of phonation, intermittent aphonia, abnormal speech rate, altered prosody, and decreased articulatory precision. The disease may flare (exacerbate) and recede (remit) spontaneously for years. In later stages, speech intelligibility may decline, and dysphagia may be present.[134] Behavioral voice treatment for this and other degenerative diseases is usually palliative, with focus on preserving functional communication. In terminal stages, cognitive decline may preclude effective behavioral compensation.

Huntington's Chorea

Huntington's chorea (HC) is a genetic autosomal dominant neurologic disease that arises from cell death in the basal ganglia and cortex. The term *chorea* means random, jerky movements, and it characterizes the debilitating loss of motor control, coordination, and balance which affects all muscles of the body in this disease.[115–118] HC usually manifests in young adulthood, although juvenile onset is also possible. Patients experience a slow, progressive decline in motor control and cognitive function. For speech and voice, early upper motor neuron signs of hyperkinetic dysarthria include strained-strangled voice and erratic involuntary phonatory bursts, grunts, and other nonspeech sounds. Behavioral voice or speech therapy is useful to forestall effects of inevitable decline and to monitor changes in speech, respiration, and swallowing. In later stages, patients lose oral, pharyngeal, and laryngeal control for speech or swallowing. If cognitive function is preserved, augmentative communication may be helpful.

Other Disorders of Voice Use

Pathologies associated with inappropriate voice maladaptations are another source of vocal pathology. Unlike organic laryngeal pathologies, disorders of voice use refer to dysphonia that occurs despite the presence of normal vocal fold structure with no evidence of neurologic disease or psychological abnormalities.

Vocal Abuse, Misuse, and Phonotrauma

These terms are subject to long-standing discussion by voice professionals who have tried to label this well-known cluster of clinical symptoms. The essential components of vocal abuse and misuse are prolonged, effortful, and maladaptive vocal behaviors, usually based on excessively loud or aggressive voice production, sharp glottal attack (voice onset), inappropriate technique for voice or singing, and aggressive laryngeal vegetative maneuvers, including throat clearing, coughing, or grunting.[1,3,13] Some forms of abuse and misuse arise from at-risk situations or environments, including occupational hazards posed by heavy voice demands in loud ambient noise or for long periods of time.[13] Vocal abuse and misuse often result from poor or ineffective training in vocal technique, including insufficient respiratory support, excessive laryngeal tension during phonation, and failure to achieve proper oral resonant focus. Across time, the cumulative effect of these poor vocal behaviors, whether produced knowingly or unknowingly, is traumatic injury to the vocal fold cover, sometimes even forming benign lesions.

Vocal Fatigue

Vocal fatigue is a frequent descriptor for another well-known set of symptoms, including deteriorated vocal quality, decreased endurance, loss of frequency and intensity control, and complaints of effortful, unstable, or ineffective voice production. Clinically, these symptoms are among the most common complaints from patients who are referred for unexplained voice disorders. Understanding vocal fatigue is complicated by our lack of thorough understanding of the pathogenesis of the complaint. Theories about the existence of muscular fatigue in the larynx have given rise to the term *laryngeal myasthenia* or *myasthenia laryngis*.[136] Yet, there is no physiological evidence to suggest that laryngeal muscles fatigue with voice tasks or that the very real symptoms of "tired voice" can be associated with either central or peripheral muscle fatigue. Other potential factors that may influence sensations of fatigue include strain of the nonmuscular laryngeal tissues (ligaments, joints, membranes), increased viscosity of the vocal fold cover caused by friction and shearing forces, loss of internal hydration and cooling in the laryngeal tissues, and loss of subglottal pressure because of respiratory fatigue.[137]

Clinically, patients with complaints of vocal fatigue will exhibit vocal folds that appear normal under indirect laryngoscopy. Symptoms of the disorder include dryness in the mouth and throat; pain at the base of tongue, throat, and neck; sensations of "fullness" or a "lump" in the throat; shortness of breath; and effortful phonation. Laryngeal imaging techniques may reveal an anterior glottal gap in the vibratory phase closure pattern, decreased amplitude, and phase asymmetry. Although the clinical signs and symptoms of vocal fatigue are well known to patients and clinicians alike, there remains a need for better clinical inclusion and exclusion criteria for this disorder. The treatment for symptoms of the disorder using physiologic voice therapy has proved effective and is described in detail in Chapter 7.

Muscle Tension Dysphonia (Primary and Secondary)

Morrison and Rammage[138–140] first described muscle tension dysphonia (MTD), a speech diagnosis characterized by variable symptoms of voice disruption in the absence of laryngeal pathology, caused by visible or palpable tension or stiffness of the neck, jaw, shoulders, and throat. Primary MTD reflects the presence of this disorder without other associated etiology (ie, without frank structural or neurological pathology). In clinical circles, primary MTD has recently supplanted the use of the term *functional dysphonia*, to place more emphasis on dysregulated (or excess) laryngeal muscle tension as the proximal cause of the dysphonia. Secondary MTD refers to maladaptive compensatory voice behaviors adopted in response to some intruding laryngeal pathology, such as a benign lesion, paresis, or other disturbance.[13,141]

Patients with MTD report periodic pain in the sites of the larynx, neck, and other areas, confirmed by laryngeal imaging studies that reveal excessive laryngeal or supraglottic tension due to medial compression or anterior to posterior glottis constriction. Also, the incidence of concomitant psychosocial stress or other interpersonal conflicts may be associated with this disorder. Common perceptual symptoms of MTD include dysphonia, vocal fatigue, loss of pitch and loudness range, reduced vocal flexibility, and strain. Behavioral voice rehabilitative therapy is useful for relieving symptoms and restoring appropriate vocal technique in patients with this disorder.

Ventricular Phonation (Plica Ventricularis)

During normal vocal fold vibration, the ventricular (false) folds are at rest, in a position superior and lateral to the true vocal folds. To achieve ventricular phonation, excessive supraglottic tension must draw the ventricular ligaments very close to midline, sufficient to allow pulmonary air to oscillate the false fold (Plate 25). This unusual approximation allows an alternate compensatory vibratory sound source for voice but is rarely produced unless the true vocal folds cannot valve normally, due to paralysis, scarring, congenital abnormalities, or other primary deficits of true vocal fold phonation.[13,142] Voice quality in ventricular phonation is always very low pitched, moderate to severely rough, and strained, with limited loudness and endurance. Patients complain of vocal fatigue due to the large effort required to create ventricular phonation. If true vocal fold vibration is physically possible, behavioral treatment will seek to practice and stabilize normal phonation. Therapy will cue higher pitch and increased loudness to trigger true vocal fold vibration, as these two vocal tasks are incompatible with ventricular phonation.

Paradoxical Vocal Fold Motion (Vocal Fold Dysfunction) or Episodic Dyspnea

Paradoxical vocal fold motion (PVFM) accurately describes the abnormal and inappropriate pattern of vocal fold adduction during inspiration, resulting in inhalatory stridor.[3,13,143–145] The condition is primarily a respiratory, not a vocal complaint, but the disorder is commonly evaluated and treated behaviorally in voice disorders clinics, even though dysphonia is seldom linked to this condition. Patients with PVFM will experience episodic shortness of breath without evidence of contributions from lower respiratory disease. Triggers for these episodes are varied, including intense exercise, psychological stress, laryngopharyngeal reflux, and environmental irritants.[146–148] Although the episodes are typically self-limiting, they have the potential to create airway distress and often frighten patients. In severe cases, the disorder may result in chronic dyspnea, requiring a tracheostomy.[3] The etiology for paradoxical vocal fold motion is unknown, but the disorder is common in adolescents, elite athletes, health care workers, and high achievers. Many patients with PVFM have laryngopharyngeal reflux and up to 50% have a history of asthma. Nonetheless, behavioral therapy for PVFM is frequently successful. Using select breathing techniques and visual biofeedback of the laryngeal image, the patient learns to interrupt the abnormal cycle of adductory inhalation and restore the correct pattern of vocal fold abduction. Depending on the patient profile, this behavioral treatment approach may be augmented with antireflux medication and psychological intervention as warranted.

SUMMARY

This chapter reviewed a large set of laryngeal pathologies that affect voice, speech, and respiration. Despite the broad range of potential etiologies, many pathologies will have similar effects on the quality, pitch, and loudness of voice production. Medical or organic contributors play a significant role in the patient population with voice disorders. By being familiar with the predisposing history, appearance, and common etiologic factors that may lead to their development, voice pathologists may plan appropriate management programs. The interaction between vocal function and laryngeal pathology, whether focal or systemic, has provided opportunity for development of new treatment approaches. Although medical diagnosis of the laryngeal pathology is the exclusive responsibility of the otolaryngologist, a voice pathologist who is well informed about the process can increase the probability of an efficacious diagnostic voice evaluation and treatment plan. Options for medical treatments, voice rehabilitation, and phonosurgery have enhanced the opportunity for voice pathologists and otolaryngologists to apply a combined team approach to diagnosis, treatment planning, and rehabilitation of voice disorders.

REFERENCES

1. Hirano M. Structure of the vocal fold in normal and disease states: anatomical and physical studies. In: Ludlow C, Hart M, eds. *Proceedings of the Conference on the Assessment of Vocal Pathology.* Rockville, MD: American Speech-Language Hearing Association; 1981:11–30.
2. Damste PH. Diagnostic behavior patterns with communicative abilities. In: Bless DM, Abbs J, eds. *Vocal Fold Physiology.* San Diego, CA: College-Hill Press; 1987:435–444.
3. Rubin JS, Sataloff RT, Korovin GS, eds. *Diagnosis and Treatment of Voice Disorders.* 2nd ed. Clifton Park, NY: Thomson Delmar Learning; 2003.
4. Herrington-Hall B, Lee L, Stemple J, Niemi K, McHone M. Description of laryngeal pathologies by age, gender, and occupation in a treatment seeking sample. *J Speech Hear Disord.* 1988;53:57–65.
5. Coyle SM, Weinrich BD, Stemple JC. Shifts in relative prevalence of laryngeal pathology in a treatment-seeking population. *J Voice.* 2001;15(3):424–440.
6. Roy N, Merrill RM, Gray SD, Smith EM. Voice disorders in the general population: prevalence, risk factors, and occupational impact. *Laryngoscope.* 2005;115(11):1988–1995.
7. Roy N, Stemple J, Merrill RM, Thomas L. Epidemiology of voice disorders

in the elderly: preliminary findings. *Laryngoscope.* 2007;117(4):628–633.

8. Titze I, Lemke J, Montequin D. Populations in the US workforce who must rely on voice as a primary tool of trade: a preliminary report. *J Voice.* 1997;11: 254–259.
9. Smith E, Lemke J, Taylor M, Kirchner H, Hoffman H. Frequency of voice problems among teachers and other occupations. *J Voice.* 1998;12:480–488.
10. Senturia B, Wilson F. Otorhinolaryngologic findings in children with voice deviations: preliminary report. *Ann Otol Rhinol Laryngol.* 1968;77:1027–1042.
11. Silverman E, Zimmer C. Incidence of chronic hoarseness among school-age children. *J Speech Hear Disord.* 1975;40: 211–215.
12. Dobres R, Lee L, Stemple J, Kummer A, Kretchmer L. Description of laryngeal pathologies in children evaluated by otolaryngologists. *J Speech Hear Disord.* 1990;55:526–533.
13. Verdolini K, Rosen C, Branski R, eds. *Classification Manual for Voice Disorders —I.* Mahwah, NJ: Lawrence Erlbaum Associates; 2006.
14. Pearson BW. Subtotal laryngectomy. *Laryngoscope.* 1981;91:1904–1912.
15. Lefebreve J. Laryngeal preservation: the discussion is not closed. *Otolaryngol Head Neck Surg.* 1999;118:389–393.
16. Colton R, Woo P, Brewer D, Griffin B, Casper J. Stroboscopic signs associated with benign lesions of the vocal folds. *J Voice.* 1995;9:312–325.
17. Wallis L, Jackson-Menaldi C, Holland W, Giraldo A. Vocal fold nodule vs. vocal fold polyp: answer from surgical pathologist and voice pathologist point of view. *J Voice.* 2004;18(1):125–129.
18. Goldman S, Hargrave J, Hillman R, Holmberg E, Gress C. Stress, anxiety, somatic complaints, and voice use in women with vocal nodules: preliminary findings. *Am J Speech Lang Pathol.* 1996;5:44–54.
19. Verdolini-Marston K, Burke MK, Lessac A, Glaze LE, Caldwell E. A preliminary study on two methods of treatment for laryngeal nodules. *J Voice.* 1995;9:74–85.
20. Roy N, Holt KI, Redmond S, Muntz H. Behavioral characteristics of children with vocal fold nodules. *J Voice.* 2007;21(2):157–168.
21. Bouchayer M, Cornut G, Witzig E, et al. Epidermoid cysts, sulci and mucosal bridges of the true vocal cord: a report of 157 cases. *Laryngoscope.* 1985; 95:1087–1094.
22. Hernando M, Cobeta I, Lara A, García F, Gamboa FJ. Vocal pathologies of difficult diagnosis. *J Voice.* 2008;22(5): 607–610.
23. Marcotullio DG. Reinke's edema and risk factors: clinical and histopathologic aspects. *Am J Otolaryngol.* 2002; 23(2):81–84.
24. Thibeault SL, Gray SD, Bless DM, Chan RW, Ford CN. Histologic and rheologic characterization of vocal fold scarring. *J Voice.* 2002;16(1):96–104.
25. Hansen JK, Thibeault SL. Current understanding and review of the literature: vocal fold scarring. *J Voice.* 2006; 20(1):110–120.
26. Ford CN, Inagi K, Bless DM, Khidr A, Gilchrist K. Sulcus vocalis: a rational approach to diagnosis and management. *Ann Otolaryngol Rhinol Laryngol.* 1996;105:189–200.
27. Crary M, Sapienza C, Cassissi N, Moore GP. A preliminary report on treatment of contact granuloma with steroid injections. *Am J Speech Lang Pathol.* 1996;7(2):92–96.
28. Emami AJ, Morrison M, Rammage L, Bosch D. Treatment of laryngeal contact ulcers and granulomas: a 12-year retrospective analysis. *J Voice.* 1999; 13(4):612–617.
29. Ylitalo R. Hammarberg B. Voice characteristics, effects of voice therapy, and long-term follow-up of contact granuloma patients. *J Voice.* 2000;14(4): 557–566.
30. Blackwell KE, Calcterra YC, Fu Y. Laryngeal dysplasia: epidemiology

and treatment outcome. *Ann Otol Rhinol Laryngol.* 1995;104:596–602.
31. Zeitels SM, Sataloff RT. Phonomicrosurgical resection of glottal papillomatosis. *J Voice.* 1999;13(1):123–127.
32. Cotton R. Prevention and management of laryngeal stenosis in infants and children. *J Pediatr Surg.* 1985;20:845–851.
33. Baker S, Kelchner L, Weinrich B, et al. Pediatric laryngotracheal stenosis and airway reconstruction: a review of voice outcomes, assessment, and treatment issues. *J Voice.* 2006;20(4):631–641.
34. Ringel R, Chodzko-Zaijko W. Vocal indices of biological age. *J Voice.* 1987;1: 31–37.
35. Woo P, Casper J, Colton R. Dysphonia in the aging: physiology versus disease. *Laryngoscope.* 1993;102:139–144.
36. Tanaka S, Hirano M, Chijiwa K. Some aspects of vocal fold bowing. *Ann Otol Rhinol Laryngol.* 1994;103:357–362.
37. Linville SE. *Vocal Aging.* San Diego, CA: Singular Publishing Group; 2001.
38. Pontes P, Brasolotto A, Behlau M. Glottic characteristics and voice complaint in the elderly. *J Voice.* 2005;19(1):84–94.
39. Bienenstock H, Ehrlich GE, Freyberg RH. Rheumatoid arthritis of the cricoarytenoid joint: a clinicopathologic study. *Arthritis Rheumat.* 1963;6:48–63.
40. Wolman L, Darke CS, Young A. The larynx in rheumatoid arthritis. *J Laryngol Otol.* 1965;79:403–434.
41. Speyer R, Speyer I, Heijnen MAH. Prevalence and relative risk of dysphonia in rheumatoid arthritis. *J Voice.* 2008;22(2):232–237.
42. Shumrick K, Shumrick D. Inflammatory diseases of the larynx. In: Fried M, ed. *The Larynx: A Multidisciplinary Approach.* Boston, MA: Little, Brown and Company; 1988:249–278.
43. Lumpkin SMM, Bishop SG, Katz PO. Chronic dysphonia secondary to gastroesophageal reflux disease (GERD): diagnosis using simultaneous dual-probe prolonged pH monitoring. *J Voice.* 1989;3:351–355.
44. Koufman JA. The otolaryngologic manifestations of gastroesophageal reflux disease (GERD): a clinical investigation of 225 patients using ambulatory 24-hour pH monitoring and an experimental investigation of the role of acid and pepsin in the development of laryngeal injury. *Laryngoscope.* 1991; 101(4, pt 2, suppl 53):1–78.
45. Kjellen G, Brudin L. Gastroesophageal reflux disease and laryngeal symptoms. Is there really a causal relationship? *Otol Rhinol Laryngol.* 1994;56: 287–290.
46. Belafsy PC, Postma GN, Koufman JA. The validity and reliability of the Reflux Finding Score (RFS). *Laryngoscope.* 2001;111(8):1313–1317.
47. Belafsky PC, Postma GN, Koufman JA. Validity and reliability of the Reflux Symptom Index (RSI). *J Voice.* 2002; 16(2):274–277.
48. Sataloff, RT. The impact of pollution on the voice. *Otolaryngol Head Neck Surg.* 1992;106:701–705.
49. Roto P, Sala E. Occupational laryngitis caused by formaldehyde: a case report. *Am J Ind Med.* 1996;29:275–277.
50. Sala E, Hytonen M. Occupational laryngitis with immediate allergic or immediate type specified chemical hypersensitivity. *Clin Otolaryngol.* 1996; 21(1):42–48.
51. Allan PF, Abouchahine S, Harvis L, Morris MJ. Progressive vocal cord dysfunction subsequent to a chlorine gas exposure. *J Voice.* 2006;20(2):291–296.
52. Gartner-Schmidt JL, Rosen CA, Berrylin R, Ferguson J. Odor provocation test for laryngeal hypersensitivity. *J Voice.* 2008;22(3):333–338.
53. Morrison M, Rammage L, Emami AJ. The irritable larynx syndrome. *J Voice.* 1999;13(1):447–455.
54. Ellis PDM, Bennett J. Laryngeal trauma after prolonged endotracheal intubation. *J Laryngol.* 1977;91:69–76.
55. Rubin AD, Hawkshaw MJ, Moyer CA, Dean CM, Sataloff RT. Arytenoid carti-

lage dislocation: a 20-year experience. *J Voice.* 2005;19(4):687–701.

56. Jafek BW, Esses BA. Manifestations of systemic disease. In: Cummings CW, Frederickson JM, Harker LA, Krause CJ, Schuller DE, eds. *Otolaryngology-Head and Neck Surgery.* St. Louis, MO: CV Mosby Company; 1986:1933–1941.
57. Abitbol J, Abitbol P, Abitbol B. Sex hormones and the female voice. *J Voice.* 1999;13(3):424–446.
58. Abitbol J, de Brux J, Millot G, et al. Does a hormonal vocal cord cycle exist in women? *J Voice.* 1989;3:157–162.
59. Higgins M, Saxman J. Variations in vocal frequency perturbation across the menstrual cycle. *J Voice.* 1989;3:233–243.
60. Davis CB, Davis ML. The effects of pre-menstrual syndrome on the female singer. *J Voice.* 1993;7:337–353.
61. Baker J. A report on alterations to the speaking and singing voices of four women following hormonal therapy with virilizing agents. *J Voice.* 1999; 13(4):496–507.
62. Jackson-Menalow C, Dzul AI, Holland R. Allergies and vocal fold edema: preliminary report. *J Voice.* 1999;13:113–122.
63. Rubin W. Allergic, dietary, chemical, stress, and hormonal influences in voice abnormalities. *J Voice.* 1987;1:378–385.
64. Millqvist E, Bende M, Brynnel M, Johansson I, Kappel S, Ohlsson A-C. Voice change in seasonal allergic rhinitis. *J Voice.* 2008;22(4):512–515.
65. Martin FG. Drugs and vocal function. *J Voice.* 1988;2:333–344.
66. Vogel D, Carter JE, Carter PB. *Effects of Drugs on Communication Disorders.* 2nd ed. Clinical Competence Series. San Diego, CA: Singular Publishing Group; 2000.
67. Ihre E, Zetterström O, Ihre E, Hammarberg B. Voice problems as side effects of inhaled corticosteroids in asthma patients—a prevalence study. *J Voice.* 2004;18(3):403–414.
68. Gallivan GJ, Gallivan KH, Gallivan HK. Inhaled corticosteroids: hazardous effects on voice—an update. *J Voice.* 2007;21(1):101–111.
69. Shemen L. Diseases of the thyroid as they affect the larynx. In: Fried M, ed. *The Larynx: A Multidisciplinary Approach.* Boston, MA: Little, Brown and Company; 1988:223–233.
70. Pennover D, Shefer A. Immunologic disorders of the larynx. In: Fried M, ed. *The Larynx: A Multidisciplinary Approach.* Boston, MA: Little, Brown and Company; 1988:279–290.
71. Dogan M, Eryuksel E, Kocak I, Celikel T, Sehitoglu MA. Subjective and objective evaluation of voice quality in patients with asthma. *J Voice.* 2007;21(2):224–230.
72. Pillsbury HC, Postma DS. Infections. In: Cummings CW, Frederickson JM, Harker LA, Krause CJ, Schuller DE, eds. *Otolaryngology-Head and Neck Surgery.* St. Louis, MO: CV Mosby Company; 1986:1919–1931.
73. Porras Alonso E, Martin Mateos A. Laryngeal tuberculosis. *Laryngol Otol Rhinol.* 2002;123(1):47–48.
74. Watson JR, Granoff D, Sataloff RT. Dysphonia due to Kaposi's sarcoma as the presenting symptom of human immunodeficiency virus. *J Voice.* 2004;18(3): 398–340.
75. Cecil M, Tindall L, Haydon R. The relationship between dysphonia and sinusitis: a pilot study. *J Voice.* 2001;15(2): 270–277.
76. Klein AM, Tiu C, Lafreniere D. Malignant mimickers: chronic bacterial and fungal infections of the larynx. *J Voice.* 2005;19(1):151–157.
77. Vrabec DP. Fungal infections of the larynx. *Otolaryngol Clin North Am.* 1993; 26:1091–1113.
78. Tashjian LS, Peacock JE. Laryngeal candidiasis. *Arch Otol.* 1984;110:806–809.
79. Aronson AE. *Clinical Voice Disorders: An Interdisciplinary Approach.* 3rd ed. New York, NY: Thieme; 1990.
80. Sapir S. (1995). Psychogenic spasmodic dysphonia: a case study with expert opinions. *J Voice.* 1995;9:270–281.

81. American Psychiatric Association. *Diagnostic and Statistical Manual of Mental Disorders*. 4th ed. Washington, DC: American Psychiatric Association; 1994.
82. Rosen CD, Sataloff RT. *Psychology of Voice Disorders*. San Diego, CA: Singular Publishing Group, Inc; 1997.
83. Baker J. Psychogenic dysphonia: peeling back the layers. *J Voice*. 1998;12(4): 527–535.
84. Butcher P. Psychological processes in psychogenic voice disorder. *Eur J Dis Commun*. 1995;30:467–474.
85. Butcher P, Elias A, Raven R. *Psychogenic Voice Disorders and Cognitive Behaviour Therapy*. San Diego, CA: Singular Publishing Group, Inc; 1993.
86. Butcher P, Elias A, Raven R, Yeatman J, Littlejohns D. Psychogenic voice disorder unresponsive to speech therapy: psychological characteristics and cognitive-behaviour therapy. *Br J Dis Commun*. 1987;22:81–92.
87. Roy N, Bless DM. Toward a theory of the dispositional bases of functional dysphonia and vocal nodules: exploring the role of personality and emotional adjustment. In: Kent RD, Ball MJ, eds. *Voice Quality Measurement*. San Diego, CA: Singular Publishing Group; 2000:461–480.
88. Roy N, Bless DM. Personality traits and psychological factors in voice pathology: a foundation for future research. *J Speech Lang Hear Res*. 2000;43:737–748.
89. Roy N, Bless DM, Heisey D: Personality and voice disorders: a superfactor trait analysis. *J Speech Lang Hear Res*. 2000;43:749–768.
90. Roy N, Bless DM, Heisey R. Personality and voice disorders: a multitrait-multidisorder analysis. *J Voice*. 2000; 14(4):521–548.
91. Roy N. Functional dysphonia. *Curr Opin Otolaryn Head Neck Surg*. 2003; 11(3):144–148.
92. Andrews ML, Schmidt CP. Gender presentation: perceptual and acoustic analysis of voice. *J Voice*. 1997;11:307–313.
93. Van Borsel J, Van Eynde E, De Cuypere G, Bonte K. Feminine after cricothyroid approximation? *J Voice*. 2008; 22(3):379–384.
94. Wilatt D, Stell P. Vocal cord paralysis. In: Paparella M, Shumrick D, eds. *Otolaryngology*. 3rd ed. Philadelphia, PA: WB Saunders; 1991.
95. Kelchner KN, Stemple JC, Gerdeman B, Le Borgne W, Adam S. Etiology, pathophysiology, treatment choices, and voice results for unilateral adductor vocal fold paralysis: a 3-year retrospective. *J Voice*. 1999;13(4):592–601.
96. Benninger MS, Gillman JB, Altman JS. Changing etiology of vocal fold immobility. *Laryngoscope*. 1998;108:1346–1350.
97. Heman-Ackah YD, Barr A. The value of laryngeal electromyography in the evaluation of laryngeal motion abnormalities. *J Voice*. 2006;20(3):452–460.
98. Sataloff RT, Mandel S, Mann EA, Ludlow CL. Practice parameter: laryngeal electromyography (an evidence-based review). *J Voice*. 2004;18(2):261–274.
99. Dursum G, Sataloff R, Spiegel J, et al. Superior laryngeal nerve paralysis and paresis. *J Voice*. 1996;10:206–211.
100. Robinson JL, Mandel S, Sataloff RT. Objective voice measures in nonsinging patients with unilateral superior laryngeal nerve paresis. *J Voice*. 2005;19(4):665–667.
101. Mygind H. Die Paralyse des M. Cricothyreoideus. *Arch Laryngol*. 1906;18: 403–418.
102. Ward PH, Berci G, Caceterra TC. Superior laryngeal nerve paralysis: an often overlooked entity. *Trans Am Acad Ophthalmol Otolaryngol*. 1977;84:78–89.
103. Sulica L. The superior laryngeal nerve: function and dysfunction. *Otolaryngol Clin N Am* 2004;37:183–201.
104. Roy N, Barton M, Smith ME, Dromey C, Merrill R, Sauder C. An in vivo model of acute ESLN paralysis: laryngoscopic findings. *Laryngoscope*. 2009; 119(5):1017–1032.
105. Roy N, Smith M, Houtz D. Laryngoscopic features of external superior

laryngeal nerve denervation: revisiting a century-old controversy. *Ann Otol Rhinol Laryngol.* 2011;120(1):1–8.

106. Eckley CA, Sataloff RT, Hawkshaw M, Spiegel JR, Mandel S. Voice range in superior laryngeal nerve paresis and paralysis. *J Voice.* 1998;12(3):340–348.
107. Robinson JL, Mandel S, Sataloff RS. Objective voice measures in nonsinging patients with unilateral superior laryngeal nerve paresis. *J Voice.* 2005;19(4):665–667.
108. Roy N, Dromey C, Smith ME, Redd J, Neff S, Grennan D. Exploring the phonatory effects of external superior laryngeal nerve paralysis: an in vivo model. *Laryngoscope.* 2009;119(4):816–826.
109. Crumley R. Unilateral recurrent laryngeal paralysis. *J Voice.* 1994;8:79–83.
110. Gardner GM, Benninger MS. Vocal fold paralysis. In: Rubin JS, Sataloff RT, Korovin GS, eds. *Diagnosis and Treatment of Voice Disorders.* 2nd ed. Clifton Park, NY: Thomson Delmar Learning; 2003:435–455.
111. Lawson G, Remacle M, Hamoir M, Jamart J. Posterior cordectomy and subtotal arytenoidectomy for the treatment of bilateral vocal fold immobility: functional results. *J Voice.* 1996;10:314–319.
112. Feehery JM, Pribitkin EA, Heffelfinger RN, et al. The evolving etiology of bilateral vocal fold immobility. *J Voice.* 2003;17(1):76–81.
113. Rubin AD, Praneetvatakul V, Heman-Ackah YD, Moyer CA, Mandel S, Sataloff RT. Repetitive phonatory tasks for identifying vocal fold paresis. *J Voice.* 2005;19(4):679–686.
114. Heman-Ackah YD, Barr A. Mild vocal fold paresis: understanding clinical presentation and electromyographic findings. *J Voice.* 2006;20(2):269–281.
115. Darley F, Aronson AE, Brown J. *Motor Speech Disorders.* Philadelphia, PA: WB Saunders; 1975.
116. Duffy J. *Motor Speech Disorders.* St. Louis, MO: Mosby; 1995.
117. Sudarsky L, Feudo P, Zubick H. Vocal aberrations in dysarthria. In: Fried M, ed. *The Larynx: A Multidisciplinary Approach.* Boston, MA: Little, Brown. 1988:179–190.
118. Griffiths C, Bough ID Jr. Neurologic diseases and their effects on voice. *J Voice.* 1989;3:148–156.
119. Mao VH, Abaza M, Spiegel JR, et al. Laryngeal myasthenia gravis: report of 40 cases. *J Voice.* 2001;15(1):122–130.
120. Aminoff M, Dedo H, Izdebski K. Clinical aspects of spasmodic dysphonia. *J Neurol Neurosurg Psychiatry.* 1978;41:361–365.
121. Cannito MP. Neurobiological interpretations of spasmodic dysphonia. In: Vogel D, Cannito MP, eds. *Treating Disordered Speech Motor Control: For Clinicians by Clinicians.* Austin, TX: Pro-Ed; 1990:275–317.
122. Schaefer SD, Finitzo-Heiber T, Gerling IJ, Freeman FJ. Brainstem conduction abnormalities in spasmodic dysphonia. In: Bless DM, Abbs J, eds. *Vocal Fold Physiology.* San Diego, CA: College-Hill Press; 1987:393–404.
123. Woodson GE, Zwirner P, Murry T, Swenson MR. Functional assessment of patients with spasmodic dysphonia. *J Voice.* 1992;6:338–343.
124. Brodnitz F. Spastic dysphonia. *Ann Otol Rhinol Laryngol.* 1976;85:210–214.
125. Tanner K, Roy N, Merrill R, Sauder C, Houtz D, Smith M. Spasmodic dysphonia: onset, course, socioemotional effects and treatment response. *Ann Otol Rhinol Laryngol.* 2011;120(7):465–473.
126. Larsson T, Sjögren T. Essential tremor: a clinical and genetic population study. *Acta Psychiatr Neurol (Scandinavia).* 1960;36(suppl 144):1–176.
127. Brown J, Simonson J. Organic voice tremor. *Neurology.* 1963:13:520–525.
128. Lundy DS, Roy S, Xue JW, Casiano RR, Jassir D. Spastic/spasmodic vs. tremulous vocal quality: motor speech profile analysis. *J Voice.* 2004;18(1):146–152.

129. Kent J, Kent RD, Rosenbek J, et al. Quantitative description of the dysarthria in women with amyotrophic lateral sclerosis. *J Speech Hear Res.* 1992;35:723–733.
130. Silbergleit A, Johnson A, Jacobsen B. Acoustic analysis of voice in individuals with amyotrophic lateral sclerosis and perceptually normal voice quality. *J Voice.* 1997;11:222–231.
131. Roth C, Glaze L, David W, Goding G. Case report: amyotrophic lateral sclerosis presenting as signs of spasmodic dysphonia. *J Voice.* 1996;10:362–367.
132. Ramig L, Countryman S, Thompson L, Horii Y. Comparison of two forms of intensive speech therapy for Parkinson disease. *J Speech Lang Hear Res.* 1995;38:1232–1251.
133. Ramig L, Countryman S, O'Brien C. Intensive speech treatment for patients with Parkinson disease: short and long-term comparison of two techniques. *Neurology.* 1996;47:1496–1504.
134. Hartelius L, Buder E, Strand E. Long term phonatory instability in individuals with multiple sclerosis. *J Speech Lang Hear Res.* 1997;40:1056–1072.
135. Dogan M, Midi I, Yazıcı MA, Kocak I, Günal D, Sehitoglu MA. Objective and subjective evaluation of voice quality in multiple sclerosis. *J Voice.* 2007; 21(6):735–740.
136. Stemple J, Stanley J, Lee L. Objective measures of voice production in normal subjects following prolonged voice use. *J Voice.* 1995;9:127–133.
137. Welham NV, Maclagan MA. Vocal fatigue: current knowledge and future directions. *J Voice.* 2003;17(1):21–30.
138. Morrison M, Rammage L. *The Management of Voice Disorders.* San Diego, CA: Singular Publishing Group; 1994.
139. Morrison M. Pattern recognition in muscle misuse: how I do it. *J Voice.* 1997;11:108–114.
140. Angsuwarangsee T, Morrison M. Extrinsic laryngeal muscular tension in patients with voice disorders. *J Voice.* 2002;16(3):333–343.
141. Altman KW, Atkinson C, Lazarus C. Current and emerging concepts in muscle tension dysphonia: a 30-month review. *J Voice.* 2005;19(2):261–267.
142. Maryn Y, DeBodt MS, Van Cauwenberge P. Ventricular dysphonia: clinical aspects and therapeutic options. *Laryngoscope.* 2003;113:859–866.
143. Christopher K, Wood R, Eckert C, Blager F, Raney R, Souhrada J. Vocal cord dysfunction presenting as asthma. *New Engl J Med.* 1983;308:1566–1570.
144. Treole K, Trudeau M, Forrest LA. Endoscopic and stroboscopic description of adults with paradoxical vocal fold motion. *J Voice.* 1999;13:143–152.
145. Andrianopoulos MV, Gallivan GJ, Gallivan KH. PVCM, PVCD, EPL, and irritable larynx syndrome: what are we talking about and how do we treat it? *J Voice.* 2000;14(4):607–618.
146. Mathers-Schmidt BA. Paradoxical vocal fold motion: a tutorial on a complex disorder and the speech-language pathologist's role. *Am J Speech Lang Pathol.* 2001;10:111–125.
147. Perkner JJ, Fennelly KP, Balkissoon R, et al. Irritant-associated vocal cord dysfunction. *J Occup Environ Med.* 1998;40(2):136–143.
148. Vertigan AE, Theodoros DG, Gibson PG, Winkworth AL. Voice and upper airway symptoms in people with chronic cough and paradoxical vocal fold movement. *J Voice.* 2007;21(3):361–383.

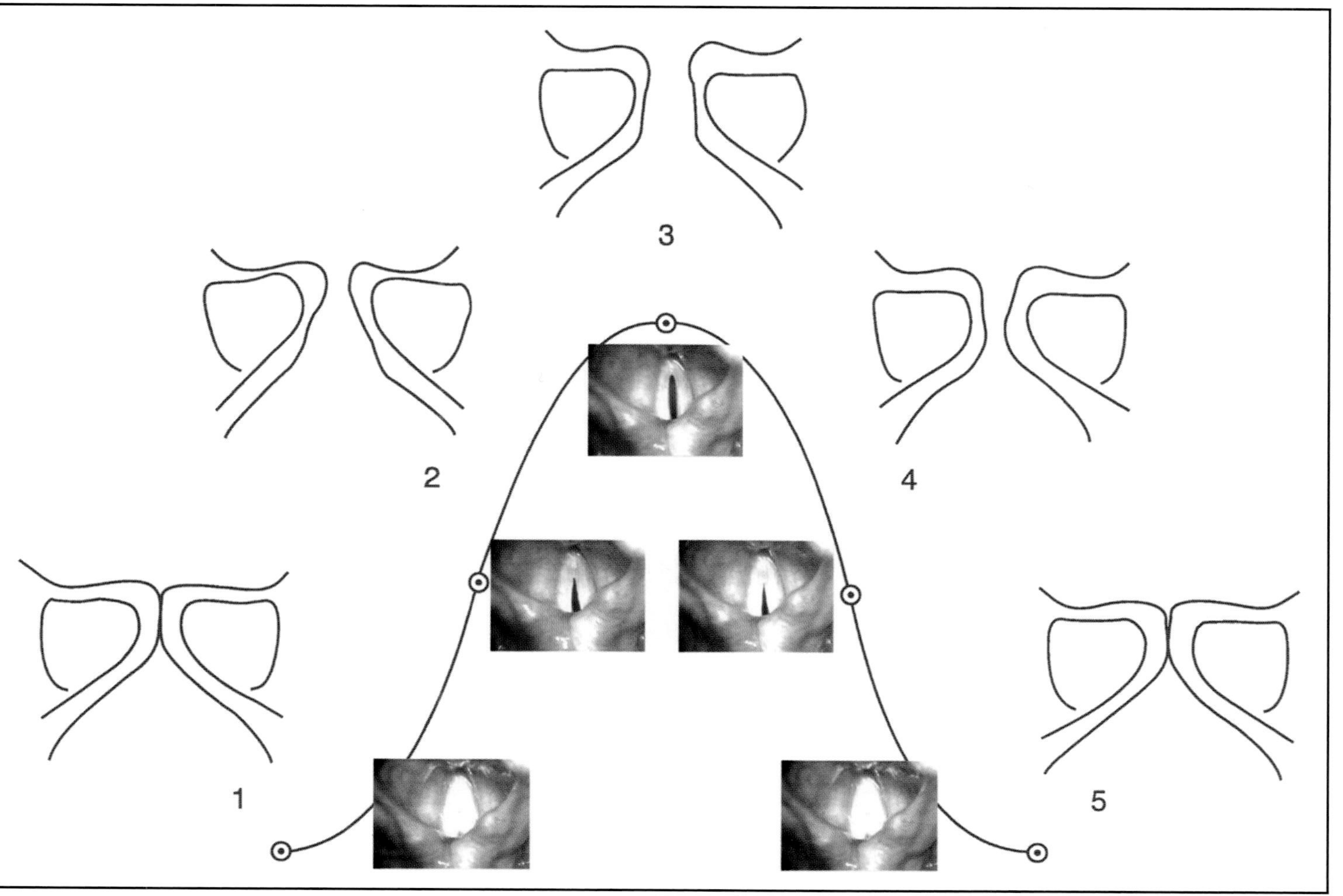

PLATE 1. Vocal fold vibratory cycle (see Chapter 2).

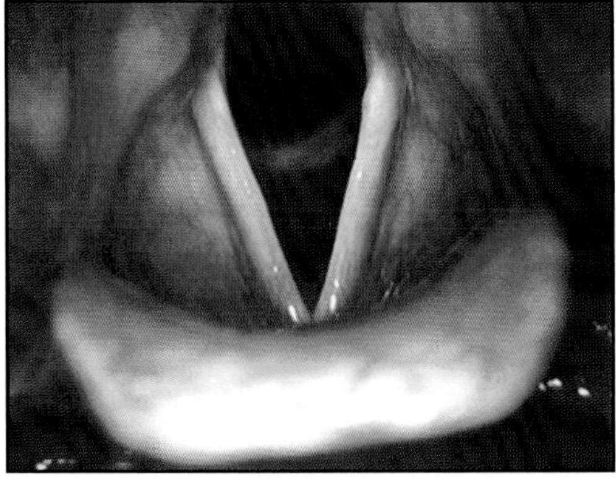

PLATE 2. Normal vocal folds (abduction) (see Chapter 4). Reprinted with permission from Jean Abitbol, MD.

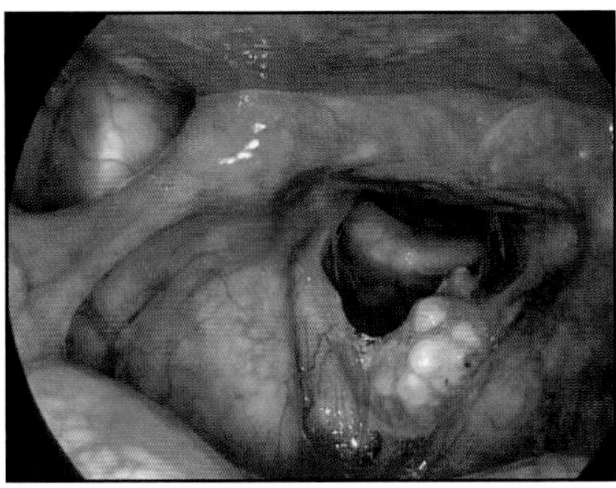

PLATE 3. Carcinoma (see Chapter 4). Reprinted with permission from Jean Abitbol, MD.

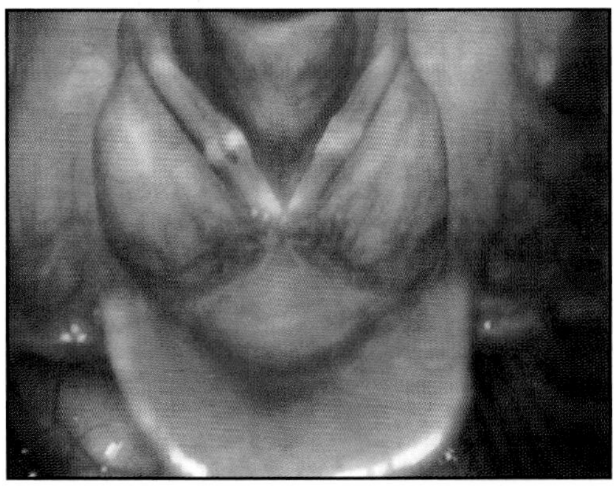

PLATE 4. Vocal fold nodules (abduction) (see Chapter 4). Reprinted with permission from Jean Abitbol, MD.

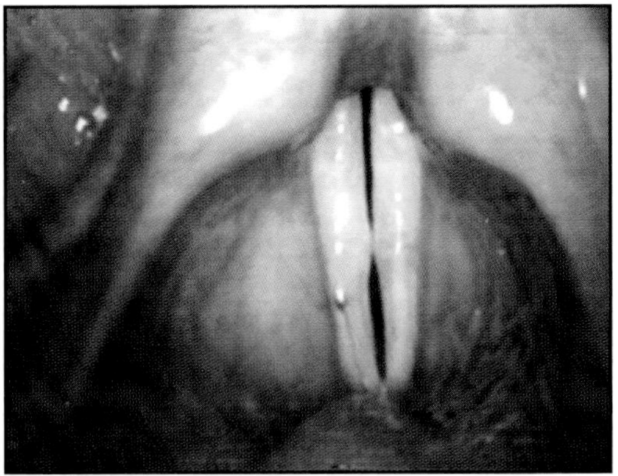

PLATE 5. Vocal fold nodules (adduction) (see Chapter 4). Reprinted with permission from Jean Abitbol, MD.

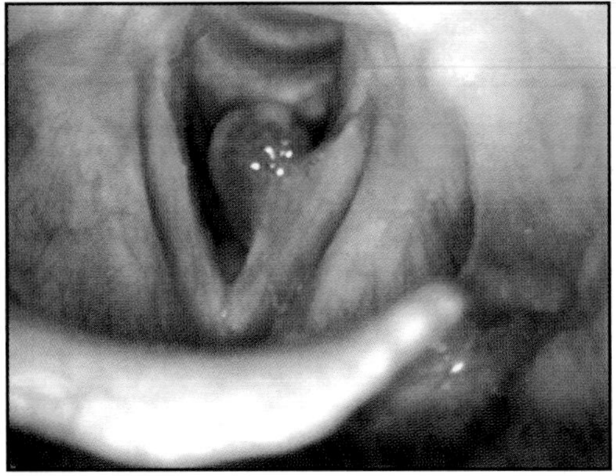

PLATE 6. Sessile polyp (see Chapter 4). Reprinted with permission from Jean Abitbol, MD.

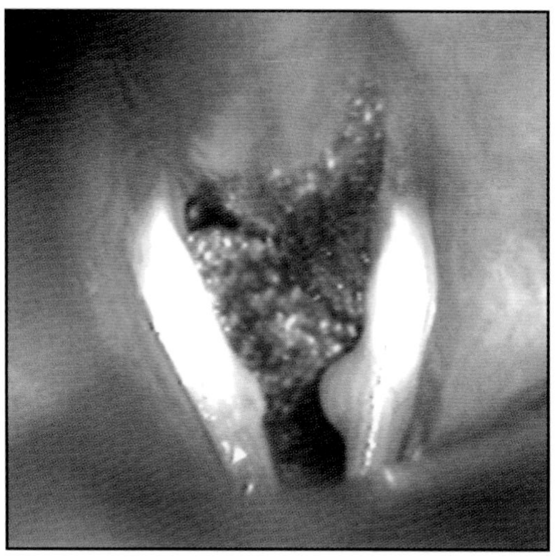

PLATE 7. Vocal fold cyst (mucosal) (see Chapter 4). Reprinted with permission from Jean Abitbol, MD.

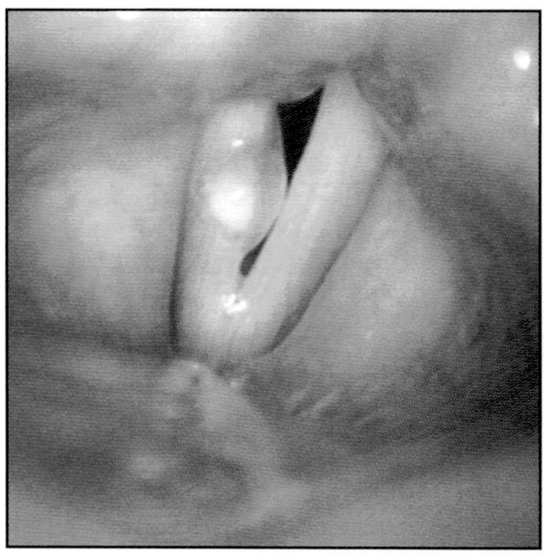

PLATE 8. Vocal fold cyst (intracordal) (see Chapter 4). Reprinted with permission from Jean Abitbol, MD.

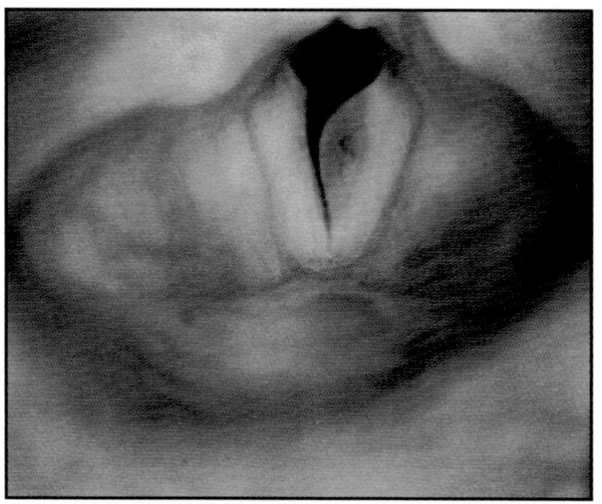

PLATE 9. Reinke's edema (early) (see Chapter 4). Reprinted with permission from Jean Abitbol, MD.

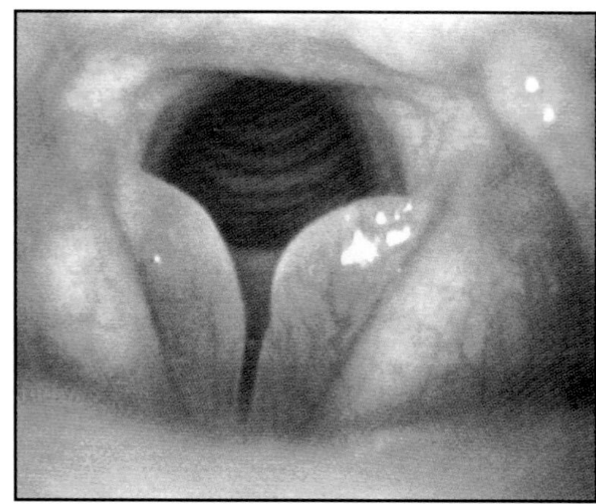

PLATE 10. Polypoid degenerations (advanced) (see Chapter 4). Reprinted with permission from Jean Abitbol, MD.

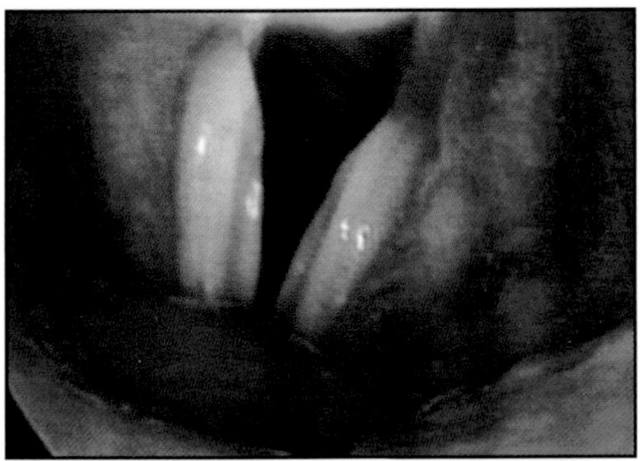

PLATE 11. Vocal fold sulcus (see Chapter 4). Reprinted with permission from Jean Abitbol, MD.

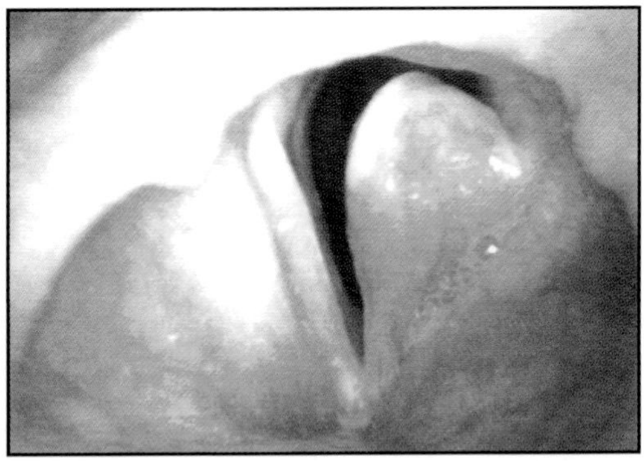

PLATE 12. Unilateral contact granulomas (see Chapter 4). Reprinted with permission from Jean Abitbol, MD.

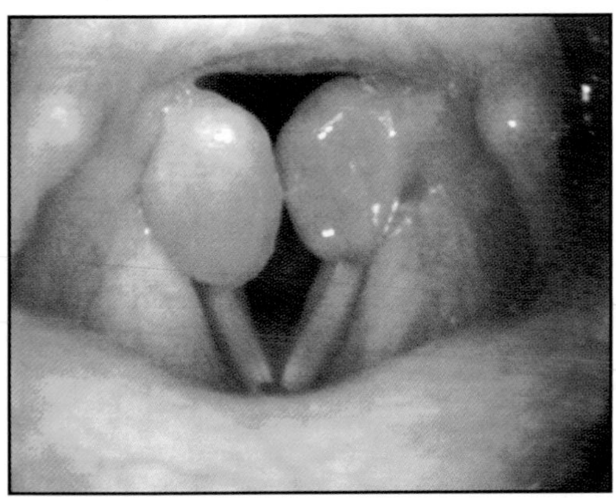

PLATE 13. Bilateral contact granulomas (see Chapter 4). Reprinted with permission from Jean Abitbol, MD.

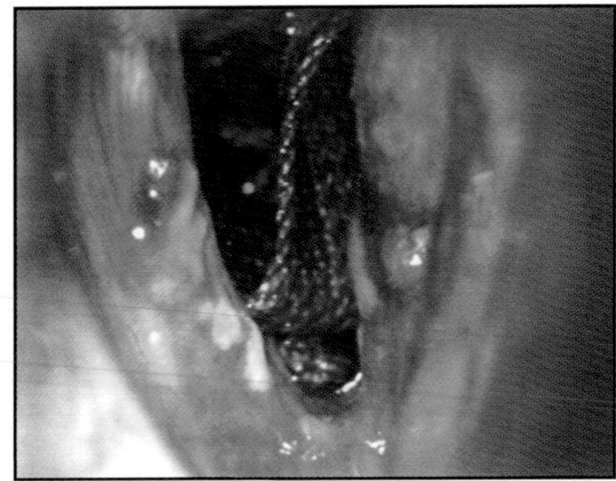

PLATE 14. Leukoplakia (see Chapter 4). Reprinted with permission from Jean Abitbol, MD.

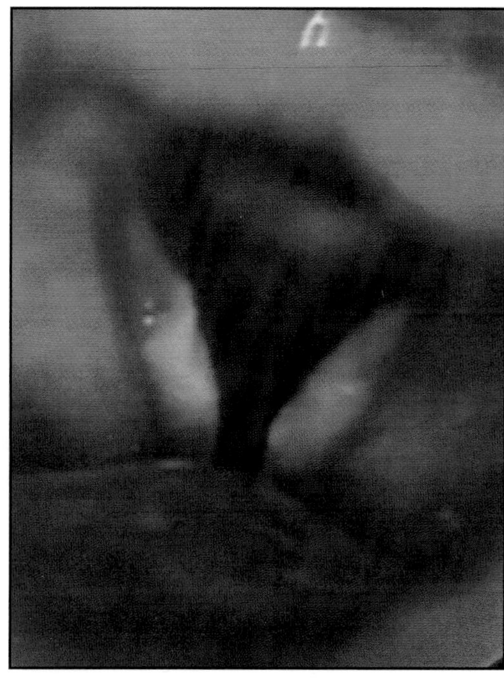

PLATE 15. Hyperkeratosis (see Chapter 4). Reprinted with permission from Jean Abitbol, MD.

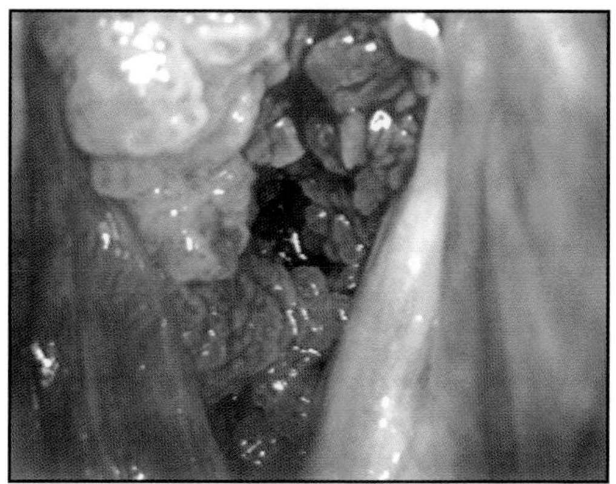

PLATE 16. Papilloma (see Chapter 4). Reprinted with permission from Jean Abitbol, MD.

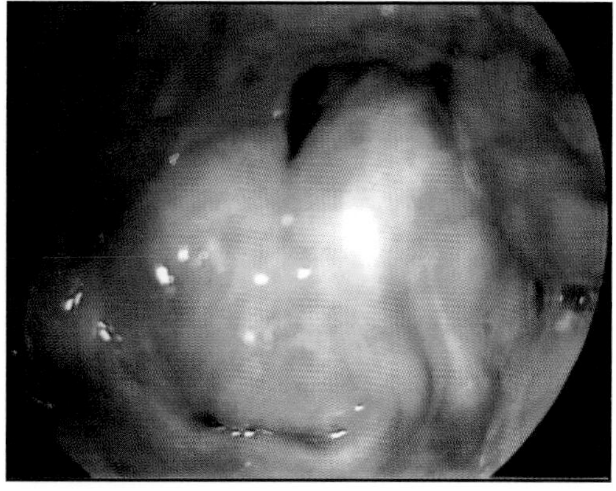

PLATE 17. Laryngeal stenosis (see Chapter 4). Reprinted with permission from Jean Abitbol, MD.

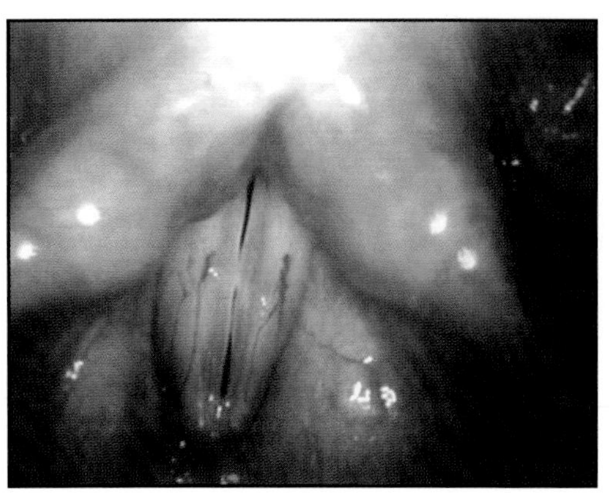

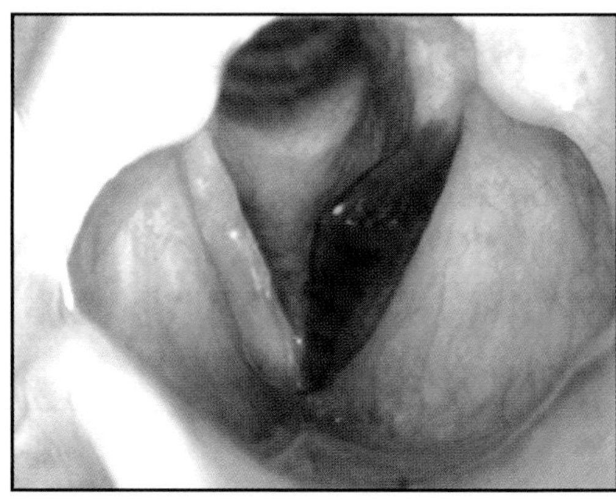

A **B**

PLATE 18. Vocal fold vascular lesions (see Chapter 4). Reprinted with permission from Jean Abitbol, MD.

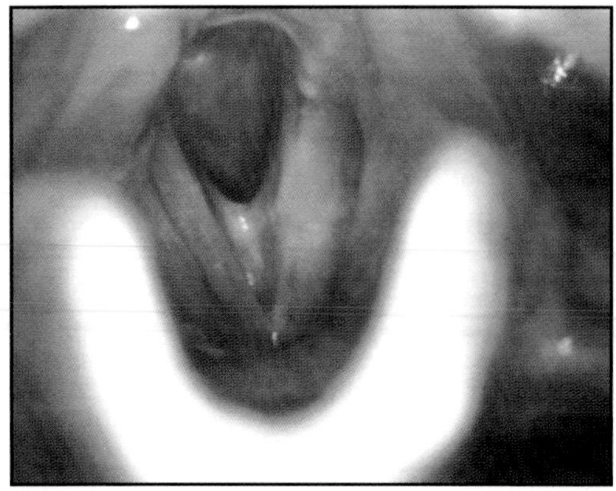

PLATE 19. Anterior congenital web (see Chapter 4). Reprinted with permission from Jean Abitbol, MD.

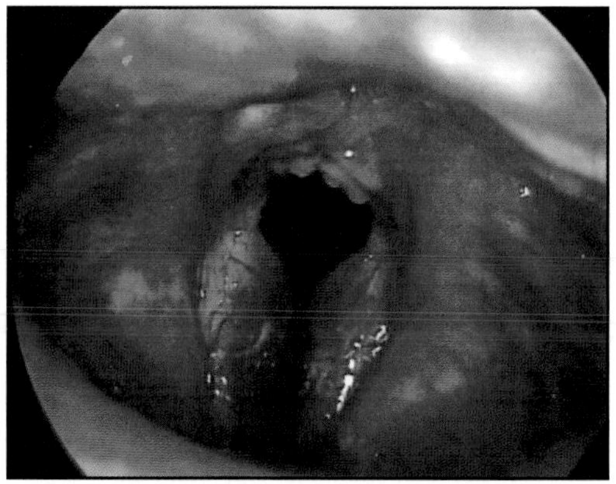

PLATE 20. Laryngopharyngeal reflux (see Chapter 4). Reprinted with permission from Jean Abitbol, MD.

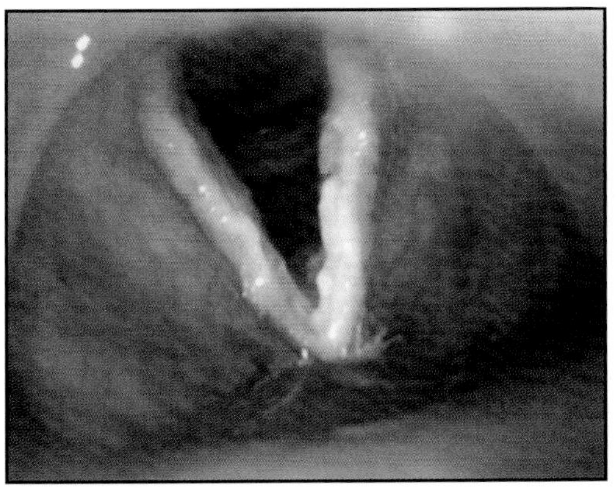

PLATE 21. Chronic laryngitis (see Chapter 4). Reprinted with permission from Jean Abitbol, MD.

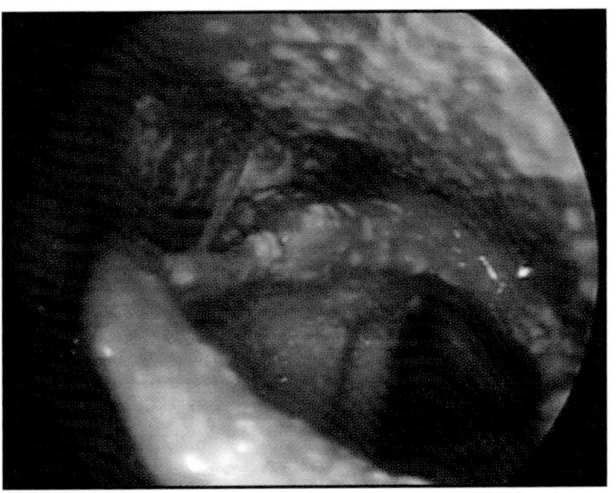

PLATE 22. Fungal infection (see Chapter 4). Reprinted with permission from Jean Abitbol, MD.

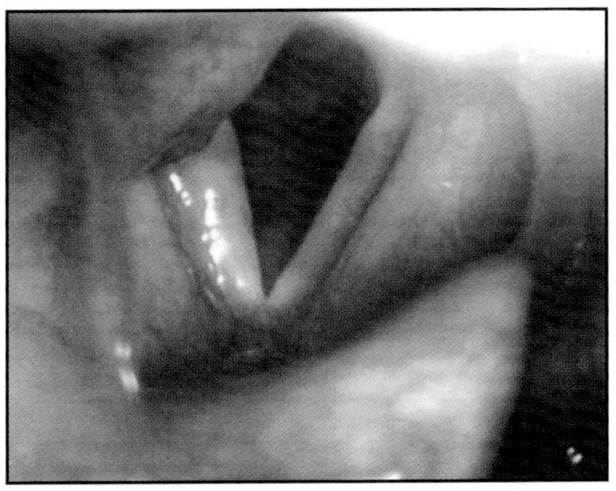

PLATE 23. Unilateral right vocal fold paralysis (abduction) (see Chapter 4). Reprinted with permission from Jean Abitbol, MD.

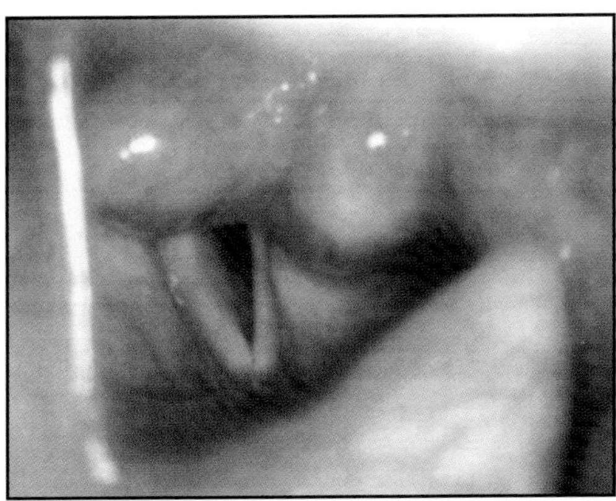

PLATE 24. Unilateral right vocal fold paralysis (adduction) (see Chapter 4). Reprinted with permission from Jean Abitbol, MD.

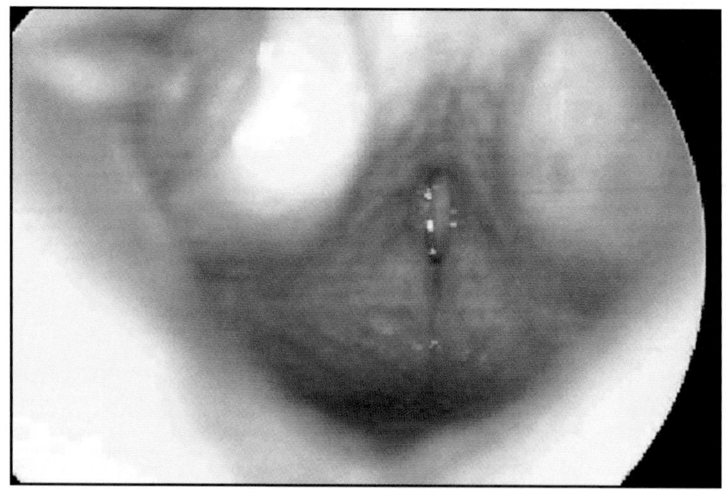

PLATE 25. Ventricular phonation (see Chapter 4). Reprinted with permission from Jean Abitbol, MD.

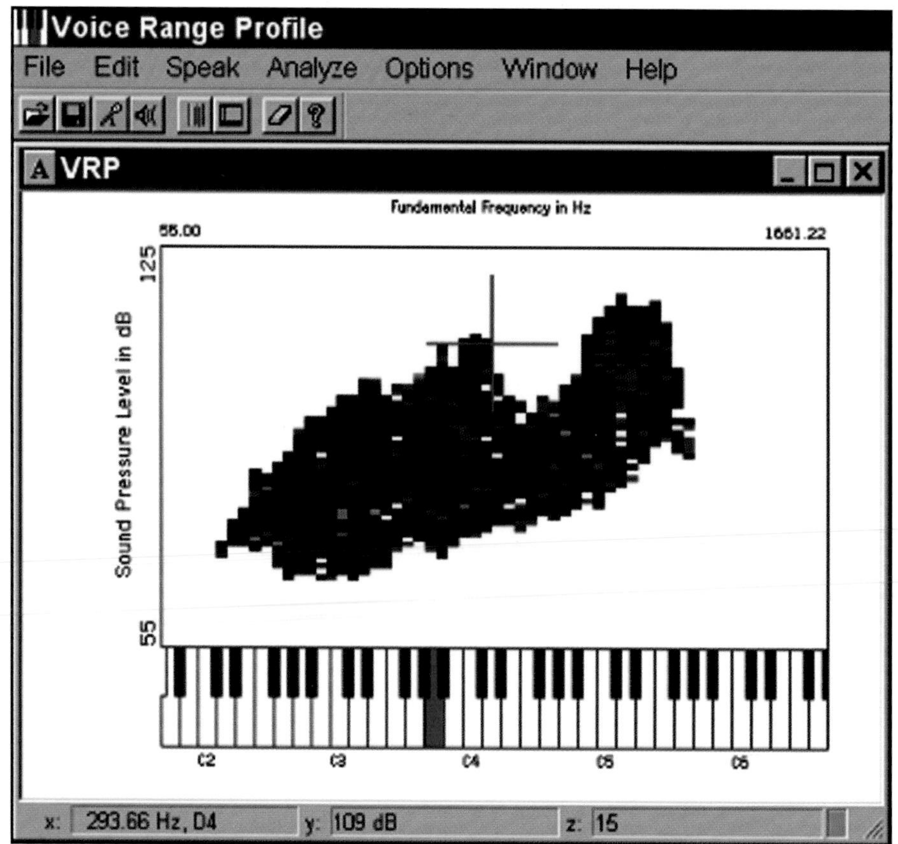

PLATE 26. Voice range profile. Plot of vowel produced at minimum and maximum intensity [decibel (dB) range on the vertical axis] across minimum and maximum frequency [hertz (Hz) and musical note range on the horizontal axis] (see Chapter 6). Image courtesy of KayPENTAX, Lincoln Park, NJ.

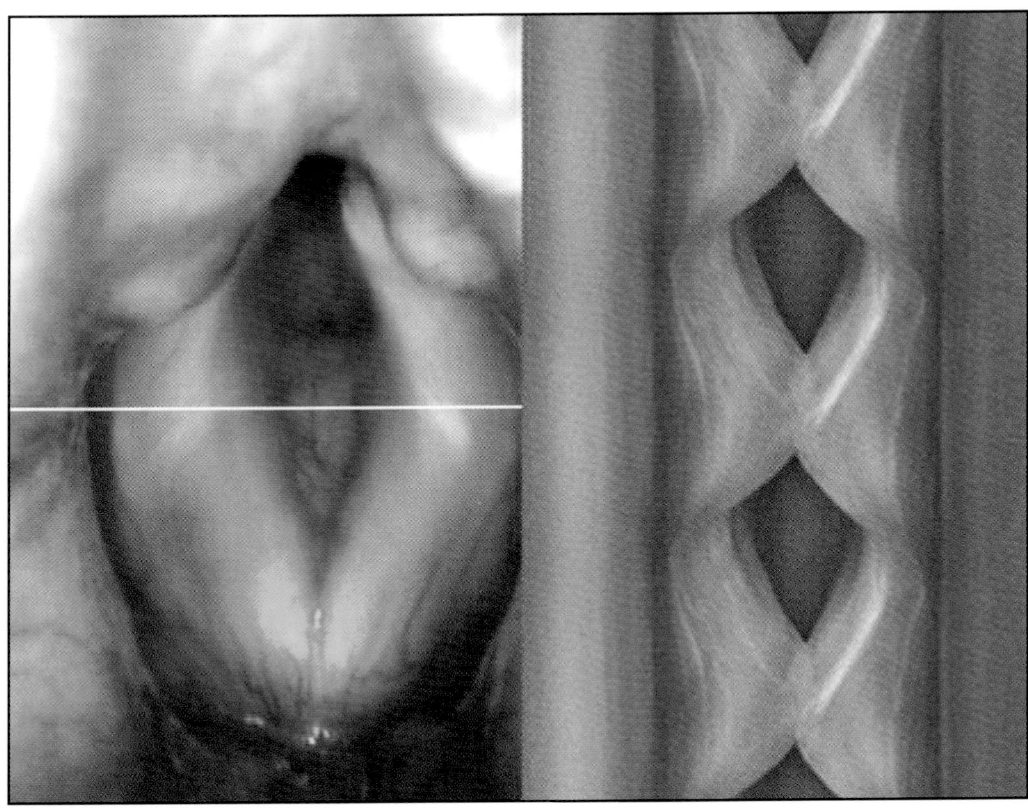

PLATE 27. Videokymographic (VKG) image of normal vocal fold vibration. The left image displays the (adjustable) location of the VKG scan line. The right image displays normal bilateral vocal fold vibration sampled at 8000 images per second (see Chapter 6). Image courtesy of KayPENTAX, Lincoln Park, NJ.

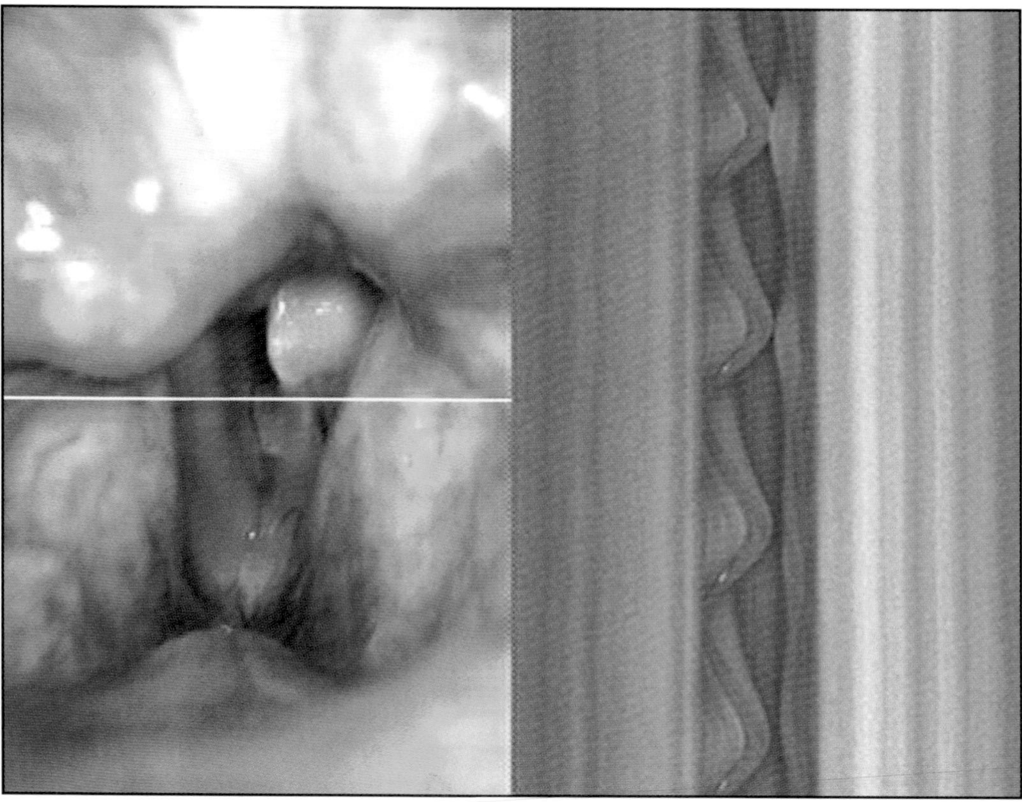

PLATE 28. Videokymographic (VKG) image of asymmetric vibration, due to the presence of a unilateral mass lesion. The left image displays the (adjustable) location of the VKG scan line. The right image displays asymmetric unilateral vocal fold vibration with contralateral adynamic tissue stiffness (see Chapter 6). Image courtesy of KayPENTAX, Lincoln Park, NJ.

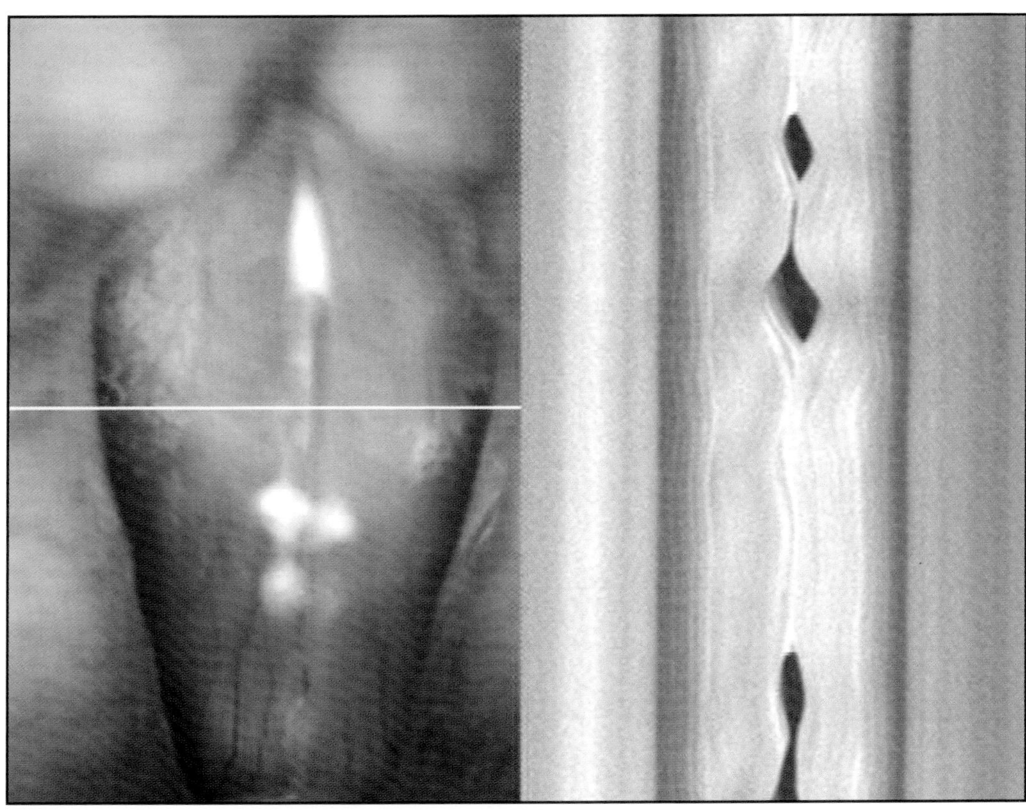

PLATE 29. Videokymographic (VKG) image of aperiodic vibration. The left image displays the (adjustable) location of the VKG scan line. The right image displays aperiodic vocal fold vibration, detected in real time by the irregular timing of tissue oscillation (see Chapter 6). Image courtesy of KayPENTAX, Lincoln Park, NJ.

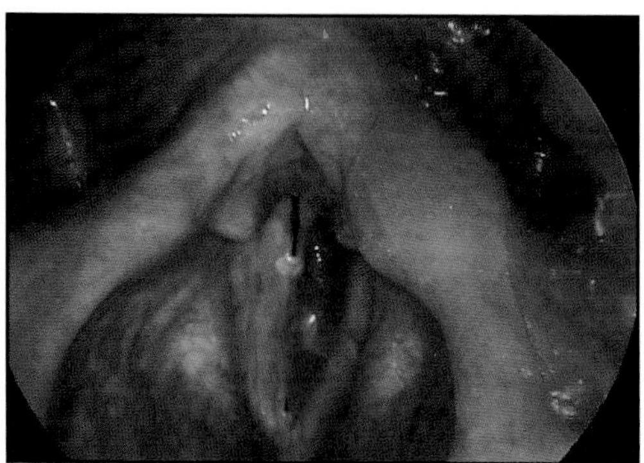

PLATE 30. Hemorrhage of the left true vocal fold during phonation (see Chapter 8). Reprinted with permission from Jean Abitbol, MD, *Atlas of Laser Voice Surgery.*

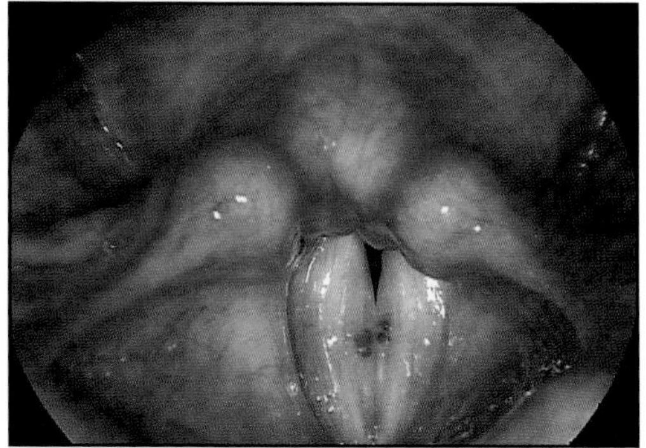

PLATE 31. Bilateral true vocal fold angiomas (see Chapter 8). Reprinted with permission from Jean Abitbol, MD, *Atlas of Laser Voice Surgery*.

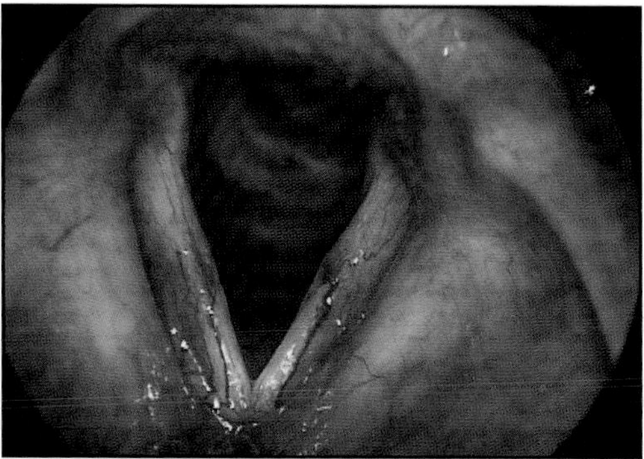

PLATE 32. Microvarices with ectasia on the left true vocal fold (see Chapter 8). Reprinted with permission from Jean Abitbol, MD, *Atlas of Laser Voice Surgery*.

5

The Diagnostic Voice Evaluation

The previous chapters of this text have described the academic areas of knowledge from a clinical perspective, which are a necessary preparation for the evaluation and treatment of voice disorders. This chapter begins our concentration on the interpersonal skills that are necessary when we assume the responsibility of guiding and helping others. These skills include listening, hearing, feeling, connecting, empathizing, motivating, encouraging, reinforcing, and rewarding. Although one may study and learn academic information and then turn it into personal knowledge, communication skills develop over a lifetime of observation and interaction. The successful voice pathologist must possess an inherent "feel" for other people and combine vast academic knowledge with the ability to communicate at both a professional and a personal level.

The primary objectives of the diagnostic voice evaluation are to discover the etiologic, physiologic, or behavioral factors associated with the development and persistence of the voice disorder; describe the deviant vocal symptoms; develop an understanding of how the disorder is affecting the subsystems of voice production, respiration, phonation, and resonance; and develop a systematic management plan. In a systematic evaluation designed to determine specific causes of disorders, voice pathologists use their knowledge of laryngeal anatomy and physiology, pathologies of the laryngeal mechanism, and common etiologic factors. Once the causes are known, the symptoms are described, and the impact on the voice-producing mechanisms is understood, a vocal management plan tailored to the individual problems and needs of each patient may be developed.

G. Paul Moore, one of the pioneers in the study of voice disorders, said that diagnosis is the process of discovering the causes of certain symptoms. Diagnosis of voice disorders ordinarily encompasses the recognition and description of individual vocal deviations and a systematic search for the factors that cause these deviations.[1]

The voice pathologist may also use the voice evaluation as a tool for patient education and motivation. Most individuals have little knowledge or understanding of voice production. The majority of patients who present with voice disorders have little understanding of the problem. During the diagnostic evaluation, the voice pathologist will find it beneficial to explain in simple terms how voice is produced and the effect that the specific pathology plays on deviant voice production. With an understanding of voice production, patients can better respond to diagnostic questions specific to discovering the etiologies of the problem. The patient who is well informed also will generally be more motivated to follow the necessary therapy regimen required to resolve the pathology. Patients who understand the causes of the disorder, are presented with a systematic management approach, and are given a reasonable estimate of the time needed for completion of the program usually develop a positive therapeutic attitude.

THE MANAGEMENT TEAM

Many components comprise the diagnostic voice evaluation, including: (1) the medical examination, (2) the patient interview, (3) the perceptual evaluation of voice, (4) the patient self-evaluation, (5) the instrumental analysis of voice (including acoustic and aerodynamic analyses), and (6) the functional evaluation of vocal fold movement. Members of our profession increasingly accomplish these diagnostic components through the teamwork of laryngologists, voice pathologists, and, when occasion dictates, other professionals such as vocal coaches, voice teachers, and other medical professionals. The laryngologist is trained to examine the laryngeal mechanism for pathology and to diagnose the voice disorder. Through the diagnosis, he or she determines whether to treat the disorder medically, surgically, or through referral for behavioral management. The voice pathologist is trained to identify the causes of the voice disorders, evaluate the vocal symptoms, and establish improved vocal function through various therapeutic methods. The vocal coach or singing instructor evaluates the efficiency and correctness of performance technique and suggests modifications as needed. Other medical professionals, such as gastroenterologists, neurologists, allergists, pulmonologists, and endocrinologists may be called upon in selected cases to aid in the evaluation process. These complementary professional relationships have significantly improved the care of patients with voice disorders.

The teamwork model for evaluating and managing voice disorders has led to the development of formal clinical voice centers. In these centers, patients have the opportunity to be evaluated by each of these core professionals during a single visit. In addition, instrumentation now permits measurement of phonation, as well as visual studies of vocal function. These more advanced laryngeal function studies are described in Chapter 6.

PATIENT PROFILE

Who are voice patients? They may be of any age, gender, race, or occupation. They may be professional voice users or Sunday morning choir members. Herrington-Hall et al[2] demonstrated this fact well in their review of patients who sought evaluation for voice disorders. The 10 most common patient occupations were retired, homemaker, factory worker, unemployed, executive or manager, teacher, student, secretary, singer, and nurse. In a follow-up study that compared results to the Herrington-Hall et al data, Coyle et al[3] reported that the 10 most common occupations among individuals seeking treatment were retired, executive or manager, homemaker, unemployed, student, teacher, clerical, factory, sales, and nurse. Based on two studies by Roy and colleagues,[4,5] it is not surprising that the "retired" category comprised the most common treatment-seeking individuals as 29% of individuals over the age of 65 years in the general population reported currently experiencing a voice disorder compared to 6% in the under 66-year-old age group. Koufman and Isaacson[6] suggested a useful four-level model of vocal usage (Table 5–1). In reviewing this model, however, the voice pathologist must not assume that a voice disorder classified in a Level IV voice user is any less important or has any less functional, financial, or emotional impact on the patient than those classified as Level I. Each patient dictates his or her own level of concern related to the effects of the voice problem.

REFERRAL SOURCES

Voice pathologists receive the majority of voice referrals from the otolaryngologist. When the referral is from elsewhere, the voice pathologist must refer the patient for an otolaryngologic examination. The importance of this medical examination for both adults and children cannot be overstated. Although Sander[7] argued against aggressively pursuing voice treatment for children, we have unfortunately seen children who were treated unsuccessfully for "hoarseness" over long periods of time before they were referred for medical evaluation. Subsequent indirect laryngoscopy revealed a small anterior web in one child and papilloma in another. Even more dramatic was the discovery of a squamous cell laryngeal carcinoma in a

Table 5–1. Levels of Vocal Usage

Description		*Examples*
Level I	Elite vocal performer	Singer, actor
Level II	Professional voice user	Clergy, lecturer, broadcast journalist
Level III	Nonvocal professional	Teacher, lawyer
Level IV	Nonvocal nonprofessional	Laborer, clerk

12-year-old girl which required a total laryngectomy. Certainly, the possibility of a life-threatening pathology is greater in the adult population, but these examples demonstrate the necessity of conducting the medical examination prior to the onset of voice therapy.

Initial identification of the voice problem may occur in several ways. From a management standpoint, it is optimal when the patient identifies the problem. Our definition in Chapter 1 established that a voice disorder may exist if the laryngeal mechanism's structure, function, or both no longer meet the patient's functional voice demands. Self-discovery and awareness of the problem often yield more motivated patients.

Friends or family members may also make an informal initial identification of vocal symptoms, or such identification may occur during a speech pathology screening in school or during a routine medical examination. When someone other than the patient identifies the symptoms, the patient may or may not consider the symptoms to be a problem. It then becomes the responsibility of the voice pathologist to educate the patient regarding the vocal dysfunction and to point out potential problems associated with the disorder.[8] The ultimate decision for treatment or management remains the individual's or, in some cases, the caregiver's choice.

The voice pathologist must also remember that the patient is the "owner" of the voice problem, and he or she is ultimately responsible for resolving the problem. The history of the medical profession has traditionally placed the responsibility of our illness and wellness squarely on the shoulders of the physician. Too often, we hear statements such as, "The doctor will take care of it. The doctor will make me better." Successful voice therapy is predicated on a motivated patient taking charge of a well-planned management program and following that program to the desired result: improved voice. The voice pathologist must not permit the patient to transfer ownership of the problem.

MEDICAL EVALUATION

A complete otolaryngologic examination involves taking a detailed history of the problem and examining the entire head and neck region. Pertinent medical history is also discussed. The examination includes otoscopic observation of the ears; examination of the oral and nasal cavities; palpation of the salivary glands, lymph nodes, and thyroid gland; and a visual examination of the larynx. The larynx is typically viewed indirectly utilizing a laryngeal mirror (Figure 5–1). To perform this examination, the laryngologist grasps the tongue and gently pulls it forward and down while placing the laryngeal mirror in the pharynx. The head mirror directs artificial light to reflect off the laryngeal mirror, illuminating the pharynx and larynx. The larynx is then viewed on the laryngeal mirror with the image of the right and left vocal folds reversed. Patients are typically asked to produce the phoneme /i/ so that the vocal fold approximation may be easily viewed. The attempt to say /i/ draws the epiglottis forward to expose the interior of the larynx. Patients with a sensitive gag reflex may have the tongue and pharynx sprayed with a topical anesthesia to suppress the reflex.

Fiberoptic laryngoscopy is also available as a simple office procedure for examining the larynx directly. When using this technique, the physician introduces a fiberoptic laryngoscope into the patient's pharynx via the nasal cavity (Figure 5–2). This device is a long, flexible tube that contains fiberoptic light bundles and a lens. A small hand control permits the physician to manipulate the flexible end of the scope. When the scope is attached to a light source,

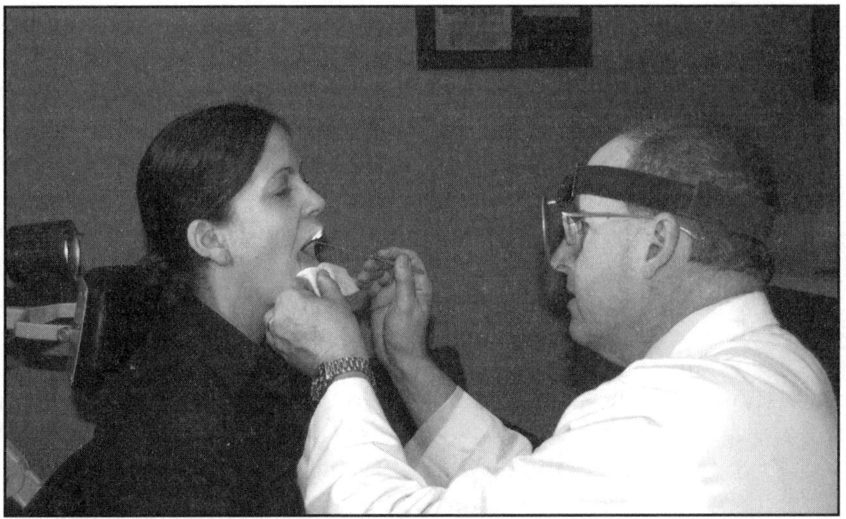

FIGURE 5–1. Indirect laryngoscopy with laryngeal mirror.

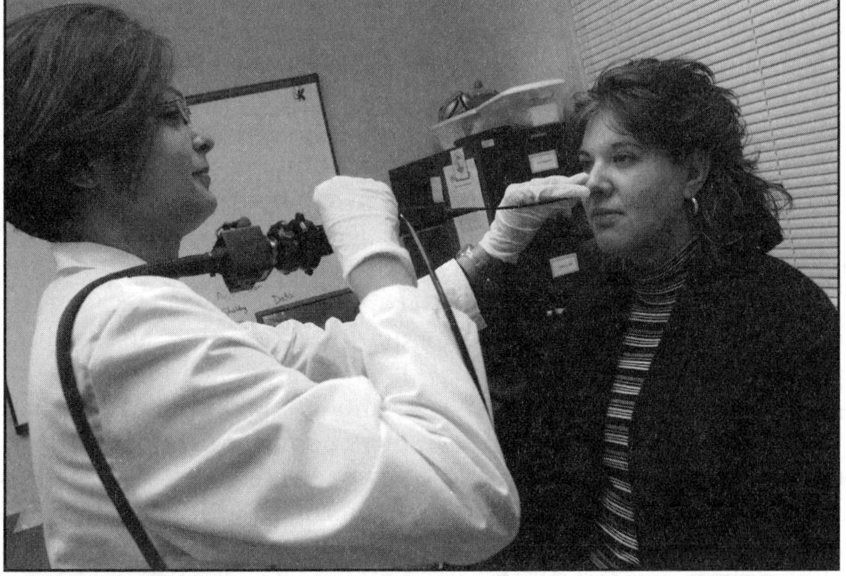

FIGURE 5–2. Flexible endoscopy.

the larynx and surrounding structures may be viewed either through an eyepiece or on a monitor when the eyepiece is attached to a digital video camera.[9] New technology continues to improve the visual image provided by fiberoptic laryngoscopy with the latest advance involving chip-in-the-tip technology. These endoscopes contain a small camera chip at the tip of the endoscope which transmits via a processor to a TV monitor and other accessories. The image is therefore transmitted along the length of the endoscope in electrical form, and there is no coherent fiber bundle to transmit the image, as in conventional fiberoptic endoscopes. The advantage of these endoscopes is that they do not contain delicate fiberoptics and are thus much more resilient. They also provide a much better picture. Fiberoptic laryngoscopy is often performed on patients who cannot tolerate indirect mirror laryngoscopy and when observation of the entire supraglottic region is desirable.

The larynx may also be viewed through direct laryngoscopy. In this surgical procedure, the patient undergoes a general anesthesia, most often in outpatient surgery. A magnifying laryngoscope is then placed in the pharynx via the oral cavity to obtain a direct microscopic view of the larynx. Biopsies and surgical excisions may also be performed through the laryngoscope.

The medical examination also may include special radiographs of the head, chest, and neck, as well as blood analyses and swallowing studies. The final result of the medical examination and studies is a diagnosis of the problem and recommendations for treatment, including medical or surgical treatment, voice evaluation and therapy, or any combination of these choices.

VOICE PATHOLOGY EVALUATION

As previously stated, the four major objectives of the diagnostic voice evaluation are to:

- Uncover etiologic, physiologic, or behavioral factors specific to the development and persistence of the voice disorder
- Describe the present vocal components
- Evaluate the effect of the disorder on respiration, phonation, and resonance
- Develop an individualized management plan.

Following referral from the otolaryngologist, the voice pathologist will begin this diagnostic process with the patient interview, the most important component of the voice evaluation.

During the interview, the voice pathologist will develop an understanding of the causes of the disorder and establish a rapport with the patient which permits the therapeutic process to proceed. The voice pathologist may use several formats to interview the patient. Some voice pathologists choose a questionnaire format that requires the patient to respond to prepared questions either prior to or during the evaluation. The answers to the prepared questions are then used to stimulate further understanding of the problem. Although helpful for the beginning clinician, we find prepared forms to be somewhat restrictive and prefer to use a less formal, yet systematic patient interview format. Goals have been established for each section of this format, and the voice pathologist makes every attempt to accomplish each goal during the interview. The suggested format that follows relates to the sample report (SR) located in Appendix 5–A.

DIAGNOSTIC VOICE EVALUATION

Referral

Goals: Establish the identity of the referral source.

The referral source should be clearly understood at the beginning of the evaluation. The major referral sources will be the otolaryngologist, other speech pathologists, physicians, voice teachers, vocal coaches, the patient's relatives and friends, or the patient may self-refer. (See SR1.)

Reason for the Referral

Goals:

1. Establish the exact reason for the patient referral.
2. Establish the patient's understanding for the referral.
3. Develop patient knowledge of the voice disorder.
4. Establish credibility of the examiner.

It is important that the voice pathologist have accurate information regarding the exact reason the patient was referred. When a physician refers the patient, the specific medical diagnosis should be reported along with the physician's expectations related to your contact with the patient. There are many reasons for patient referrals. These may include preoperative audio recording of the voice, laryngeal function studies (see Chapter 6), evaluation without management, preoperative trial voice therapy, postoperative evaluation and treatment, or a complete diagnostic voice evaluation with the appropriate management plan. In our practice, patients often are referred only for a laryngeal videostroboscopic evaluation. Understanding the physician's expectations will avoid confusion and will help to maintain the necessary cooperative working relationships. (See SR2.)

It also is desirable to ensure that the patient understands the reason for the referral for "speech therapy." Voice therapy suffers from poor patient adherence, and several studies have documented a high dropout rate from therapy.[10,11] The literature documents that there is an improved likelihood that the patient may follow through with the recommendation for voice therapy if these three key elements occur: (1) communication between the physician, speech language pathologist, and patient is open and optimized; (2) the expected outcome from therapy is discussed prior to the initiation of therapy; and (3) the patient's readiness for change is determined and addressed early in the therapy process. Quite often, the patient is confused about the purpose of being evaluated by a "speech therapist." This confusion may be addressed by simply asking the patient, "Do you understand why Dr A referred you here?" When confusion is evident, explain the voice pathologist's role along with the 4 major goals you intend to accomplish during the evaluation. As patients better understand the process and procedures, the more reliable they become in communicating pertinent information throughout the evaluation.

It may also be helpful to educate the patient about the voice disorder before proceeding. There are differing opinions regarding explanation of diagnosis and treatment processes. Some believe in cognitive simplification of therapy and increased self-awareness through vocal work with little explanation of the actual therapy process. This author (JCS) believes it is desirable at this time to establish the patient's understanding of the referral for speech therapy. A typical dialogue between a patient (*PT*) and voice pathologist (*VP*) might be as follows:

VP: Do you understand what vocal nodules are and how they might develop?

PT: Dr A said that they're like bumps on my vocal cords and that I got them 'cause I holler too much.

VP: That may be, but there are many reasons why nodules may develop. Let's talk about it. When Dr A looked down your throat with his mirror, he was essentially looking at 2 solid shelves of muscle tissue, 1 on each side, each covered by a soft, pliable, and flexible mucous membrane covering. (It is helpful to schematically draw the vocal folds or to show a picture so that patients may be able to visualize the anatomy. Use of the patient's own stroboscopic video is extremely helpful if available.) These shelves are the vocal cords, or folds, and we're looking straight down on top of them in this picture. The point where the 2 folds meet at the front is inside the V of your Adam's apple. Can you feel yours? Now, the space between the vocal folds is called the glottis, and the tube below the folds is the windpipe or trachea. This, of course, is the airway where air travels to the lungs as we breathe.

Attached to the back of each vocal fold, we have 2 cartilages, 1 here and 1 here. These cartilages serve as the points of attachment for the vocal folds and for other muscles responsible for opening and closing the vocal folds. When the vocal folds are approximated, air pressure from the lungs may build beneath the folds. When the pressure is great enough, the air will blow the folds apart and begin the vibration, which we hear as voice.

If the muscles pull too hard and the air pressure is too great, such as when we shout, talk loudly over noise, or even when we cough, this excessive tension and pressure will cause the vocal folds to bang and rub together. (Demonstrate with hand clapping movements.) If this banging and rubbing occurs frequently, the impact will eventually cause some swelling or edema of the vocal folds that will usually cause a temporary hoarseness. We have all experienced this kind of hoarseness, maybe at a party or a sporting event. In a day or two, this hoarseness goes away. But if whatever caused the hoarseness persists, the folds may remain edemic and will eventually begin to try to protect themselves from further damage. In your case, they've done this by developing, layer by layer, small callous-like structures on the point of the vocal folds where they hit the hardest. These growths are called *vocal nodules*.

As you have experienced, the nodules have caused a change in your voice. Because of the edema and the presence of the nodules, your voice may have dropped in pitch; because the nodules cause gaps to occur on either side of them when the vocal folds close to vibrate, a greater amount of air escapes, causing you to sound breathy. You've also probably noticed that when you do a lot of talking, your voice weakens, and it becomes quite an effort just to talk. By the end of the day, some people report being worn out from the effort and simply do not feel like talking anymore.

One final point: Vocal nodules are not a cancerous type of growth and do not eventually lead to cancer. Many people do not understand this, so I think it is important to mention. Does this information help you to better understand what vocal nodules are and how they affect voice?

PT: Yes, now I do. I am glad that you mentioned the part about cancer. I have to admit that I was worried about that. But, what do you think caused my nodules? I really don't raise my voice that much.

VP: That's what we're here today to try and find out. I'm going to ask you many questions. I need to get to know you and how you use your voice in all situations. From that information, we will try to determine specifically what caused your nodules, how the nodules currently affect your efforts to talk, and then develop a plan to attempt to resolve them. Any questions?

This type of discussion goes far in developing your credibility as the person who is qualified to help resolve this disorder. The voice pathologist will have managed to develop a high level of trust before the actual diagnostic questioning regarding the history of the problem begins.

History of the Problem

Goals:

1. Establish the chronologic history of the problem.
2. Seek etiologic factors associated with the history.
3. Determine patient motivation for resolving the problem.

This section of the evaluation is designed to yield an exact history of the disorder from the onset of vocal difficulties, through the development of the problem over time, and ending with the patient's current vocal experiences. All questions are designed to yield information regarding the causes of vocal difficulties. Finally, the patient's motivation for seeking vocal improvement is determined. (Please refer to SR3.) A list of appropriate questions might include the following:

- Let's go way back. When did you first begin to notice some change or difficulty in your voice?
- Was that the first time that you ever experienced vocal difficulties?
- How did the problem progress from there?
- What finally made you decide to see your doctor about it?
- What did the doctor tell you?
- How did the doctor treat the problem?
- Did your family doctor refer you to the ear, nose, and throat doctor?
- Has anyone else in your family ever experienced a voice problem?
- Does your voice follow a pattern? For example, is it better in the morning than in the evening, or vice versa?
- Do you get more hoarse simply by talking normally?
- Have you ever lost your voice totally?
- Do you have any occasion to raise your voice, to talk over noise, or to shout?
- Are you required to talk to anyone who is hard of hearing?
- Do you have a pet?
- As I have never heard your voice before, I don't know what your normal voice sounds like. I have a 6-point

scale where (0) represents perfectly normal voice and (5) represents as hoarse as you have ever been with this current problem. Where are you on that scale today?

- The effort to talk is sometimes a real problem for people. On a scale of 0 to 7 with 0 being no effort and 7 being extreme effort to talk, how much effort does it take you to make your voice work throughout the day.
- How much does this problem actually bother you? Is it causing any daily problems at home or on your job?
- What is your interest in pursuing voice therapy?

Questions similar to these will lead the voice pathologist along the trail of the development of the voice disorder. The answers will also provide the examiner with an idea of the severity level of the problem as perceived by the patient and the motivation to follow the course of treatment necessary for improvement. On rare occasions, patients have at this point expressed a disinterest in continuing with the diagnostic process. Usually, they have discovered that the problem is not of sufficient concern to them to proceed. A common example is patients who, once they understood that they did not have cancer, were not interested in the consequences of their dysphonia. Although it is the voice pathologist's responsibility to inform the patient and attempt to motivate the patient to seek positive change, the ultimate decision of following through with treatment rests with the individual.

Medical History

Goals:

1. Seek medically related etiologic factors.
2. Establish awareness of patient's basic personality.

The medical history seeks out any medically related factors that may have contributed to the development of the present voice disorder. Utilizing our knowledge of medically related etiologies, the voice pathologist asks questions regarding past surgeries and hospitalizations. Chronic disorders are probed along with the use of medications. Smoking, alcohol, and drug use histories are also explored, and the patient's current hydration habits are discussed.

The medical history also helps the voice pathologist establish how patients "feel" about their physical and emotional well-being. This may be accomplished by asking patients whether, on a day-to-day basis, they feel "excellent, good, fair, or poor." The response to this question will often provide this insight. For example, some patients report lengthy medical histories with many chronic disorders that would give them the right to feel "poorly." Nonetheless, they may still indicate that on a day-to-day basis, they feel "good." Other patients, with unremarkable medical histories, may report feeling only "fair" or "poor." Following up with "Why" is important in this situation.

The answer to this simple question helps the voice pathologist learn the basic personality of the patient. A negative response provides the voice pathologist with an excellent opportunity to pursue the line of questioning further. For example, your response may be, "Oh, why do you feel only fair?" This is often a pivotal moment in the evaluation process, and, more often than not, patients share many important details related to their emotional well-being. These details may be related to marriage, family, job, or friends. Patients with voice disorders often share their emotions and concerns with voice pathologists because we are the first people to ask and show an interest. Handling this information and guiding the patient appropriately become a major responsibility. (See SR4.)

Social History

Goals:

1. Develop knowledge of the patient's home, work, social, and recreational environments.
2. Discover emotional, social, and family difficulties.
3. Seek additional etiologic factors.

The social history is the final opportunity to gather information about the patient and the patient's home, work, recreational and social environments, and lifestyle that may contribute to the development of the voice disorder. All questions probe for answers to possible etiologic factors. For example:

- Are you married, single, divorced, or widowed?
- How long have you been married, single, widowed, or divorced?
- Do you live alone or with other people?
- Do you have children? What are their ages? How many are still at home?
- Does anyone else live in your home? Parents, aunts, friends?
- Do you work outside of the home? Where? How long?
- What kind of work do you do? Specifically, what do you do in your job?
- How much talking is required, and how much is social?
- Does your husband/wife work? Where? How long? What shift?
- When you are not working, what do you enjoy doing (ie, clubs, hobbies, groups, organizations, sports, other social activities)?
- Are you involved in any hobbies or activities where you are in contact with dust, fumes, chemicals, or paints?
- Sometimes stress and tension may contribute to the development of voice problems. In all of these activities and relationships that we've discussed, are there any issues that you think might contribute to this type of tension or stress?
- When you have a lot of stress or tension, who helps you or takes care of you? (Persons who say "no one" are often at risk for emotional stress.)

As you begin the questioning related to the social history, you may find it helpful to explain to patients the need to get to know who they are and what they do in order to find the causes of their vocal difficulties. You want the patient to understand that even if some of the questions seem personal, they are necessary when trying to discover all possible causes. You should not be surprised when patients open up to you with many personal, family, social, marital, or work problems. When you develop credibility and gain the patient's trust, you often receive such important information. (See SR5.)

Oral-Peripheral Examination

Goals:

1. Determine the physical condition of the oral mechanism.

2. Observe areas of the upper body for tension during breathing, speaking, and rest.
3. Check for swallowing difficulties.
4. Check for laryngeal sensations.

A routine oral-peripheral examination should be conducted to determine the condition of the oral mechanism in its relation to the patient's speech and voice production. The exam allows the voice pathologist to observe the patient's laryngeal area and whole-body tension. This is accomplished through visually observing posture and neck muscle tension, as well as carefully digitally manipulating the thyroid cartilage. When tension is not present, the thyroid cartilage may be rocked gently back and forth in the neck. Laryngeal hyperfunction often contributes to laryngeal strap muscle tension, which precludes this rocking motion. The muscle tension often causes laryngeal area muscle aches or discomfort. Patients should be asked about laryngeal sensations because common symptoms associated with voice disorders include throat dryness, tickling, burning, aching, lump-in-the-throat, or thickness sensations. Finally, voice pathologists also should ask their patients whether any swallowing difficulties are present. This information will determine whether the swallowing function is affected by or is affecting vocal production. (See SR6.)

Auditory-Perceptual Voice Assessment

Goals:

1. Describe the present vocal components.
2. Examine inappropriate use of vocal components.

The direct evaluation of voice is conducted to describe the present condition of voice production and to determine whether any vocal components are being used in a habitually inappropriate manner, contributing to the development or maintenance of the pathology. Each vocal component may be examined separately following a general subjective description of voice quality.

Through the patient interview, the examiner has had an adequate sample of conversational voice to make a subjective description of the patient's voice quality. Several formal voice rating scales have been developed and utilized for perceptually judging voice quality.[12–15] One method used to report the degree of baseline dysphonia uses a 6-point, equal-appearing interval scale where: (0) is normal, (1) mild, (2) mild to moderate, (3) moderate, (4) moderate to severe, and (5) severe dysphonia. This scaled description is followed, for the future reference of the examiner, by a descriptive characterization of the voice, including descriptive terms such as hoarseness, harshness, breathiness, raspiness, glottal fry, low pitch, and so on. (See SR7.) This subjective scale is somewhat problematic as the results may not be readily shared with other professionals.

Attempts have been made to improve the reliability of auditory-perceptual evaluations of voice with the development of more formalized evaluation tools. One such tool is the GRBAS scale. GRBAS was developed by the Committee for Phonatory Function Tests of the Japan Society of Logopedics and Phoniatrics.[11] This scale evaluates 5 components of voice production: grade (G), rough (R), breathy (B), aesthenic (A), and strained (S). Each component is rated on a 4-point scale where "0" is normal, "1" is slight, "2" is moderate, and "3" is extreme.

Grade (G) represents the overall degree of hoarseness of voice abnormality. Rough (R) represents the perceptual impression of the irregularity of vocal fold vibrations. It corresponds to the irregular fluctuations in the fundamental frequency, the amplitude of vibration, or both. Breathy (B) represents the perceptual impression of the extent of air leakage through the glottis. Aesthenic (A) denotes weakness or lack of power in the voice. Strained (S) represents the perceptual impression of vocal hyperfunction.

In an attempt to further improve the perceptual evaluation of voice, a committee of the American Speech-Language-Hearing Association Special Interest Division 3, Voice and Voice Disorders, developed the Consensus Auditory-Perceptual Evaluation of Voice (CAPE-V).[16] The CAPE-V uses a 100-mm visual analog scale to assess voice quality at the vowel, sentence, and conversational speech levels. The parameters of voice assessed include overall severity, roughness, breathiness, strain, pitch, and loudness. Areas for describing additional features such as diplophonia, fry, falsetto, asthenia, aphonia, pitch instability, tremor, wet/gurgly, or other relevant terms are provided (Appendix 5–B). The CAPE-V is this author's audioperceptual evaluation tool of choice.

As with all perceptual rating scales, GRBAS and the CAPE-V are subjective and depend on the trained clinical ear. Securing an audio recording of the pretreatment voice using a standard reading passage, such as The Rainbow Passage[17] (Appendix 5–C) for posttreatment comparison is advisable at this time. Following the perceptual description of voice production, each vocal property may then be individually reviewed including the following:

- **Respiration:** This includes a description of:
    1. Conversational breathing patterns, including supportive or nonsupportive
    2. Locus of respiration such as clavicular, thoracic, or abdominal-diaphragmatic breathing
    3. Breath holding or shallow breathing
    4. Coordination of respiration and phonation.

In addition, the s/z ratio may be formally tested in cases where vocal nodules are known to be present on the vocal folds.[18] The presence of laryngeal mass lesions will yield a longer voiceless /s/ than the voiced /z/ because of the inability of the folds to adequately approximate. Generally, ratios greater than 1:4 are considered abnormal. Several trials of each phoneme are conducted, and the patient is encouraged each time to give maximum effort in sustaining for as long as possible. In addition, they are coached to produce maximum inhalation. The usefulness of this method is most likely restricted to screening patients with vocal nodules.

Maximum phonation time (MPT) is also measured at a modal pitch level. MPT is often negatively affected by laryngeal pathology caused by inefficient vocal fold vibration. Therefore, pretest and posttest MPT measures may be used as a tool to demonstrate voice improvement. However, phonatory airflow volume during MPT tasks is not well-correlated with actual measures of pulmonary function. For this reason, phonatory volume should not be accepted as an accurate estimate of lung volume. (See SR8.)

- **Phonation:** Subjective observations regarding the actual voice onset, phonatory register, and strength of phonatory adduction may be made through critical listening. These observations may include the presence of hard glottal attacks, glottal fry, breathiness, or overly compressed adduction. These phonatory symptoms may be observed conversationally throughout the evaluation. The symptoms may also be rechecked by having the patient say the alphabet slowly and then more rapidly. These observations should be formally documented using an audioperceptual rating scale such as the Consensus Auditory Perceptual Evaluation of Voice (CAPE-V), previously discussed. (See SR9.)
- **Resonance:** The term *resonance* refers to the location of amplified sound transmission in the upper aerodigestive tract. Terms like *hypernasal* and *assimilative nasality* are used when describing the quality of sound as a result of the extent of sound transmission in the nasal cavity and are most often used in reference to persons with velopharyngeal incompetence or insufficiency. Cul-de-sac resonance may occur when the tongue is held in a posterior fashion and the sound is primarily focused in the oral pharyngeal port. This type of resonance is most often associated with hearing loss, velopharyngeal incompetence, and has been noted in patients with significant compensatory posterior tongue carriage in the absence of a pathological cause. Hyponasality is the sound associated with an upper respiratory infection and stuffy nose. Often called denasal, the patient with hyponasality should be referred to the otolaryngologist for follow-up of the presence of nasal obstruction. Finally, the term *resonance* in voice often means the place in the hypopharynx for primary sound transmission, or what people refer to as focus of the voice. There remains no standardized method to identify tone focus/resonance of voice transmission. The evaluation of resonance is auditory perceptual. Many voice pathologists believe that resonance is sensed as the place where the voice emanates or where the patient senses vibration of sound. (See SR10.)
- **Pitch:** The patient's present pitch range is tested by singing up and down the scale from midrange voice in whole notes until the highest and lowest attainable notes have been identified. Usually, patients can benefit from both models and multiple trials to achieve best performance. Conversational inflection and pitch variability are also described. (See SR11.)
- **Loudness:** The appropriateness of the patient's speaking loudness level and the variability of loudness, as observed during the interview, are described. It is also important to test the patient's ability to increase subglottic air pressure. This may be accomplished by asking the patient to shout "Hey!" We have found that the ability to produce a solid phonation during a shout, in the presence of a dysphonic conversational voice, is a positive prognostic sign. When the patient is able to override the dysphonia with increased intensity (which is determined by the ability of the folds to approximate tightly to

increase subglottic air pressure), the disorder appears to respond more quickly to remediation methods. In contrast, determining the patient's ability to produce voice softly will demonstrate the efficiency or lack of efficiency of the vocal fold vibration. Additionally, if there is a vocal fold tissue pliability issue, the patient may complain that there are places in the vocal range that require greater loudness/effort to produce the sound. One simple task is to ask the patient to sing up the scale while maintaining steady-state loudness. If the patient reverts to a louder sound at the higher notes, ask the patient to produce the same notes cueing them with "softer, softer, softer." If the patient is unable to produce sound softly, there is likelihood that an adynamic area is present on the vocal folds that does not vibrate, thus requiring greater subglottal pressures to initiate and maintain vocal fold vibration. (See SR12.)

- **Rate:** The rate of a patient's speech may contribute to the development of laryngeal pathology. This is especially true for the individual who speaks with an exceptionally fast rate of speech. As observed during the diagnostic workup, the speech rate may be described as normal, fast, or slow. The rate may also be judged to be monotonous, and like pitch and loudness, rate may contribute to a lack of speech and voice variability. (See SR13 and Appendix 5–D.)

In reviewing each component of voice production, the voice pathologist must not only continually make note of the patient's current vocal behaviors but must also probe for the best voice possible. Voice probing is a form of trial diagnostic therapy and can be done through reading, singing, chanting, or counting while shaping and experimenting with alternative methods of voice production. Habitual vocal habits and potential abilities are often not the same. The use of negative practice, even during this probing stage, can be revealing to the patient. In the end, the voice pathologist seeks to understand the performance gap between what the patient does habitually and what he or she potentially can do.

Patient Self-Analysis of the Voice Disorder

This chapter has been designed to demonstrate to the voice pathologist the steps of the diagnostic voice evaluation. Another important aspect of the evaluation process is to gain an understanding of the functional impact of the voice disorder on the individual in daily life. Those in clinical practice know that different patients will perceive similar voice disorders differently. For example, a singer with vocal nodules may be devastated by the effect that the nodules have on the voice, whereas a computer programmer may not consider the mild hoarseness to be a problem. One method of gaining this functional measure is through the use of validated tools that measure the patient's self-assessment of the voice disorder. One such tool is the Voice Handicap Index (VHI), a test battery that has been statistically validated and is used widely in voice centers[19] (Appendix 5–E).

This instrument, completed before and after treatment by the patient, permits an understanding of the handicapping nature of the voice disorder as perceived by the patient. The 30-item VHI examines self-perceived voice severity as related to functional, physical, and emotional issues. The functional scale includes statements that describe the impact of the patient's voice disorder on daily activities. The physical scale contains statements representing self-perceptions of laryngeal discomfort and voice output characteristics. The emotional scale consists of statements representing the patient's affective responses to the voice disorder. A 5-point scale is used to rate each statement as it reflects the patient's experience with the voice disorder. The scale has the words "never" and "always" anchoring each end, and the words "almost never," "sometimes," and "almost always" appearing in between. An "always" response is scored 4 points, a "never" response is scored 0, and the remaining options are scored between 1 and 3 points. The ratings of the 30 statements are totaled for both pretreatment and posttreatment scales. Any shift of 18 points or more represents a significant shift in the patient's psychosocial functioning, as related to the voice disorder.

Other scales that measure the handicapping effects of voice disorders include Voice-Related Quality of Life (V-RQOL),[20] the Voice Activity and Participation Profile (VAPP),[21] and the Voice Symptom Scale (VoiSS).[22] In addition, population-specific tools have been developed including the Voice Handicap Index-Singers (VHI-S),[23] the Pediatric Voice Handicap Index (p-VHI),[24] the Voice Outcome Survey (VOS)[25] for use with individuals with unilateral vocal fold paralysis, the Pediatric Voice Outcome Survey (PVOS)[26] for use with children with a tracheotomy or with a history of tracheotomy, and a variety of head and neck cancer instruments.

We have found the use of the various quality of life tools to be an extremely valuable addition to the voice evaluation protocol. It provides great insight into the patient's perception of the voice disorder and serves as a natural point of departure in discussing the disorder and its impact on the patient.

Impressions

Goal: To summarize the etiologic factors associated with the development and maintenance of the individual's voice disorder.

The impressions section of the diagnostic evaluation summarizes the causes of the voice disorder as determined through the evaluation. These causes are listed in order of perceived importance as they relate first to the initiation of the problem and second to the maintenance of the problem. Recall that the precipitating factor may not be the same as the maintenance factor. (See SR14.)

Prognosis

Goal: To analyze the probability of improvement through voice therapy.

The prognosis for improving many voice disorders through voice therapy generally is good. Nonetheless, many factors influence prognosis including the patient's motivation, interest, time available, ability to follow instructions, and physical and emotional status, to name a few. The prognosis statement permits the voice pathologist to give a subjective opinion regarding the chances for improved voice production based on the diagnostic information. A reasonable time frame for expected completion of the management program should also be stated. (See SR15.)

Recommendations

Goal: Outline the management plan.

The management plan is then briefly outlined based on the etiologic factors discovered during the evaluation and the medical examination. The outline will include the therapy approaches to be utilized and any additional referrals. (See SR16.)

Additional Considerations

The evaluation format we have presented is semistructured. The basic questions remain the same from patient to patient, but the answers given by individual patients dictate the direction in which the questions will proceed and the order in which each diagnostic section is reviewed. Although the beginning clinician may choose a more structured format, such as a questionnaire, the semistructured method is preferred because it allows a more patient-direct approach to diagnosis.

The diagnostic report should include only the information pertinent to the development and maintenance of the voice disorder, as well as the projected plan of care. Referring physicians are not interested in the patient's life history. Most physicians turn directly to the sections on impressions and recommendations, which justifies the need for a detailed explanation of the problem and the plan of care.

Some voice pathologists prefer to audio-record the entire diagnostic session for later review. This review may help determine the exact vocal components produced during the evaluation and serves as a record of baseline voice quality. Even when the entire diagnostic session is not recorded, recording of a standard speech sample is necessary for later reference. It is not unusual for the voice pathologist and the patient to forget the actual severity of the baseline voice quality. Audio recordings serve as an objective reminder and should be used liberally throughout the treatment course.

Finally, the American Speech-Language-Hearing Association mandates that patients who undergo speech, language, and voice evaluations must have a current hearing screening. Audiometric evaluation is important for the patient with a voice disorder. The inability to monitor voice well may result in the use of inappropriate vocal components. Severe voice disorders are often observed in the hard-of-hearing and deaf populations.

SUMMARY

Diagnosis is probably the most important single aspect of a remedial program.[27(p108)] A systematic diagnostic voice evaluation is important for all types of voice disorders, with minor modifications in the format made as needed to accommodate individual patients. The major goals are as follows:

- Discover the causes of the voice disorder.
- Describe the present vocal components.

- Evaluate the effect of the disorder on respiration, phonation, and resonance.
- Determine the direction for intervention, if warranted.

Finally, the diagnostic voice evaluation teaches and educates the patient about the disorder. In this manner, the evaluation tool may be viewed in its own right as a primary therapy tool.

The goal of describing the vocal components has been greatly enhanced with the use of more objective procedures and techniques for assessing voice function. Chapter 6 introduces instrumental voice measurement techniques, including acoustic analysis, aerodynamic measurement, and laryngeal imaging. When combined with findings from the patient interview, the audio-perceptual evaluation of voice, and the patient self-assessment, these instrumental techniques greatly enhanced the evaluation of voice disorders.

REFERENCES

1. Moore P. *Organic Voice Disorders*. Englewood Cliffs, NJ: Prentice-Hall; 1971.
2. Herrington-Hall BL, Lee L, Stemple JC, Niemi KR, McHone MM. Description of laryngeal pathologies by age, sex, and occupation in a treatment-seeking sample. *J Speech Hear Disord*. 1988;53(1):57–64.
3. Coyle SM, Weinrich BD, Stemple JC. Shifts in relative prevalence of laryngeal pathology in a treatment-seeking population. *J Voice*. 2001;15(3):424–440.
4. Roy N, Merrill RM, Gray SD, Smith EM. Voice disorders in the general population: prevalence, risk factors, and occupational impact. *Laryngoscope*. 2005;115(11):1988–1995.
5. Roy N, Stemple J, Merrill RM, Thomas L. Epidemiology of voice disorders in the elderly: preliminary findings. *Laryngoscope*. 2007;117(4):628–633.
6. Koufman JA, Isaacson G. The spectrum of vocal dysfunction. *Otolaryngol Clin North Am*. 1991;24(5):985–988.
7. Sander EK. Arguments against the aggressive pursuit of voice therapy for children. *Lang Speech Hear Serv Sch*. 1989;20:94–101.
8. Blood GW, Mahan BW, Hyman M. Judging personality and appearance from voice disorders. *J Commun Disord*. 1979;12(1):63–67.
9. Yanagisawa E, Yanagisawa R. Laryngeal photography. *Otolaryngol Clin North Am*. 1991;24(5):999–1022.
10. Hapner E, Portone-Maira C, Johns MM, 3rd. A study of voice therapy dropout. *J Voice*. 2009;23(3):337–340.
11. Portone C, Johns MM, 3rd, Hapner ER. A review of patient adherence to the recommendation for voice therapy. *J Voice*. 2008;22(2):192–196.
12. Gelfer M. Perceptual attributes of voice: development and use of rating scales. *J Voice*. 1988;2:320–326.
13. Hirano M. *Clinical Examination of Voice*. New York, NY: Springer-Verlag; 1981.
14. Wilson D. *Voice Problems of Children*. 2nd ed. Baltimore, MD: Williams and Wilkins; 1979.
15. Wilson F. The voice disordered child: a descriptive approach. *Lang Speech Hear Serv Sch*. 1970;4:14–22.
16. American Speech-Language-Hearing Association. *Consensus Auditory-Perceptual Evaluation of Voice (CAPE-V): purpose and Applications*. Rockville, MD: American Speech-Language-Hearing Association; 2002.
17. Fairbanks G. *Voice and Articulation Handbook*. New York, NY: Harper & Row; 1960.
18. Eckel FC, Boone DR. The s/z ratio as an indicator of laryngeal pathology. *J Speech Hear Disord*. 1981;46(2):147–149.

19. Jacobson B, Johnson A, Grywalski C, et al. The Voice Handicap Index (VHI): development and validation. *Am J Speech Lang Pathol*. 1997;6(3):66–70.
20. Hogikyan ND, Sethuraman G. Validation of an instrument to measure voice-related quality of life (V-RQOL). *J Voice*. 1999;13(4):557–569.
21. Ma E, Yiu E. Voice activity and participation profile: assessing the impact of voice disorders on daily activities. *J Speech Lang Hear Res*. 2001;44:511–524.
22. Deary I, Wilson J, Carding P, MacKenzie K. VoiSS: a patient-derived voice symptom scale. *J Psychosom Res*. 2003;54:483–489.
23. Cohen SM, Jacobson BH, Garrett CG, et al. Creation and validation of the Singing Voice Handicap Index. *Ann Otol Rhinol Laryngol*. 2007;116(6):402–406.
24. Zur KB, Cotton S, Kelchner L, Baker S, Weinrich B, Lee L. Pediatric Voice Handicap Index (pVHI): a new tool for evaluating pediatric dysphonia. *Int J Pediatr Otorhinolaryngol*. 2007;71(1):77–82.
25. Gliklich R, Glovsky R, Montgomery W. Validation of a voice outcome survey for unilateral vocal cord paralysis. *Otolaryngol Head Neck Surg*. 1999;120:153–158.
26. Hartnick C. Validation of a pediatric voice quality-of-life instrument. *Arch Otolaryngol Head Neck Surg*. 2002;128:919–922.
27. Moore GP. *Organic Voice Disorders*. Englewood Cliffs, NJ: Prentice-Hall; 1971.

Appendix 5–A
Sample Report

Name:

Type of Case: Bilateral vocal fold nodules

Age: 58 years

Address:

Date of Birth: 2-14-50

Phone:

Date: 4-22-13 Examiner: JCS

SR1 **Referral:** The patient was referred by, __________ MD, otolaryngologist, Lexington, KY.

SR2 **Reason for Referral:** The patient was referred for both evaluation and treatment with a diagnosis of small, bilateral vocal fold nodules and possible reflux laryngitis.

SR3 **History of the Problem:** The patient reported first experiencing vocal difficulties in April 2012. At that time, she contracted a cold that created an excessive amount of coughing and throat clearing. She then experienced dysphonia, which persisted after the cold symptoms resolved. Another cold was experienced over the Labor Day weekend, at which time the patient became aphonic for 2 days. This motivated her to seek the medical examination. The patient reported that her voice quality is currently better in the morning and worsens with use as the day progresses. An increased amount of hoarseness has been noted following church choir rehearsals. Motivation for modifying these vocal difficulties appeared to be high because of the patient's vocal needs in her work setting.

SR4 **Medical History:** The patient was hospitalized in 1979 for a tonsillectomy and in 2004 for a complete hysterectomy. Chronic disorders reported by the patient included excessive sinus drainage, which creates coughing and throat clearing and nightly heartburn, which is exacerbated by stress and nervousness. The patient reported that she presently takes no medications and that she stopped smoking 3 weeks prior to this evaluation. Her liquid intake was poor and consisted of mostly caffeinated products. She previously smoked 1 package of cigarettes per day for 32 years. On a day-to-day basis, the patient reported that she generally felt "good."

SR5 **Social History:** Mrs. __________ was divorced in 1984 and has 4 children, ages 30, 31, 32, and 35 years. One child and two grandchildren presently are living in her home. She is an employee of __________ city government as an Equal Employment Opportunity program manager. This position involves managing a federal woman's job program, career counseling of female employees, and the conduction of management relations seminars. Much speaking is required on a daily basis, which the patient continued during the initial cold and the onset of dysphonia.

Nonwork interests and activities include playing the piano, singing in the church choir, teaching Sunday School to preschoolers, conducting church youth meetings, sewing, and reading. The patient reported that singing, teaching Sunday school, and the youth meetings all tax her voice, creating increased dysphonia. Mrs. __________ also admitted to some shouting at her grandchildren in the home environment. Other than job tension, no emotional difficulties were reported.

SR6 **Oral-Peripheral Examination:** The structure and function of the oral mechanism appeared to be well within normal limits for speech and voice production. Laryngeal sensations reported included dryness, burning, occasional pain, and a "lump-in-the-throat feeling." The patient reported having difficulty swallowing pills. Food and liquids were swallowed well. Laryngeal area muscle tension was not noted subjectively.

Voice Evaluation

SR7 **General Quality:** The patient demonstrated a mild dysphonia characterized by breathiness and intermittent glottal fry phonation. She further reported that the voice quality worsened with use and toward the end of every day.

SR8 **Respiration:** A supportive, thoracic breathing pattern was demonstrated. The patient was able to sustain the /a/ for 14 seconds, the /s/ for 27 seconds, and the /z/ for 22 seconds.

SR9 **Phonation:** Occasional glottal fry phonation and breathiness were noted. No hard glottal attacks were observed.

SR10 **Resonance:** Normal.

SR11 **Pitch:** The patient demonstrated an almost 2-octave pitch range with good inflection and variability noted conversationally. Habitual pitch level was within normal limits for the patient's gender and age.

SR12 **Loudness:** Loudness was appropriate for the speaking situation. The patient was readily able to increase loudness to a shout.

SR13 **Rate:** Normal.

SR14 **Impressions:** It is my impression that this patient presents with a voice disorder with a primary etiology of voice abuse. These include the abusive behaviors of:

1. Coughing and throat clearing that have persisted since recovering from the April cold
2. Straining the voice while singing
3. Raising the voice during youth meetings and in her home.

Secondary precipitating factors include:

1. The contribution of laryngopharyngeal reflux
2. Poor hydration
3. The necessity to speak excessively on a daily basis in the presence of the current dysphonia

4. The use of breathy phonation
5. General weakness and imbalance of the laryngeal musculature.

SR15 **Prognosis:** The prognosis for modifying these etiologic factors and resolving the laryngeal pathology is good based on the small size of the nodules, the continued fluctuation of the voice quality, and the patient's apparent desire to return to normal voicing. Estimated time for completion of the vocal management program is 8 to 10 weeks.

SR16 **Recommendations:** It is recommended that the patient enroll in a weekly voice therapy program with therapy focusing on:

1. Vocal hygiene counseling
2. Elimination of the abusive behavior of habit throat clearing
3. Vocal function exercises designed to balance respiration, phonation, and resonance
4. Formal hydration program.

In addition, the patient will return to her family physician to discuss the possibility of being placed on an antireflux regimen.

Appendix 5–B
Consensus Auditory-Perceptual Evaluation of Voice (CAPE-V)

Name: ______________________________ **Date:** ____________

The following parameters of voice quality will be rated upon completion of the following tasks:

1. Sustained vowels /a/ and /i/ for 3- to 5-seconds duration each.
2. Sentence production
   a. The blue spot is on the key again.
   b. How hard did he hit him?
   c. We were away a year ago.
   d. We eat eggs every Easter.
   e. My mama makes lemon muffins.
   f. Peter will keep at the peak.
3. Spontaneous speech in response to "Tell me about your voice problems." or "Tell me how your voice is functioning."

Legend: C = Consistent
I = Intermittent
MI = Mildly deviant
MO = Moderately deviant
SE = Severely deviant

SCORE

Overall Severity ______________________________ C I ____/100
MI MO SE

Roughness ______________________________ C I ____/100
MI MO SE

Breathiness ______________________________ C I ____/100
MI MO SE

Strain ______________________________ C I ____/100
MI MO SE

Pitch (Indicate the nature of the abnormality):

____

______________________________ C I ____/100
MI MO SE

SCORE

Loudness (Indicate the nature of the abnormality):

____

____ **C I** ____**/100**

MI MO SE

____ **C I** ____**/100**

MI MO SE

____ **C I** ____**/100**

MI MO SE

COMMENTS ABOUT RESONANCE NORMAL OTHER (Provide description):

____

____

ADDITIONAL FEATURES (for example, diplophonia, fry, falsetto, asthenia, aphonia, pitch instability, tremor, wet/gurgly, or other relevant terms)

____

Clinician: ________________________________

Printed in the USA

Appendix 5–C
The Rainbow Passage

When the sunlight strikes raindrops in the air, they act like a prism and form a rainbow. The rainbow is a division of white light into many beautiful colors. These take the shape of a long round arch, with its path high above, and its two ends apparently beyond the horizon. There is, according to legend, a boiling pot of gold at one end. People look, but no one ever finds it. When a man looks for something beyond his reach, his friends say he is looking for the pot of gold at the *end of* the rainbow.

Passage is reprinted from: Fairbanks G. *Voice and Articulation Handbook*; 1960, p. 127.

Appendix 5–D
Vocal Component Checklist

Breathing Pattern	Clavicular		☐
	Thoracic		☐
	Abdominal-diaphragmatic		☐
	Supportive ☐ Nonsupportive ☐		
	/s/_____ ☐ /z/_____ ☐		
Phonation	Voice onset:	hard glottal attack	☐
		aspirate attack	☐
		static attack	☐
	Registration:	glottal fry	☐
		loft	☐
		modal	☐
Resonance	Hypernasal		☐
	Denasal		☐
	Cul-de-sac		☐
	Assimilative		☐
	Normal		☐
Pitch	High		☐
	Low		☐
	Poor variability		☐
	Normal		☐
Loudness	Too loud		☐
	Too soft		☐
	Poor variability		☐
	Normal		☐
	Ability to shout		yes ☐ no ☐
Rate	Too fast		☐
	Too slow		☐
	Poor variability		☐
	Normal		☐

Appendix 5–E
Voice Handicap Index (VHI)

Instructions: These are statements that many people have used to describe their voices and the effects of their voices on their lives. Circle the response that indicates how frequently you have the same experience.

		Never	Almost Never	Sometimes	Almost Always	Always
Fl.	My voice makes it difficult for people to hear me.	0	1	2	3	4
P2.	I run out of air when I talk.	0	1	2	3	4
F3.	People have difficulty understanding me in a noisy room.	0	1	2	3	4
P4.	The sound of my voice varies throughout the day.	0	1	2	3	4
F5.	My family has difficulty hearing me when I call them throughout the house.	0	1	2	3	4
F6.	I use the phone less often than I would like.	0	1	2	3	4
E7.	I'm tense when talking with others because of my voice.	0	1	2	3	4
F8.	I tend to avoid groups of people because of my voice.	0	1	2	3	4
E9.	People seem irritated with my voice.	0	1	2	3	4
P10.	People ask, "What's wrong with your voice?"	0	1	2	3	4
F11.	I speak with friends, neighbors, or relatives less often because of my voice.	0	1	2	3	4
F12.	People ask me to repeat myself when speaking face-to-face.	0	1	2	3	4
P13.	My voice sounds creaky and dry.	0	1	2	3	4
P14.	I feel as though I have to strain to produce voice.	0	1	2	3	4

		Never	Almost Never	Sometimes	Almost Always	Always
E15.	I find other people don't understand my voice problem.	0	1	2	3	4
F16.	My voice difficulties restrict my personal and social life.	0	1	2	3	4
P17.	The clarity of my voice is unpredictable.	0	1	2	3	4
P18.	I try to change my voice to sound different.	0	1	2	3	4
F19.	I feel left out of conversations because of my voice.	0	1	2	3	4
P20.	I use a great deal of effort to speak.	0	1	2	3	4
P21.	My voice is worse in the evening.	0	1	2	3	4
F22.	My voice problem causes me to lose income.	0	1	2	3	4
E23.	My voice problem upsets me.	0	1	2	3	4
E24.	I am less outgoing because of my voice problem.	0	1	2	3	4
E25.	My voice makes me feel handicapped.	0	1	2	3	4
P26.	My voice "gives out" on me in the middle of speaking.	0	1	2	3	4
E27.	I feel annoyed when people ask me to repeat.	0	1	2	3	4
E28.	I feel embarrassed when people ask me to repeat.	0	1	2	3	4
E29.	My voice makes me feel incompetent.	0	1	2	3	4
E30.	I'm ashamed of my voice problem.	0	1	2	3	4

Note. The letter preceding each item number corresponds to the subscale. *E*, emotional subscales; *F*, functional subscales; *P*, physical subscale. Reprinted with permission from "The Voice Handicap Index (VHI): Development and validation" by B. Jacobson, A. Johnson, C. Grywalski, A. Silbergleit, G. Jacobson, and M. S. Benninger. *American Journal of Speech-Language Pathology*, *6*, 66–70.

6

Instrumental Measurement of Voice

INTRODUCTION TO INSTRUMENTATION IN VOICE ASSESSMENT

Instrumental measures of vocal function contribute to the voice evaluation by augmenting information from case history, audioperceptual judgments, and behavioral observations of voice. The most common instruments in a clinical voice laboratory measure 1 of 3 features: the acoustic signal, aerodynamic changes in pressure or flow, or visual images of vocal fold vibration. All 3 approaches are indirect measures of voice production through which voice clinicians and researchers make inferences about underlying laryngeal and vocal fold physiology. If used appropriately, instrumental measures provide critical information about the respiratory, laryngeal, and phonatory behaviors in voice production.

In the past 3 decades, both technologic and professional efforts have prompted a rapid explosion of new technology designed to measure voice. As the speed, memory, and affordability of digital microprocessing capabilities have increased, researchers have developed more powerful voice measurement tools that can capture the voice signal or record the vocal fold vibratory image accurately. The collaborations between voice pathologists, scientists, and otolaryngologists have fostered advances in voice laboratory development, protocols, and interpretation.[1–8] The purpose of this chapter is to examine measurement instruments common to clinical voice laboratories and to discuss the scientific principles that underlie their development, application, and interpretation.

Speech and voice analysis tools are often promoted as "objective," because the instruments provide documentable or numeric measures, as in the case of a recorded image or an airflow rate. However, the utility of any tool is only as appropriate as the user's knowledge; without careful attention to correct task protocol, calibration, analysis, and interpretation, instruments do not ensure better measurement reliability or validity. Often, product developers and vendors are our best allies in understanding the optimal applications of clinical voice measurements. Reputable vendors consult regularly with (or are themselves) speech scientists and clinicians who understand what tools can and cannot do, including the technical limits and the practical threats to valid interpretation. Some companies promote best practices through sponsored continuing education opportunities and published reports in peer-reviewed journals or newsletters.

To be useful, clinical instruments must contribute to the diagnosis, etiology, severity, prognosis, or measurable change in the voice disorder.[2–4,8] The validity of instrumental measures in clinical problem solving can be appraised on 4 levels: (1) detection, (2) severity, (3) diagnosis, and (4) treatment. In essence, can the voice measurement validly and reliably:

- Identify the existence of a voice problem (detection)?
- Assess the severity or stage of progression of the voice problem, thereby potentially serving as a treatment outcomes tool?
- Identify the differential source of the voice problem (diagnosis)?
- Serve as a primary treatment tool, for behavioral modification, biofeedback, or patient education (treatment)?

Evaluating an instrument's efficacy is complicated by the large number and variety of clinical voice instruments, many using dissimilar equipment or software and analysis routines. This disparity limits comparisons between voice laboratories and across equipment. For example, a recent study measured normal speech samples using two different commercial acoustic analysis programs to see whether the results were directly comparable. Some values, such as fundamental frequency and harmonics-to-noise ratio, were strongly correlated between programs, but other measures were not. Although the absolute values were not consistently comparable, both program analyses correctly identified these speech samples as normal, based on equipment-based norms.[9] This outcome underscores the recognized need for an adequate normative base that is specific to both equipment and recording protocol. The National Center for Voice and Speech, the American Speech-Language-Hearing Association's (ASHA's) Special Interest Group 3 (Voice and Voice Disorders), commercial vendors, and other research groups have contributed to the evidence pool in using vocal function measures, including detailed standards in calibrating, recording, analyzing, and interpreting vocal function measures.[5–8,10,11]

CLINICAL UTILITY

Voice pathologists have limited time to select and perform the large number of vocal function measures available (Table 6–1). Choosing equipment can be particularly confusing because of the broad range of measurement capabilities and analysis routines. Some priorities for deciding which clinical laboratory measurement tools are as follows.[3,12,13]

Table 6–1. Instrumental Measures in the Voice Laboratory

Technique	*Information*
Laryngeal imaging	Gross structure and movements Vibratory characteristics Vibratory onset and offset (real time imaging only)
Acoustic recording and analysis	Fundamental frequency Intensity Signal/harmonics-to-noise ratio Perturbation measures Spectral features
Aerodynamic measurement	Airflow rate and volume Subglottal (intraoral) pressure Phonation threshold pressure Laryngeal resistance
Inverse Filter	Glottal waveforms of acoustics or airflow
Electroglottography (EGG)	Measure of vocal fold contact area
Electromyography (LEMG)	Direct measures of muscle activity

- How is the instrument used? Will it serve clinic, research, or teaching purposes?
- What analysis capabilities are desired? Are multiple vocal function measures to be integrated (eg, acoustic, aerodynamic, electroglottography [EGG], and imaging)?
- What restraint does the instrument impose on the patient and the speech product? Does the equipment (eg, a tight-fitting face mask) or speech task (eg, sustained /i/ vowel) limit or alter the voice production? Can the speech sample represent (or approximate) typical behavior, or can other evaluation procedures compensate for this factor?
- Are the measures valid? Have the recording procedures and analysis routines been shown to reflect the underlying truths of the speech behavior? Have they been cross-validated with existing measures?
- Are the measures reliable? Have they been used to establish normative values specific to this equipment? How do these data compare with measures collected in other laboratories?
- Are there clinical macros that increase the user friendliness of the standard clinical analysis protocol? Does equipment cost, speed, or technical support limit the feasibility of the measure?
- Is the equipment easy to maintain and calibrate? What user strategies will help avoid instrumental artifact or measurement error?

Although no measurement technique will satisfy all of these criteria, clinicians must know these limits to avoid inappropriate or misleading interpretations. All noninvasive voice laboratory measurements are merely *indirect* estimates of vocal function. (The few direct measures of vocal function, such as direct measures of tracheal pressure or percutaneous laryngeal electromyography of muscle activity, are beyond the scope of voice pathology practice and require collaboration with an otolaryngologist or neurologist.) Indirect measures must be cross-validated carefully with a perceptual and visual monitor of speech and voice behaviors. Consider, for example, a patient who is referred for evaluation of incomplete glottic closure. The patient sounds severely breathy and has limited phonation time, apparently caused by excessive glottal airflow leak. If airflow measurements were to fall within a normal range, that information would be a complete mismatch with other clinical impressions. A knowledgeable user will ask other questions to reconcile the discrepancy. Was the airflow mask applied securely? Was the airflow device calibrated accurately? Although instrumental measures will not always support our clinical and perceptual biases, they should not automatically override experienced clinical judgment.

Recently, statistical advances have made it possible to evaluate the predictive power of many vocal function measures simultaneously, for comparison with perceptual or self-rating measures.[14,15] For example, 4 vocal function measures form the Dysphonia Severity Index (DSI), a derived value based on multivariate analysis of over 1000 normal and pathologic voices.[16] Maximum phonation time, highest fundamental frequency, lowest intensity, and jitter were selected on the basis of their linear correlation to the perceptual judgment of normal, mild, moderate, or severe vocal hoarseness taken from rating "G" (Grade) on the GRBAS scale.[1] The DSI has successfully discriminated between organic and nonorganic etiologies in a large patient population.[17] Another mathematical algorithm based on four different acoustic measures (jitter, shimmer, standard deviation of fundamental frequency, and glottal-to-noise excitation ratio) classified 120 voices as "healthy" or "hoarse" with 80% accuracy.[18] Another study examined whether acoustic measures (fundamental frequency, jitter %, shimmer %, signal-to-noise ratio, mean root-mean-square intensity, or fundamental frequency standard deviation) or physiologic measures (aphonic periods or breath groups) could predict patient self-ratings on the Voice Handicap Index (VHI).[14,19] No relationship was determined for any single measure in those comparisons, which suggests that a combination of values may improve discrimination between normal and disordered voice quality. Other investigators believe that vowel-based acoustic measures are inherently flawed, as disordered voice quality is always judged in connected speech contexts. Instead, they examined long-term average spectral acoustic measures taken from a standard reading passage to predict ratings of voice severity and pleasantness, and to discriminate normal from dysphonic voice quality. Their results showed that acoustic measures in isolation had only limited success in predicting severity or pleasantness ratings for dysphonic speakers. Moreover, when audioperceptual judgments and acoustic measures were used together, classification of normal versus dysphonic voice rose to 100%.[20] Currently, no single vocal function measure appears to be able to identify dysphonia accurately and consistently. Nonetheless, these complex statistical models are encouraging us to consider the predictive power of various combinations of acoustic, aerodynamic, or other instrumental measures in classifying normal versus disordered voice.

BASICS OF TECHNICAL INSTRUMENTS

Clinicians who use voice laboratory instrumentation will benefit from some general principles of electronics, physics, and digital processing to help understand the science and artifact of signal measurement and analysis.[7,21] Essentially, speech and voice measures rely on three events: signal detection, signal manipulation or conditioning, and signal reconversion. In these three processes, the physical phenomenon, whether it be a sound (eg, sustained vowel), an image, or a physiologic event (eg, air pressure, muscle movement) is:

- Detected and input by a device, such as a microphone, camera, electrode, pressure transducer, or flow meter
- Manipulated in some manner, such as filtering, amplification, or digitization, for use with a specific type of equipment or analysis routine
- Reconverted for output and display in some readable form, such as a numerical value, oscilloscope tracing, pixel display, or speaker.

Because most instrumental measures rely on a series of inputs and outputs between electronic or digital components and computers, the quality of the professional data acquisition hardware and software does affect the integrity of the voice quality recording and analysis.[22] Moreover, faulty connections between components or computer interface incompatibility between different hardware and software versions may potentially distort the signal. Reputable vendors can familiarize users with the technical requirements and recommended coupling devices needed to avoid transmission error.

MICROPHONES AND RECORDING ENVIRONMENT

For acoustic measurement, signal detection begins with a microphone. Vibrating sound waves oscillate against an internal diaphragm or other sensing device that connects electronically to an amplifier and, eventually, to an output device, such as a monitor, oscilloscope, or speaker. The free-field, sound pressure level energy excites the microphone's internal diaphragm, changing acoustic sound energy into mechanical energy, and then changing it again into electronic energy for transmission through the system. The process of changing energy from one form to another is called *transduction*, and any device that converts the energy is called a *transducer*. This electrical energy can then be connected to other clinical instruments for recording and subsequent analysis.[7]

To ensure reliable speech and voice recordings, microphones should conform to recommended technical standards, including a professional-grade, condenser-type microphone with unidirectional or cardioid filtering characteristics.[11,23] The microphone should be positioned off center from the mouth to avoid excessive aspirate noise, at a constant mouth-to-microphone distance of approximately 3 to 8 cm for sustained vowels, although longer distances may be acceptable for connected speech tasks. Environmental noise matters, too; ambient noise degrades the accuracy of acoustic perturbation measures.[24] Therefore, recordings should always be conducted in a quiet environment, preferably with a minimum signal-to-noise ratio of 42 dB.[11,23,24]

Following are definitions of some of the most common technical specifications for microphones:

- *Amplification* means increasing the magnitude of a signal, while keeping the waveform shape intact. A larger signal magnitude may be necessary for signal analysis or playback.
- *Gain* is the exact magnitude of the amplification, usually expressed as ratio of signal input to signal output (after amplification).
- Amplifier *linearity* is the degree to which gain is constant across all input magnitudes. If the amplifier gain across a speech signal is not equal across all frequencies (ie, nonlinear), then signal distortions result because some frequencies will be amplified more than others.
- *Peak clipping* is a signal distortion that occurs when amplification (gain) exceeds the linear limits of the microphone. The amplitude peaks of the waveform are cut off or flattened, and the resulting acoustic signal is both incomplete and inaccurate.
- *Frequency response* is the range of frequencies that can be detected by a component. If the frequency range is too small to accommodate the entire speech signal, then the signal will be distorted. A common frequency response is 20 to 20,000 kHz and can apply to microphones, recording devices, sound cards, and speakers.
- *Filters* reshape the acoustic waveform to eliminate selected energy above or below a certain frequency range. Three common types of filters used in speech processing are low pass, high pass, and band pass. Low-pass filters allow energy in the lower frequencies to pass through (high-frequency energy excluded). High-pass filters allow the high-frequency energy to pass through (excluding low-frequency energy). Band-pass filters will admit energy only within a certain range (band), excluding frequencies above and below.[21]

DIGITAL SIGNAL PROCESSING

Speech and voice signals travel in sound pressure waves, composed of a series of air molecule compressions and rarefactions, radiated from lips, teeth, and mouth. Sound waves are analog signals because they are continuous and time varying. To convert this continuous analog signal into a digital format for computer recording and speech processing, it must be divided into small, discrete bits of information that can accurately represent the waveform numerically. This process is called *digitization* and is achieved by analog-to-digital (A/D) processing. Frequency and intensity are two important parameters that must be converted accurately if the digital signal is to represent the analog waveform. The time-varying changes (seen on the horizontal axis) represent the frequency contour. The signal height (displayed on the vertical axis) represents amplitude. The A/D conversion uses two key operations, sampling and quantization, to assign numeric values that represent both the time-varying frequency and amplitude height changes in the speech and voice signal.[21]

When the continuous waveform is divided into discrete numeric values, the intervals between points are eliminated. Therefore, it is critical that the sampling rate must be high enough to detect the frequency contour accurately. If the spacing between sampled points is too large, this undersampling can lead to an artifact known as *aliasing*, where high-frequency information is misrepresented. In the past decade, advances in microprocessing speed and power have produced sampling rate capabilities that are sufficiently high to accommodate digital conversion for speech and voice. Recommendations for sampling rates in speech acoustic analysis begin at a minimum of 20 kHz (sufficient to sample frequencies of interest up to 10 kHz),[21] and currently, most digitizing routines adopt sampling rates up to 100 kHz.

Quantization is the process that converts amplitude height into discrete numerical values in a manner similar to the sampling process. The varying signal waveform is divided into small increments of amplitude height, and each increment is assigned a numeric value. Like sampling rate, it is important that sufficient quantization levels (variations in height) are available to accurately convert the signal. The number of quantization levels available is determined by conversion "bits." A minimal standard for speech and voice digitization is 16 bits of amplitude quantization, which is equivalent to 65,536 different amplitude increments or levels. Together, sampling and quantization operations determine the adequacy of the conversion from a continuous analog signal to a digitized waveform.[21]

ACOUSTIC MEASUREMENTS

Acoustic measures can provide objective and noninvasive analyses of vocal function, if they are recorded and interpreted carefully. Figure 6–1 shows an acoustic analysis system for recording, storing, and analyzing the speech signal.

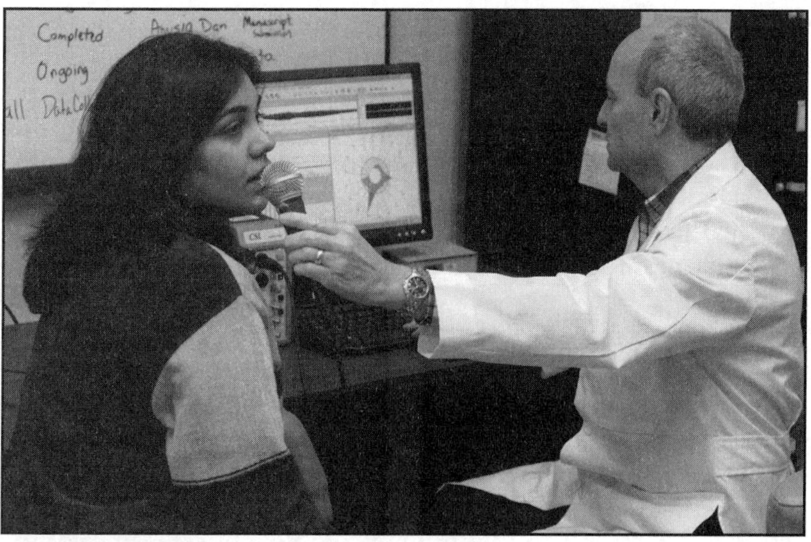

FIGURE 6–1. Acoustic analysis system for recording, storing, and analyzing the speech signal.

To validate the clinical utility of a specific acoustic measure, users must gather adequate normative information using a standard protocol to determine whether the acoustic measure(s):

- Can discriminate between normal and disordered voice quality
- Correlate with audioperceptual judgments of voice quality
- Are sufficiently stable to assess change in performance across time.

Before one can answer these questions, it is important to recognize that there are a large (and ever-increasing) number of acoustic measures, most of which are mathematical derivations of 5 common measures:

1. Fundamental frequency, which is an acoustic measure of the perceptual judgment of pitch
2. Intensity, which is an acoustic measure of the perceptual judgment of loudness
3. Perturbation measures, which assess the cycle-to-cycle variation in the acoustic waveform for either frequency or intensity
4. Ratio of signal (or harmonic) energy-to-noise, which reflects the relative contribution of periodic and aperiodic (noisy) components of the acoustic signal
5. Spectral features, which represent vocal tract harmonic energy.

Although there are normative data that delineate boundaries of normal and abnormal acoustic values, the agreement between acoustic measures and audio-perceptual ratings of voice quality remains inconsistent.[25–32] Historically, studies attempted to identify which acoustic measure(s) best predicted perceptual dysphonia. Although acoustic measures have become more accurate with better signal detection and processing techniques, they still fail to serve as reliable predictors of normal and disordered voice. As discussed earlier, new statistical models analyze many acoustic and physiologic measures simultaneously to identify a cohort of useful predictors. This elusive connection may also be improved if the reliability of perceptual judgments can be improved, using different psychometric techniques, such as averages from multiple listening trials and standard scores.[33]

Lack of clinical and technical standards has also limited the utility of acoustic measures, due to variations in elicitation techniques, recording tasks, speech sample lengths, and number of samples needed for reliability. Nonetheless, acoustic measures appear to be reasonably successful in measuring vocal change across time within a patient's course of evaluation and treatment. Comparison of pre- and posttreatment acoustic measures may serve 2 purposes. At evaluation, acoustic measures provide indirect evidence of the severity of the voice problem, even if they cannot pinpoint the specific etiologies or pathologies. At follow-up, these measures help evaluate the effects of the rehabilitation plan.[34–41]

Pitch Detection Algorithm

A starting point for acoustic analysis is to determine the fundamental frequency of a given signal. This process is known as *pitch detection*. In normal speakers, the digitized acoustic waveform reveals a complex, but quasiperiodic repetition of pitch periods across time. Pitch detection identifies and extracts the pitch of an acoustic signal, through 1 of 3 mathematical approaches. Peak-picking identifies the highest point of amplitude excursion in successive periods and calculates the distance between "peaks" to reveal the pitch period (Figure 6–2). Zero crossing uses a similar technique by identifying the point of waveform crossing on the horizontal axis. When the waveform pattern is noisy or deteriorated, as in a severely dysphonic voice, the amplitude peaks and axis-crossing points can be highly irregular and difficult to detect, making both methods particularly susceptible to error.[5–7,11,21] A third method, waveform matching, uses many points to identify the shape of a whole pitch period, tracking the entire shape of successive waveforms. The pitch period is calculated using mathematical autocorrelation of the shape and length of successive waveforms across cycles, with interpolation between samples to detect variability or waveform deviations. Waveform matching appears to be more valid because it is resistant to error from fluctuations in peak amplitude or axis crossing.[11,35,42] In acoustic analysis, any acoustic measures that rely on pitch detection will be susceptible to mathematical error whenever the pitch period cannot be detected reliably.

Fundamental Frequency

Once the pitch period (T) is detected, then fundamental frequency (F0) can be calculated from the reciprocal (F0 = 1/T). Fundamental frequency is the rate of vibration of the vocal folds and is expressed in hertz (Hz) or cycles per second. Recall that fundamental frequency is the acoustic measure of an audioperceptual correlate, pitch. Several frequency measures are useful in assessing vocal function. The mean fundamental frequency can be measured during sustained vowels or extracted from connected speech. Fundamental frequency range measures the highest and lowest pitch a patient can produce. A large range may indicate better vocal flexibility. For example, patients with vocal

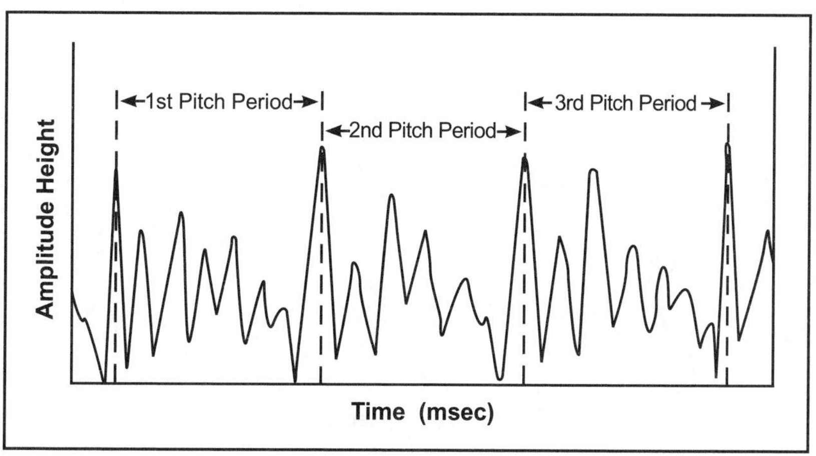

FIGURE 6–2. Fundamental frequency. Detecting fundamental period in an acoustic waveform using the peak picking method.

nodules often exhibit increased fundamental frequency and frequency range following successful rehabilitation.

When comparing fundamental frequencies across time, recall that the hertz units are scaled exponentially. For example, the perceptual difference in pitch between 200 and 400 Hz is far greater than the perceptual difference between 600 and 800 Hz. Therefore, it is misleading to compare the absolute change in hertz; rather it is best to report both pre- and posttreatment values. A better approach is to normalize the hertz value to notes on the musical scale, so they can be expressed as a number of notes, or semitones.[1] Finally, consider that fundamental frequency does covary with intensity, so clinicians should always control the intensity when measuring fundamental frequency production. Other factors that will affect fundamental frequency include the speech sample (sustained vowel or connected speech) and the vowel type (high or low). Most protocols recommend multiple trials to determine the stability of repeated productions and to establish a consistent baseline for future measures.[38–40]

Intensity

Vocal intensity (I0), the acoustic correlate of loudness, is referenced to sound pressure level (SPL), measured on the logarithmic decibel (dB) scale, and is represented on the acoustic waveform by amplitude height (Figure 6–3).

Both habitual intensity and intensity range (maximum and minimum) are useful clinical measures of vocal function, reflecting vocal fold adduction and phase closure. Intensity measurements can be made with a number of different instruments, including sound level meters, acoustic analysis programs, and some aerodynamic measurement devices. Certain recording artifacts may confound intensity measurement, including ambient noise or an inconsistent mouth-to-microphone distance. Other technical problems may interfere if the microphone or sound card has a limited dynamic range that is not calibrated for the full range of vocal loudness (eg, from <60 dB to over 100 dB SPL).[5,11,22–24] As for all acoustic measures, clinicians must adopt a standard, well-

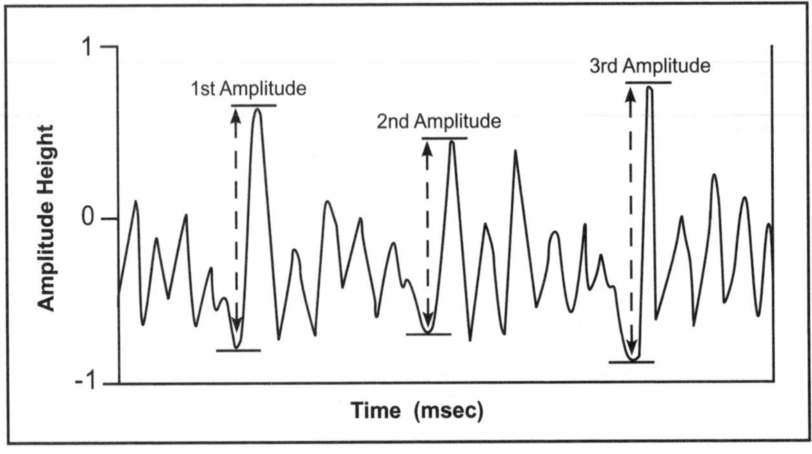

FIGURE 6–3. Intensity. Measuring amplitude height in an acoustic waveform.

monitored elicitation protocol to minimize error. The speech sample should include both habitual and maximal speech tasks, such as sustained vowels at softest possible loudness, shouting "Hey!" as loudly as possible, and connected speech at habitual loudness. Clinician models and multiple trials may be needed to ensure a true "minimum" or "maximum" loudness effort.

Voice Range Profile, Phonetogram, and Physiologic Frequency Range of Phonation

The voice range profile (VRP) (Plate 26), the phonetogram, and the physiologic frequency range of phonation (PFRP) are 3 names given to a similar clinical task that assesses both fundamental frequency and intensity at an individual's absolute minimum and maximum capabilities.[43–46] A patient produces his or her lowest fundamental frequency at minimum loudness, followed by the same frequency at maximum loudness, and continues up the frequency range to the absolute highest production. Many software programs now provide semiautomatic cue tones, semitone by semitone, which the patient matches. The patient's minimum and maximum intensity for each frequency are plotted on a matrix, with frequency on the horizontal axis and intensity on the vertical axis.

The resulting plot is an ellipse-shaped frequency-intensity profile, with dimensions expressed in semitones. Collecting the complete VRP can be time consuming and fatiguing, so some patients receive an abbreviated protocol. However, the complete profile is a thorough description of the patient's physiologic limits of frequency and intensity, especially useful for monitoring vocal range in professional voice users.[1,3,5,43–46] The speech range profile (SRP) is a briefer alternative protocol that constructs a frequency and intensity contour based on a short reading passage. Rather than accessing physiologic limits, the SRP measures habitual frequency and intensity ranges. The SRP has been proposed as a viable screening tool for discriminating normal and dysphonic speakers.[47]

Perturbation Measures

Perturbation is defined as the cycle-to-cycle variability in a signal and can only be measured from sustained or extracted vowel segments. Two common perturbation measures are jitter (cycle-to-cycle variation in frequency) and shimmer (cycle-to-cycle variation in amplitude). There are many different mathematical calculations for jitter and shimmer, usually specified by 3 general parameters[7,8,11]:

1. Length of the voice analysis window, as perturbation measures can be calculated in either short- or long-term averages.
2. Absolute or relative measurement units, as perturbation measures can be reported as an absolute amount, a ratio, or a percentage of the whole voice segment.
3. Statistical emphasis, as perturbation measures are reported as means (eg, central tendency) and coefficients of variation (eg, variability).

There is no agreement among voice laboratory users about optimal perturbation measures. Although improvements in technical capabilities have made it easier to capture normal and disordered acoustic waveforms reliably for acoustic perturbation analysis, this lack of comparable and agreed upon normative measures has impeded cross-comparison of studies conducted in different sites with different equipment.[11,25,35,36,48]

To improve technical standards in acoustic analysis, a group of voice scientists, acoustic engineers, product developers, and clinicians produced a summary statement (National Center for Voice and Speech, 1995) of recommendations for measuring vocal pitch, perturbation, and other acoustic analyses.[11] Algorithms are based on assumptions of a quasiperiodic, stable sound source, but disordered voices certainly may violate that premise. To alleviate this artifact, voice waveforms can be inspected visually and classified as type I, II, or III, based on their suitability for acoustic perturbation analysis. Type I waveforms are quasiperiodic, mostly continuous, and contain a single cluster of dominant fundamental frequency values. Clinically, type I voice usually represents a normal voice or a mild impairment that does not include obvious perceptual deviations or distortions. Type I voice is acceptable for perturbation analysis.[11] Type II waveforms display random or periodic modulations that fluctuate too much to allow an acoustic analysis program to detect a single, recurring fundamental frequency. This aperiodicity or variability in the waveform may result in either multiple or intermittent fundamental frequencies. Clinically, this type II signal can arise from both disordered productions (such as glottal fry, vocal tremor, intermittent aphonia, or roughness) or from intentional modulations (such as vibrato). Type II voice precludes reliable acoustic perturbation analysis because of excessive noise, variations, and aperiodicity. Therefore, type II voice analysis should be limited to spectral analysis or other visual displays.[11] Finally, type III waveforms display random, aperiodic signals that have no identifiable fundamental frequency pattern whatsoever. Clinically, these voices are severely impaired and contain large noisy components caused by breathiness, roughness, or a combination of perceptual distortions. Type III voices are not suitable for instrumental acoustic analysis and can only be assessed using audioperceptual judgments.[11]

Other clinical guidelines for acoustic recording protocols emerged from the consensus conference and from methodological research. For example, acoustic assessment should include multiple trials to consider individual variability and establish a stable baseline performance; the number of trials must represent the speech behavior adequately. Occasionally, a patient's first trial will be too loud or too high pitched because of unfamiliarity with the task or test anxiety. The voice pathologist must observe the patient's production carefully to elicit representative productions and monitor the interactions of fundamental frequency, intensity, and perturbation values, as each can influence the others. For example, frequency rises with increased intensity; perturbation values decrease with increased fundamental frequency, and all vary with the vowel selection.[38,40,49,50] Certainly, the clinician cannot hold frequency and intensity constant in all clinical measures, but these values should be documented to help account for differences in pre- and posttreatment comparisons. Sustained or extracted vowel samples are the most reliable speech tasks for acoustic analysis, but long-term averaged samples from connected speech are also possible, although they appear to be less reliable in discriminating pathologic voice.[51] In both conditions, the length of window analysis must be sufficient to preserve the validity of acoustic measurement.[34,35] Improvements in perturbation values across a pre- and posttreatment period are viewed favorably, but it is impossible to assign a direct association between any single perturbation measure and perceptual changes in voice quality. Consequently, perturbation measures, like all instrumental data, should be interpreted in context with other clinical impressions and cross-validating data.

Signal (or Harmonic)-to-Noise Ratios

Acoustic analysis programs often derive some measure of the ratio of periodic or harmonic signal energy to the aperiodic or noise energy in the voice waveform. Normal voices are mostly periodic and have high signal or harmonic energy. Dysphonic voices have large aperiodic or noisy components, due to roughness, which reflects aperiodic vocal fold vibration, or breathiness, which reflects turbulent noise. A signal (or harmonic)-to-noise ratio captures the relative contributions of all periodic to aperiodic (noise) energy in the speech signal. Thus, a high signal (or harmonic)-to-noise ratio (eg, SNR or HNR) represents a high-quality periodic signal, as is common in normal voice quality.[6,7,9] Dysphonic voices exhibit greater amounts of random spectral noise, and thus, a lower signal (or harmonic)-to-noise ratio. Some calculations invert the ratio and assign noise or aperiodic energy to the numerator and periodic or harmonic signal energy to the denominator (ie, noise-to-harmonic ratio, or NHR). For these calculations, normal voice should produce a low NHR to reflect the relatively small amount of noise in the overall signal. SNR, HNR, and NHR specify the magnitude of separation between the periodic or harmonic energy to the magnitude of noise energy and may be calculated using sustained tones or connected speech. Some ratios are expressed in decibels, others as a percentage.[7] As with other acoustic measures, this variability limits comparisons across laboratories, so its clinical value is strongest when applied to clinical pre- and posttreatment probes.

Spectral Analysis

Spectral analysis is useful to assess the interaction between the glottal sound source (vocal folds) and supraglottic (vocal tract) influences.[6,7,21] A sound spectrogram is a graphic display of the speech signal, plotting frequency and intensity in the time domain. Time is represented on the horizontal axis, frequency on the vertical axis, and sound intensity by the gray or color scale.

The spectrogram (Figure 6–4) displays both the glottal and supraglottal influences, such as vowel type, voiced and voiceless transitions, aspirate noise, or other coarticulatory features. Both formant frequency energy (concentrations of harmonic energy in the vocal tract) and noise components (aperiodicity, transient or turbulent noise) of speech production are presented in this 3-dimensional scale. The lowest energy band always represents the fundamental, with formant energies in the higher frequencies above. The sound spectrogram

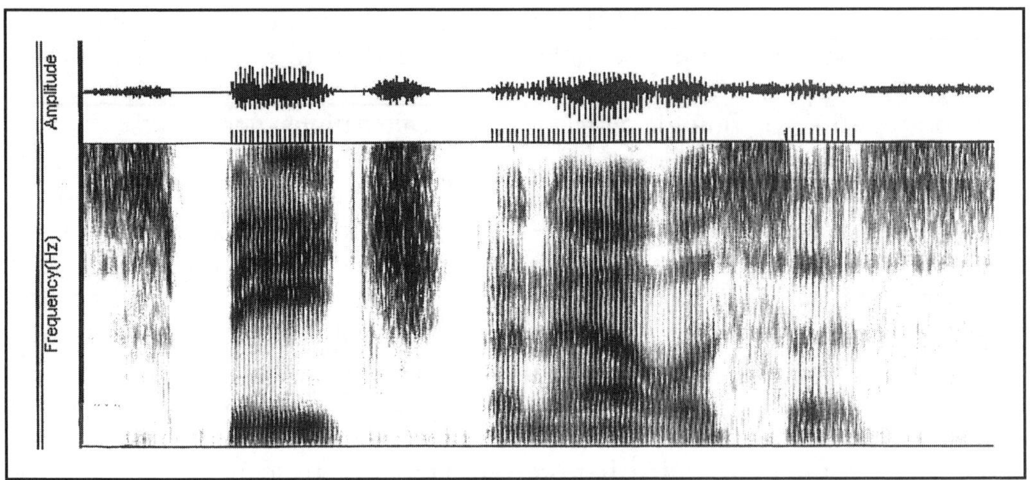

FIGURE 6–4. Wideband spectrogram. Upper waveform displays the acoustic signal for the sample phrase "speech analysis," with the spectrogram displayed. Note the formant concentrations (*darker horizontal bands*) produced during the vowel segments.

can be displayed in wide or narrow bandwidths. In wideband spectrograms (which include most of the harmonic spectrum), the fundamental and first formant may be too close to separate visually. Narrowband spectrograms (which exclude higher frequencies) are useful for observing the spectral energy of the fundamental in detail. The stronger the formant energy, the darker the gray scale bands; lighter or diffuse gray bands suggest a noisier signal and poorly identified formant energies. In this manner, the spectrogram provides a visual representation of the harmonic-to-noise ratio of a speech production.[6,7,21]

A second form of spectral analysis is the line spectrum. Where the sound spectrogram displays the acoustic spectrum across time, the line spectrum is a plot in the frequency domain. The spectrum plots all harmonic energies (frequencies) at a single time point on the horizontal axis, with amplitude on the vertical axis.

Because a line spectrum (Figure 6–5) displays harmonics at only one moment in time, it is useful to compare multiple spectra to observe changes in formant patterns across a speech sample.[6,7,21] Advanced spectral analysis routines, such as fast Fourier transform (FFT) and linear predictive coding (LPC), have been applied to line spectra to identify formant characteristics of the vocal tract. FFT analysis achieves this formant analysis by dividing the complex speech waveform into individual harmonics. These harmonic amplitudes are plotted in a series of adjacent peaks that represent individual amplitude heights across all resonant frequencies in that single moment of speech production. LPC analysis produces a smoothed trajectory line above the FFT peaks that identifies the vocal tract formants created by the sum of individual harmonics. The LPC analysis is useful in identifying the major formant energy concentrations at any given point in the speech sample. For both FFT and LPC analyses, microprocessing capabilities have increased the speed and accessibility of spectral processing. Nonetheless,

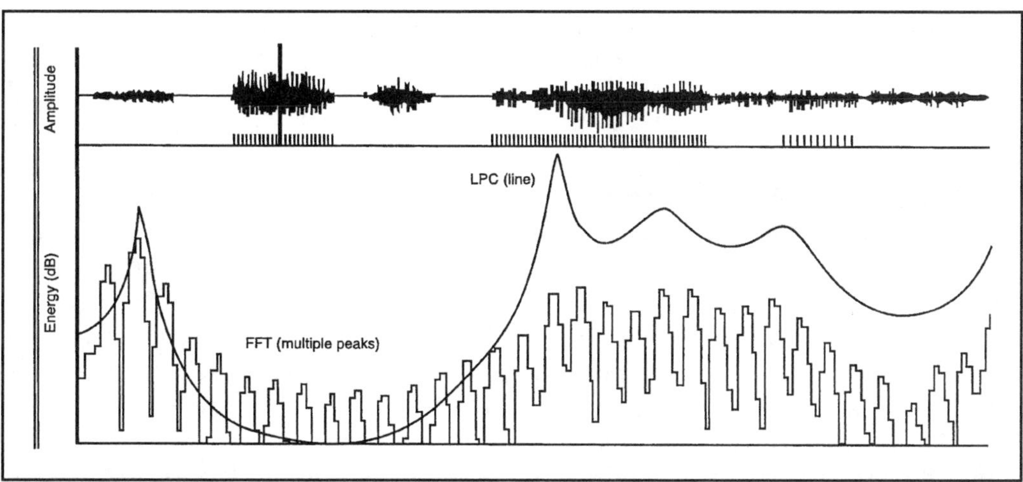

FIGURE 6–5. Same acoustic waveform as that shown in Figure 6–4, with a line spectrum displayed below. LPC and FFT formant tracings correspond to a single spectral moment extracted from the midpoint of the /i/ vowel (*see vertical cursor bar on acoustic waveform*).

as with other forms of acoustic analysis, FFT and LPC routines are highly sensitive to noise and other signal artifacts. To avoid error, care must be taken to ensure that a clean, undistorted signal is presented to the system for analysis.[6,7,21]

A third form of voice spectral analysis that has been explored is the cepstrum. Recall that a Fourier transformation changes a spectrogram (in the time domain) to a spectrum (in the frequency domain). A second Fourier transformation on the spectrum converts the plot to the quefrency domain (where quefrency = 1/frequency, or the inverse of frequency). This mathematic transformation alters the spectrum plot of all harmonic amplitude peaks to a cepstrum plot, which emphasizes the peaks of the strongest harmonics, including the fundamental frequency. One measure, cepstral peak prominence (CPP), compares the amplitude height of the cepstral peak to the linear regression of all frequencies in the voice signal (Figure 6–6). These cepstral peaks represent the magnitude of harmonic energy that rises above random aperiodic background noise in the voice signal. The sharper the cepstral peak prominence, the stronger is the periodic energy in the voice signal. Conversely, very noisy voice signals will have a flat cepstral peak prominence.[52–54] Moreover, because cepstral measures are based on peak-to-average calculations, they do not rely on pitch detection algorithms, as do acoustic perturbation measures (eg, jitter and shimmer), and can be used when the fundamental frequency cannot be identified accurately (eg, type II and III voices). A number of variations on cepstral analysis have been explored, and none has emerged as an agreed-on approach to measuring dysphonic voice quality. But, cepstral analysis has been shown to correlate with perceptual judgments of breathy and rough voices.[32,52–55] Furthermore, a recent meta-analysis of the acoustic analysis of voice literature revealed that measures of the amplitude of the cepstral peak prominence in relation to extraneous cepstral components surfaced as a generally robust acoustic measure that strongly correlated with listener judgments of dysphonia severity.[56]

Cepstral Spectral Index of Dysphonia (CSID)

Recently, an acoustic analysis tool known as the Cepstral Spectral Index of Dysphonia (CSID) (KayPentax, Lincoln Park, NJ) has been developed which automatically provides an objective estimate of dysphonia severity produc-ed via multiple regression formulae that incorporate measures from both spectral and cepstral analyses. While spectral analysis provides information regarding the component frequencies of a complex waveform (like voice) and their relative amplitudes, the cepstrum graphically displays the extent to which the dominant rahmonic (an anagram of harmonic, the cepstral peak often associated with the vocal fundamental frequency) is individualized and emerges out of the background noise level (Figure 6–6). In a variety of studies, Awan and colleagues showed that CSID measures correlated well with audio-perceptual judgments of dysphonia severity across heterogeneous voice qualities and severities in both connected speech and sustained vowels.[57–59] Thus, it appears to be a promising tool not only to objectively discriminate normal from disordered voices, but to also track change after treatment. Unlike time-based measures (ie, jitter and shimmer), the CSID does not require a quasiperiodic voice signal to permit valid analysis; thus it is extremely attractive as a potentially objective treatment outcomes measure.

AERODYNAMIC MEASURES

Two aerodynamic measurements, subglottic pressure and transglottic flow, assess physiologic vocal function indi-

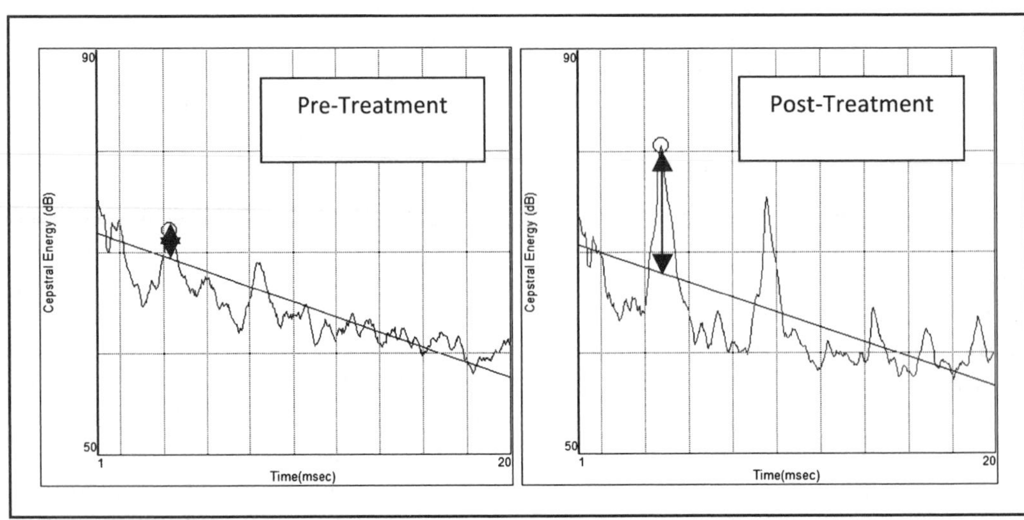

FIGURE 6–6. Two cepstral frames from a female patient's sustained vowel production, before and after voice therapy.

rectly and noninvasively. Both measures reveal information about the laryngeal valving mechanism, based on the interchange of pressure and flow during vocal fold vibration.[1,3,4,6–8,60–64] Additional derived measures that integrate pressure and flow in a single mathematic ratio have also been examined, such as glottal power, laryngeal resistance, vocal efficiency, and others.[1,6–8,65–68] Like acoustic measures, aerodynamic measures are usually recorded during a consistent speech task designed to standardize (pressure or flow) behaviors across individuals and capture transient changes in speech pressure or flow reliably. Some tasks probe minimal or maximal performance; others assess typical or mean activity. For example, phonation threshold pressure is defined as the minimum subglottal pressure needed to initiate vocal fold vibration, measured at the quietest possible initiation of voicing.[69–70] In contrast, transglottal flow can be captured during either sustained vowels or longer windows of connected speech and in different pitch and loudness contexts.[6,7,60–64] Figure 6–7 displays an aerodynamic recording system for measurement of airflow during voice production.

Aerodynamic measures are subject to the same constraints as other instruments, including technological error, intrasubject variability, and difficulty comparing similar measures collected using diverse recording protocols.[61,64,71–73] Nonetheless, measures of intraoral pressure, transglottal flow, and derived measures have been used to discriminate normal and disordered vocal function, assess disorder severity, and even indicate the etiology of dysphonia. For example, an excessive average flow rate usually reflects an underlying glottal incompetence, whereas increased subglottic pressure measures are often associated with hyperfunctional voice

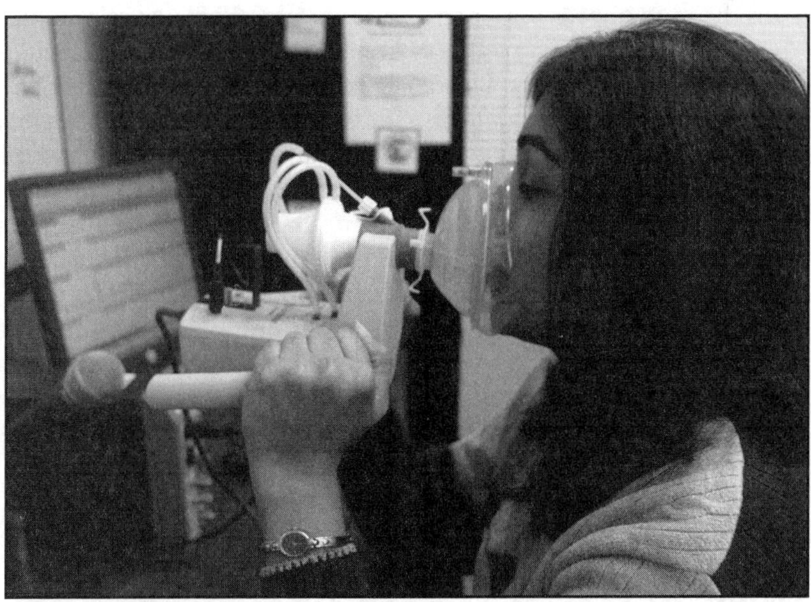

FIGURE 6–7. An aerodynamic recording system for measuring airflow and pressure during speech production.

use patterns.[60,71] When aerodynamic measures provide a real-time visual display, clinicians can also use them as primary feedback tools in behavioral therapy. Most pressure and flow measures are reported in standard units that can be referenced to normative data and (assuming careful calibration to avoid artifact) allow comparison across instruments and clinical sites.[58,60,67–69]

Calibration

Aerodynamic equipment that measures pressure and flow requires regular calibration, due to fluctuating environmental influences, such as atmospheric pressure and temperature. Two simple instruments measure static pressure and static flow for calibration. The pressure meter is called a U-tube manometer and consists of a glass tube shaped into a long U standing upright with a calibrated index visible on its side. The tube is filled with water or mercury, depending on the type of pressure measurement needed. Pressure is applied to one side of the U, and the displaced amount of liquid is read directly off the contralateral side in appropriate units (cm H_2O or mm Hg).[7] Airflow rate can be similarly measured, using a rotameter, which is a tall glass tube with a port at its base and a small float inside. When airflow is blown into the port, the float rises to the level that corresponds with the flow rate, which can be read directly (in mL or cc per second) from the index on its side. Because these two devices can only measure static sustained pressure and flow, they are not clinically applicable to rapid and transient voice and speech measures. However, when used with a compressed air source, they serve as external calibration measures for pressure and flow instruments.[7]

Pressure, Flow, Resistance, and Ohm's Law

Instruments that measure speech aerodynamics exploit the integral and predictable relationship between pressure, flow, and resistance. Recall that molecules in fluid (air or water) will always flow from a region of higher density (ie, tight, compressed) to lower density (ie, more space). Imagine 100 hot and crowded people huddled together in a small room. Suddenly, a small door opens to the outside. People start pushing toward the door, trying to get outside. The flow of people spreading out into a wider space mimics the activity of compressed molecules or electrons; if given an outlet, no matter how small, molecules will always move from regions of high concentration to regions of lower concentration. This molecular activity is *flow*; when electrons do the same, it is called *current*. Current (for electrons) and flow (for molecules) are analogous. Resistance is the impediment to flow, whether molecular or electronic. In the crowded room, the outflow of people is limited by the physical constraints of the walls and small door (resistance), which pose a restriction to the natural tendency of people who wish to spread out.

Flow (and current) will only occur when there is an asymmetry in the molecular (or electron) concentration (low versus high). The concentration difference between two points creates a driving pressure and a potential for molecular flow. In aerodynamic terms, this asymmetry is represented as differential pressure, which is defined as the difference in pressure between two points, and thus the potential to do work. In the electronic form, this potential is called *voltage*. Consider again the image of crowded people pushing up against the door jam, trying to ease through the small opening. The pressure just inside the doorway is far greater than the pressure just outside of it, where unconstrained people wander about freely. The relative pressure inside (p1) versus outside (p2) is a differential pressure, created by the flow asymmetry on either side of a known resistance, in our example, the walls around the small doorway.

The relationship between differential pressure, flow, and resistance has been clarified in the electrical principle known as Ohm's law, which states that:

Voltage [E] is equal to Current [I] times the Resistance [R]

or E = IR

Restated in aerodynamic terms:

Differential Pressure [p1 versus p2] is equal to Flow [V] times the Resistance to flow [R]

or [p1 − p2] = VR

This means that if we know the value of the two separate pressure points (p1 and p2) and the value of the resistance, we can solve the equation algebraically to calculate the magnitude of flow:

V = [p1 − p2]/R

See Figure 6–8 for a visual graphic of this relationship between pressure, flow, and resistance.

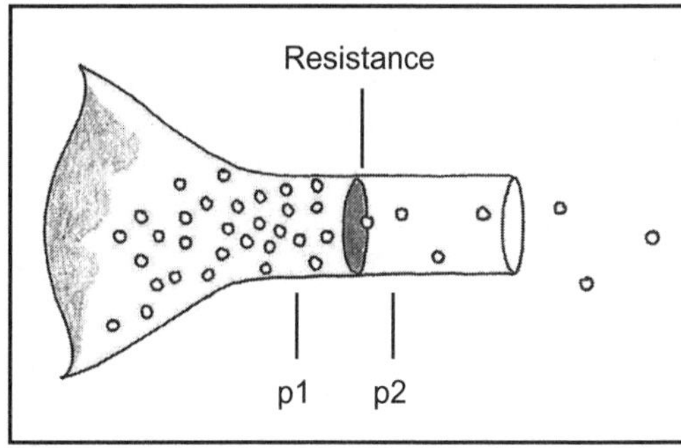

FIGURE 6–8. Flow, resistance, and differential pressure. As flow passes through a known resistance, it creates a pressure change (p1 versus p2).

Airflow Equipment

The most common airflow device is the pneumotachograph, which uses the principle of differential pressure across a known resistance to estimate flow rate. A pneumotachograph is essentially a metal tube with a mechanical resistance (usually a wire mesh screen or a series of small tubes) inside. As airflow is blown through the tube, differential pressures are measured at sites directly upstream (p1) and downstream (p2) from the resistance. Recall from Ohm's law that flow is calculated using the differential pressure divided by the resistance. Flow divided by time equals flow rate. Another device used to measure airflow is the warm wire anemometer. Flow passes over a warm wire in this instrument, cooling the wire and changing its electrical resistance with the change in temperature. The change in resistance in the wire is proportional to the flow, and flow rate can be calculated from that change.[7,64]

To measure airflow, some airflow mouthpiece or face mask must be coupled to the equipment. Flow masks must be airtight to avoid measurement error, but this creates an artificial sensation of "backpressure," which may cause the patient to perform differently. Occasionally, patients require coaching to produce a natural and comfortable voice sample that represents free speech conditions. Rothenberg developed a mask with wire mesh screen vents that serve as the resistance.[60] The pressure drop is calculated from pressure inside the mask relative to atmospheric pressure (outside the mask), and the signal can be inverse filtered to remove vocal tract influence and reveal the glottal airflow waveform. The circumferential venting also alleviates the backpressure artifact and provides the speaker with more natural acoustic feedback. Patient comfort and compliance are critical to eliciting as natural speech as possible, repeated in enough trials to achieve a stable baseline.

Flow Measurement

Two basic airflow measurements are used in speech production: average flow rate and flow volume. To measure average flow, the airflow mask or mouthpiece is secured firmly. The patient takes a comfortable breath and produces a steady vowel at normal pitch and loudness for at least 5 to 10 seconds. If a real-time display is available, the clinician can inspect the pattern of average flow, whether stable, falling, or irregular. In normal speakers, average flow rates are approximately 80 to 200 mL/s. Patients with respiratory compromise or neurologic disease may exhibit unstable or irregular patterns of average flow. Patients with severely hyperfunctional voice or glottal fry will demonstrate very minimal airflow rates, as low as 10 to 15 mL/s. Conversely, patients with primary glottal incompetence, such as vocal fold paralysis, may generate average airflow rates as high as 400 to 600 cc/s, accompanied by short vowel durations.

Volume is the general term describing the total amount of flow used during a given speech task. Volume is generally measured in liter or milliliter units. When total volume of airflow is measured during a maximum sustained vowel production, the resulting measure is usually called *phonatory volume*. Note that this measure is slightly different from vital capacity, a respiratory measure of the volume of air exhaled during a maximal forced exhalation. In both measures, the patient begins the task by breathing in as deeply and completely as possible. To measure vital capacity, the patient exhales as rapidly and completely as possible, while the volume of air is recorded. For phonatory volume, the volume of air is measured during the sustained vowel, held as long as possible. For adults, normal phonatory volume amounts range from 1500 mL to nearly 4000 mL, depending on the patient's gender and body size. This technique allows a gross estimate of a patient's breath supply for voice and speech, but it is not an accurate estimate of pulmonary function or other respiratory measures, such as tidal volume (the amount of air in an average breath). Because the amount of air needed for connected speech and voice is very small relative to total lung capacity, most voice patients will not need comprehensive pulmonary function testing to verify sufficient breath support for speech. However, patients who have respiratory compromise or obvious shortness of breath should be referred for qualified pulmonary function testing.

Subglottal Air Pressure Measurement

Pressure is defined as the force per unit area, acting perpendicular to the area. In phonation, respiratory (subglottal) pressure acts as a force building up below the adducted vocal folds, rising until it overcomes vocal fold resistance and sets the folds into oscillation. Subglottal air pressure is the power supply, but vocal fold valving characteristics, such as tissue viscosity and adductory closure force, will dictate how much subglottal effort is needed to initiate phonation. Actual subglottal pressure can only be measured directly through an invasive procedure that requires a needle puncture into the trachea directly below the vocal folds. The needle is attached to a pressure transducer that calculates units of tracheal pressure directly. However, this technique is never used clinically.[7]

Instead, a noninvasive, indirect approach has been used to estimate subglottal pressure clinically. This method measures intraoral pressure during production of the unvoiced bilabial plosive consonant /p/. Theoretically, this intraoral pressure is a feasible analog to subglottal pressure if the following assumptions are met:

- Oral /p/ plosive constriction creates a momentary airtight seal, with a continuous opening from the lungs to the lips. (Note that velopharyngeal incompetence [leak] would violate this assumption.)
- Vocal folds are open so that the oral pressure produced in the plosive production is equivalent to the tracheal driving pressure that would be available to set the vocal folds in oscillation.[64,65]

Using this intraoral method, subglottic pressure is estimated from repeated production of an unvoiced plosive + vowel syllable (eg, /pi/). An oral tube placed between the closed lips and connected to a pressure transducer records the intraoral pressure. Usually, dual channel recordings will allow simultaneous airflow measurements to verify that during pressure peaks, airflow is at zero (Figure 6–9).

Procedures for recording intraoral pressure are specific and must be followed carefully. The oral catheter is sealed behind the lips but not occluded by the tongue or by saliva. Tube length and diameter of the tube can influence the pressure measurement, so it is important to follow equipment guidelines. The velum must be closed, and if nasal air leak is suspected, it is appropriate to use nose clips. Clinicians must model and monitor the rate and loudness of the /pi/ syllable train, to keep elicitation cues stable and constant. If the syllable train is produced too quickly, pressure peaks may be artificially lower than actual driving pressure. If /pi/ productions are too loud, pressure peaks may be artificially high. When these considerations are met, the peak intraoral pressure recorded during the plosive /p/ production is a reasonable estimate of tracheal pressure.[65] Currently, this is the most feasible clinical approach to collecting subglottal pressure data.

Phonation Threshold Pressure

A special application of subglottal pressure estimates has gained increasing attention in clinical voice pathology. Titze first defined the concept of phonation threshold pressure (PTP), which is the minimal driving pressure required to set the vocal folds into oscillation.[6,69,70] PTP is thought to be a potentially important predictor of the structure and function of the vocal fold

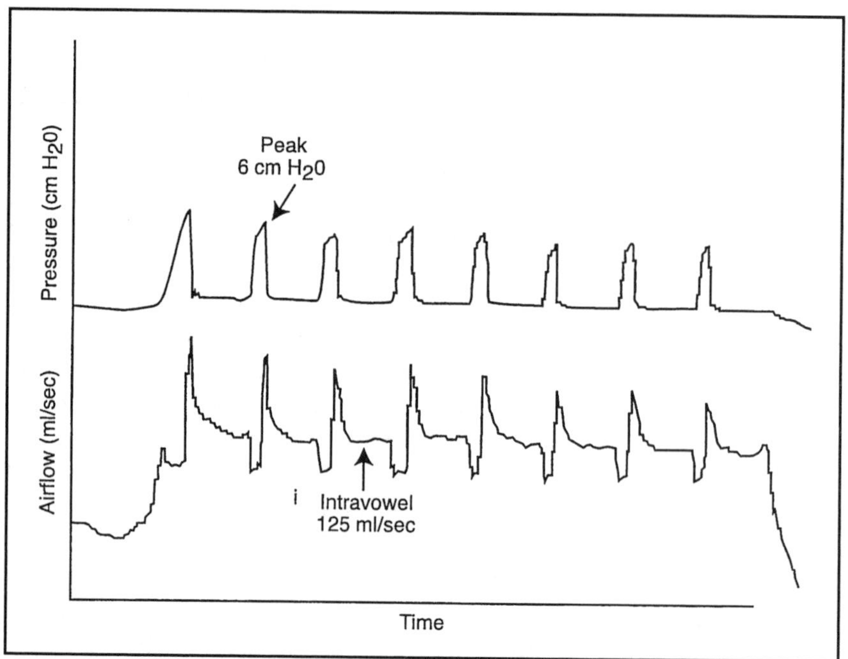

FIGURE 6–9. Simultaneous pressure (*upper trace*) and airflow (*lower trace*) recordings in a repeated /pi/ task. Note the reciprocal timing of pressure and flow peaks. Pressure peaks just before the aspirate airflow peak for /p/. During vocalic /i/, pressure is zero, while mean flow rate is quasilevel.

vibratory capabilities. The measure has been estimated indirectly using intraoral pressure during a repeated syllable /pi/ production at the minimal loudness possible for phonation. Titze has defined the theoretical relationship between phonation threshold pressure and the presumed vocal fold tissue properties that affect PTP.[6,69] To summarize, phonation threshold pressure is affected by the following:

- Prephonatory glottal width
- Thickness of the vocal fold edge
- Amount of tissue damping (gradual loss of oscillation amplitude)
- Mucosal wave velocity[6,70]

Theoretically, the healthier are the vocal folds, the lower PTP needed to power vibration. In conditions most favorable for decreased PTP, the prephonatory glottal width is small, the vocal fold edge is relaxed and rounded, tissue damping is minimal (ie, vocal fold flexibility is great), and mucosal wave velocity is decreased. For most speakers, these conditions for lower PTP are present during low fundamental frequency voice. In general terms, PTP can be interpreted as a measure of the effort needed to begin phonation. PTP appears to correlate directly with changes in vocal fold hydration, whether systemic or superficial.[74–78] PTP increases when subjects have undergone "dehydrating" conditions, but decreases again after rehydration is accomplished. This PTP effect is even more prominent in individuals with chronic vocal fatigue, or in normal speakers who have undertaken vocally fatiguing tasks. The fact that PTP increases with fatigue suggests that the measure is sensitive to even transient increases in vocal fold edema, represented by increases in tissue viscosity and vocal fold damping in Titze's model. Because individuals with voice disorders frequently report greater effort in "turning on the voice," this measure may prove to be an important clinical probe for assessing effects of treatment or phonosurgical results.[74–78]

Laryngeal Resistance

Derived measures that combine measures of pressure and flow in a ratio or product have also been examined.[1,6,7,65] Laryngeal resistance is the quotient of peak intraoral pressure (estimated from production of an unvoiced plosive /p/) divided by the peak flow rate (measured from production of a vowel /i/) produced in a repeated train of /pi/ syllables. This measurement is intended to reflect the overall resistance of the glottis and serve as an estimate of the laryngeal valving function, whether too tight (hyperfunctional), too loose (hypofunctional), or normal.[65–68] Laryngeal resistance and other derived ratios (eg, glottal power) have been used in experimental settings to examine the relationship between pressure and flow in vocal fold vibration. However, because derived measures integrate 2 covarying measures, their magnitude can be difficult to interpret without reference to the individual contributions of pressure and flow. For example, increased laryngeal resistance values might be attributable to excessive subglottal pressure, insufficient transglottal flow, or both.

Inverse Filter

Inverse filtering is a special analysis technique that can be applied to either acoustic or aerodynamic signals for specialized analysis of the glottal waveform (Figure 6–10).

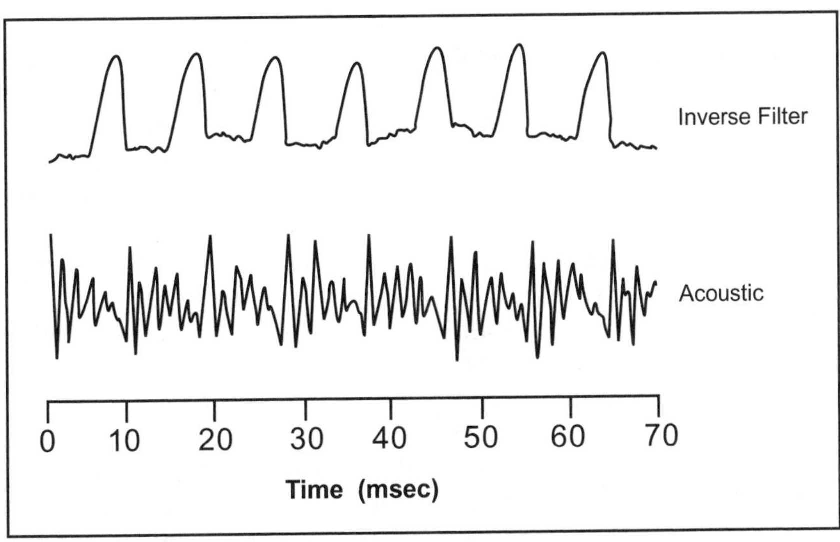

FIGURE 6–10. Sample acoustic waveform (*lower trace*) with simultaneous inverse filter waveform (*upper trace*).

Because all speech signals (acoustic and aerodynamic) are measured at the mouth, the resulting waveform is a product of 2 components: the glottal sound source and the resonance characteristic from the vocal tract. Inverse filtering is a technique that theoretically isolates these two components. Through mathematical filtering, the effects of the supraglottic (vocal tract) influences can be removed to reveal the real-time patterns of the glottal acoustic or airflow waveform as it alternates from open to closed phases with vocal fold vibration. Measures of interest often are the slope or rate of waveform opening and closing, because the shape and timing of the inverse filtered waveform directly reflect the vocal fold vibratory patterns. Inverse filtering techniques yield a wide range of possible calculations, including ratios of opening or closing time to the total period and shape changing features, such as waveform minima or peaks.[79]

One aerodynamic measure, maximum flow declination rate (MFDR), refers to the negative slope of the glottal airway waveform.[80,81] MFDR correlates strongly with intensity, because it relates to vibratory amplitude and glottal phase closure, as is needed for loud productions. The steeper the MFDR slope, the higher is the vocal intensity. Men, women, and children appear to make different physiologic adjustments during soft, habitual, and loud productions, and MFDR exhibits these gender- and age-based differences.[82] One analysis compared 78 different computations of the inverse filtered glottal source spectrum to determine which measure best represented shape and slope of glottal pulses. Not surprisingly, there was considerable overlap among the various glottal source spectrum measures, but none emerged as strong predictors of variation in spectral slope, nor of perceptual voice quality.[83] Inverse filtering separates glottal and vocal tract influences from real-time measures of vocal function, such as acoustics, airflow, and electroglottography, but its applications warrant further investigation.

LARYNGEAL IMAGING

Laryngeal imaging provides more information about the severity and possible etiology of a voice disorder than other instrumental measures. This visible evidence of the laryngeal structure, movement, and function during voice and vegetative gestures surpasses other approaches to instrumental voice evaluation or remediation planning.[84–86] Current digital processing and laryngeal imaging capabilities allow the clinician to view and record images from flexible or rigid endoscopes on a monitor to provide a bigger, brighter, and longer look at the larynx which is available to compare with follow-up images. Three kinds of imaging techniques are used to assess voice disorders: stroboscopy, kymography, and high speed. Each has different advantages, limits, and interpretive power for voice pathologists who treat patients and scientists who study vocal function.[1–4,10,84]

Images from each device allow users to make visual perceptual judgments about vocal fold appearance, movement, and vibratory pattern and their associated impact on voice production. However, all endoscopic imaging techniques are limited to indirect visual perceptual measures of vocal function, observable only through the optic filter of a magnifying camera lens, light source, digital processor, and pixels on a monitor. Consequently, variables such as lighting, color, lens focus and angle, lens-to-object distance, and system resolution all contribute to the adequacy and accuracy of the resulting image.[87] Despite significant advances in digital imaging technology, visual artifacts and distortions are possible and must be prevented through careful operations such as focus and white balance.

Experience with laryngeal imaging has taught us that individual subject variability is large, so there is a critical learning curve to understanding what "normal" looks like. Moreover, all image interpretations involve visual perceptual judgments, subject to the same threats of bias and unreliability as other perceptual measures. Although it is easier to feel confident about visual perceptual judgments made on a bright, centered, magnified, and focused recording of a complete protocol with sufficiently long task samples, not every patient will be able to produce such a recording, due to anatomic limits, gag reflex, dysphonia severity, or lack of task compliance.[84] In the clinical setting, it is common for the professional to know the clinical history of the patient before interpreting the visual recording, which can also bias the visual judgments. Two strategies may alleviate this risk. First, a group strobe review opportunity allows other otolaryngology and voice pathology staff to view and interpret each other's recordings and confirm findings. Second, many image devices incorporate concurrent dual-channel recordings of acoustic (eg, frequency and intensity) and physiologic (eg, electroglottographic) measures, to cross-validate perceptual judgments of vocal fold movement and vibratory pattern with other physiologic measures (Figure 6–11).[88]

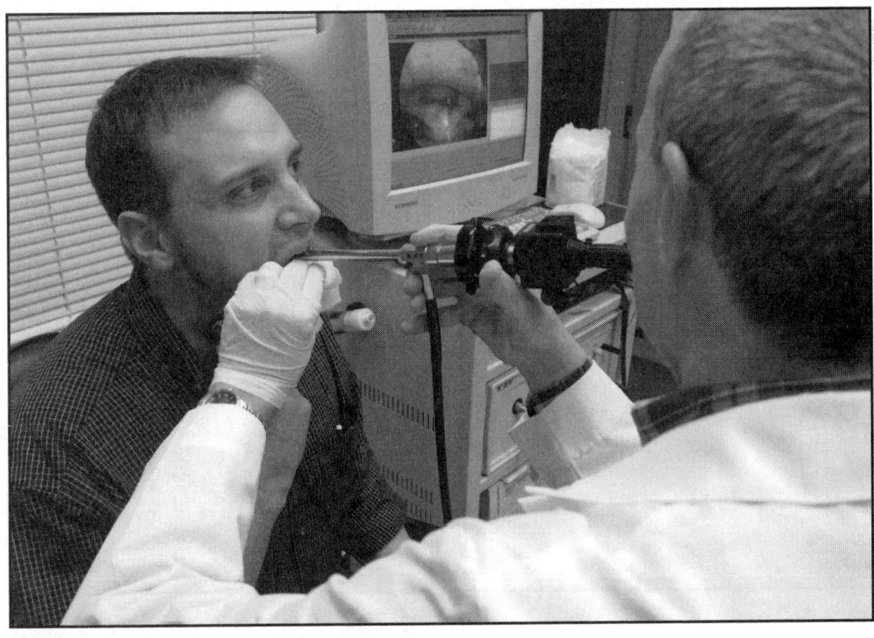

FIGURE 6–11. A stroboscopic unit used for laryngeal imaging.

Endoscopy

Three different endoscopes are used for laryngeal imaging. Two rigid scopes vary by angle of insertion. The 90-degree scope is inserted parallel to the floor; the 70-degree scope is canted downward onto the tongue. The flexible scope is inserted into the nasal passage and advanced until it drapes downward over the velum in the pharynx (Figures 6–12, 6–13, and 6–14).

Rigid endoscopy allows a close view of the larynx and vocal folds and supplies better lighting to the image because of larger fiberoptic bundles. But, to draw the epiglottis forward and view the vocal folds, the speech sample is limited to a sustained /i/ vowel, often produced at pitches higher than conversational connected speech and certainly in a posture unnatural for speech (eg, mouth open, tongue and neck extended). Rigid endoscopy avoids some of the optical artifacts common in flexible imaging because of its larger magnification and a stable lens-to-object distance and is advantageous whenever a complete view of the vocal folds (from anterior commissure to arytenoid cartilage) can be recorded. If the patient has a hypersensitive gag reflex, then the patient can be relaxed through coaching. The resulting vibratory image allows optimal views of the superior surface of the vocal folds, but it is never

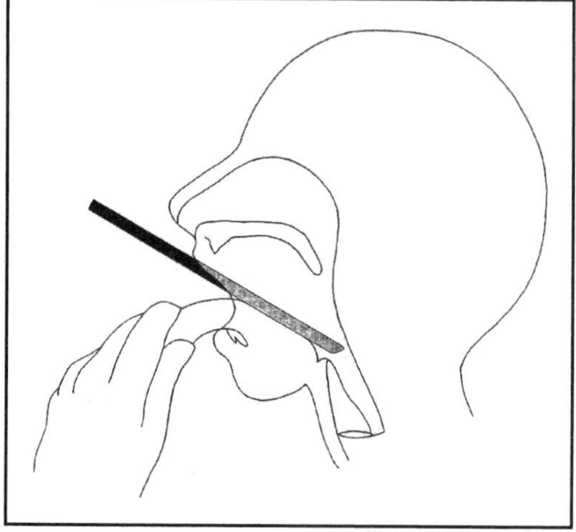

FIGURE 6–13. Seventy-degree endoscope position.

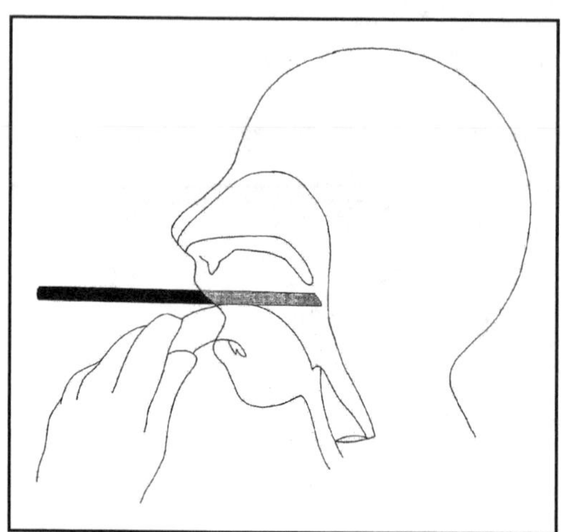

FIGURE 6–12. Ninety-degree endoscope position.

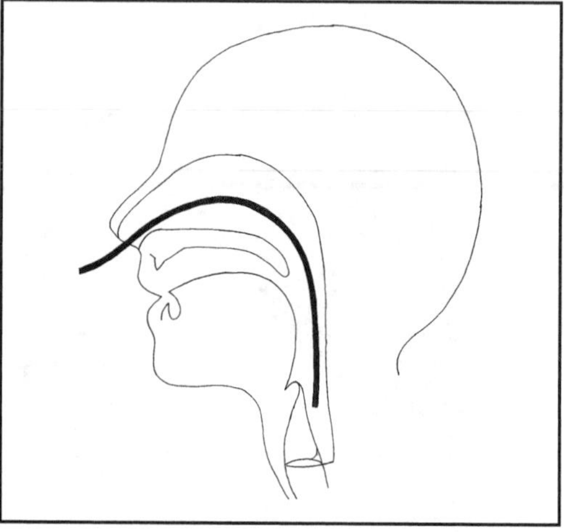

FIGURE 6–14. Flexible endoscope position.

fully representative of vibration during habitual speech. Task-based artifacts are an inherent limit of rigid endoscopy, but the tradeoff is a superior, stable view.[84]

Flexible endoscopy provides the opportunity for viewing the larynx during connected speech tasks and allows a broader view of the vocal tract and supraglottic region. But, it yields a darker image due to the smaller diameter of the fiberoptic light bundle, although new distal chip cameras and lighting filters improve this flaw. Flexible endoscopy is slightly more invasive than rigid endoscopy and is limited by disruptive vertical movements as the patient alters position of the velum or swallows. It is more difficult to achieve a stable image, especially during connected speech.[84,89,90] Nonetheless, patients often can make use of the onscreen image of the velum or vocal fold movements as a primary biofeedback treatment. In general, fiberoptic endoscopy is preferred whenever:

- Rigid endoscopy is not possible because of anatomic limits or patient tolerance.
- Connected speech, vocal tract movement, or velopharyngeal function is of special interest, as for patients with a motor speech disorder, cleft palate or velopharyngeal inadequacy, or professional voice users.
- Visual biofeedback of vocal fold, vocal tract, or velar movements would be a helpful adjunct to the treatment plan.

Approximately 5% to 10% of all patients may require intraoral topical anesthesia to suppress the gag reflex to tolerate the rigid examination. Topical anesthetic with or without lubrication and decongestant is used commonly in flexible endoscopy. The use of topical anesthesia does not alter the resulting visual image of the larynx,[91] but it should not be administered without medical oversight, including a standing order from a physician and in a setting that is prepared to handle the remote possibility of allergic complications.[84,92–95] The participation of speech-language pathologists in laryngeal endoscopy was clarified in a joint position statement approved by the American Speech-Language-Hearing Association (ASHA) and the American Academy of Otolaryngology-Head and Neck Surgery (Appendix 6–A).[92] Using rigid and flexible endoscopy is part of the speech-language pathology scope of practice and is included in ASHA's Preferred Practice Patterns for Speech Language Pathology (Appendix 6–B).[93] However, with this specialized practice come certain responsibilities that compel clinicians to seek appropriate academic preparation and technical competence before using these procedures independently. In 2004, ASHA's Special Interest Division 3 (Voice and Voice Disorders) prepared both a Vocal Tract Visualization and Imaging: Position Statement[94] and a comprehensive report of Knowledge and Skills for Speech Language Pathologists with Respect to Vocal Tract Visualization and Imaging[95] to advise voice pathologists who use these techniques. Both are available at http://www.asha.org/policy. These guidelines provide a thorough overview of criteria required to perform these procedures safely. Regardless of the instruments, setting, or techniques, it is universally recommended that voice pathologists receive mentored training with an experienced clinician, examining at least 20 normal subjects. This effort will instill confidence and ensure competence before attempting to examine a patient. The clinician and mentor must adhere to skill-based criteria to determine when independent endoscopy can be performed competently.[84] State licensure guidelines, institutional endoscopy boards, and individual practice patterns may also contribute to decisions about who may perform endoscopy, with what instruments, and in what settings. Overall, patient safety and professional standards must take precedence over other concerns.

Stroboscopy

Stroboscopy is a special lighting technique that has been used for 3 decades to approximate the appearance of vocal fold vibration. Based on the principle of Talbot's law, stroboscopy relies on an optical phenomenon called "persistence of vision" of the human retina. This law describes the physiologic limits of the retina, which can only perceive a maximum of 5 separate images per second, at a rate not faster than 0.2 seconds per image. If separate images are presented at this speed, then the eye will perceive each image independently, but if images are presented at faster rates, they will be visually "fused" and appear to be one continuous, moving image. When a strobe light illuminates the vocal folds at a flash rate faster than 5 images per second, separate images taken from flashpoints along the waveform are perceived as continuous motion.[7,10,84]

Human vocal folds vibrate at rates from approximately 60 (low bass) to greater than 1400 (whistle register) Hz. Therefore, the vocal folds oscillate at rates far faster than can be perceived by the naked eye. Stroboscopic light flashes sample these quasiperiodic waveforms to create a composite vibratory cycle, taken from many single points along multiple waveforms. Because the accuracy of the strobe flashing rate depends on stable pitch tracking from the contact microphone, an aperiodic or aphonic voice cannot trigger the strobe light consistently. When this occurs, the image will flicker in a rapid, irregular fashion and is not a valid representation of the vocal fold vibratory pattern.[84]

The strobe unit has 2 lighting sources: a steady halogen light and a flashing xenon light. The steady light illuminates the larynx and vocal folds, similar to the otolaryngologist's indirect mirror examination. This view is helpful for looking at gross structures, vocal fold adduction and abduction, and if white balanced, color or tissue variations on the surface of the vocal folds. The steady light does not allow the clinician to observe vocal fold vibration. The xenon light produces the strobe flash. Xenon lights contain xenon gas, and the brightness of the light source dissipates, slowing after about 50 hours of use, gradually darkening the image, instead of burning out all at once.[84] Because most examinations use only approximately 3 to 5 minutes of actual strobe light, each bulb is capable of illuminating hundreds of exams. The timing of the xenon strobe flash is triggered by the fundamental frequency of the voice, as detected by a contact microphone placed tightly over the thyroid lamina. The strobe flash pulses are short (<40 microseconds) and are triggered under two operating modes to create either a still or traveling image of the vocal folds. In the still mode, the strobe flashes occur at exactly the same point within the vibratory cycle, and the resulting image appears stable or "locked." In the traveling mode, the strobe flashes occur at progressively different points within each vibratory cycle, and the resulting image appears as a slow-moving wave of vibration (Figures 6–15 and 6–16).

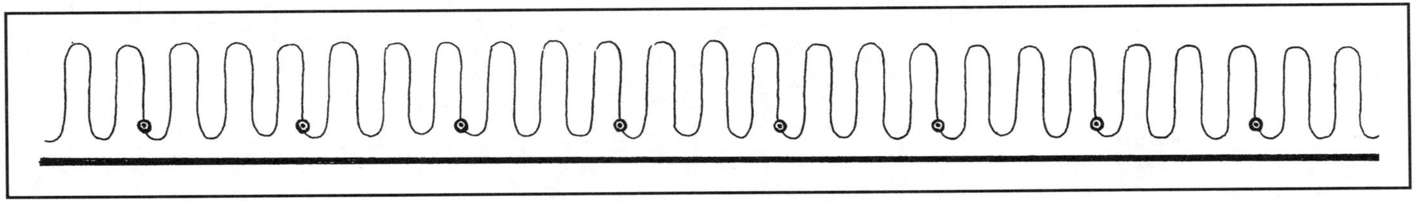

FIGURE 6–15. Strobe flashing at the same point in the vibratory cycle: still (*locked*) image.

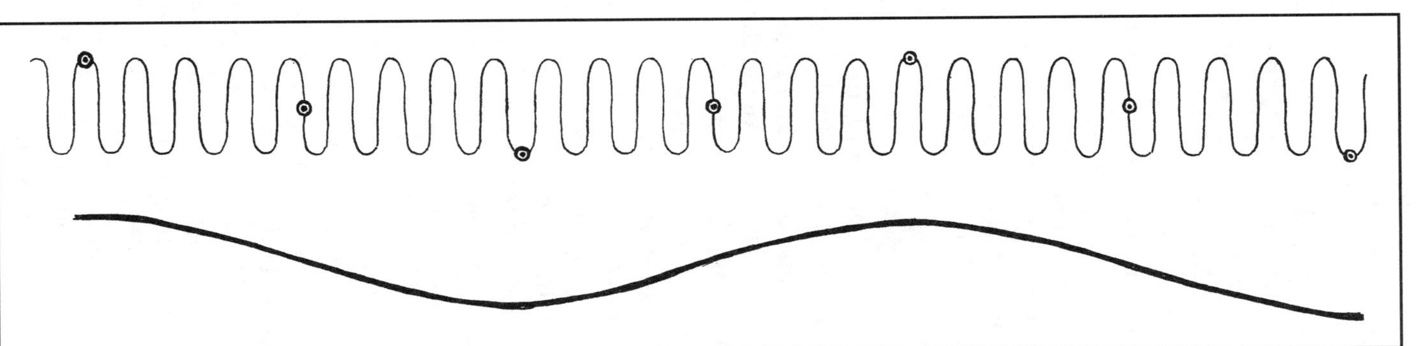

FIGURE 6–16. Strobe flashing at different points in the vibratory cycle: traveling wave.

To achieve this apparent (not real!) slow motion, the contact microphone detects the fundamental frequency and triggers the strobe light to flash at a phase point that is slightly faster than the fundamental frequency. Each flash supplies 1 image, taken at 1 phase point of the whole cycle. Each successive flash captures a phase point that is slightly ahead of the previous flash, but taken from a different cycle of vibration. This series of separate images, sampled from different points of vocal fold vibration, appears to the viewer's eye to be a continuous cycle of vibration. Thus, stroboscopy is not real-time slow motion, but rather a composite of separate flashes, triggered across many waveforms. In fact, the number of actual vocal fold vibratory cycles between flashes can range from less than 10 to over a 100, depending on the fundamental frequency.[84,96]

Moreover, similar cautions apply to stroboscopy as were pertinent to acoustic waveform analysis. Because the accuracy of the strobe flash trigger is based on the fundamental frequency, the more periodic the voice source, the more regular the strobe flash point, to produce an accurate representation of underlying vocal fold vibration. Strobe flash precision depends on stable pitch tracking from the contact microphone, so a very aperiodic or aphonic voice—as is common with dysphonia—will introduce error. Thus, poor tracking may produce an image that fails to capture the actual vocal fold vibratory function accurately. Unfortunately, voice pathologists often examine patients whose voices are incapable of stable fundamental frequencies. Under those conditions, the resulting stroboscopic image is likely to result from strobe flash points triggered aperiodically at various places in the glottic cycle because of the irregular fundamental frequency. Obviously, the composite vibratory image may be substantially different from the real-time vocal fold vibration, and clinicians have reason to be suspicious of any visual perceptual judgments for those images.[84,95]

High-Speed Digital Imaging

High-speed digital imaging allows direct recording of true vocal fold vibration, using a very bright xenon light source (300 W) and a rigid endoscope to create a magnified, high-resolution, 3-dimensional image of vocal fold vibration. High-speed imaging samples vocal fold vibration at acquisition rates ranging from 2000 to 10000 cycles per second. Recently, digital high-speed color imaging techniques have been introduced with sampling rates of 4000 Hz.[96] Recall that vocal fold vibration ranges from approximately 60 (low bass) to 1400 (high soprano) Hz. Thus, the sampling rate in high-speed imaging is fast enough to allow real-time recording of actual vocal fold oscillation, including phonatory onset (initiation) and offset (ending), sustained voice, and changes in pitch and loudness. Unlike stroboscopy, high-speed imaging does not rely on fundamental frequency to create the image. This means that any patient's voice, regardless of the dysphonia severity, can be recorded accurately with high-speed imaging.[96] Figure 6–17 displays a montage comparison of the laryngeal images captured during 2 cycles of high-speed digital imaging compared to the 4 flash points (only one-half of a cycle) captured during the same time period of stroboscopic imaging. This illustrative figure and the accompanying schematic drawing

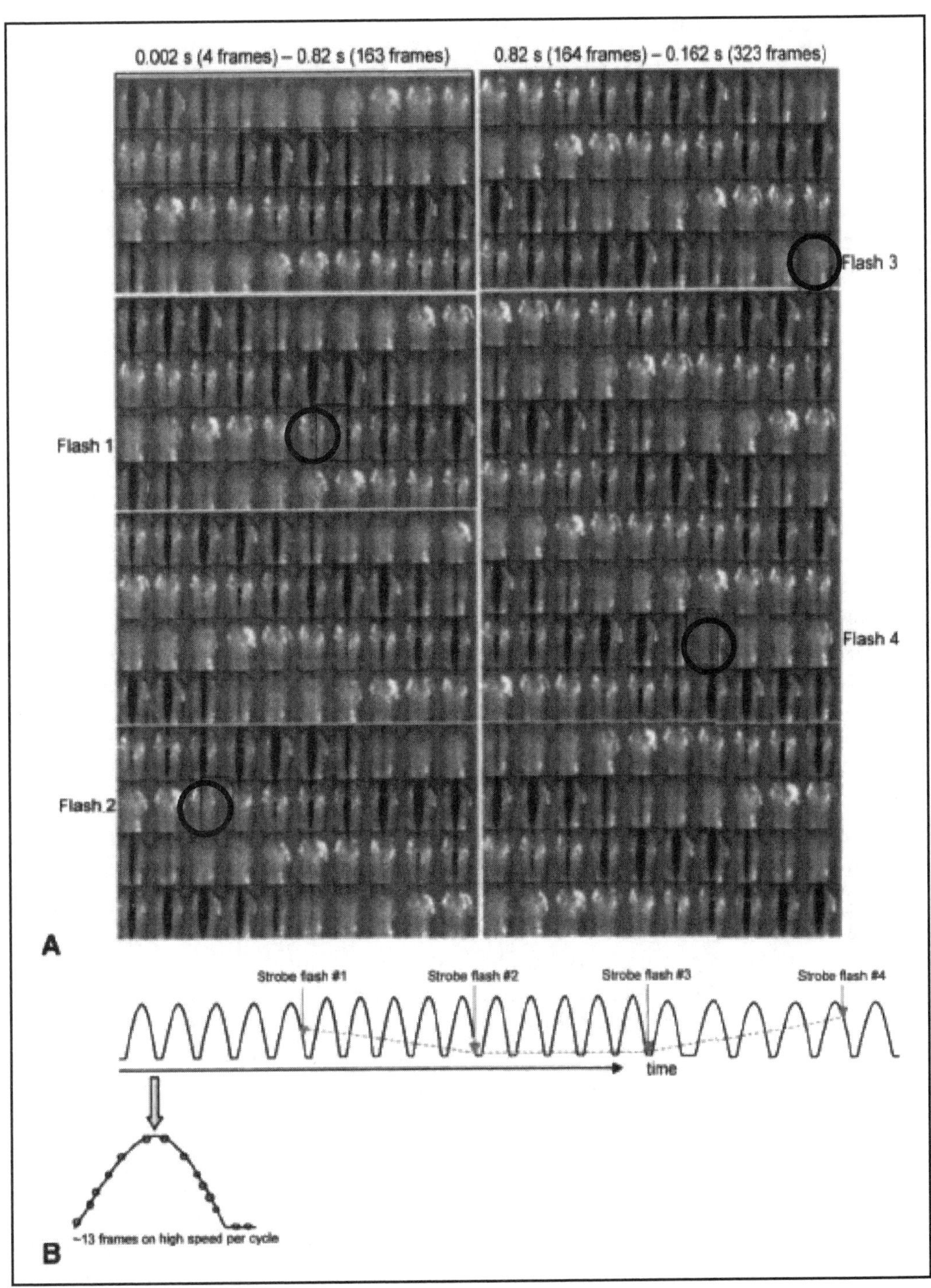

FIGURE 6–17. Image montage comparing frames of vocal fold vibration captured using high-speed digital imaging into frames detected using stroboscopy flashes (*circled*) during the same time period. The line tracings below (**A** and **B**) display the flash points in the vibratory cycle for both high-speed digital imaging (13 frames/cycle) and stroboscopy (4 flashes yield one partial composite cycle). Reprinted with permission from the original article: Patel R, Dailey S, Bless D. Comparison of high-speed digital imaging with stroboscopy for laryngeal imaging of glottal disorders. *Annals of Otology, Rhinology, and Laryngology*, 2008;17(6):413–424.

illustrate how little waveform activity is actually captured using stroboscopic imaging to estimate the vibratory cycle (Figure 6–17).

Imaging samples from 252 patients representing 3 different disorders types (epithelial, subepithelial, and neurologic) were compared using high-speed and stroboscopic imaging. Each was analyzed for visual perceptual judgments of vibratory features of vocal fold edge, glottal closure, phase closure, vertical level, vibratory amplitude, mucosal wave, phase symmetry, tissue pliability, and glottal cycle periodicity. High-speed imaging successfully recorded all disordered samples, but 63% of the stroboscopic recordings could not be interpreted due to severity of the dysphonia, with largest difficulty seen in the neurologic group (74%), followed by epithelial (58%), then subepithelial (53%) disorders.[96]

The impact of so many frames of vibratory movement brings on a novel problem: how to analyze and interpret so much information? High-speed digital imaging of the vocal fold vibratory pattern requires a computer program to be able to extract the image, detect the vibratory edge, and produce motion tracings for subsequent analysis. The sheer size of the high-speed data set also poses a challenge in developing software to process these recordings efficiently and accurately, so that the information can be used clinically.[97,98] New statistical algorithms have been developed for this purpose, with future goals of being able to autoprocess high-speed digital image recordings by plotting and analyzing vibratory motion traces captured in real-time imaging.[97–99] High-speed recordings have also been analyzed for comparison to simultaneous acoustic measures to cross-validate image findings in normal and abnormal voices and measure quantitative differences between normal, diplophonic, and other vibratory patterns.[97]

Kymography

Kymography is another real-time imaging technique that uses a camera to scan a single horizontal line of vocal fold vibration at a sampling rate of 8000 lines/s. Like high-speed imaging, kymography uses a bright light source to illuminate and does not rely on fundamental frequency tracking. However, unlike a high-speed image, the kymographic image is limited to the spatial and temporal changes of a single horizontal line of bilateral vocal fold movement. The scan line is usually directed at the midline juncture of the membranous folds, where maximum mucosal wave and amplitude are present. However, the line could be directed to any point of interest along the vocal folds, such as the anterior or posterior commissure. The resulting image is a diamond-shaped display of the glottic open and closing phases recorded from the exact point of the scan line. The real-time series of subsequent opening and closing cycles are connected in a vertical column, so that the viewer can appreciate bilateral tissue excursion across several cycles. These stacked images reveal cycle-to-cycle variability, left- or right-sided asymmetry, mucosal wave and amplitude, open or closed phase timing, phonatory onset and offset movements, and upper and lower vocal fold margin changes. In some videokymographic images, it is even possible to capture small oscillations of the ventricular folds, a feature that is never visible under stroboscopic light. Figure 6–18 presents a schematic comparison of stroboscopic and videokymographic images.

One disadvantage of the technique is that videokymography never allows a complete view of the vocal folds at once because the image is limited to the bilateral tissue motion recorded from the scan line. To counteract this constraint, it is useful to record lines from several different points of interest on the vocal folds, such as the anterior commissure, midline juncture, and posterior junction of the cartilaginous and membranous folds.[100,101]

In Plates 27 and 28, the left image displays the scan line location used to extract the videokymographic image. The right image displays the resulting real-time tissue vibration, extracted from the horizontal scan line as indicated. Plate 27 exhibits normal bilateral

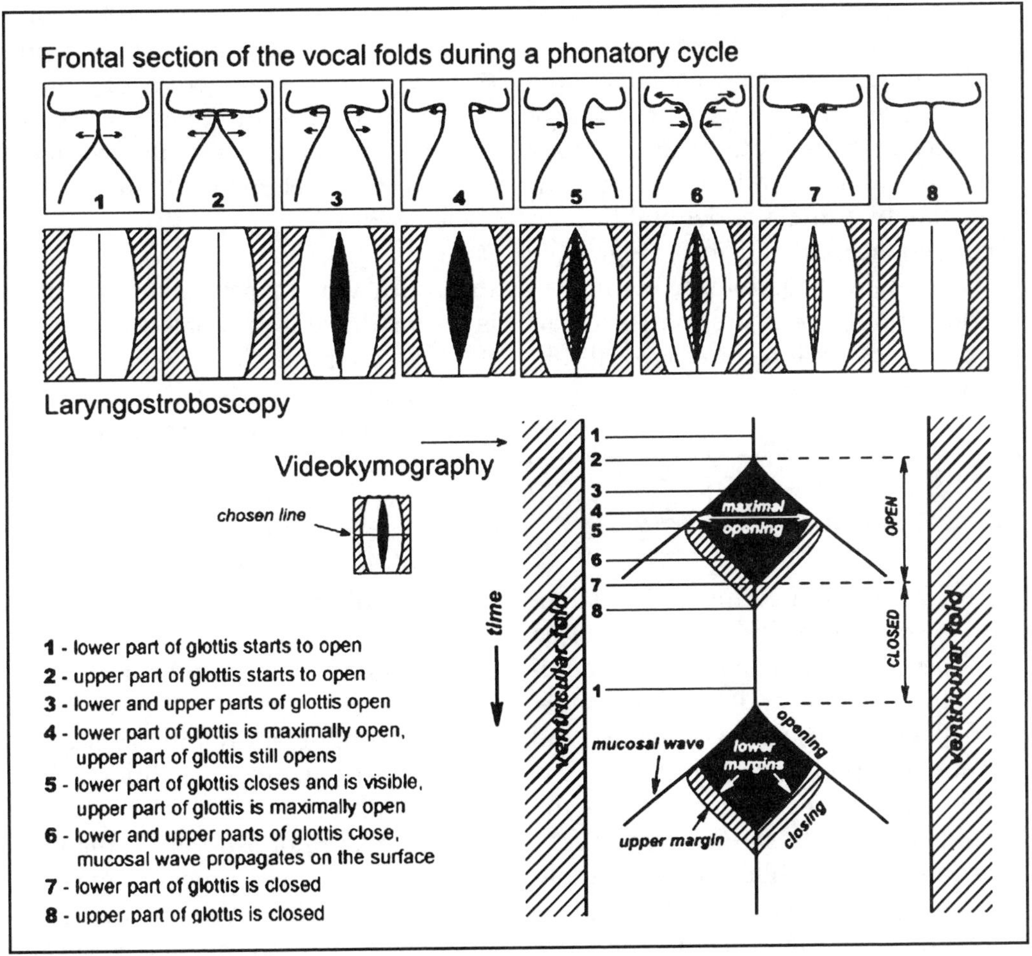

FIGURE 6–18. Schematic comparison of characteristic features of normal vocal fold vibration in stroboscopy and videokymography. From Svec JC. *On vibration properties of human vocal folds: Voice registers, bifurcations resonance characteristics, development and application of videoymography*. Doctoral dissertation, University of Groningen, The Netherlands, 2000. Used with permission of the author.

mucosal wave, consistent with healthy folds. Plate 28 exhibits asymmetric unilateral right vocal fold vibration with stiff, nonvibrating left vocal fold vibration due to the presence of a large unilateral lesion. Finally, Plate 29 displays bilaterally aperiodic and out-of-phase vibration, despite apparently normal vocal fold tissue.

Although kymography has been present in research laboratories for over a decade, recent advances in digital instruments and processing have improved the image clarity, processing speed, and clinical convenience of the technique. The strongest advantage of kymography is its real-time image of vocal fold oscillation; an obvious constraint is its small recording window of only a single horizontal line. To accommodate that deficit, kymographic recordings are synchronized with electroglottography, which provides a real-time cycle-to-cycle record of vocal fold contact area.[100,101]

Criteria for Laryngeal Imaging

Is imaging warranted for every patient with a voice disorder? The answer to this question will depend on the medical delivery model and ultimately must be decided by the professionals who use and interpret these techniques. Certainly, permanent documentation of the vocal pathology or status of vocal fold function is worthwhile. However, more critical rationales for using these diagnostic tools will help justify their use to both patients and insurers. Repeatedly, imaging (especially, stroboscopy, which is most common clinically) has been shown to contribute significantly to accurate medical diagnoses of laryngeal lesions and voice disorders.[84–86,96,98]

The following are some questions for consideration:

- What information does laryngeal imaging provide that is not available in the otolaryngologist's indirect examination? Voice pathologists have recognized the unique importance of assessing the vibratory pattern of phonation, an event that cannot be seen without the special lighting techniques of stroboscopy, high-speed imaging, or kymography.
- How might knowledge of the vibratory image influence or change either the diagnosis or the treatment plan, whether medical, surgical, or behavioral?

In an era when documentation alone is an insufficient rationale for referral, the following criteria have been developed and used by otolaryngologists and voice pathologists to clarify the need for imaging techniques:

- To assess patients with persistent dysphonia (greater than 3 weeks' duration) unexplained by an indirect exam (normal or inconclusive)
- To evaluate patients who are professional voice users and have noted changes or deterioration in voice performance (eg, range, quality, stability, or endurance)
- Whenever phonosurgery is planned, to allow adequate preoperative vocal fold imaging and postoperative assessment of tissue recovery and healing
- To clarify the etiology of the voice disorder, whenever organic or functional contributors are unclear

- To determine an optimal management plan, whether medical, surgical, or rehabilitative.

Endoscopic Imaging Techniques

Rigid Scope

The patient is seated comfortably in a supportive chair, with hips back into the seat and leaning slightly forward. The patient is instructed to open the mouth, relax the tongue, and begin saying a prolonged /i/ sound. With a 70° endoscope, the clinician inserts the scope directly in the center of the mouth, pressing firmly down on the tongue and angling the endoscope backward beginning at middorsum, until the larynx comes into view on the monitor. The endoscope does not go very far; in most patients, the angle of insertion will bring the vocal folds into viewing range easily. With a 90° endoscope the clinician holds the scope parallel to the floor in the center of the mouth, above the tongue and advances it under the velum drape and nearly to the posterior pharyngeal wall. In both cases, care should be taken to avoid touching the back of the pharynx or faucial pillars with the endoscope, which may elicit a gag reflex. The endoscope position should be stable and firm because light and inconsistent pressure on the tongue may also trigger a gag.[84]

Flexible Endoscope

The patient is seated upright in a supportive chair. If possible, determine from prior endoscopic imaging records whether the right or left nasal passage is more amenable to flexible scoping, to avoid touching large nasal turbinates or a deviated septum. Topical anesthetic, decongestant, lubrication, or a combination are applied to the left or right nares via spray, atomizer, wooden cotton swab, or drip, according to individual setting practice patterns. The flexible endoscope is advanced gently into the inferior meatus, simultaneously observing progress on the monitor, until the tip reaches the curve of the velum. Using the flexible angle control, curve the scope down toward the vocal tract and advance the tip until it hovers in the laryngeal vestibule, behind the epiglottis and above the vocal folds. If the image is foggy, the patient can swallow to warm the endoscope tip.[84,87]

Patient Comfort

Some "tips of the trade" can assist clinicians in achieving a full view of the larynx and vocal folds, and ensure patient comfort:

- The patient should breathe gently through the mouth during the examination. It is usually helpful to have the patient keep the eyes open during the exam. If possible, ask the patient to observe the imaging simultaneously (via second monitor or a well-placed mirror). Otherwise, an interesting photograph or other visual distraction may help relax the patient during endoscopy.
- Warm the endoscope tip to reduce fogging. During the exam, intermittent fogging can be removed by touching the tip of the endoscope to the buccal mucosa.
- The rigid endoscope tip can be positioned forward or back in the mouth,

angled upward or down, and rotated laterally in either direction. Clinicians should learn to rotate the scope in any of these three planes to obtain the optimal view. An optimal view is one in which the vocal folds are large enough to be clearly visible and centered on the screen. When the image is angled or otherwise distorted on the monitor, it may be impossible to judge movement patterns accurately, and an artificial left-right imbalance may appear. Adjust the endoscope to achieve a stable vertical level (lens-to-object distance) on the left versus right side, working toward achieving a full image (anterior commissure to posterior rim of the glottis), as well as a clear, well-lit, and well-focused image.

- The recorded sample should be long enough (5 seconds or longer) to allow sufficient successive strobe images or recording. If the images are fleeting and cannot be sustained, the vibratory pattern cannot be assessed reliably.
- If mucus obscures the vocal fold images, the patient can perform a gentle glottal stop or throat clear. Mucus seems to settle on lesion sites, so it is important to clear it to appreciate the underlying vocal fold mucosa.

Recording Protocol

The laryngeal image recording protocol must accommodate individual patient needs, but generally includes the following:

- A full face recording with a connected speech sample (eg, counting, standard passage, and sustained vowels) allows the clinician to assess overall perceptual quality and free-field speech and voice behaviors. In a busy clinic, it also helps match a "face" to the "larynx."
- Sustained /i/ vowel productions bring the epiglottis forward and allow the clinician to view the vocal folds during vibration. In early trials, a full view is easier to achieve during higher pitched /i/ productions. The patient can be cued to decrease pitch once the clinician obtains a satisfactory view. The sustained vowels should include habitual and range tasks of pitch and loudness capabilities.
- Laryngeal diadochokinesis, using repeated /i i i i/ and /hi hi hi hi/, is used to observe the glottic closure pattern and rapid abduction and adduction of the vocal folds.
- Vegetative maneuvers (including inhalation, rest breathing, coughing, laughing, and throat clearing) allow the clinician to observe the laryngeal valve function and help identify any structural or movement problems.
- Multiple trials of all speech tasks are necessary. These maneuvers are necessary, if possible, to assess individual variability. Occasionally, the patient's tolerance for scoping will not allow for repeated trials, but alternatively, some patients improve noticeably after a second or third attempt.

Visual Perceptual Judgments

Both steady light and vibratory (stroboscopy, high-speed imaging, or kymography) light observations can be made from the recorded image. Although a variety of rating scales and schemes exist, some consensus has been achieved about the salient features for visual perceptual judgments (Table 6–2).[10,84]

Steady light observations include the following:

- Structural appearance of the entire larynx: The vocal folds, epiglottis, posterior glottic rim, ventricular folds, and piriform sinuses should be explored under steady light along with movement (abduction and adduction) of the vocal folds to reveal any gross asymmetry or abnormality.
- Glottic closure pattern: If glottic closure is incomplete, gaps are noted as irregular, hourglass, posterior, anterior, or spindle shaped (bowing). Note that glottic closure judgments must be made during vibratory samples, for comparison with steady light image; often, slight gaps that are apparent during vibratory closure patterns are not seen in steady light.
- Supraglottic hyperfunction: These observations include medial compression of the lateral ventricular folds, the anterior-to-posterior "squeeze" of the epiglottis and arytenoids, or a circular narrowing and lowering of the entire laryngeal vestibule. This

Table 6–2. Visual Perceptual Judgments of Laryngeal Imaging

Gross Observations	Glottic closure (static)
	Supraglottic hyperfunction
	Mucus
	General appearance and movement
Vibratory Features	Glottic closure (vibratory)
	Phase closure
	Symmetry
	Amplitude
	Mucosal wave
	Stiffness/nonvibrating portion/adynamic segment
	Periodicity
Real-Time Imaging	Vibratory onset and offset
Other Observations	Patient tolerance
	Endoscope type
	Topical anesthesia
	Perceptual quality
	Fundamental frequency and Intensity: range and habitual
Drawing/Sketch	Ad- and Abduction Pattern
	Midline closure pattern (adduction)
	Lateral excursion of the vocal folds (abduction)
	Sites of notable features (eg, hemorrhage, lesions, mucus, etc)

tension is especially notable in contrast to relaxed, open postures during quiet breathing.

- Mucus presence: Tacky, pooling, or strands of mucus may signal a tissue irritation or lesion in the same location.

The vibratory image allows visual perceptual judgments of the shape-changing and timing factors that occur during phonation. In real-time imaging (high speed and kymography), the sampling rate is large enough that phonation onset and offset can be observed directly. Visual perceptual vibratory judgments include the following:

- Glottic closure pattern as compared to steady light impressions. Phase closure is the relative ratio of glottis-open to glottis-closed within a single vibratory cycle.
- Mucosal wave reflects the overall flexibility of the vocal fold during vibration. Absence of mucosal wave, called nonvibrating portion, stiffness, or adynamic segment, can be described in terms of its location and extent of the vocal fold.
- Amplitude reflects the medial to lateral excursion of the vocal fold from midline.
- Symmetry refers to the shape-changing relationship between left and right vocal folds. Across cycles, do both folds move in the same manner at the same time? Is the shape of the glottic space between the vocal folds symmetric, cycle after cycle?
- Periodicity or regularity is a timing characteristic and refers to the cycle-to-cycle stability of the vocal fold oscillation. This judgment is difficult to make without real-time recording of vibration. A gross estimate of periodicity can be made using stroboscopy if the image can be set to "locked" phase, so that the strobe flash triggers at the exact same phase point across samples. If vocal fold vibration is periodic, the image will be still, hence the term *locked*. If vibration is aperiodic, the image will appear to be "jumpy" or unstable.

As for all perceptual ratings, it is difficult to achieve reliability in visual perceptual judgments of laryngeal images. Scheduling regular strobe review sessions with otolaryngology and voice pathology colleagues is highly recommended, to increase intra- and interjudge reliability and reduce internal bias in making visual perceptual judgments of the laryngeal image, whether real time or stroboscopic. Rating schemes may be tailored to individual needs, but for consistency across settings, ratings should include most of the visual perceptual features listed in Table 6–2.

In addition to minimizing interpretive error, test-retest reliability is essential to allow useful comparison of pre- and posttreatment laryngeal images. To improve the comparability of separate recordings, it is first essential to employ the identical examination protocol in follow-up sessions, using the same endoscope and equipment, speech sample and task order, and cuing the patient to vocalize at the same fundamental frequency and intensity. Second, using the pretest image (on a split screen or cameo inset image, if possible), verify that the relative position of the larynx on the monitor is framed as closely as possible to the prerecording image, to achieve similar endoscope position or angle, white balance and lighting, magnification, and lens to object distance. New image calibrating software programs in development for use with digital images can add precision to test-retest protocols, allowing users to measure select anatomic landmarks or lesion size for comparison across recordings.

Laryngeal imaging offers extraordinary diagnostic and rehabilitative opportunities for voice pathologists. Current digital technology has improved the resolution and the convenience of these tools considerably in the past decade. Although the techniques require special experience, a commitment to skill-based competencies, and additional professional liabilities, professionals who use imaging technique consistently reap the benefits of this visual information.

ELECTROGLOTTOGRAPHY (EGG)

Electroglottography is a noninvasive tool that uses electrical current passing through the neck to measure vocal fold contact across time. Two electrodes are placed on either side of the thyroid alae, with a small electrical current passing through as the vocal folds vibrate. The electrodes measure the variable resistance as the vocal folds vibrate. Because tissue conducts the electrical current better than air does, the resistance increases when the vocal folds are opening or opened and decreases during the closing or closed phase. The EGG waveform displays this variable resistance and serves as a real-time analog of the vocal fold vibratory pattern, with peaks and troughs representing maximum points of open and closed phases.[102–104] The technique is subject to artifact, however, because variations in tissue thickness, electrode placement, mucous interference, and laryngeal movements can produce errors in this measure. Using a dual-channel EGG (with two electrodes positioned vertically on each side of the thyroid) can reduce some of this error and achieve better representation of the upper and lower vocal fold contact area. EGG has been used in combination with other vocal function measures, such as acoustics, airflow, and inverse filtering.[8,73,79,105] A most useful application of EGG is as a simultaneous glottal contact area to cross-validate stroboscopic flash pulses, thus offering a real-time monitor of the vibratory phase points across the stroboscopic image.[88] EGG is also used with kymography and high-speed imaging.[96,100] Recently, EGG was used to predict the likelihood of abnormal laryngeal electromyography (LEMG) in patients with suspected paresis. Findings revealed that normal EGG recordings can rule out the need for LEMG, based on the strong negative probability of finding abnormal laryngeal muscle activity if the EGG waveform is normal.[106]

LARYNGEAL ELECTROMYOGRAPHY (LEMG)

Electromyography is a direct measure of laryngeal muscle activity and function, and because it is an invasive procedure, it must be performed by a neurologist or otolaryngologist. Needle electrodes are inserted percutaneously into the laryngeal muscles, and the pattern of electrical activity is studied.[1,106–114] Because the placement of the electrodes cannot be seen directly in laryngeal muscles, insertions are essentially "blind." A series of vocal tasks are used to confirm electrode placement in the correct muscles.[107–110] To verify correct placement in the cricothyroid muscle, for example, the LEMG activity should be active as soon as the patient produces a high pitch but should be entirely "quiet" (inactive) during rest breathing. Electrical activity for the thyroarytenoid muscle is strongest during firm glottal stop productions. LEMG electrical signals recorded from the muscles are interpreted as normal or pathologic based on four basic features: timing (onset and offset) of muscle activity, and the pattern, number, and amplitude of muscle action potentials.[107] The widest clinical application of LEMG is in providing diagnosis and prognosis for suspected vocal fold movement disorders, including paralysis, paresis, dystonia, and other neuromuscular disorders and for discriminating vocal fold paralysis from mechanical fixation of the cricoarytenoid joint.[111,112] In a retrospective study of 37 LEMG studies, 10 (27%) studies influenced a change in the medical treatment plan.[109]

NORMATIVE INFORMATION

Normative information is essential to establish the clinical utility of instrumental measures of voice. Equipment-based norms are used to compare individual results to normal and pathologic groups. Ideally, normal databases should report demographics of their sample populations to account for factors that influence the instrumental results, such as gender, age, health history, and local dialect. Elicitation techniques and sample tasks may vary across studies, as well as equipment and analysis routines. These factors limit the ability to compare different findings. A practical solution may be to collect "local norms," by measuring a large group of normal speakers as a reference sample. Such findings could be interpreted with maximum confidence if data were collected using the same equipment, recording protocols, and other methods common to that clinical laboratory. Published normative information is available on fundamental frequency, intensity, and aerodynamics (Tables 6–3, 6–4, 6–5, and 6–6). Normative standards for acoustic perturbation measures or signal/harmonic-to-noise ratios cannot be compared easily across sites due to differences in recording techniques, analyses, units of measurement, and equipment variables. However, acoustic analysis programs have begun to include normal and disordered speaker databases specific to their technology and equipment as part of the system package. Nonetheless, the emerging normal database for instrumental measures of voice must continue to expand with cooperative contributions across laboratories.

ELECTRICAL SAFETY

If possible, clinicians who are working in clinical voice laboratories should seek professional advice from biomedical technology services to assist with accurate equipment setup. These personnel can provide electronic safety checks, recommend strategies to troubleshoot equipment problems, and ensure that voice laboratory procedures meet appropriate institutional standards. Some general recommendations for electronic

Table 6–3. Normative Fundamental Frequency

	Mean (Hz)	*Minimum (Hz)*	*Maximum (Hz)*
Children[a] 6–10 years			
Boys (*n* = 59)	226	179	272
Girls (*n* = 62)	238	193	294
Adults[b]			
Males (*n* = 58)	106	77	482
Females (*n* = 61)	193	137	634

[a]Adapted with permission from Glaze LE, Bless DM, Milenkovic PH, Susser RD. Acoustic characteristics of children's voice. *J Voice*. 1988;2(4):312–319.

[b]Adapted with permission from Bless DM, Glaze LE, Biever-Lowery DM, Campos G, Peppard RC. Stroboscopic, acoustic, aerodynamic, and perceptual attributes of voice production in normal speaking adults. In: Titze IR, ed. *Progress Report 4*. Iowa City, IA: National Center for Voice and Speech; 1993:121–134.

Table 6–4. Normative Intensity

	Mean	*Range*
Children[a] 6–10 years (*n* = 97)	70 dB	60–99 dB
Adults[b]		
Males (*n* = 58)	70 dB	<60–110 dB
Females (*n* = 61)	68 dB	<60–106 dB

[a]Adapted with permission from Glaze LE, Bless DM, Susser RD. Acoustic analysis of vowel and loudness differences in children's voice. *J Voice*. 1990;4(1):37–44.

[b]Adapted with permission from Bless DM, Glaze LE, Biever-Lowery DM, Campos G, Peppard RC. Stroboscopic, acoustic, aerodynamic, and perceptual attributes of voice production in normal speaking adults. In: Titze IR. ed. *Progress Report 4*. Iowa City, IA: National Center for Voice and Speech; 1993:121–134.

Table 6–5. Normative Airflow Rate

	Mean	*Range*
Adults[a]		
Males (*n* = 67)	119 cc/s	40–320
Females (*n* = 78)	115 cc/s	50–220

[a]Adapted with permission from Bless DM, Glaze LE, Biever-Lowery DM, Campos G, Peppard RC. Stroboscopic, acoustic, aerodynamic, and perceptual attributes of voice production in normal speaking adults. In: Titze IR, ed. *Progress Report 4*. Iowa City, IA: National Center for Voice and Speech; 1993:121–134.

Table 6–6. Normative Intraoral Pressure Estimates

	Normal *(cm H_2O)*	***Soft*** *(cm H_2O)*	***Loud*** *(cm H_2O)*
Adults[a]			
Males (*n* = 25)	5.91	4.79	8.39
Females (*n* = 25)	6.09	4.79	8.46
	Normal *(cm H_2O)*	***Low Pitch*** *(cm H_2O)*	***High Pitch*** *(cm H_2O)*
Adults[b]			
Males (*n* = 25)	6.3	7.0	7.5
Females (*n* = 20)	5.8	6.7	6.1

[a]Adapted with permission from Holmberg EB, Hillman RE, Perkell JS. Glottal airflow and transglottal air pressure measurements for male and female speakers in soft, normal, and loud voice. *J Acoust Soc Am.* 1988;84:511–529.

[b]Adapted with permission from Holmberg EB, Hillman RE, Perkell JS. Glottal airflow and transglottal air pressure measurements for male and female speakers in low, normal and high pitch. *J Voice.* 1989;3(4):294–305.

setup and safety apply to all settings. Cables and wiring should be sufficiently strong and devoid of any breaks or weaknesses to allow accurate transmission of the current (signal) and should be checked periodically for line continuity.

Discard equipment that shows signs of distressed wiring (cracks, taped connections, breaks in insulation seal). The wiring and electrical connections between the many components in a voice laboratory should be appropriately labeled and stored off the ground. Wires that are repeatedly pulled, bent, stretched, stepped on, or rolled over will be damaged easily, which creates unnecessary repair expense and a potential electrical hazard. Usually, cables should be coaxial or triaxial and well insulated to avoid functioning as an antenna by picking up extraneous electrical signals or 60-cycle (60 Hz) noise from other electrical equipment in the room (eg, lights, lamps, heating units, etc). Cables should also be long enough to connect various components without being overly long. The longer the cable, the greater the resistance along its path, and the greater the likelihood for increased error to be transmitted.[7]

Patients must be protected from inappropriate grounding and low-resistance current. Equipment should be stored on nonmetal racks, if possible. If water is used in the laboratory, it should not be exposed to electrical wiring. Always use grounded (3-prong) plugs for all electrical equipment. Never use a 2-prong adapter to override a 3-prong plug in an ungrounded outlet. Fuses should be replaced carefully, using the exact size and strength recommended by the manufacturer. If a piece of equipment blows fuses repeatedly, the source of electrical overload must be examined and repaired. Fuses should never be replaced with a larger size to avoid blowout; this tactic only masks the real problem and can create dangerous electrical safety conditions.

HYGIENIC SAFETY

All laboratory equipment that comes in contact with patients must be sterilized as recommended by the manufacturer. Whenever possible, disposable items should be used (eg, airflow tubes), despite the increased expense and waste. Most facilities have medical hygiene standards committees that can ensure compliance with the institutional requirements for safe precautions and equipment sterilization. The clinician, too, must practice stringent and rigid adherence to hygiene. Voice laboratories must adhere to Universal Precautions guidelines, as established by Occupational Safety and Health Administration (OSHA).[84] This includes thorough hand washing before and after having contact with a patient and using gloves during any procedure that puts the clinician's hands or equipment (eg, endoscope) in contact with any mucous membrane of the mouth, nose, throat, or ears. In some circumstances, additional guidelines are appropriate to protect patients or clinicians from infectious disease transmission by wearing eye shields or surgical masks. Whenever a patient is immunocompromised or otherwise at risk for transmission of airborne disease, it is appropriate to secure qualified advice from health care professionals to ensure safe precautions.

Routine cleaning should be performed to maintain hygiene in the clinical voice laboratory, including equipment, racks, furniture, floors, and handwashing area. Sterilize all equipment according to both institutional and product guidelines. Wash and soak rigid and flexible endoscopes in an antimicrobial solution after every use. Verify with biomedical safety personnel that any updates in Universal Precautions or institutional guidelines are routinely shared with the voice laboratory staff, to ensure full compliance with current recommended standards.

THE CLINICAL VOICE LABORATORY

The data generated by instrumental measures of voice have contributed greatly to our understanding of phonatory function and the complex relationship between laryngeal anatomy, physiology, and voice quality. Instrumental data must be paired with clinical impressions and audioperceptual judgments of voice quality to be used meaningfully. Multiple sources of complementary information improve our ability to observe and monitor vocal capabilities in normal and professional speakers and voice production limits in patients with disorders. Better recording devices have enhanced acoustic, aerodynamic, imaging, and other physiologic measures of vocal function, signal processing techniques, and analysis routines. Voice pathologists have recognized the clinical applications of these measurement tools and integrated instrumental measurements in the assessment and management of patients with voice disorders. Nonetheless, interpretation must always be done with care, and users must be knowledgeable about the risks of artifact and error to ensure valid application of these measures. Normative information must be collected within each voice lab setting and compared to larger pools of standard equipment and software-based databases, as we continue to improve our ability to recognize normal from disordered vocal function.

Despite immense progress over the past 3 decades, the clinical utility of the voice laboratory is still emerging. Currently, instrumental measures offer varying success at detecting pathology, assessing vocal severity, and contributing to accurate diagnoses. [114] In the rehabilitation process, however, voice pathologists use instrumental measures as a primary treatment tool to display, instruct, motivate, and justify treatment needs. For example, instrumental feedback may assist a patient in achieving target behaviors. Repeated pretest and posttest measurements may reinforce the patient's progress. Finally, vocal function measures offer a means to document the pathology that may be far more convincing than perceptual judgments of voice quality alone. Ultimately, the goal of the clinical voice laboratory is to inform patients, clinicians, and scientists about the nature and limits of human voice production. As new and better tools are refined, as normative information continues to accrue, and as equipment becomes increasingly accessible, these instrumental measures will improve our ability to do so.

GLOSSARY

Acoustics

Acoustic Waveform

Cepstrum: The mathematic inverse (Fourier transform) of the acoustic spectrum, to highlight the peaks of the strongest harmonic energies in the acoustic signal.

Frequency: The rate of vibration, represented by a number of waveform periods per unit time, for example, hertz as the number of cycles per second.

Fundamental frequency: The lowest periodic waveform of vocal fold vibration. Fundamental frequency is the reciprocal of the pitch period ($F = 1/T$).

Harmonics (signal)-to-noise ratio: The mathematical ratio of periodic energy (signal) to random or aperiodic energy (noise) in a given signal.

Intensity: Sound energy present in a signal, represented by waveform amplitude.

Jitter: Also known as pitch perturbation; a measure of cycle-to-cycle variability in fundamental frequency. Can be expressed in absolute measures or as a percentage referenced to the fundamental frequency.

Perturbation: Measures of variability or instability in a quasiperiodic waveform.

Pitch: The perceptual correlate of the fundamental frequency, based on a judgmental rating from low to high.

Pitch detection algorithm (PDA): A mathematical equation designed to detect the fundamental frequency of a speech waveform. Several methods are used commonly: zero-crossing, peak-picking, and waveform matching with autocorrelation.

Pitch period: The length of time for one waveform of vocal fold vibration. The pitch period is the reciprocal of fundamental frequency ($T = 1/F$).

Semitone: A unit devised for comparison of frequencies (eg, 200 to 400 Hz represents a 12-semitone range). The semitone scale includes all of the notes (sharps and flats included) on the musical scale, and is logarithmic.

The semitone scale reflects perceptual attributes of the human ear, as the difference in hertz between semitones lower on the musical scale is smaller than semitones that reflect higher frequencies.

Shimmer: Also known as amplitude perturbation; a measure of the cycle-to-cycle variability on waveform amplitude.

Spectrogram: A visual display of a speech signal across time (horizontal axis), giving information about frequency (vertical axis) and intensity (gray or color variation) in the display.

Spectrum: A plot of signal energy (intensity) by frequency at a single point in time.

Signal Processing

Amplification: Increasing the amplitude of a signal to increase the "gain" (measurable or detectable changes) in time-variation for purposes of recording, playback, data measurement, or signal processing.

Analog-to-digital (A/D) processing: Conversion of an analog signal to digital form, using a computer hardware device (A/D board or converter). An analog signal is time-and-amplitude varying and continuous. Digital processing, or digitization, divides the signal into discrete bits of information which are encoded numerically.

Filters: A method of including (passing) and excluding (filtering) specified levels of energy in the signal, usually in the course of signal processing. A low-pass filter excludes energy at high frequencies, a high-pass filter excludes energy at low frequencies, and a band-pass filter excludes energies higher or lower than a specified band of frequencies.

Quantization: The division of amplitude in an analog signal into discrete numeric values. The greater the quantization levels, the more adequately the amplitude waveform is represented.

Sampling rate: The number of samples per second of a digital signal. The greater the sampling rate, the more information obtained for signal processing.

Transducer: A device that converts energy from one form to another, for example, flow or pressure into an electrical signal.

Aerodynamics

Pressure

Differential pressure: Referenced to some other pressure (eg, between two measured sites, such as left and right nares).

Driving pressure: Flow of a gas from higher to lower regions of molecular concentration.

Intraoral pressure: Obtained from the closed oral cavity when the vocal folds are abducted, as in an unvoiced plosive consonant; an indirect estimate of subglottal pressure.[61]

Phonation threshold pressure: The minimal pressure needed to set the vocal folds into oscillation, considering variables of tissue damping, mucosal wave, vocal fold thickness, prephonatory glottal width, and transglottal pressure.[6]

Pressure: Force per unit area acting perpendicular to the area.

Subglottal pressure: Measured directly from the lung pressures below the glottis, when the vocal folds are adducted.

Subglottic pressure: Estimated clinically using intraoral pressure peaks produced during an unvoiced plosive consonant; a measure of the tracheal (respiratory) driving pressure used during phonation.

Airflow and Volume

Flow: The movement of a quantity of gas through an area.

Flow rate (volume velocity): Speed (and direction) of flow per unit time.

Flow volume: Quantity of flow.

Pneumotachograph: A differential pressure-sensing device that measures the drop in pressure when airflow passes across a known mechanical resistance (eg, wire-mesh screen or narrow tubes).

Rotameter (flow meter): Airflow measurement device; a cylindrical tube with a ball "float" within and an external measurement index. As flow passes through the bottom of the tube, the float rises to a level corresponding to the flow rate.

U-tube manometer: Pressure measurement device; a bent glass tube with external measurement index, filled with liquid (usually water or mercury). As pressure is applied to one side of the U, the direct reading can be taken from the liquid displacement on the other side.

Warm-wire anemometer: Flow measurement device; as airflow passes over (and cools) the warm metal wire, its electrical resistance changes, and flow magnitude can be predicted from the change in resistance of the wire.

Imaging

High-speed imaging: An imaging technique capable of capturing fast movements (eg, vocal fold vibration) at greater than 2000 images per second. Because vocal folds vibrate at much slower rates, high-speed laryngeal imaging records real-time vocal fold vibratory movement.

Kymography: An imaging technique capable of capturing one line (window) of vocal fold vibration (eg, a bilateral point at midline) at a sampling rate of 8000 images per second.

Stroboscopy: An imaging technique that captures discrete and distant flashes of vocal fold vibration, triggered by a light synchronized in phase with the fundamental frequency. These separate images are joined in a composite sequence and appear to the naked eye as one continuous vibrating image.

Talbot's law: Persistence of vision on the retina; the human retina cannot perceive more than 5 separate images per second (each image "rests" 0.2 seconds on the retina) and, when presented in succession, are fused into one apparent continuous image. Thus, a series of still images presented at this rate (or faster) will be perceived visually as a connected, moving image.

Vibratory Features

Amplitude: The lateral excursion of the vocal folds.

Mucosal wave: The movement of the vocal fold cover in lateral, longitudinal, and vertical waveform motion.

Periodicity: Regularity of the timing of successive cycles.

Phase closure: Ratio of open to close phase of the glottis during one full vibratory cycle.

Stiffness/nonvibrating portion/adynamic segment: Commonly expressed as a percentage of the full length of the membranous portion of the vocal fold.

Symmetry: The extent to which the left and right vocal folds appear to move as mirror images; changes in phase are identical.

Vibratory onset and offset: The behavior of the vocal folds at the initiation and ending of phonation. This feature can only be seen in real-time imaging techniques, such as kymography or high-speed imaging.

REFERENCES

1. Hirano M. *Clinical Examination of Voice.* New York, NY: Springer-Verlag; 1981.
2. Sataloff RT, Spiegel JR, Carroll LM, Darby KS, Hawkshaw MJ, Rulnick RK. The clinical voice laboratory: practical design and clinical application. *J Voice.* 1990;4(3):264–279.
3. Bless DM. Assessment of laryngeal function. In: Ford CN, Bless DM, eds. *Phonosurgery.* New York, NY: Raven Press; 1991:91–122.
4. Hicks DM. Functional voice assessment: what to measure and why. In: *Assessment of Speech and Voice Production: Research and Clinical Applications.* Bethesda, MD: National Institute on Deafness and Other Communicative Disorders; 1991:204–209.
5. Titze IR. Towards standards in acoustic analysis of voice. In: Titze IR, ed. *Progress Report Four.* Iowa City, IA: National Center for Voice and Speech; 1993: 271–280.
6. Titze IR. *Principles of Voice Production.* Englewood Cliffs, NJ: Prentice-Hall; 1994.
7. Baken RJ. *Clinical Measurement of Speech and Voice.* San Diego, CA: Singular Publishing Group; 1997.
8. Behrman A, Orlikoff R. Instrumentation in voice assessment and treatment: what's the use? *Am J Speech Lang Pathol.* 1997;6(4):9–16.
9. Smits I, Ceuppens P, De Bodt MS. A comparative study of acoustic voice measurements by means of Dr. Speech and Computerized Speech Lab. *J Voice.* 2005;19(2):187–196.
10. Bless DM, Glaze LE, Biever-Lowery D, Campos G, Peppard RC. Stroboscopic, acoustic, aerodynamic, and perceptual attributes of voice production in normal speaking adults. In: Titze IR, ed. *Progress Report 4.* Iowa City, IA: National Center for Voice and Speech; 1993:121–134.
11. Titze I. *Workshop on Acoustic Voice Analysis: Summary Statement.* Iowa City, IA: National Center for Voice and Speech; 1995.
12. Read C, Buder EH, Kent RD. Speech analysis systems: a survey. *J Speech Hear Res.* 1990;33(2):363–374.
13. Read C, Buder EH Kent RD. Speech analysis systems: an evaluation. *J Speech Hear Res.* 1992;35(2);314–332.
14. Wheeler KM, Collins SP, Sapienza CM. The relationship between VHI scores and specific acoustic measures of mildly disordered voice production. *J Voice.*2006;20(2):308–317.
15. Askenfelt A, Hammarberg B. Speech waveform perturbation analysis: a perceptual-acoustic comparison of seven measures. *J Speech Hear Res.* 1986;29(1): 50–64.
16. Wuyts FL, De Bodt M, Molenberghs G, et al. The dysphonia severity index: an objective measure of vocal quality based on a multiparameter approach. *J Speech Lang Hear Res.* 2000;43:796–809.
17. Hakkesteegt MM, Brocaar MP, Wieringa MH, Feenstra L.The relationship between perceptual evaluation and objective multiparametric evaluation of dysphonia severity. *J Voice.* 2008; 22(2):138–145.
18. Linder R, Albers AE, Hess M, Pöppl SJ, Schönweiler R. Artificial neural network-based classification to screen for dysphonia using psychoacoustic scaling of acoustic voice features. *J Voice.* 2008;22(2):155–163.

19. Jacobson B, Johnson A, Grywalski C, Silbergleit A, Jacobson G, Benninger MS. The Voice Handicap Index (VHI): development and validation. *Am J Speech Lang Pathol.* 1997;6:66–70.
20. Eadie T, Doyle P. Classification of dysphonic voice: acoustic and auditory perceptual measures. *J Voice.* 2005; 19(1):1–14.
21. Kent RD, Read C. *The Acoustic Analysis of Speech.* San Diego, CA: Singular Publishing Group; 1992.
22. Deliyski DD, Evans MK, Shaw HS. Influence of data acquisition environment on accuracy of acoustic voice quality measurements. *J Voice.* 2004; 19(2):176–186.
23. Titze IR, Winholtz WS. Effect of microphone type and placement on voice perturbation measurements. *J Speech Hear Res.* 1993;36(6):1177–1190.
24. Deliyski DD, Shaw HS, Evans MK. Adverse effects of environmental noise on acoustic voice quality measurements. *J Voice.* 2005;19(1):15–28.
25. Hill DP, Meyers AD, Scherer RC. A comparison of four clinical techniques in the analysis of phonation. *J Voice.* 1990;4(3):198–204.
26. Hillman RE, Holmberg EB, Perkell JS, Walsh M, Vaughn C. Phonatory function associated with hyperfunctionally related vocal fold lesions. *J Voice.* 1990;4(1):52–63.
27. Kempster G, Kistler DJ, Hillenbrand J. (1991). Multidimensional scaling analysis of dysphonia in two speaker groups. *J Speech Hear Res.* 34(3): 534–543.
28. Wolfe V, Cornell R, Palmer C. Acoustic correlates of pathologic voice types. *J Speech Hear Res.* 1991;34(3):509–516.
29. Wolfe V, Fitch J, Cornell R. Acoustic prediction of severity in commonly occurring voice problems. *J Speech Lang Hear Res.* 1995;38(2):273–279.
30. Martin D, Fitch J, Wolfe V. Pathologic voice type and the acoustic prediction of severity. *J Speech Lang Hear Res.* 1995; 38(4):765–771.
31. Rabinov C, Kreiman J, Gerratt B, Bielamowicz S. Comparing reliability of perceptual ratings of roughness and acoustic measures of jitter. *J Speech Lang Hear Res.* 1995;38(2):26–32.
32. Hillenbrand J, Houde R. Acoustic correlates of breathy voice quality: dysphonic voices and continuous speech. *J Speech Lang Hear Res.* 1996;39(2): 311–321.
33. Shrivastav R, Sapienza CM, Nandur V. Application of psychometric theory to the measurement of voice quality using rating scales. *J Speech Lang Hear Res.* 2005;48:323–335.
34. Karnell MP. Laryngeal perturbation analysis: minimum length of analysis window. *J Speech Hear Res.* 1991;34(3): 544–548.
35. Scherer R, Vail V, Guo C. Required number of tokens to determine representative voice perturbation values. *J Speech Lang Hear Res.* 1995;38(6):1260–1269.
36. Titze IR, Liang H. Comparison of Fo extraction methods for high-precision voice perturbation measurements. *J Speech Hear Res.* 1993;36(6):1120–1133.
37. Bielamowicz S, Kreiman J, Gerratt B. Voice analysis systems for perturbation measurement. *J Speech Lang Hear Res.* 1993;39(1):126–134.
38. Garrett KL, Healey EC. An acoustic analysis of the fluctuations in the voices of normal adult speakers across three times of day. *J Acoust Soc Am.* 1987;82:58–62.
39. Nittrouer S, McGowan RS, Milenkovic PH, Beehler D. Acoustic measurements of men's and women's voice: a study of context effects and covariation. *J Speech Hear Res.* 1990;33(3):761–775.
40. Stone RE, Rainey CL. Intra- and intersubject variability in acoustic measures of normal voice. *J Voice.* 1991;5(3): 189–196.
41. Pausewang Gelfer M. Fundamental frequency, intensity, and vowel selection: effects on measures of phonatory stability. *J Speech Lang Hear Res.* 1995; 38(6):1189–1198.

42. Milenkovic PH. Least mean squares of waveform perturbation. *J Speech Hearing Res.* 1987;29(4):529–538.
43. Titze IR. Acoustic interpretation of the voice-range profile (phonetogram). *J Speech Hear Res.* 1992;34(5):21–35.
44. Akerlund L, Gramming P, Sundberg J. Phonetogram and averages of sound pressure levels and fundamental frequencies of speech: comparison between female singers and nonsingers. *J Voice.*1992;6:55–63.
45. Schutte HK, Seidner W. Recommendation by the Union of European Phoniatricians (UEP): standardizing voice area measurement/phonetography. *Folia Phoniatr.* 1983;35:286–288.
46. Behrman A, Agresti CJ, Blumstein E, Sharma G. Meaningful features of voice range profiles from patients with organic vocal fold pathologies. *J Voice.* 1996;12:540–550.
47. Ma E, Robertson J, Radford C, Vagne S, El Halabi R, Yiu E. Reliability of speaking and maximum voice range measures in screening for dysphonia. *J Voice.* 2007;21(4):397–406.
48. Carson P, Ingrisano DR, Eggleston KD. The effect of noise on computer-aided measures of voice: a comparison of CSpeech and the Multi-Dimensional Voice Program software using the CSL 4300B Module and Multi-Speech for Windows. *J Voice.* 2003;17(1):12–20.
49. Higgins M, Netsell R, Schulte L. Vowel-related differences in laryngeal articulatory and phonatory function. *J Speech Lang Hear Res.* 1998;41(4):712–724.
50. Glaze LE, Bless DM, Susser RD. Acoustic analysis of vowel and loudness differences in children's voice. *J Voice.* 1990;4(1):37–44.
51. Parsa V, Jamieson DG. Acoustic discrimination of pathological voice: sustained vowels versus continuous speech. *J Speech Lang Hear Res.* 2001;44:327–339.
52. Heman-Ackah YD. Reliability of calculating the cepstral peak without linear regression analysis. *J Voice.* 2004; 18(2):203–208.
53. Heman-Ackah YD, Michael DD, Goding GS. The relationship between cepstral peak prominence and selected parameters of dysphonia. *J Voice.* 2002; 16(1):20–27.
54. Awan SN, Roy N. Acoustic prediction of voice type in women with functional dysphonia. *J Voice.* 2005;19(2):268–282.
55. Martin D, Fitch J, Wolfe V. Pathologic voice type and the acoustic prediction of severity. *J Speech Hear Res.* 1995; 38(4):765–771.
56. Maryn Y, Roy N, De Bodt M, Van Cauwenberge P, Corthals P. Acoustic measurement of overall voice quality: a meta-analysis. *J Acoust Soc Am.* 2009;5: 2619–2634.
57. Awan SN, Roy N, Jette M, Meltzner GS, Hillman RE. Quantifying dysphonia severity using a spectral/cepstral-based acoustic index: Comparisons with auditory-perceptual judgments from the CAPE-V. *Clin Linguist Phon.* 2010;24:742–758.
58. Awan SN, Roy N. Acoustic prediction of voice type in adult females with functional dysphonia. *J Voice.* 2005;19: 268–282.
59. Peterson E, Roy N, Awan S, Merrill R, Banks R, Tanner K. Toward validation of the Cepstral Spectral Index of Dysphonia (CSID) as an objective treatment outcomes measure. *J Voice.* 2013; 27(4):401–410.
60. Rothenberg M. Measurement of air flow during speech. *J Speech Hear Res.* 1977;2(1),155–176.
61. Scherer RC. Aerodynamic assessment in voice production. In: *Assessment of Speech and Voice Production: Research and Clinical Applications.* Bethesda, MD: National Institute on Deafness and Other Communicative Disorders; 1991:42–49.
62. Schutte HK. Integrated aerodynamic measurements. *J Voice.* 1992;6(2):127–134.
63. Kitajima K, Fujita F. Clinical report on preliminary data on intraoral pressure in the evaluation of laryngeal pathology. *J Voice.* 1992;6(1):79–85.

64. Miller CJ, Daniloff R. Airflow measurements: theory and utility of findings. *J Voice.* 1993;7(1):38–46.
65. Smitheran J, Hixon YJ. A clinical method for estimating laryngeal airway resistance during vowel production. *J Speech Hear Dis.* 1981;46(1):138–146.
66. Melcon M, Hoit JD, Hixon TJ. Age and laryngeal airway resistance during vowel production. *J Speech Hear Dis.* 1989;54(2):282–286.
67. Hoit JD, Hixon TJ. Age and laryngeal airway resistance during vowel production in women. *J Speech Hear Res.* 1992; 35(2):309–313.
68. Finnegan E, Luschei E, Barkmeier J, Hoffman H. Sources of error in estimation of laryngeal airway resistance in persons with spasmodic dysphonia. *J Speech Lang Hear Res.* 1996;39(1): 105–113.
69. Titze IR. (1991). Phonation threshold pressure: a missing link for glottal aerodynamics. In: Titze IR, ed. *Progress Report 1.* Iowa City, IA: National Center for Voice and Speech; 1991:1–14.
70. Fisher K, Swank P. Estimating phonation threshold pressure. *J Speech Lang Hear Res.* 1997;40(5):1122–1129.
71. Holmberg EB, Hillman RE, Perkell JS. Glottal airflow and transglottal air pressure measurements for male and female speakers in soft, normal and loud voice. *J Acoust Soc Am.* 1988;84: 511–529.
72. Weinrich B, Salz B, Hughes M. Aerodynamic measurements: normative data for children ages 6:0 to 10:11 years. *J Voice.* 2005;19(3):326–339.
73. Higgins MB, Netsell R, Schulte L. Aerodynamic and electroglottographic measures of normal voice production: intrasubject variability within and across sessions. *J Speech Hear Res.* 1994; 37(1):38–45.
74. Verdolini-Marston K, Titze IR, Drucker DG. Changes in phonation threshold pressure with induced conditions of hydration. *J Voice.* 1990;4(2):141–151.
75. Fisher KV, Ligon J, Sobecks JL, Roxe DM. Phonatory effects of body fluid removal. *J Speech Lang Hear Res.* 2001; 44:354–367.
76. Verdolini K, Min Y, Titze IR, et al. Biological mechanisms underlying voice changes due to dehydration. *J Speech Lang Hear Res.* 2002;45:268–281.
77. Sivasankar, Mahalakshmi, Fisher, Kimberly V. Oral breathing challenge in participants with vocal attrition. *J Speech Lang Hear Res.* 2003;46:1416–1427.
78. Tanner K, Roy N, Merrill RM, Elstad M. The effects of three nebulized osmotic agents in the dry larynx. *J Speech Lang Hear Res.* 2007;50:635–646.
79. Fritzell B. Inverse filtering. *J Voice.* 1992;6(2):111–114.
80. Stathopoulos ET, Sapienza CM. Developmental changes in laryngeal and respiratory function with variations in sound pressure level. *J Speech Lang Hear Res.* 1997;40:595–614.
81. Titze IR. Theoretical analysis of maximum flow declination rate versus maximum area declination rate in phonation. *J Speech Lang Hear Res.* 2006;49: 439–447.
82. Sapienza C, Stathopoulos E. Comparison of maximum flow declination rate: children versus adults. *J Voice.* 1994; 8(3):240–247.
83. Kreiman J, Gerratt BR, Antoñanzas-Barroso N. Measures of the glottal source spectrum. *J Speech Lang Hear Res.* 2007; 50:595–610.
84. Hirano M, Bless DM. *Videostroboscopic Examination of the Larynx.* San Diego, CA: Singular Publishing Group; 1993.
85. Colton R, Woo P, Brewer D, Griffin B, Casper J. Stroboscopic signs associated with benign lesions of the vocal folds. *J Voice.* 1995;9(3):312–325.
86. Woo P, Colton R, Casper J, Brewer D. Diagnostic value of stroboscopic examination in hoarse patients. *J Voice.* 1991; 5(3):231–238.
87. Hibi SR, Bless DM, Hirano M, Yoshida T. Distortions of videofiberoscopy

imaging: reconsideration and correction. *J Voice.* 1988;2(2):168–175.

88. Karnell MP. Synchronized videostroboscopy and electroglottography. *J Voice.* 1989;3(1):68–75.
89. Yanagisawa E. Fiberoptic and telescopic videolaryngoscopy—A comparative study. In: Baer T, Sasaki C, Harris K, eds. *Laryngeal Function in Phonation and Respiration.* Boston, MA: College-Hill Press; 1987:475–484.
90. Casper JK, Brewer DW, Colton RH. Pitfalls and problems in flexible fiberoptic videolaryngoscopy. *J Voice.* 1988;1(4): 347–352.
91. Peppard RC, Bless DM. The use of topical anesthesia in videostroboscopic examination of the larynx. *J Voice.* 1991; 5(1):57–63.
92. American Speech-Language-Hearing Association. The roles of otolaryngologists and speech-language pathologists in the performance and interpretation of strobovideolaryngoscopy. Retrieved November 7, 2013, from http:// www.asha.org/policy.
93. American Speech-Language-Hearing Association. Preferred practice patterns for the profession of speech-language pathology. Retrieved November 7, 2013, from http://www.asha.org/policy.
94. American Speech-Language-Hearing Association. Vocal tract visualization and imaging: position statement. Retrieved November 7, 2013, from http://www.asha.org/policy.
95. American Speech-Language-Hearing Association. Knowledge and skills for speech-language pathologists with respect to vocal tract visualization and imaging. Retrieved November 7, 2013, from http://www.asha.org/policy.
96. Patel R, Dailey S, Bless D. Comparison of high-speed digital imaging with stroboscopy for laryngeal imaging of glottal disorders. *Ann Otol Rhinol Laryngol.* 2008;117(6):413–424.
97. Yan Y, Damrose E, Bless D. Functional analysis of voice using simultaneous high-speed imaging and acoustic recordings. *J Voice.* 2007;21(5):604–616.
98. Yan Y, Ahmad K, Kunduk M, Bless D. Analysis of vocal-fold vibrations from high-speed laryngeal images using a Hilbert transform-based methodology. *J Voice.* 2005;19(2):161–175.
99. Zhang Y, Bieging E, Tsui H, Jiang JJ. Efficient and effective extraction of vocal fold vibratory patterns from high-speed digital imaging. *J Voice.* 2008. doi:10.1016/j.jvoice.2008.
100. Svec JG, Sram F, Schutte HK. Videokymography in voice disorders: what to look for? *Ann Otology Rhinol Laryngol.* 2007;116(3):172–180.
101. Qui Q, Schutte HK. A new generation videokymography for routine clinical vocal fold examination. *Laryngoscope.* 2006;116(10):1824–1828.
102. Childers DG, Alsaka YA, Hicks DM, Moore GP. Vocal fold vibrations: an EGG model. In: Baer T, Sasaki C, Harris K, eds. *Laryngeal Function in Phonation and Respiration.* Boston, MA: College-Hill Press; 1987:11–202.
103. Colton RH, Contour EG. Problems and pitfalls of electroglottography. *J Voice.*1990;4(1):10–24.
104. Orlikoff R. Scrambled EGG: the uses and abuses of electroglottography. *Phonoscope.* 1998;1(1):37–53.
105. Vieira M, McInnes F, Jack M. Comparative assessment of electroglottographic and acoustic measures of jitter in pathological voices. *J Speech Lang Hear Res.* 1997;40(2):170–182.
106. Mayes RW, Jackson-Menaldi C, DeJonckere PH, Moyer CA, Rubin AD. Laryngeal electroglottography as a predictor of laryngeal electromyography. *J Voice.* 2007. doi:10.1016/j.jvoice.2007.03.005.
107. Hirose H. Electromyography of the laryngeal and pharyngeal muscles. In: Cummings CW, Frederickson JM, Harker LA, Krause CJ, Schuller DE, eds. *Otolaryngology-Head and Neck Surgery.* St. Louis, MO: CV Mosby; 1986:1823–1828.

108. Ludlow CL. Neurophysiological assessment of patients with vocal motor control disorders. In: *Assessment of Speech and Voice Production: Research and Clinical Applications.* Bethesda, MD: National Institute on Deafness and Other Communicative Disorders; 1991:161–171.
109. Kotby M, Fadly E, Madkour O, et al. Electromyography and neurography in neurolaryngology. *J Voice.* 1992; 6(2):159–187.
110. Koufman J, Walker. Laryngeal electromyography in clinical practice: indications, techniques, and interpretation. *Phonoscope.* 1998;1(1):57–70.
111. American Association of Electrodiagnostic Medicine. Laryngeal electromyography: an evidence-based review. *AAEM Practice Topic Electrodiagn Med. Muscle Nerve.* 2003;28:767–772.
112. Rubin AD, Praneetvatakul V, Heman-Ackah Y, Moyer CA, Mandel S, Sataloff RT. Repetitive phonatory tasks for identifying vocal fold paresis. *J Voice.* 2005;19(4):679–686.
113. Heman-Ackah YD, Barr A. The value of laryngeal electromyography in the evaluation of laryngeal motion abnormalities. *J Voice.* 2006;20(3):452–460.
114. Roy N, Barkmeier-Kramer J, Sivasankar M, et al. Evidence-based clinical voice assessment: a systematic review. *Am J Speech Lang Pathol.* 2013;22(2):212–226.

Appendix 6–A
Joint Statement: ASHA and AAO-HNS

The Roles of Otolaryngologists and Speech-Language Pathologists in the Performance and Interpretation of Strobovideolaryngoscopy

American Academy of Otolaryngology Voice and Swallow Committee and ASHA Special Interest Division on Voice and Voice Disorders

This joint statement regarding the use of strobovideolaryngoscopy has been developed by the American Academy of Otolaryngology Voice and Swallow Committee and the Special Interest Division on Voice and Voice Disorders of the American Speech-Language-Hearing Association.

Strobovideolaryngoscopy (including rigid and flexible endoscopy) is a laryngeal imaging procedure that may be used by otolaryngologists and other voice professionals as a diagnostic procedure. Physicians are the only professionals qualified and licensed to render medical diagnoses related to the identification of laryngeal pathology as it affects voice. Consequently, when used for medical diagnostic purposes, strobovideolaryngoscopy examinations should be viewed and interpreted by an otolaryngologist with training in this procedure. Speech-language pathologists with expertise in voice disorders and with specialized training in strobovideolaryngoscopy are professionals qualified to use this procedure for the purpose of assessing voice production and vocal function. Within interdisciplinary settings, these diagnostic and vocal function assessment procedures may be accomplished through the combined efforts of these related professionals. Strobovideolaryngoscopy may also be used as a therapeutic aid and biofeedback tool during the conduct of voice treatment. Care should be taken to use this examination only in settings that assure patient safety.

Note. From American Speech-Language-Hearing Association. (1998). *The Roles of Otolaryngologists and Speech-Language Pathologists in the Performance and Interpretation of Strobovideolaryngoscopy* [Relevant paper]. Available from http://www.asha.org/policy.

Appendix 6–B
Vocal Tract Visualization and Imaging: Position Statement

Ad Hoc Committee on Advances in Clinical Practice

It is the position of the American Speech-Language-Hearing Association (ASHA) that vocal tract visualization and imaging for the purpose of diagnosing and treating patients with voice or resonance/aeromechanical disorders is within the scope of practice of the speech-language pathologist.

The practice of speech-language pathology is dynamic and changing. The scope of practice grows along with advances in technology enabling practitioners to provide new and improved methods of diagnosis and treatment. By identifying vocal tract visualization and imaging as within the scope of practice, it is not intended to limit any other new or emerging areas from being developed by speech-language pathologists or others to help improve treatment and diagnosis of voice and resonance/aeromechanical disorders.

If practitioners choose to perform these procedures, indicators should be developed, as part of a continuous quality improvement process, to monitor and evaluate the appropriateness, efficacy, and safety of the procedure conducted.

Note. From American Speech-Language-Hearing Association. (2004). *Vocal Tract Visualization and Imaging: Position Statement* [Position statement]. Available from http://www.asha.org/policy.

7

Survey of Voice Management

The extensive diagnostic voice evaluation has provided the voice pathologist with answers to what has caused the voice disorder and a description of the current vocal symptoms. The answers to the etiologic questions include primary causes as well as secondary etiologic factors. In addition, an understanding of the present vocal physiology and the relationship of respiration, phonation, and resonance has been established. A systematic management approach must now be initiated with the purpose of modifying or eliminating the etiologic factors and improving voice by rebalancing the three subsystems of voice production. This chapter is designed to survey the basic philosophies of voice treatment and to introduce the reader to some specific voice therapy techniques. In addition, the evidence that supports the use of the various techniques will be examined. Although the information contained in this chapter is by no means an exhaustive presentation of all voice therapy approaches, the survey is a useful point of departure for the study of voice management.

VOICE THERAPY ORIENTATIONS

As stated in Chapter 1, the management of voice disorders by "speech correctionists" began in the 1930s. Since that time, a rich and interesting history of voice therapy approaches has evolved, leading to several philosophical orientations of therapy. These orientations include hygienic, symptomatic, psychogenic, physiologic, and eclectic voice therapies.[1]

Hygienic Voice Therapy

Hygienic voice therapy often is the first step in many voice therapy programs. As discussed in Chapter 3, many etiologic factors contribute to the development of voice disorders. Poor vocal hygiene may be a major developmental factor. Some examples of behaviors that constitute poor vocal hygiene include shouting, talking loudly over noise, screaming, vocal noises, coughing, throat clearing, and poor hydration. When the inappropriate hygienic behaviors are identified, appropriate treatments can be devised for modifying or eliminating those behaviors. Once modified, voice production has the opportunity to improve or return to normal.

When poor vocal hygiene behaviors are modified, vocal symptoms may improve without direct manipulation of the voice subsystems (respiration, phonation, resonance). A common example is the reduction of the abusive behavior of shouting in children who have nodules. By eliminating the shouting behavior, the nodules are given an opportunity to resolve, and the voice may improve. If the compensations in the voice subsystems that resulted from the presence of the nodules have not habituated, improvement may result without the need for direct modification of the voice components, such as inappropriate pitch, breathiness, glottal attacks, and so on.

Hygienic voice therapy presumes that many voice disorders have a direct behavioral cause. This therapy strives to instill healthy vocal behaviors in the patient's habitual speech patterns. Good vocal hygiene also focuses on maintaining the health of the vocal fold cover through adequate internal hydration and diet. Once identified, poor vocal hygiene habits can be modified or eliminated leading to improved voice production.

Research Evidence and Vocal Hygiene

Thomas and Stemple[2] presented a comprehensive review of the research evidence supporting the use of the major voice therapy orientations. Despite the fact that hygienic methods have been a mainstay of voice therapy from the earliest days to the present, few studies have systematically investigated the efficacy of vocal hygiene therapy alone as a means of managing functional voice disorders. More common in the literature have been studies using vocal hygiene training as a control against which other more *direct* therapy methods are measured. In their review, Thomas and Stemple examined the evidence supporting vocal hygiene in several categories including:

- individual vocal hygiene training[3–9]
- group vocal hygiene training[10–15]
- specific vocal hygiene targets
  - ☐ Hydration[12,16–20]
  - ☐ Silent cough[21–23]
  - ☐ Voice rest/modified voice rest[21,24–31]

The major conclusions drawn from this review raised questions regarding the sufficiency of a vocal hygiene training as a stand-alone therapy. Results from many of the reviewed studies point to a superiority of direct treatments over hygiene approaches for treating voice disorders and call into question the degree of change possible with vocal hygiene when used alone.[5,6,9]

Studies examining the potential for *group-based* hygiene training for altering vocal behaviors have raised questions regarding the effectiveness of this form of treatment. Studies have demonstrated changes in *knowledge level* following training; however, such changes have not translated into changes in *behavior*.[10–15] As a result, the benefit of group hygiene training for preventing and managing voice disorders has not yet been clearly demonstrated.[2]

An exception to the above statement involves research related to hydration. Several well-controlled studies have identified reductions in phonation threshold pressure[17–19] as well as improvement in vocal endurance[32] following hydration conditions. Unfortunately, only one study has demonstrated the benefit of hydration in subjects with diagnosed voice disorders.[20] Nonetheless, hydration studies provide evidence to suggest that increased hydration may yield reduced phonatory effort along with enhanced vocal endurance, important considerations for the treatment of voice disorders.

A review of the above studies suggests that vocal hygiene training lacks adequate scientific evidence to support its use as a *primary* mode of voice treatment, but it should be considered as part of a larger, more comprehensive voice therapy program.

Symptomatic Voice Therapy

The focus of symptomatic voice therapy is on the modification of the deviant vocal symptoms or perceptual voice components that were identified during the diagnostic voice evaluation. Aberrant symptoms include a pitch that is too high or low, voice that is too soft or loud, breathy phonation, or the use of hard glottal attacks or glottal fry among others. Daniel Boone[24] was the first voice pathologist to organize previous literature and introduce this symptomatic therapy orientation to our profession. Symptomatic voice therapy is based on the premise that most voice disorders are caused by the functional misuse of the voice components including respiration, phonation, resonance, pitch, loudness, and rate. When identified through the diagnostic process, the misuses are eliminated or reduced through various voice therapy facilitating techniques. Boone[24(p11)] stated:

> In the voice clinician's attempt to aid the patient in finding and using his best voice production, it is necessary to probe continually within the patient's repertoire to find that one voice that sounds "good" and which he is able to produce with relatively little effort. A voice therapy facilitating technique is that technique which, when used by a particular patient, enables him easily to produce a good voice. Once discovered, the facilitating technique and resulting phonation become the symptomatic focus of therapy . . . This use of a facilitating technique to produce a good phonation is the core of what we do in symptomatic voice therapy for the reduction of hyperfunctional voice disorders.

Boone's original facilitating techniques included:

- altering of tongue position
- change of loudness
- chewing exercises
- digital manipulation
- ear training
- elimination of abuses
- elimination of hard glottal attack
- establishment of new pitch
- explanation of the problem
- feedback
- hierarchy analysis
- negative practice
- open-mouth exercises
- pitch inflections
- pushing approach
- relaxation
- respiration training
- target voice models
- voice rest
- yawn-sigh approach

As you read through this chapter, many of these approaches are described in detail, as they continue to be well utilized in the treatment of voice disorders. To summarize symptomatic voice therapy, we conclude that:

- The voice pathologist evaluates the presence of deviant voice components.
- The voice pathologist constantly probes for the "best" voice in the presence of the disorder.
- When the best voice is found, facilitating techniques are used to stabilize the improved voice production.

Symptomatic voice therapy assumes voice improvement through direct symptom modification.

Research Evidence and Symptomatic Voice Therapy

Many efficacy studies related to symptomatic treatment have failed to isolate a specific facilitating method for investigation. The studies have, rather, examined comprehensive symptomatic programs composed of a variety of facilitating methods. For the purpose of examining the evidence supporting this method of treatment, a therapy method was considered "symptomatic" if it aligned closely with one of the traditional facilitating methods listed above, or if it focused on the modification of an isolated vocal symptom for correction of voice.[2] Individual facilitating methods of pushing,[33,34] humming,[35] chewing,[36–38] yawn-sigh,[39–42] feedback (EMG,[43–46] acoustic and aerodynamic,[47,48] stroboscopy[49,50]), change of loudness,[51–53] inhalation phonation,[40,54,55] digital manipulation,[40,55] relaxation,[43,56,57] establishment of a new pitch,[40,58] amplification,[53,59] and comprehensive symptomatic programs with multiple methods employed[60–63] were reviewed.

The review of symptomatic therapies revealed concerns related to efficacy research within this therapy orientation. The majority of studies cited above demonstrated a lack of rigor in their research design. As a result, many of the facilitating methods within the symptomatic model have been supported by limited evidence. Although the studies provide early evidence for the use of a method, firm efficacy conclusions cannot be derived from these studies. Second, few of the above studies examined the efficacy of *specific* symptomatic techniques. Authors reported on the efficacy of *comprehensive* voice therapy protocols, but examinations of specific components of those protocols were few. Finally, the literature search demonstrated that no published evidence exists for many of the traditional symptomatic methods proposed by Boone and others.

At present, only one symptomatic method has been examined through multiple group studies. Promising lines of research have emerged suggesting the benefit of various forms of biofeedback for relaxing the laryngeal musculature. Systems offering feedback on laryngeal function, acoustic/aerodynamic output, and muscle effort appear efficacious. Recent advances in instrumentation perhaps will allow for the future development of even more sophisticated biofeedback methods.

The paucity of research evidence in support of symptomatic voice therapy does not mean that the approaches used in this method are not effective. The methods have been used successfully for many years. However, to *prove* the efficacy of these approaches, research in this area must advance on 2 fronts. First, the theoretical foundations of symptomatic methods must be examined. As sophisticated instrumentation was not available when symptomatic therapy emerged, the physiologic underpinnings of many symptomatic methods have not been demonstrated. Researchers should employ the advanced instrumentation now available in the field to examine the physiology behind these conventional methods. Second, the symptomatic methods must be examined more fully for their clinical efficacy. Future studies must advance beyond previous work by isolating specific facilitating methods for examination and employing more rigorous group research designs.

Psychogenic Voice Therapy

Psychogenic voice therapy is based on the assumption of underlying emotional or psychosocial behavioral causes for the voice disturbance. The relationship of emotions to voice production has been well documented in the literature starting as early as the mid-1800s to the present.[64–66] West, Kennedy, and Carr[67] and Van Riper[68] discussed the need for emotional retraining in voice therapy, whereas Murphy[69] and Brodnitz[70] presented excellent information related to the psychodynamics of voice production. In her comprehensive discussion of voice therapy and children, Moya Andrews[71] presented a compelling argument for examining the psychodynamics of a child's speaking environment when treating voice disorders in this population.

Aronson[72(p131)] first articulated his description of a psychogenic voice disorder when he stated that:

> A psychogenic voice disorder is broadly synonymous with a functional one but has the advantage of stating positively, based on the explanation of its causes, that the voice disorder is a manifestation of one or more types of psychological disequilibrium, such as anxiety, depression, conversion reaction, or personality disorder, which interfere with normal volitional control over phonation.

Aronson,[73] Case,[74] and Colton and Casper[75] further discussed the need for determining the emotional dynamics of the voice disturbance from the interactive perspectives of emotions as a cause for voice disorders and voice disorders as the cause of emotional disequilibrium.

In other words, psychogenic voice therapy focuses on identification and modification of the emotional and psychosocial disturbances associated with the onset and maintenance of the voice problem. When the psychogenic causes are resolved, the voice disorder dissipates. Voice pathologists must develop and possess superior interviewing and counseling skills, as well as the skill to know when the emotional or psychosocial problem is in need of more intensive evaluation and therapy by other professionals.

Research Evidence to Support Psychogenic Voice Therapy

Although it is well understood that emotions, personality, and psychological disorientation may play a vital role in the development and maintenance of voice disorders, there have been no studies designed to determine the efficacy of counseling, either by a speech-language pathologist or other health care providers, in resolving voice disorders. Further research is needed in the area of the contribution of emotions and personality to voice disorders as related to direct treatment, as described by Aronson.[72]

Physiologic Voice Therapy

Physiologic voice therapy includes voice therapy programs that have been devised to directly alter or modify the physiology of the vocal mechanism. Normal voice production is dependent on a balance among airflow, supplied by the respiratory system; laryngeal muscle strength, balance, coordination, and stamina; and coordination among these and the supraglottic resonatory structures (pharynx, oral cavity, nasal cavity). Any disturbance in the physiologic balance of these vocal subsystems may lead to a voice disturbance.

Disturbances may be in respiratory volume, power, pressure, and flow. Disturbances may also manifest in vocal fold tone, mass, stiffness, flexibility, and approximation. Finally, the coupling of the supraglottic resonators and the placement of the laryngeal tone may cause or be perceived as a voice disorder. The overall causes may be mechanical, neurologic, or psychological. Whatever the cause, the management approach is direct modification of the inappropriate physiologic activity through exercise and manipulation.

Inherent in physiologic voice therapy is a holistic approach to the treatment of voice disorders. They are therapies that strive to balance the 3 subsystems of voice production at once, as opposed to working directly on single voice components, such as pitch or loudness. Examples of physiologic voice therapy include vocal function exercises (VFEs),[76] resonant voice therapy (RVT),[77] the accent method of voice therapy,[78] and the manual laryngeal musculoskeletal reduction technique (MLMRT).[79]

Research Evidence and Physiologic Voice Therapy

Physiologic approaches to the management of voice emerged at a time of increased interest in efficacy research. The timing of the emergence of the 2 areas has resulted in a solid base of work. A number of well-controlled studies have been conducted that have demonstrated the efficacy of the accent method,[78,80–82] vocal function exercises,[83–87] RVT,[37,59,87–89] and the MLMRT.[79,90,91] A review of the above studies demonstrates support for physiologic approaches along both theoretical and clinical lines. The development of specialized instrumentation for viewing and measuring voice production has allowed the physiologic approaches to be examined from a physiologic, or theoretical, standpoint. Researchers have confirmed the physiology behind a number of these methods and arrived at conclusions regarding their potential benefit. Physiology studies, although not true efficacy studies, provide evidence in support of the theory behind the methods. Second, the majority of the physiologic approaches have been supported through stringent clinical research. Most methods have been investigated using at least one well-controlled group study; others possess lines of clinical research that have developed over a number of years.

Evidence suggests that physiologic methods of therapy enjoy greater scientific support than the other methods of voice treatment. Multiple, well-controlled group studies have emerged demonstrating the efficacy of physiologic treatments. On the other hand, evidence for other forms of therapy has lacked in strength and consistency. Hygiene methods, although subjected to group study, have not consistently emerged as efficacious. In addition, psychogenic voice therapy and the majority of facilitating methods under the symptomatic model have not received sufficient research attention.

Eclectic Voice Therapy

Eclectic voice therapy is the combination of any and all of the orientations of voice therapy. Successful voice therapy depends on the voice pathologist using all of the voice therapy techniques that seem appropriate for individual patients. Many patients may share the same diagnosis, but the etiologies and personalities, vocal needs, emotional reactions, compensatory responses, and motivations of their voice problems may be different. Because of these differences, the same pathologies may require different management approaches. Therefore, the voice pathologist is advised not to adhere to any one philosophical orientation of voice therapy but to learn a broad range of management approaches. Utilizing a case study format, let us examine a composite patient with a voice disorder from the perspective of each voice therapy orientation.

Case Study 1

The patient was a 48-year-old woman who was diagnosed by the laryngologist as having moderate, bilateral Reinke's edema, with the left fold suggesting a more severe draping, polypoid degeneration. The patient was referred for a voice evaluation and a trial voice therapy program. If short-term therapy was not successful in improving her vocal fold condition and voice quality, then the patient would be scheduled for surgical intervention.

History of the Problem

The patient was referred to the otolaryngologist by her internist when, during a regular physical examination, she noticed that the patient's voice quality "sounded as deep as a man's." The patient stated that her voice had always been deep and that she really did not think that there was much of a problem. When the otolaryngologist told her that she had vocal fold polyps, however, she became concerned enough to throw her cigarettes in the exam-room trash can and, by the time of the voice evaluation, had not smoked for 2 weeks. She reported that her voice quality was essentially the same throughout the day, although it tended to become "huskier" toward the end of a workday.

Medical History

The patient reported undergoing thyroid surgery 5 years ago during which her left thyroid lobe was excised. In addition, she underwent a tonsillectomy and an appendectomy as a teenager. She had also been hospitalized for chronic depression on 2 occasions. The last hospitalization lasted for 3 weeks and occurred 18 months ago. The patient continued to be treated for depression with medication and remained in bimonthly counseling.

Chronic medical conditions included asthma and frequent bronchitis; high blood pressure; elevated blood sugar; and rheumatoid arthritis. Daily medications were taken for depression, "nerves" (a sleep aid), thyroid, high blood pressure, and pain associated with the arthritis. Until 2 weeks prior, she had smoked 1½ to 2 packages of cigarettes per day for approximately 30 years. Her liquid intake was poor, consisting of approximately 3 cups of caffeinated coffee and 4 cans of caffeinated soda per day. Chronic throat clearing was noted throughout the evaluation. The patient indicated that on a day-to-day basis she felt "fair-to-poor" because of stress, fatigue, and arthritis pain.

Social History

The patient had been married for 29 years but recently had been separated from her husband for 3 months, causing much stress and tension. She had 3 grown children. The middle child, a 26-year-old son, had divorced recently and temporarily moved back into the house. Again, the patient pointed to the stress of this situation. The patient was not reticent to talk about her depression and indicated that an unhappy marriage and the feeling of an unfulfilled life were the causes.

A factory that made latex gloves for medical use had employed the patient for 6 years. She indicated that her specific job was in the "powder room" where the gloves were filled with powder and packaged. Apparently, the powder dust caused much coughing during the day. In addition, the packaging machines were noisy, requiring the workers to talk loudly to be heard. Most talking on the job was social among 8 people who worked in a large, well-ventilated room.

Nonwork activities included walking her 2 dogs nightly, talking on the telephone with her daughter, and actively shopping at yard sales and flea markets with a close friend. However, all of these activities were curtailed when she did not feel well physically and emotionally.

Oral-Peripheral Examination

The structure and function of the oral mechanism appeared to be well within normal limits for speech and voice production. The patient reported laryngeal sensations of dryness and occasional thickness. She demonstrated laryngeal area muscle tension and neck tension.

Voice Evaluation

The patient's voice quality was described as mild-to-moderately dysphonic, characterized by low pitch, increased loudness, and husky hoarseness.

- Respiration: Patient demonstrated a thoracic, supportive breathing pattern. She tended to speak at the end of her respiratory volume, especially toward the end of phrases.
- Phonation: A slight breathiness was noted during conversational voice. Occasional glottal fry was noted toward the end of phrases.
- Resonance: Normal
- Pitch: Patient demonstrated an unusually low pitch conversationally.
- Loudness: Patient spoke unusually loud for the speaking situation.
- Rate: Normal

Acoustic measures and aerodynamic analyses revealed the following:

- fundamental frequency = 136 Hz (low for gender)
- frequency range = 106 to 320 Hz (limited for gender)

- jitter percent /a/ = 0.56 (normal <1.04%)
- shimmer dB /a/ = 0.67 (abnormally high >0.35 dB)
- intensity (habitual) = 78 dB (normal to loud)
- airflow volume = 2300 mL (within normal limits [WNL])
- airflow rate = 180 mL/s, all pitches (WNL 75–200 mL/s)
- phonation time = 12.7 s (low)
- subglottic air pressure = 8.6 cm H_2O (high 5–7 cm H_2O)

Laryngeal videostroboscopic observation revealed a moderate bilateral vocal fold edema, worse left than right. Prominent blood vessels were noted bilaterally. Glottic closure was complete with mild ventricular fold compression. The amplitude of vibration was moderate-to-severely decreased left and moderately decreased right. The mucosal wave was severely decreased bilaterally. The open phase of the vibratory cycle was slightly dominant, while the symmetry of vibration was irregular by 50%. In short, the patient demonstrated an edematous, stiff, out-of-phase vocal fold vibratory pattern.

Impressions

The patient presented with a voice disorder secondary to many possible etiologic factors:

- long-term cigarette smoking
- laryngeal area muscle tension
- harsh employment environment in terms of dust and talking over noise
- poor hydration and large caffeine intake
- asthma and frequent bronchitis
- prescription medications causing mucosal drying
- frequent coughing and throat clearing
- emotional instability
- talking too loudly in general conversation
- using a low pitch

Recommendations

Recommendations based on the selected therapy orientations are as follows.

Hygienic Voice Therapy. The general focus would be to identify the primary and secondary behavioral causes of the voice disorder and to modify or eliminate these causes. The primary causes would include:

- smoking
- laryngeal dehydration from poor hydration, caffeine intake, and prescription drugs
- voice abuse such as talking loudly over noise at work, coughing, and throat clearing
- inhalation of large quantities of powder.

Therapy would focus on modification or elimination of the primary etiologic factors. The patient would be supported in her effort to stop smoking, encouraged to begin a hydration program and to reduce caffeine intake, given vocal hygiene counseling in an effort to reduce vocally abusive habits, and encouraged to wear a mask to filter her breathing at work. The secondary causes of tension, low pitch, and increased loudness would be expected to spontaneously improve as the primary causes were modified and the vocal fold condition improved.

Symptomatic Voice Therapy. The general focus would use facilitating techniques to:

- raise pitch
- reduce loudness
- reduce laryngeal area tension and effort

This direct symptom modification would follow an explanation of the problem and would run concurrently with modification of the vocally abusive behaviors including:

- smoking
- caffeine intake
- coughing and throat clearing

Psychogenic Voice Therapy. The general focus would explore the psychodynamics of the voice disorder. This exploration would include the following:

- Detailed patient interview to determine the cause and effects of stress, tension, and depression
- Determination of the exact relationship of emotions on voice problems
- Counseling of the patient regarding the effects of the emotions on voice problems
- Reduction of musculoskeletal tension caused by emotional upheaval
- Support of ongoing psychological counseling

The secondary focus would deal with modification or elimination of the abusive behaviors including:

- smoking
- caffeine intake
- coughing and throat clearing

Inappropriate use of pitch and loudness would most likely be viewed as obvious symptoms of the voice problem. As the psychodynamics improve, the voice symptoms would be expected to improve.

Physiologic Voice Therapy. The general focus would be to evaluate the present physiologic condition of the patient's voice production and develop direct physical exercises or manipulations to improve that condition. This patient demonstrated increased mass and stiffness of the vocal folds impairing the physical dynamics of vocal fold vibration. She was required to build greater subglottic air pressure to initiate and maintain vibration that required a borderline high airflow rate. This increased pressure caused her to speak too loudly in conversation. She also attempted to overcome these problems by making physical adjustments, such as increasing supraglottic tension in an effort to maintain her voice. When added to the mucosal and muscular stiffness, vocal hyperfunction was the result. The primary management program would therefore include vocal function exercises and resonant voice therapy designed to rebalance the 3 subsystems of voice production.

The secondary focus would include the following:

- Implementation of hydration program and decreasing of caffeinated products to improve the mucous membrane of vocal folds
- Discussion of the potential impact of her medications with the patient's physician
- Elimination of habit coughing and throat clearing

Eclectic Voice Therapy. It is obvious in the review of these orientations that each management approach has certain strengths, as well as inherent weaknesses. It also is obvious that the orientations must overlap to be effective. You will be able to best treat your patients with the understanding and use of all of these orientations. Therefore, eclectic voice therapy is obviously the treatment of choice with any patient with a voice disorder. This particular patient would best be served when the management plan included:

- elimination or modification of the vocal abuses and attention to the mucosal covering of the vocal folds
- symptom modification as required
- attention to the psychodynamics of the problem
- direct physiologic exercise

The remainder of this chapter presents specific treatment strategies categorized under the major therapy orientations including hygienic, symptomatic, psychogenic, and physiologic voice therapies. Also included are voice therapy strategies used with special populations.

HYGIENIC VOICE THERAPY

Treatment Strategies for Vocally Traumatic Behavior

Hyperadduction of the vocal folds is vocally traumatic, especially when the trauma occurs frequently. Some common vocally traumatic behaviors that may be modified through voice therapy include shouting, loud talking, screaming, producing vocal noises, and habitual throat clearing. There are many opportunities for voice trauma among both adults and children. Homemakers may shout at their children for discipline, factory workers talk loudly over noise for extended periods of time, and teachers and lecturers may talk too loudly with inappropriate tone focus on a routine basis. Most children shout and make vocal noises. They shout during unsupervised play; they are encouraged to shout while participating in team sports; and they shout when they are angry. Even artistic voice users exhibit vocally "aggressive" productions in voiceover advertisements, character voices, music videos, and other media images. Both adults and children also are susceptible to the development of throat clearing, either primarily as the result of frequent colds or allergies or secondary to the development of laryngeal pathologies. Let us examine some of the techniques used for modifying these vocally traumatic behaviors through vocal hygiene counseling.

Vocal Hygiene Therapy Approaches

The most effective way of dealing with voice abuse and misuse (sometimes called *phonotrauma*) is through vocal hygiene counseling. Once the abusive vocal behaviors have been identified, the first step of this approach is patient education. Patient education involves making the patient aware of the effects that trauma has on the laryngeal mechanism by utilizing graphic pictures and descriptions of the anatomy and physiology. The most effective educational tool is the patient's own video of the stroboscopic evaluation, if available. When not available, a quick Internet search will yield multiple videos of laryngeal pathology which can be used for demonstration. It is easier for patients to resolve their vocal problems when they truly understand the cause-and-effect relationships that may be displayed visually.

After the general phonotraumatic behaviors have been identified and explained in detail, it is important to determine exactly why the patient presents with these specific behaviors. If the trauma is caused by shouting, for example, the voice pathologist will want to know when and why it occurs and whether the patient feels it is required. Once these factors are determined, the treatment plan will involve eliminating the traumatic behaviors that can be eliminated, modifying the traumatic behaviors that cannot be totally eliminated to reduce the impact on the vocal mechanism, and manipulating the environment to secure more favorable voicing conditions.

We may synthesize the vocal hygiene approach to a 4-step outline:

1. Identify the vocally traumatic behaviors
2. Describe the effects on the voice-producing mechanisms
3. Define *specific* occurrences of the behaviors
4. Modify the behaviors.

Let us examine several cases in the context of the vocal hygiene therapy approach.

Case Study 2: The Homemaker

A 35-year-old patient was referred with the diagnosis of bilateral vocal fold nodules. She had a several-year history of intermittent dysphonia that became persistent approximately 3 months before the voice evaluation. She reported that her voice was better in the morning than in the evening and that she had never experienced aphonia.

The patient's medical history was unremarkable except for a large intake of caffeine and little other liquid. She had never smoked and had always lived in a nonsmoking environment. Socially, she was a homemaker with 3 sons, ages 3, 8, and 12 years. She enjoyed crafts, decorating her newly purchased Victorian home, and until recently, sang soprano in the church choir. Her voice problem now precluded singing. Her 2 oldest sons played soccer, and her oldest son also played baseball and basketball. The patient's husband was a manufacturer's representative and was on the road 3 out of 5 working days. The patient admitted to frequent shouting when disciplining her children and cheering loudly during their many sporting events.

The patient's voice quality during the evaluation was moderately dysphonic, characterized by low pitch and a breathy hoarseness. This was consistent with the overall hoarseness rating on the CAPE-V of 67 mm. Respiration was thoracic and supportive for conversational voice. She was able to sustain the /z/ for 7 seconds and the /s/ for 21 seconds. Phonation was characterized by voice breaks and the production of occasional glottal fry. A limited pitch range was demonstrated with the habitual pitch located near the bottom of the range. Limited inflection was noted conversationally. Resonance was back-focused, and the loudness level was appropriate for the speaking situation. She was able to readily increase the loudness level to a shout. Rate was normal. The phonotraumatic behavior of throat clearing was noted throughout the evaluation. The patient complained that her voice quality worsened with use, suggesting laryngeal fatigue.

Instrumental measures yielded the following:

- fundamental frequency = 168 Hz (low <180 Hz)
- frequency range = 156 to 460 Hz (very limited for soprano)
- jitter percent = 0.57% (WNL <1.04%)
- mean intensity = 68 dB SPL (sound pressure level) (WNL)
- shimmer dB = 0.47 dB (high >0.35 dB)
- airflow volume = 3200 mL (WNL)
- airflow rate = 235 mL/s (high >200 mL/s)
- maximum phonation time = 13.6 s (low)
- subglottic air pressure = 5.2 cm H_2O (normal 5–7 cm H_2O)

Vocal traumas are common in many homemakers.[92,93] Homemakers often shout for disciplinary purposes and call their children home from long distances. Traumatic voice behaviors in the home that may not be easily recognized include calling or reprimanding a pet, shouting from one room to another, calling someone to the telephone, talking to a spouse or relative who is hard of hearing, and talking loudly over the noise of the children, television, or music and video players. By discussing the specific situations that relate to the patient, the voice pathologist and the patient may devise alternatives to the traumatic behaviors. The alternatives may be as simple as turning the volume down on electronic devices when speaking or as creative as blowing a whistle to call the children home for dinner. Some patients are advised not to answer when someone calls from another room but rather to make the caller seek them or to go to the caller before replying. Again, once the specific traumatic behaviors are identified, most motivated patients are able either to eliminate them or devise creative nontraumatic alternatives to aid in their own treatment processes.

The homemaker in Case Study 2 developed vocal nodules as a result of shouting in the home situation and at sporting events. She maintained inappropriate vocal health through habitual throat clearing, laryngeal dehydration, and laryngeal muscle strain. Following the 4-step vocal hygiene plan, this problem was managed as follows:

1. Identify the traumatic behavior:
   - shouting
   - throat clearing
   - caffeine intake
   - laryngeal muscle strain
2. Describe the effect:
   - accomplished with illustrations, as well as the patient's own stroboscopic evaluation
3. Define specific occurrences:
   - shouting to discipline children and at sporting events
   - chronic habitual throat clearing
   - heavy caffeine intake
4. Modify the traumatic behaviors:
   - attempt to discipline through discussion and behavioral consequences
   - substitute a mechanical noise maker for vocal enthusiasm at sporting events
   - eliminate habitual throat clearing through a behavior modification program (discussed later this chapter)

- introduce a formal hydration program {6 to 8 glasses [240 mL (8 oz)] of water or juices per day}.

Case Study 3: The Noisy Job Environment

Communication often is difficult and potentially vocally traumatic for people who work in noisy job environments. In these situations, the vocal trauma usually takes the form of loud talking or shouting over noise for extended periods of time. In defining specific occurrences, it is necessary to determine how much talking is job related—how much is necessary for the worker to carry out the duties of the job, and how much is simply social discourse. Unnecessary communication may certainly be reduced, but this is not the total answer. The clinician will also want to know the type of noise, whether constant or intermittent, to determine if there are more appropriate times than others to talk.

Strategies for modifying this behavior may include moving as far away from the noise sources as possible, shielding the voice with the body by turning away from the noise source, and wearing ear protectors so background noise is masked and the speaker is better able to hear his or her own voice. Another beneficial principle to teach patients who must talk in noisy environments is to "make the listener strain to hear you; do not strain your voice to be heard by the listener." Describing the Lombard effect,[94] in which the speaker will always talk slightly louder than the noise source, is often helpful for patients. Many patients do not realize how loudly they are talking in the noisy background because of the Lombard effect. Patients may also use electronic amplification of the voice. Personal amplifiers that fit in shirt pockets or attach to belts are available at reasonable prices and have been shown to be very effective for reducing vocal loudness for improving voice.[53] Finally, the most drastic step in working with a patient with a voice disorder caused by a noisy environment is to explore the possibility of removing the patient through job transfer to a less noisy environment.

For example, a 50-year-old male with a diagnosis of a postsurgical left unilateral vocal fold polyp was referred for voice evaluation and treatment. He worked as a foreman at a local automobile assembly plant. Being a nonsmoker, the polyp development was thought to be associated with his need to speak loudly in the work environment. The following vocal hygiene plan was developed during the diagnostic evaluation:

1. Identify the traumatic behavior:
   - talking loudly over noise on a daily basis
2. Describe the effect:
   - accomplished with video and discussion of physiology
3. Define specific occurrences:
   - discussing daily work duties with 22 workers
   - reporting daily activities to a supervisor
   - social discussions
4. Modify the traumatic behaviors:
   - meet with workers, 2 to 4 at a time, in office away from noise source
   - make inspections on the line, then ask workers to come into the office as needed
   - decrease social conversations
   - make workers strain to hear
   - explore the use of personal amplification

Case Study 4: The Public Speaker

Excessive loud talking with inappropriate tone focus and breath support by teachers, lecturers, politicians, preachers, actors, and other professional voice users may often be the cause of vocal dysfunction. These inappropriate vocal behaviors or misuses may lead to vocal fatigue and, in some cases, to vocal fold mucosal changes, including edema and mass lesions. In the early stages of the problem, the public speaker often will describe to the voice pathologist, in a perfectly normal voice, extreme vocal difficulties that occurred during presentations or lectures. The history of the problem normally includes strong voice in the morning that weakens as the day progresses.

Some of these patients report that by the end of the day they are "lucky to have any voice at all."

As the voice is tested during the diagnostic session, there is a good chance that findings will be normal and that the phonotraumatic behaviors will not be evident. Clinicians should secure an audio recording of the public-speaking voice to determine the presence of vocal trauma during the presentation. This is easily accomplished by having the patient ask a lecture participant to record 10-minute samples at both the beginning and the end of a presentation.

If it is determined, after reviewing the recording, that excessive loudness, inappropriate pitch, and poor tone focus are causing strain of the vocal mechanism, then the need to define the specific situation is present. For example, how large is the room? Are the acoustics adequate? How many people are being addressed? Is amplification available? What is the seating arrangement in relation to the podium? How many hours of public speaking are done each day? When do breaks occur? What is the subject matter?

After defining the situations, the occurrences, and the specific environment of the speaker, modifications are made. These may include moving the lecture site closer to the audience, using amplification, building vocal time-outs into daily lesson plans, or simply talking more softly while monitoring the back row of the audience to see if the speaker can still be heard.

For example, a 32-year-old female was referred for voice evaluation and treatment with the diagnosis of bilateral vocal fold edema and erythema. She was experiencing daily voice fatigue as she lectured to her classes. The patient was a new college professor who taught courses in special education and remedial reading. The following vocal hygiene plan was developed during the diagnostic evaluation:

1. Identify the traumatic behaviors:
   - excessive loudness during lectures
   - use of a high pitch
   - poor tone focus
2. Describe the effect:
   - accomplished with videostroboscopy of own vocal folds and discussion of physiology
3. Define specific occurrences:
   - during 9 hours of lecture per week to an average class size of 25 students
   - during occasional (average once per month) guest lectures that involved half-day workshops
4. Modify the traumatic behaviors:
   - ask the students to sit in the front of the room

- build in more classroom discussion and less straight lecture
- have more audience participation during workshops
- use amplification whenever possible

Case Study 5: Phonotrauma in Children

By far the most common cause of voice disorders in children is phonotraumatic behavior,[95] including the potentially traumatic behaviors of shouting, crying, loud talking, vocal noises, and throat clearing. Most children shout, and some shout more than others. Part of the natural childhood expression is through shouting. The problem, of course, arises when children who traumatize their vocal folds develop laryngeal pathologies such as vocal fold nodules or chronic vocal fold edema.

When laryngeal pathologies occur, traditional management approaches have focused on ways of reducing or eliminating the traumatic behaviors through behavior modification programs.[96] These programs involve identifying the specific vocal trauma and then charting their occurrences on daily graphs prepared by the voice pathologist. Reduction in the occurrences is recorded in some manner, and the child is given a physical reward for the reduction of the offending behaviors. Although this approach has proved to be successful with many children, its limited scope proves less than adequate for many others. We suggest that other vocal hygiene questions must be considered when planning management strategies for vocally traumatic behaviors of children. These questions include the following:

- How does the child shout?
- Why does the child shout?
- Does the child make vocal noises?
- Does nonplay shouting occur?
- Has the laryngeal pathology created a physiologic imbalance of the vocal mechanism?
- Does habitual throat clearing occur?

We examine each question individually.

How Does the Child Shout? Why, if most children shout, do some children develop laryngeal pathology and others do not? We might speculate that some children simply shout more than others do; or children are differentially susceptible to the development of laryngeal pathology; or maybe some vocal mechanisms are not as resilient as are others. Another reason that appears clinically significant is that different children shout in different ways. Some of the shouting behaviors may be more physiologically balanced and supported than others, and therefore not as traumatic to the vocal mechanism.

These speculations have led us to attempt a treatment strategy that has yielded successful results. That strategy is to *teach the child how to shout*. We believe that it is not practical or totally fair to ask a child to stop all shouting behaviors. Rather than trying to extinguish all shouting (especially during play), it is possible and effective to teach children to shout using a low-pitched voice with improved breath support and adequate forward focus. Using lower pitch reduces the natural stiffness and tension of the vocal folds inherent to higher pitch, thus reducing the glottal impact. This may be accomplished by teaching the child to use a "grown-up voice," "daddy's voice," or a "papa bear voice," depending on the child's age.

With older children, we simply explore their lower pitch range and choose a pitch level in the lower midportion of the range. The patient practices speaking at that level in a comfortable conversational loudness level and then is instructed in gradual steps to increase the loudness level without increasing pitch until an appropriate "shout" is attained. At the same time, respiratory support, using abdominal breathing patterns, is established. As the pitch and loudness are modified, a forward focus tone placement is established to further reduce glottal impact and to enhance loudness (Forward Focus or resonant voice exercises are discussed later in this chapter.) This method also works well with cheerleaders who develop voice disorders.

Why Does the Child Shout? This question explores the psychodynamics of the shouting behaviors. Andrews[71,97] explained the importance of modifying the psychosocial aspects of the child's shouting behavior for the more direct therapy interventions to be successful. The exploration and modification of these behaviors must involve cooperation of the parents. At times, major changes in family interactions must be developed. Reactions to the child who is vocally abusive often require major modifications in interpersonal strategies of parents and siblings. In extreme cases, family counseling may be helpful in developing more appropriate family psychodynamics.

Does the Child Make Vocal Noises? A traumatic vocal behavior that can be overlooked is the production of vocal noises. Many children make vocally traumatic noises during play, but unless children are specifically asked about vocal noises during the voice evaluation, they will remain undetected. Some favorite noises include machine guns, cars, trucks, motorcycles, sirens, various character voices, and animal noises. Each year there appears to be a popular new set of noises that most often are influenced by popular toys, movies, television shows, or video games. Modification or elimination of these abusive noises is often desirable as a part of the treatment plan. Various mouth sounds and whistles that do not involve phonation may serve as acceptable substitutions. Extinguishing these phonotraumatic behaviors rarely proves to be difficult as play behavior is quickly modified through natural maturity.

Does Nonplay Shouting Occur? Another factor that needs to be identified and modified is nonplay shouting. Again, it is extremely helpful to have a parent involved in the entire management process. If such cooperation is available, parent education may help to modify occurrences of shouting in the home, such as shouting from room to room, calling people to the telephone, and arguing with brothers and sisters. Suggestions for the parent may include not responding when the child calls from another room, forcing the child to physically seek the person being called; not shouting for the child and expecting a response; and attempting to control vocal sibling arguments. Without the parent's cooperation, nonplay shouting will probably continue, ideally with a modified low-pitched, abdominal-breath-supported, forward-focused shout.

Does Habitual Throat Clearing Occur? Many patients present with habitual throat-clearing behavior. As a primary etiology, throat clearing most commonly develops as a result of mucous drainage caused by colds, flu, and allergies or as a secondary symptom of laryngopharyngeal reflux. Although drainage is not detrimental to the laryngeal mechanism, the throat-clearing habit that results is potentially abusive because of the mechanical impact of the vocal folds and the grinding of the posterior laryngeal structures. In addition, acid burning caused by reflux in the posterior larynx may create a globus sensation, or "lump in the throat" feeling leading to habitual throat clearing. The behavior often continues even after the medical condition has resolved because of the inherent edema and irritation that lead to yet more throat clearing, simply as a result of habit. At times, this cycle continues until laryngeal pathology results.

Throat clearing may also develop secondary to laryngeal pathologies. This behavior occurs especially in the presence of mass lesions and vocal fold edema. Many patients report that they "feel" something in their throats that they try to clear. Some patients clear their throats to prepare the voice for phonation before they talk; others have no or little awareness of their throat clearing habit.

The importance of eliminating this behavior cannot be overstated. We have seen clinical cases in which all etiologic factors except throat clearing were resolved, and the phonotraumatic nature of this behavior alone maintained the pathology. The techniques for significantly reducing throat clearing apply to both children and adults. The following example is a management approach that is appropriate for all ages; the language used will vary, of course, with the age of the patient.

> Throat clearing is one of the most traumatic things you can do to your vocal folds. When you clear your throat like this (demonstrate), you create an extreme amount of movement of your vocal folds, causing them to slam and rub together (demonstrate using your hands). You should understand that it is not unusual for you to have developed this habit. The majority of patients we see with your type of voice problem also have this habit. Sometimes people do not even know that they are doing it. But often they say that they feel something in their throat, like phlegm or mucus. Most of the time, however, when you clear your throat, there is simply nothing there. The only thing you have accomplished is to create more vocal fold trauma.
>
> We have demonstrated to you with a recording of this evaluation that often when you clear your throat, it occurs right before you begin to speak. Also, you are clearing many more times than you realized. This is a sign that throat clearing is very much a habit. Like all habits, it is difficult to break. We are, therefore, going to try to make it easier by giving you a substitute habit that will take the place of throat clearing, accomplish the same thing as throat clearing, and will not hurt your vocal folds. This substitute, nonabusive habit is a forceful swallow. If you do, in fact, occasionally have an increased amount of mucus on your vocal folds, a forceful swallow will accomplish the same thing as throat clearing, minus the vocal fold trauma. The only difference is that throat clearing actually feels good. It psychologically gives you more relief than the forceful swallow, even though it physically accomplishes no more. It is your goal to overcome this psychological dependence. Understand that this habit is harmful, and it must be broken.
>
> To break this habit, you need to tell everyone in your family and any friends who are around you often (and whom you feel comfortable in telling)

that you are not permitted to clear your throat anymore. When these "helpers" hear you clear your throat, and they will, they are to immediately point it out to you. Your task then is to "swallow hard." Obviously, it will not be necessary to swallow, because you just cleared your throat. Nonetheless, this is your first step in substituting the forceful swallow for the throat clearing.

After your family and friends have pointed out your throat clearing to you several times, you will begin to catch yourself. You will clear your throat and almost immediately think "OOPS! I am not supposed to do that." Your response again should be to swallow forcefully. When you have caught yourself clearing your throat several times, you will begin to halt yourself just prior to clearing. Once again, you will substitute the swallow, but this time the throat clearing was stopped. By the time you have reached this point, you will be very close to breaking the habit totally. The final goal will be met when you realize that you are swallowing many fewer times than the number of times you used to clear your throat.

I want you to work very hard on this problem. I think you will be very surprised just how quickly you are able to break this habit. As a matter of fact, the majority of our patients have significantly reduced the habit within 1 to 2 weeks. Most patients, though, cannot do it alone. So please, find other people to help you by having them point out when this occurs.

Following this explanation, the patient typically will clear his or her throat more times than usual. The voice pathologist immediately points out each event, and the forceful swallow substitution is initiated. Great gains in habit modification often are made during this initial session.

Zwitman and Calcaterra[98] made another suggestion for modifying throat clearing. These authors suggested a "silent cough" substitution for this behavior. The silent cough is accomplished by breathing deeply and forcing air strongly through abducted vocal folds. This technique also reduces the abuse of coughing. A modified Valsalva maneuver may also be used as a throat clearing substitution. The patient is instructed to lightly approximate the vocal folds as if lifting an object. The impounded subglottic air is then sharply released without vocalization.

As stated previously, several factors must be considered when planning therapy strategies for children with vocally traumatic behaviors. Charting and graphing may certainly serve as a positive behavior modification approach in modifying or eliminating traumatic vocal events; however, many more factors may be considered and other approaches utilized. A summary of a vocal hygiene plan for phonotraumatic children would be as follows:

1. Identify the traumatic behaviors:
   - Shouting
   - Loud talking
   - Vocal noises
   - Throat clearing
2. Describe the effect:
   - Use pictures, diagrams, drawings, and video of the pathology. (Do not hesitate to give simple explanations of anatomy and physiology to children.)
3. Define specific occurrences of the behaviors:
   - These may be distinctly different with every child. No 2 children will follow the exact same management plan as the specific occurrences will vary.

- Psychodynamics of the behavior must also be described.

4. Modify the traumatic behaviors:
    - Teach the child how to shout
    - Modify or eliminate vocal noises
    - Eliminate nonplay shouting
    - Eliminate throat clearing

Case Study 6: Can We Always Expect Success?

Vocal trauma may occur in many settings under many different circumstances. These settings might include nightclubs, bars, bowling alleys, swimming pools, auction houses, sporting events, work environments, homes, schools, and churches. Wherever we communicate, the possibility of voice misuse is present. The lifestyles of patients often dictate the ease or difficulty they will have in attempting to make vocal modifications. Some patients are not willing to modify their lifestyles even for the health of the laryngeal mechanism. Voice pathologists must realize that their own concern for the patient's voice disorder does not always match that of the patient. For example, the patient who enjoys "getting rowdy" in bars may not respond well to the voice pathologist's greatest efforts for vocal reeducation. The patient who enjoys bowling in winter leagues may continue to bowl and abuse the voice by laughing, talking, and shouting above the noise level, as well as drinking dehydrating liquids and perhaps smoking. These are the patients who provide us with interesting challenges, but we must remember that the ultimate responsibility for change rests with the patient. The following is an interesting example of the patient who failed to respond to a 4-step vocal hygiene counseling program.

The patient was a 30-year-old female who was referred for evaluation and treatment with the diagnosis of chronic vocal fold edema. The patient reported experiencing intermittent dysphonia for several years, but the dysphonia became persistent about 6 months prior to the evaluation. The diagnostic evaluation yielded the following management plan:

1. Identify the phonotrauma:
    - shouting
    - straining the singing voice
2. Describe the effect:
    - accomplished with illustrations and review of stroboscopic examination
3. Define specific occurrences:
    - shouting to discipline her children
    - straining the voice during church singing on Sunday mornings and Wednesday evenings
4. Modify the behaviors:
    - discussed various other strategies for disciplining children
    - patient agreed to discontinue singing until her voice improved
    - singing without strain would then be discussed

The patient's voice quality during the evaluation was moderately dysphonic, characterized by a low pitch, glottal fry phonation, pitch breaks, and breathiness. No significant change or improvement in voice quality was observed during a 3-week period of therapy sessions, which were held weekly. The patient denied shouting at her children and singing in church during this time.

Also during this period an interesting pattern of dysphonia was noted. The patient reported experiencing severe dysphonia and almost total aphonia every Sunday night and Thursday morning. When the patient was seen in therapy on Wednesdays, the original moderate dysphonia was noted. Further questioning yielded the true cause of the patient's disorder.

As you may have guessed, she attended church services on Sunday mornings and Wednesday evenings. Although she refrained from singing, she joined the many people in the congregation who responded with vigorous vocal enthusiasm to the preacher's message. The need to add this behavior to those requiring modification was explained to the patient.

Although she made concentrated efforts to reduce her vocal enthusiasm during the church service, she had little success in doing so. Final attempts were made to counteract these periods of extreme vocal trauma through direct symptom modification and attempting to train a more healthy vocal focus. Because of the frequency of the trauma, however, this also proved unsuccessful. The patient eventually was terminated from therapy with no improvement noted in her vocal condition. This patient made an informed decision that her enthusiastic vocal behaviors during the church service were more important to her than improving the quality of her voice.

Can we always expect success? Yes! Otherwise, we may be guilty of a self-fulfilling prophecy. Will we succeed with all patients? The answer, unfortunately, is no. But only a concerted effort for a reasonable period of time will give us that answer.

Hydration

The vocal hygiene program not only considers elimination and modification of traumatic vocal behaviors, it must also attend to the health of the tissue lining of the true vocal folds and larynx. Internal hydration is an important component of good vocal hygiene.[32,99–101] In our clinical experience, most of the patients who present with voice disorders are not well hydrated. It has been demonstrated that phonation threshold pressure is increased under experimentally induced laryngeal dehydration.[100] Increased phonation threshold pressure translates to increased effort by the patient to produce voice. Over an extended period of time this increased effort may lead to voice fatigue, laryngeal pathology, or both.

We recommend that most of our patients begin a formal hydration program. Various recommendations have been made regarding the appropriate amount of liquid intake per day. The 2 most common recommendations include drinking 8, 240-mL (8 fl oz) glasses of water per day or drinking half of an individual's body weight in ounces. So, if a person weighs 63 kg (140 pounds), she/he would drink 2100 mL (70 fl oz) of water per day. The appropriate amount of hydration will vary as determined by body size and physical activity. Increased physical activity would require a greater intake of fluid. It is explained to the patient that what is swallowed does not touch the vocal folds. Rather the liquid and food is diverted around the vocal folds by the epiglottis and collects in the piriform sinus cavity and then enters the esophagus. Should any of the swallowed substance mistakenly enter the larynx, a spontaneous protective cough would be initiated (as if it went down the wrong pipe). The importance of liquid intake is based on the need for whole-body hydration. It is explained that the vocal folds must be well lubricated for them to function normally. Secretory glands that lie in the ventricles and below the folds and mucus from the lungs provide this lubrication. The whole body must be well hydrated; otherwise, the fluid secreted by the glands to the vocal folds will demonstrate increased viscosity. In other words, thick, sticky mucus will cover the vocal folds and interfere with vibration.

In this dehydrated state, patients often feel the sticky mucus and assume that sinus drainage is causing this problem. Often, the natural reaction is to take a dehydrating medication to reduce the mucus. Of course, this only exacerbates the problem. Another negative result may be the development of a throat-clearing habit.

When patients understand the importance of adequate hydration to maintaining a healthy vocal mechanism, they most often respond well by conforming to a hydration program. It is requested that the patient significantly reduce caffeine and alcohol intake, as these are both diuretics and contribute to dehydration. Patients are instructed to find a receptacle with a known liquid volume. Each day they are requested to gradually increase their liquid intake from the receptacle until they reach and then maintain the required liquid intake. Improved laryngeal hydration often leads directly to improved voice quality, as well as reduction in the physical sensations in the throat as reported by patients.

Confidential Voice

Initiation of a vocal hygiene program may require short-term vocal conservation especially when the vocal fold injury is recent, or the patient has just had vocal fold surgery. Colton and Casper[75] suggested the term "confidential voice" to describe an easy, quiet, breathy voice, as if speaking confidentially to someone at close range. When the voice is produced in this manner, the vocal folds have small amplitudes of vibration, and they do not strike each other forcefully. Confidential voice therapy (CVT) does not involve a single procedural protocol from start to finish for all patients. Rather, the voice pathologist adapts CVT to fit the patient's particular need. The clinician will demonstrate to the patient how to produce quiet, easy, breathy voice. Whispered voice is not desirable. The main challenge to the patient is remembering to use the confidential voice in all speaking situations. The confidential voice is usually used in therapy for only a short period of time. After some recovery has been achieved, other therapy approaches are used to complete the voice recovery.

SYMPTOMATIC VOICE THERAPY

Chapter 3 describes the components of voice that include respiration, phonation, resonance, pitch, loudness, and rate. The inappropriate use of any one vocal component or combination of components may lead directly to the development of a voice disorder. Voice disorders may occur in patients who simply have faulty vocal habits and use, for example, a functionally breathy voice, soft voice, or voice that is too high or too low in pitch. Other patients may use the resonance system inefficiently or may focus the laryngeal tone inappropriately, whereas others talk either too fast or too slow. When inappropriate vocal components are used, direct symptomatic voice therapy may be in order.

It is important to understand, however, that inappropriate vocal components may also be the *result* of laryngeal pathologies and not their cause. A patient with Reinke's edema may have a voice quality that is breathy and low in pitch for example. Although the components of pitch and respiration are inappropriate, they are not the primary causes of the voice disturbance, just merely 2 of the symptoms. Modification of the primary etiology (such as smoking in the case of Reinke's edema) is the first line of treatment, with symptom modification following only when necessary. We now examine symptom modification approaches for the primary components of voice production.

Therapy Approaches for Respiration

In reviewing the literature related to the role of respiration or breathing training in voice therapy, it becomes evident that a primary debate, which appeared in the early part of the 20th century, continues to this day. The debate questions whether respiratory control of voice production should be considered automatic and essentially ignored, or should direct respiratory training be part of a voice therapy program? As we travel through the literature, some authors give direct respiratory exercises and breathing training and some do not. Some authors state that few voice patients have breathing patterns so faulty that they interfere with normal phonation. However, it is evident that some laryngeal pathologies certainly alter normal respiration.[24,68,72,74,102–106]

The current conclusion that we have drawn from this debate is that respiratory training, whether direct or indirect, is a primary part of improving the disordered voice. The justification for this conclusion is that most therapy techniques modify air pressures and airflow in an attempt to bring about efficient voice production. Respiration is one of the three major subsystems responsible for the production of voice. Because physiologic balance of respiration, phonation, and resonance is the ultimate goal of voice therapy, the respiratory component cannot be ignored.

Symptomatic voice therapy techniques concentrate on direct modification of breathing for voice production. Breathing modifications most often are needed in individuals who talk with decreased breath support and professional speakers and singers who may require greater breath support during presentations than during normal conversational speech.

Limited Breath Support

Patients who continue to talk following the normal expiration of air are talking with limited breath support. Because this type of phonation requires increased laryngeal muscle tension, this behavior may strain the vocal mechanism and lead to the development of a voice problem. Suggestions for reducing this behavior include the following:

- Identification: Identify the problem for the patient and describe its effect in detail, utilizing illustrations and descriptions of vocal fold anatomy and physiology.
- Ear training: Monitor the patient's respiration strategy utilizing audio-recorded samples of the voice.

- Component modification:
  - ☐ Practice breathing for voice by saying as many numbers as possible on a normal expiration. Stop before any force or strain is evident.
  - ☐ Mark a paragraph with phrase markers (Appendix 7–A). Read the paragraph aloud with normal inhalations occurring at each phrase marker.
  - ☐ Audio record an open discussion between the voice pathologist and the patient during the structured therapy period. Monitor the recording for inappropriate breathing patterns.
  - ☐ Stabilization: Ask the patient to monitor the voice daily during nontherapy conversational times. A good time to do this may be during dinner with the family.

Abdominal/Diaphragmatic Breathing Patterns

Some patients, especially those who use their voices for some type of public speaking, request strategies for learning "diaphragmatic breathing." Although the diaphragm is always active during respiration, some individuals use a greater amount of thoracic or chest breathing during respiration for speech. Chest breathing patterns may be adequate for voice support, although a more efficient means of breathing for speech can be achieved when the abdominal/diaphragmatic movements predominate over other respiratory chest wall movements.

A suggested approach for training this method follows:

> By utilizing a box diagram (Figure 7–1), describe the various means of air exchange, including clavicular, thoracic, and abdomino/diaphragmatic. The voice pathologist may say, "There are three ways in which air may be made to flow into the lungs. All three ways require some expansion of the thoracic cavity, where the lungs are located. The least efficient way to expand the cavity is to raise the top of the box or the shoulders. This allows for poor cavity expansion and would require much vocal effort and tension given the small amount of the air that enters the lungs. This type of breathing pattern is seldom used. The most common way of expanding the cavity is to raise the sides of the box, or the rib cage. This larger expansion normally allows enough air to be inhaled to support voice during normal conversational speech. If you watch people breathe in this manner as they talk, you will notice an increased chest and neck tension.
>
> "The most efficient method of air intake for the support of voice is through the downward contraction of the bottom of the box, or the diaphragm, and the outward expansion of the abdomen. The diaphragm is the dome-shaped elastic muscle that forms the bottom of the thoracic cavity. When it contracts downward, the abdomen is forced outward, and the cavity expands to its maximum extent without an unacceptable elevation of the chest. This expansion permits a greater flow of the air into the lungs. The air may then be used to better support your voice."

Following this explanation, the patient is asked to place one hand on the chest and the other hand on the upper abdominal wall. When inhaling, the abdominal wall will expand outward while the chest remains in a nearly fixed position with only minimal movement. Contraction of the diaphragm cannot be seen. The patient is asked to breathe in this manner without phonation while

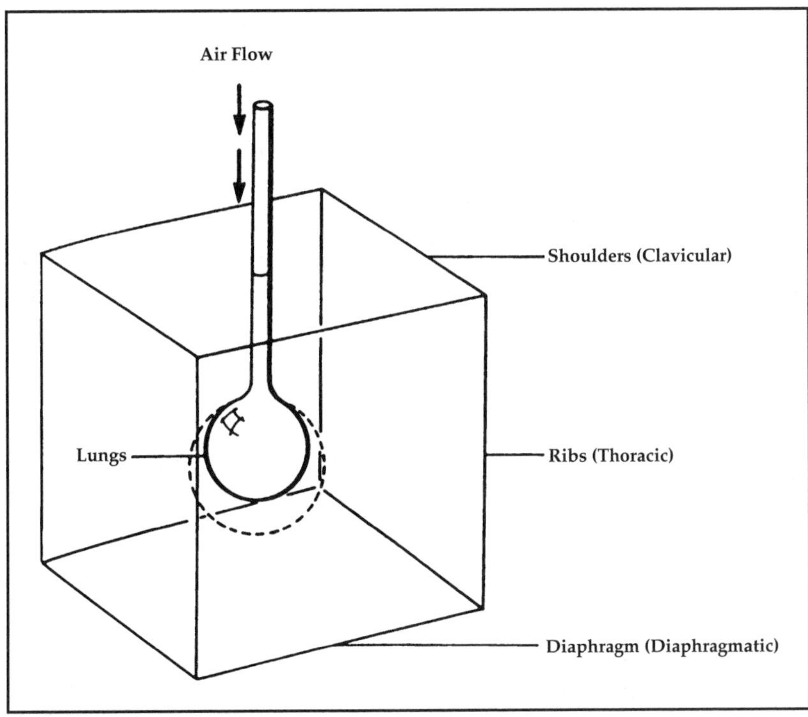

FIGURE 7–1. Box diagram representing breathing patterns.

observing the proper hand movement on both inhalation and exhalation. Practice is then gradually expanded, utilizing vowels, words, phrases, paragraph reading, and conversational speech, timed to the breathing pattern. The public speaking voice may also be practiced in the therapy session utilizing the new breathing method.

A variation of this method for training appropriate breathing is to ask the patient to lie down in a supine position. A book then may be placed on the abdomen while the patient is asked to observe the natural movement of the abdomen during breathing. As the patient inhales, the book will rise. The opposite movement will be observed during exhalation. As in the previous example, the patient is asked to breathe in this manner without phonation and then gradually introduce the voice component. This technique is simply used to introduce the patient to proper abdominal movement during respiration. The voice pathologist must understand that breathing in a supine position is different physiologically than breathing in an upright position.

Therapy Approaches for Phonation

Symptomatic voice therapy may be used to modify inappropriate components of phonation. Inappropriate phonatory habits include hard glottal attacks, glottal fry phonation, and breathy phonation. As usual, the first step in modifying these behaviors involves identifying the presence of these behaviors to the patient. This may be accomplished by evaluating audio-recorded samples of the voice. The impact of the vocal trauma should also be identified through illustrations and discussion of the effects on the voice-producing mechanisms. Finally, the specific misuse should be described in detail as follows.

Hard Glottal Attack

A hard glottal attack is made when subglottic air pressure, or air that you build up below your vocal folds, is increased to a very high pressure level just before you say a word that begins with a vowel sound. Then, when you say that word, the vocal folds literally blow apart (demonstrate a hard glottal attack) like this. This action is very harsh on the vocal folds. It causes them to squeeze together very hard to maintain the high air pressure. Then when the vowel sound is produced, they rub and bang together as the pressure is released.

Another way of describing this behavior is to use the example of a garden hose:

> A typical garden hose is attached to a faucet at one end and has a spray nozzle at the other end. When the nozzle is closed and the water is turned on at the faucet, a tremendous amount of pressure builds up through the whole system, with the greatest amount of pressure at the nozzle. If the nozzle is suddenly opened and then closed, the water gushes out and then slams against the nozzle valve when closed. If the nozzle were slightly open and the water was controlled at the faucet, however, the entire system would remain relaxed and little pressure would be exerted on the valve. We can relate the pressure in the hose to the air pressure you use for voice and the nozzle to your vocal folds. What you need to do is to learn how to produce words that begin with vowel sounds without building up that pressure.

The patient is then taught to produce a soft glottal attack or an easy onset by initiating phonation with the sound /h/, utilizing vowels such as h-a, h-i, h-e. h-o, vowel-consonant combinations such as h-it, h-at, h-ot, and progressing through words, phrases, paragraph reading, and conversation. The /h/ is extinguished as soon as possible in the process. Negative practice is effective as a stabilization strategy.

Glottal Fry Phonation

Glottal fry is the lower register of voice produced at the bottom of the normal pitch range.[107] It may be recognized as an aperiodic staccato sound and is produced on tightly approximated vocal folds with just the free edges vibrating. Aerodynamic measures reveal that glottal fry is produced with extremely reduced airflow (10–20 mL/s). We often observe glottal fry phonation at the end of phrases, as patients drop breath support, and in the voices of patients who complain of voice fatigue. Glottal fry during voice production has become somewhat common as a voicing technique in popular culture. Extended use of glottal fry phonation may lead to vocal dysfunction and should be modified. Because it often occurs in conjunction with the use of an inappropriately low pitch, modification of glottal fry is made by training a slight increase in pitch and loudness. The increase in pitch and loudness requires improved respiratory support, which explains why this technique eliminates the glottal fry. Another technique for modifying glottal fry phonation is the use of resonant voice therapy, which is described later in this chapter.

Breathy Phonation

Some patients have the habit of speaking with an incomplete adduction of the vocal folds, yielding a weak, breathy voice. A weak, breathy speaking voice may also be the result of disengaging the thyroarytenoid muscles and speaking in a falsetto voice. Although some actors cultivate this type of voice to project an image of sultriness or sexiness, it is a vocal misuse. Its prolonged use can lead to vocal dysfunction.

Again, therapy would begin with identification of the problem and education of the effects that breathy phonation may have on the vocal mechanism. When phonation is breathy, causing wastage of air during phonation, the vocal folds are forced to vibrate inefficiently. The inherent poor breath support impairs vocal quality by causing secondary abusive glottal or supraglottal tension.

The major symptomatic therapy approaches for modifying the breathy voice involve training the patient to produce a more firm or engaged vocal fold approximation. The specific approach used will depend on the severity of the breathiness:

- Mild breathiness may be modified through patient education and often through the use of a more precise articulation, especially on the plosive sounds /p/, /t/, and /k/.
- Training the speaker to increase vocal intensity may often modify a moderate amount of breathiness. A slightly louder voice will force the vocal folds to approximate more firmly, thus decreasing the wastage of air.
- Ear training, using an audio recording to compare the breathy voice to the louder voice, and negative practice are excellent modification approaches.
- A more than moderate amount of breathiness may require these approaches, as well as a more rigorous therapy approach. This may include actually teaching the patient to approximate the vocal folds utilizing the previously described "misuse" of hard glottal attacks. Hard glottal attacks will give the patient an awareness of vocal fold approximation and muscle engagement. The vowels produced in this manner will have clearer tones that can be compared to the patient's breathy tones. An even more rigorous approach would be the use of pushing exercises. These exercises combine the isometric pushing of the arms at the same moment of phonation. These simultaneous activities create firmer adduction of the vocal folds through overflow muscular tension, thus decreasing breathiness. Once the clearer tone is experienced and stabilized, the glottal attack and pushing strategy are quickly extinguished so as not to develop a vocal hyperfunction habit. (A complete description of glottal attack and pushing exercises is provided under voice therapy for vocal fold paralysis later in this chapter.) As a rule, we do not typically endorse the use of glottal attack and pushing exercises as a primary therapy approach. The use of these techniques has potential to lead to vocal hyperfunction. In this case, however, these techniques are used as a means

for educating the patient as to the physical sensation and the improved sound of well-approximated and engaged vocal folds. In further discussion, the reader will see that we use these approaches as teaching tools when dealing with other types of voice problems caused by glottal insufficiency.

Therapy Approaches for Resonance

Functionally inappropriate resonance may be one of the more difficult properties of voice to modify. Thus far in our discussion, we have been concerned with functional voice behaviors. When considering therapy for resonance disturbances, it is important for voice pathologists to be certain that the disorder is, in fact, functional and not organic in origin. There are many organic causes for resonance disturbances including various palatal clefts, insufficient functioning of the velopharyngeal port, surgical trauma, and neurologic diseases and disorders. These organic causes are determined through medical examination, flexible videoendoscopy, cinefluoroscopy, and manometric measures. The major characteristic of *functional* resonance disorders is the lack of consistency in the resonance quality and positive stimulability for more normal resonance characteristics.

Typical speech resonance patterns vary greatly from one geographic location to another. For example, resonance judged appropriate in the eastern states may not be acceptable in the Midwestern states. These qualities often change naturally as speech and voice patterns are assimilated into the local patterns, or they may need to be modified through therapy. Another common cause of functional resonance disturbances is structural oral-pharyngeal change following tonsillectomy and adenoidectomy.

Treatment of organic resonance problems is usually limited to surgical and orthodontic or prosthodontic procedures followed by therapy. These may include the closing of clefts, the creation of pharyngeal flaps for inadequate velar closure, or the molding and fitting of prosthetic obturators to provide posterior velar competence. An interdisciplinary group of professionals that comprise a Cleft Palate/Craniofacial Anomaly Team most often provides evaluation and treatment of organic resonance disturbances. Team members may include a speech-language pathologist, audiologist, orthodontist, prosthodontist, otolaryngologist, and oral and plastic surgeons. Voice/speech therapy often follows medical treatment to guarantee that the combined treatments achieve maximum gain.

The voice pathologist is most concerned with modifying both functional hypernasality and hyponasality, as well as dealing with the more common use of an inappropriate tone focus. Treatment of resonance and focus problems often proves difficult and requires all the creative skills available. No management approach can be generalized to any population with a resonance disturbance. Techniques that work to improve voice quality for an individual may not work for others with the same problem.

For functional hypernasality and denasality problems, the direction of voice therapy is to boldly manipulate articulation, mouth opening, vocal tract postures, and phonation in as many combinations as prove necessary to locate the most efficient resonant quality. Use of imagery, modeling, imitation, and negative practice are all strategies that may assist patients in achieving consistently appropriate resonance.

Hypernasality

- *Identification:* As usual, the first step in the modification of any vocal property is to identify the problem and describe it in detail to the patient. Illustrations demonstrating the relationships between the resonance cavities are helpful. Audio-recorded samples of the patient's voice compared to the voices of other individuals of similar age are helpful for ear training.
- *Articulation therapy:* Often, maximizing the strength and precision of articulatory movements and decreasing any articulation errors will increase the intelligibility of the speech and decrease the perception of hypernasality.[108,109] Increasing articulatory precision will involve activating all the articulators in a somewhat exaggerated manner, with special emphasis placed on a wider mouth opening, thus decreasing the contribution of the nasal cavity in the treatment of the glottal sound.[96]
- *Pitch and loudness modification:* Boone[110] discussed the positive decrease in the amount of nasal resonance in some patients who were taught to speak with increased intensity at a lower pitch level. Activation of the glottal tone through increased loudness focuses more of the speech energy into the oral cavity, decreasing the contribution of nasal resonance.
- *Nonspeech phonation:* The patient plays with the voice, making various nonspeech vocal sounds, such as animal and engine noises. If any of the nonspeech sounds demonstrate reduced nasality, then work from this sound by comparing it to the hypernasal sounds, training similar sounds, and expanding into speech sounds.
- *Utilize articulation deep test:* The deep test of articulation is used to determine if any sounds in any phonetic contexts are made with normal or near-normal levels of nasal resonance. If so, these phoneme productions are expanded into similar sound clusters, then words, phrases, and conversational speech.
- *Do the obvious:* The patient's ability to produce a voice "as if you have a cold" is explored. Some patients with functional hypernasality can easily produce a denasal voice quality when speaking in this manner. They simply were not aware that a slight modification of the "cold" voice would yield the normal nasal resonance. It pays to explore this ability early in the therapy program.
- *Negative practice:* Negative practice may also be an effective therapy tool used with resonance disorders. When the patient first produces new normal resonance, purposeful productions of the same sounds utilizing the "old" hypernasal voice may reinforce and strengthen the use of normal resonance. The patient's ability to use both voices upon dismissal from therapy shows a true mastery of the therapeutic goals.
- *Instrumental feedback:* Many of the explorations mentioned above may be aided by instrumental assessment and biofeedback. The Nasometer (Figure 7–2; Kay Elemetrics Corporation) is an instrument that measures and visually demonstrates the degree of nasalance on a computer screen. This instrument provides for excellent patient monitoring and feedback, as

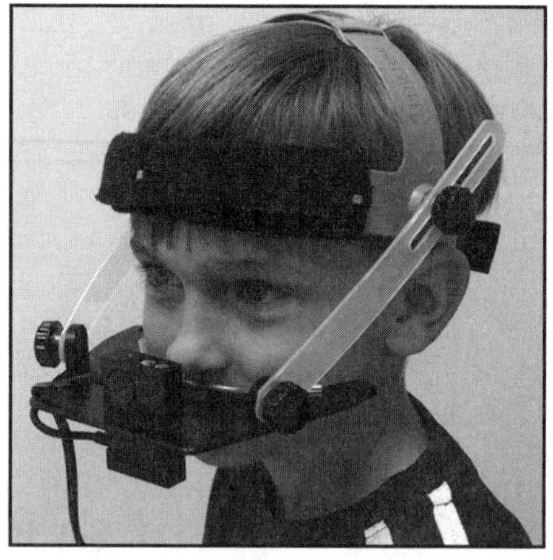

A

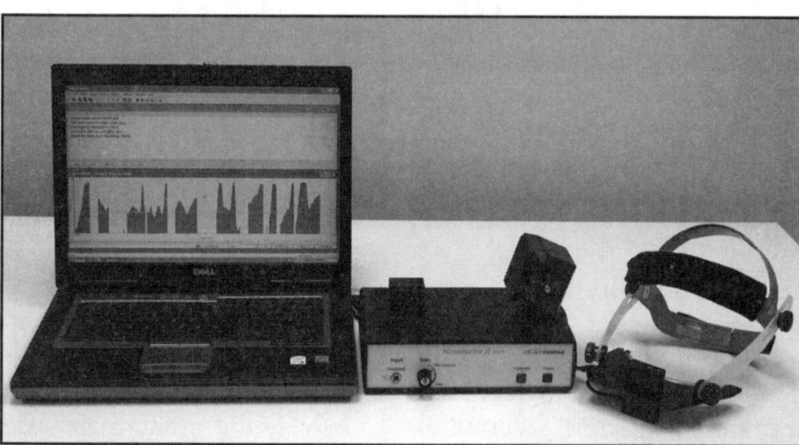

B

FIGURE 7–2. Nasometer (Courtesy of KayPentax).

well as is a useful resonance evaluation tool.

Denasality

Functional denasality may occasionally occur, especially following the removal of nasal obstructions. Wilson[96] suggested that the patient's auditory feedback system does not quickly adjust as he or she continues to attempt to maintain the status quo, even though the nasal cavity is no longer obstructed. Once the disorder has been identified and described in detail, approaches used to modify the behavior include the following:

- Utilizing the normal nasal sounds: In this approach, the voice pathologist should determine the patient's ability to produce /m/, /n/, and /ng/ with normal resonance. If this is possible, /m/ and /n/ may be combined with vowel sounds and expanded through words, phrases, and so on. If the nasal sounds are also produced with the denasal quality, attempts may be made to train nasalization of /m/ using the singing voice.

- Humming, with the lips closed in the /m/ position, forces the production of more nasal resonance. These productions may be slowly modified by opening the mouth while humming and saying /ma/; expanding to other vowel sounds; eliminating the hum; and then expanding into other sounds, words, phrases, and so on.
- Utilizing hypernasal resonance: Some patients who demonstrate a functional denasal voice are readily able to produce an exaggerated hypernasal voice quality. If this is so, then different gradients of velar closure may be demonstrated and stabilized, leading to normal velopharyngeal functioning.
- Nonspeech phonation: Explained under hypernasality, this approach may also be an effective means of initiating normal voice resonance.
- Negative practice: (Explained under hypernasality.)

Tone Focus

Focus refers to the resonance of the voice in the supraglottic vocal tract. Constriction of the supraglottic airway at any point will alter the focus of voice production. When the vocal tract is relaxed and open without supraglottic constriction, the glottal sound source can resonate freely and maximally, creating what is called a "forward focus" or "placement" of tone. The ideal placement of this tone is forward, as this placement allows the voice to resonate fully throughout the pharyngeal, nasal, and oral cavities without effort or tension. Tension at any point in the vocal tract will alter both the free resonance of the tone and voice quality. In addition to changing the quality, less than ideal tone placement may result in voice that fatigues easily and lacks flexibility and vibrancy.

Poor tone focus may be observed in patients who functionally constrict the pharynx, retract the tongue, and elevate the larynx as the habitual manner in which voice is produced. Poor tone focus also may be the result of laryngeal pathologies that, when present, force the patient to constrict the upper airway to compensate for the presence of the pathology. This constriction often leads to what is commonly termed a *back-focused tone*. The voice qualities associated with several laryngeal pathologies commonly present with a backward tone focus. These pathologies include edema and mass lesions of the vocal folds which require the patient to constrict the supraglottic structures as compensation for the presence of the increased mass; bowed vocal folds and other incomplete glottic closures caused by presbylaryngeous, paresis, or paralysis; and adductor spasmodic dysphonia, which forces the patient to tense the vocal mechanism as a means of pushing the voice through the spasms. As the inappropriate focus becomes habituated, direct voice therapy approaches commonly must be utilized to reintroduce a more ideal and less tense placement of the tone.

Following is a therapy approach that we have found useful for improving tone focus using nasal sounds and sensory feedback to "tune the patient in" to the nebulous concept of focus:

- *Patient education:* We begin by teaching the patient about the concept of resonance by demonstrating how one sentence may be said with various resonance characteristics. Patients are made aware of how celebrity impersonators change the resonance of the voice to sound like other people. The concepts of frontal, back, and mid-focus are introduced by first demonstrating a tight, constricted, back-focused phrase that the patient is asked to imitate. Because this type of tone placement often is implicated as the problem, most patients, although somewhat embarrassed, are able to produce this voice. Second, a breathy, poorly focused tone is imitated followed by an exaggerated, almost nasal forward focus. It is explained to the patient that, although the ultimate goal was not to talk in a nasal quality, practicing this placement would help to approximate the desired focus. Practice of this exaggerated forward placement would be a step toward learning the desired placement:

- *Nasalized phrase production:* The clinician instructs the patient to slowly and softly chant the following phrases, exaggerating the vowel sounds, on a comfortable pitch level slightly above the fundamental frequency:

  OH MY OH MY OH MY OH MY . . .

  OH ME OH ME OH ME OH ME . . .

  OH NO OH NO OH NO OH NO . . .

  OH MY NO OH MY NO OH MY NO . . .

  OH ME OH MY OH ME OH MY . . .

  The forward resonance of each phrase is exaggerated to the extreme, and the clinician instructs the patient to feel and sense the energy of the tone in the nose, on the lips, in the front of the face, and so on. Audio recordings of the phrases are made for both the clinician and the patient, and ear training is accomplished as needed.

  Once the phrases are produced to the satisfaction of the voice pathologist, negative practice is used. The patient is asked to alternate between forward and back focuses to demonstrate the mastery of the focus technique on these simple phrases.

- Introduce intensity and rate variations: Using the same phrases, the clinician asks the patient to chant each phrase multiple times using the following routine:

  Very slow and very soft

  Faster and louder

  Fast and loud

  Slower and softer

  Very slow and very soft

  Changing the rate and loudness of the chanted phrases adds a new dimension to the exercise that forces the patient to concentrate on maintaining the forward placement even as the intensity and rate are increased and decreased. The pitch remains the same.

- Introduce inflected phrase and normal speech: When the patient has succeeded in mastering the first 3 steps, the practice phrases may be modified from the single pitch chant to a more "sing-song" or overinflected vocal presentation and then directly into a normally spoken phrase:

  soft and slow

  louder and faster

  exaggerated inflection

  normal speech

The proper focus of the tone is closely monitored during each of the steps utilizing the phrases. Negative practice is judiciously used throughout each session. Some patients move quickly through each of these steps and master a forward focus with ease. Others require many therapy sessions to master the appropriate focus. The final step is to expand the ability to produce a forward focus from these phrases into expanded phrases and sentences, paragraph reading, and conversational speech.

Other clues to help make patients aware of forward focus include playing a comb wrapped with waxed paper with the lips. The lips are made to vibrate by phonation, and the comb resonates this vibration making patients more aware of the forward placement of the tone. Make a motorcycle noise by vibrating the lips together (this technique works well with children) and trilling the tongue on the top of the alveolar ridge while moving the lips to shape different sounds.[111]

The above therapy techniques isolate the resonance component of voice production. Later in this chapter, resonance will be integrated with phonation and respiration in a holistic voice therapy program known as RVT.

Therapy Approaches for Pitch

Pitch levels that are either too high or too low are represented in many different types of laryngeal pathologies. The decision to modify pitch should be based on whether it is a primary etiologic factor (the actual cause of the voice disorder) or whether it is merely a symptom of the pathology. If an inappropriate pitch is present because of laryngeal pathology, it is likely to reach a normal level without direct component modification once the pathology is resolved. Direct pitch modification can be somewhat difficult and has the potential of causing laryngeal harm if the new pitch level is trained artificially high or low. Let us examine some of the more common reasons for the use of inappropriate pitch levels and identify those that may benefit from direct symptom modification.

Increased vocal fold mass as a result of edema and mass lesions of the vocal folds may cause a lowering of the fundamental frequency. The primary etiology is whatever caused the pathology. If the cause proved to be the inappropriate use of pitch, therapy would focus on direct pitch modification.

An example of inappropriate pitch as a primary cause of laryngeal pathology would be the use of a pseudoauthoritative voice. Conscious efforts by both men and women to sound more authoritative or self-assured by using a forceful deep voice, especially in work settings, may lead to the development of a voice disorder. In this case, the therapy of choice would be a direct symptom modification approach, as well as a discussion of why the need to use this voice is perceived by the patient.

Another example of an intentional pitch modification occasionally seen in therapy is the patient who is trying to "save" the voice. These are patients who are experiencing some vocal difficulties. In an attempt to counteract these difficulties, they try to "save" the voice by habitually lowering the pitch and loudness. These patients have the misconception that by talking in this manner, they are reducing the impact of whatever is causing the vocal difficulty. In reality, just the opposite is true. Habitual use of an inappropriately low-pitched voice may be a vocal misuse and can lead to the development of pathology. Direct pitch modification is then in order.

Patients who develop a hormonal imbalance after surgery, because of malfunction of the endocrine system, or as a side effect to medications present an interesting problem. These factors often cause a permanent change in the vocal folds, causing a permanent pitch modification. In this etiologic scenario, laryngeal pathology is not likely to occur unless the patient's auditory feedback system attempts to modify the pitch level back to the original level. Counseling against direct pitch modification is often the treatment of choice here.

Emotional and physical disturbances often will lead to a voice of depression. The way a person "feels" physically and emotionally may be directly reflected in the vocal quality. People who are depressed, agitated, upset, physically ill, mourning, or going through other emotional conflicts often have a low-pitched, poorly supported voice quality. The primary etiology is the emotional stress, but secondary use of the inappropriate pitch may lead to vocal dysfunction.

Two other factors that lead to the inappropriate use of pitch are whole-body and laryngeal fatigue. The person who is constantly fatigued is likely to use poor breath support and permit the pitch level to lower. Fatigue may also affect the components of respiration and loudness. Sensations of general and laryngeal fatigue often lead to an "effort" to talk. As a result, patients often drop the pitch and respiratory support, which actually exacerbates the problem. These patients are encouraged to "energize" the voice with increased loudness and breath support, which will increase the pitch to a more appropriate level.

Upward pitch changes may also cause voice problems. Recall that as vocal intensity increases, so does the frequency level. This problem may be remediated through direct pitch modification. Finally, pitch change may be desirable in transgendered individuals. Let us now look at some therapy approaches for pitch modification.

Case Study 7: The Pseudoauthoritative Voice

A 25-year-old male with the diagnosis of a right contact ulcer without evidence of reflux was referred for evaluation and treatment. Voice quality during the evaluation was mildly dysphonic, characterized by low pitch, glottal fry phonation, inappropriate loudness (too loud for the speaking situation), and breathiness. The patient reported experiencing vocal difficulties soon after beginning a new job as a bank manager trainee 5 months prior to the evaluation. Other than occasional shouting at sporting events, no other phonotrauma was identified. Results of the evaluation revealed that the patient's contact ulcer was likely the result of using a loud, low-pitched, pseudoauthoritative voice in his work setting. Being in his first position of authority, the patient attempted to project a "strong" image. Inappropriate use of the low, loud voice involved posterior laryngeal tension that led to the development of the pathology. The treatment plan involved 3 major steps:

- The first step was to identify the causes and to explain to the patient in detail the nuances of the contact ulcer and what led to its development. When dealing with a male patient, it generally is not wise to explain that the pitch must be raised. The mental impression he gains would be that of a major pitch modification, when, in fact, a minor modification is needed. It is better to explain that he is talking at the bottom of his voice range and that therapy will be designed to return the voice to its normal level. Audio-recorded samples were then used to demonstrate the vocal symptoms in question. The voice pathologist also imitated examples of the voice components.

- The second step was an attempt to identify a more appropriate pitch level. As previously stated, this is somewhat risky with the pathological voice. However, a higher pitch that is comfortable for the patient, and produced with little effort, will normally prove adequate. Cooper[103] suggested having the patients say, in a natural conversational voice, "um-hum" as if answering "yes" to a question. The "hum" part of the production is usually produced in a relaxed tone near the patient's most comfortable pitch.
- The third step was to match the appropriate pitch level to a musical note on a pitch pipe, which served as a reference note for the rest of the therapy process. The patient was then asked to match that level while repeating single-syllable words and short phrases. The phrases were gradually lengthened, and inflectional patterns were introduced. Sentences, paragraph reading, and conversational speech marked his progress, which was monitored with immediate audio replays (Facilitator by Kay Elemetrics Corporation) and by audio-recorded samples. Negative practice was also used. It is positive for a patient to have total control of the voice, and negative practice helps the patient meet this goal.

Case Study 8: The Voice Saver

The patient was a 31-year-old male who was referred for evaluation and treatment with the diagnosis of mild, bilateral vocal fold edema. The patient had only recently begun experiencing vocal difficulties. As a young assistant pastor of a large parish, he was required to hold meetings, counsel youth, visit the sick and elderly, teach a Bible studies class, and deliver a sermon 1 Sunday per month. He noticed 4 weeks prior to the evaluation that his voice routinely tired and became hoarse every day in the early afternoon. The patient denied any vocal abuse and did not feel that he gave enough group presentations to cause the vocal problem. His medical history was unremarkable, and the social history did not yield evidence of the typical forms of phonotrauma except for throat clearing, which was noted throughout the evaluation.

The patient's voice quality during the evaluation was described as moderately dysphonic, characterized by low pitch, low-intensity, glottal fry phonation, and an unusual amount of breathiness. The use of these inappropriate voice components could account for the patient's voice difficulties, but the severity of voice quality did not fit the observations made through the laryngeal videostroboscopy or the diagnosis of mild edema.

The patient therefore was asked if this voice was typical of his voice when it would fatigue. "Oh, no!" he replied, and to the voice pathologist's surprise, his reply was in a normal voice. "I'm talking down like that to save my voice."

Further questioning revealed that the patient had a chest cold for 2 weeks prior to the onset of his daily voice fatigue. Much coughing and throat clearing during the cold was reported. When the cold subsided, the throat clearing persisted, continuing the mild edema of the vocal folds and an imbalance of voice subsystems. Introduction of the "saving" voice only caused more vocal dysfunction. Successful therapy focused on vocal hygiene counseling, elimination of throat clearing, and balancing of the voice subsystems through Vocal Function Exercises. Attempts to "save" the voice were extinguished.

It is said that experience is the best teacher. After that experience, we have found several patients who were trying to "save" the voice in much the same manner. This especially seems to occur in people who do a great deal of talking or singing on a daily basis. They report that they begin to experience laryngeal fatigue and therefore let the voice drop lower in pitch, decreasing the phonatory effort and respiratory support. This, of course, is a misuse of the vocal components that may lead to an imbalance in the 3 subsystems of voice production, thus accelerating sensations of laryngeal fatigue.

The most positive short-term approach to counteract fatigue is to train the patient to use more breath support for voice, slightly increase the loudness, and maintain the higher, more appropriate pitch level. Even though this requires more perceived physical effort, the improved balance of the vocal components will often reduce the sensations of fatigue and refresh the voice production.

Case Study 9: Emotional Voice Changes

The patient was a 23-year-old woman who was referred for evaluation and treatment, with a diagnosis of mild-to-moderate vocal fold edema. The patient's voice quality during the evaluation was a mild dysphonia, characterized by low pitch, low intensity, and breathiness. She reported that she began experiencing vocal difficulties just 1 month prior to the evaluation, and the usual diagnostic questions were posed, probing for the etiologic factors associated with the development of the disorder. No form of vocal trauma could be identified, and the medical history was unremarkable.

Questions regarding her social history, specifically, "How long have you been married?" elicited an emotional and tearful response, however. This line of questioning was followed. The patient volunteered that just prior to the onset of her vocal difficulties she discovered that her husband of 11 months had been unfaithful. Rather than confront him with this information, she remained silent and was contemplating divorce.

The relationship of emotional tension and depression on the vocal components and the resulting voice quality were explained. Often, the patient's understanding of why the voice lowers, weakens, becomes breathy, and tires easily is enough to relieve the additional anxiety of the vocal problem. In all cases, the need for further counseling is determined, and the appropriate referrals are made. This particular patient was referred for family counseling to attempt to resolve the primary cause of her laryngeal pathology. Direct vocal component modification was not appropriate or necessary in this situation.

Therapy Approaches for Gender Reassignment Voice Change

The voice pathologist may be called on to aid in the feminization of the male-to-female transsexual voice and speech patterns. Individuals who desire gender reassignment therapy and surgery are often referred to "gender dysphoria" clinics. The programs these clinics offer include step-by-step procedures leading to the final surgical modifications necessary to accomplish the permanent gender reassignment. The procedures also include psychological counseling, electrolysis for the removal of body hair, and hormone treatments to enhance female characteristics. In addition, patients are required to live the part of the desired gender for 1 year prior to surgery.

The effects of hormones administered for the purpose of feminization are minimal as related to voice change. Therefore, the individual is required to make numerous changes to create a more feminine speech pattern. The patient must elevate the fundamental frequency, modify the resonance characteristics, and alter inflection and intonation patterns, precision of articulation, and even type of vocalized pauses.[112–114] It is desirable to modify these speech and voice characteristics even prior to the gender reassignment surgery.

Pitch modification is actually the first and easiest part of the feminization of the voice. We choose to test the entire frequency range of the patient and then attempt to place the new fundamental frequency as close to the comfortable midrange as is possible. In the normal laryngeal mechanism, pitch modification is potentially harmful if muscle tension results. Tension is monitored throughout therapy to ensure that voice misuse does not occur. The new pitch range is defined on a monitoring instrument (in our case, a KayPentax Visi-Pitch), and the patient practices producing words, phrases, sentences, paragraph readings, and conversations until the pitch level is habituated. At the same time, a slightly breathy phonation is taught, and when necessary, the patient is taught to retract the tongue slightly, which also tends to elevate the larynx in the neck. These slightly altered tongue and larynx positions tend to shorten the length of the vocal tract and reduce the available area for supraglottic resonance, which tends to feminize the voice.[114]

Along with direct modification of the voice and vocal tract, patients must learn to increase their rate of speech and lengthen their pauses, while at the same time increasing the precision of articulation.[115,116] Because female speakers use increased intonation, inflection patterns also must be increased through practice with the voice pathologist. Finally, vocalized pauses, coughing, and throat clearing must be modified. A harsh, low-pitched "uh" or throat clearing sound would certainly destroy the effect of the new voice and speech production. Patients must be trained to produce these sounds within a new acceptable range. Although the need for voice modification is of major importance for successful gender reassignment, other factors related to body affect and image are also important. Please see *Voice and Communication Therapy for the Transgender/Transsexual Client* by Adler, Hirsch, and Mordaunt (2006, Plural Publishing, Inc., San Diego, CA).

Therapy Approaches for Loudness Modification

Functional misuse of the intensities of voice may lead to the development of vocal dysfunction. The vocally traumatic behaviors of shouting and loud talking have been previously discussed under Vocal Hygiene. Habitual misuses of conversational voice levels that are either too loud or too soft also may lead to vocal difficulty. The first step in dealing with patients with either of these behaviors is to refer them for a complete hearing evaluation. The voices of patients with sensorineural hearing loss often are produced with too much intensity, caused by the inability to monitor the voice adequately. Those with conductive hearing losses may talk too softly, caused by the ability to hear through bone conduction and their inability to monitor competing background noise. When an auditory disorder has been ruled out or treated, several intensity modification approaches may be followed:

- Make the patient aware of the problem by utilizing the diagnostic voice evaluation audio recording. Compare the patient's vocal intensity to that of the voice pathologist on the recording. Use illustrations and discussion to explain what effect the inappropriate use of loudness has had on the laryngeal mechanism.
- Raise the patient's awareness level regarding how people react to the voice. For example, if the patient talks too loudly, do people back away, look away, or cut the patient short? Does the patient perhaps project an overbearing image? People who talk too softly frequently may be asked to repeat themselves, may be ignored, or may project a bashful or backward image.
- Practice direct manipulation of many different intensities. Record these using short phrases for ear training purposes.
- Utilize a hand-held sound level meter (many Apps are available for this purpose) or another commercial intensity monitor (such as a Visi-Pitch) to stabilize productions at a reasonable intensity level. Habituate this level through words, phrases, paragraph readings, and conversational speech.

Therapy Approaches for Rate Modification

Seldom is the rate of a patient's speech deviant enough to cause laryngeal pathology. If rate becomes inappropriate enough to create a voice disorder, it is typically because the rate is too fast. Speaking with too fast a rate may create vocal hyperfunction. A modification approach for reducing rate follows:

- Make the patient aware of the problem by reviewing the voice on the diagnostic evaluation recording and comparing it to the rate of the voice pathologist on the same recording. Use illustrations of vocal fold anatomy and discussion of physiology to explain how a faster rate creates vocal hyperfunction.
- Many patients who attempt to slow the rate of speech attempt to accomplish this by pausing longer between words and phrases. Although this is helpful, it is more effective to have the patient exaggerate vowel prolongation in words within moderately long phrases. This exercise is totally opposite their normal habit.
- From deliberate vowel prolongation in phrases, the patient may move into reading song lyrics and poetry. The inherent rhythms and inflectional patterns are ideal for indirectly teaching timing and melody, both of which are lacking.
- When the patient has sufficiently mastered the reading of lyrics and poetry at an appropriate rate, begin paragraph readings of prose material. Monitor progress through audio recordings or the use of a Facilitator (KayPentax), a device specifically developed for speech and voice feedback.

- Begin negative practice. Listen to audio recordings of the same material read by the patient at an increased rate and at a normal rate.
- Stabilize the new rate in structured conversational speech within the therapy setting. Use negative practice and expand the physical settings until the new rate is stabilized.

Treatment Approaches for Laryngeal Area Muscle Tension

Laryngeal muscle tension may be intermittent, as may occur when someone shouts or clears the throat. It may also be a persistent general laryngeal area muscle tension. The term *muscle tension dysphonia* (MTD) has been used as a descriptor for chronic laryngeal area muscle tension. This tension may be either the cause of a voice disorder or the result of compensations made for the presence of a disorder. Several symptomatic therapy techniques that may be used to reduce persistent laryngeal area muscle tension are progressive relaxation, chewing exercises, the yawn-sigh facilitating technique, and EMG biofeedback:

- *Progressive relaxation:* Reduction of whole-body tension may serve as an indirect method of reducing laryngeal area tension. Progressive relaxation techniques presented by Jacobson[117] are designed to teach patients to recognize the differences between muscles that feel tense and muscles that feel relaxed. The most popular exercise involves alternately tensing and relaxing all the muscles from the scalp to the toes. This technique may prove helpful in reducing whole-body and laryngeal area tension for patients who are diagnosed with MTD.
- *Chewing exercises:* In 1952, Froeschel[118] described the chewing method for laryngeal tension reduction. This method is based on the theory that phonating during vegetative chewing will relax all the structures involved in articulation, resonance, and phonation. Wilson[96] described a detailed approach in utilizing the chewing method with children. Using this technique, patients are taught to imagine they are chewing food. They are encouraged to utilize a wide excursion of their jaws and tongues while simulating chewing food. When a relaxed chewing method has been achieved, vocalization of a neutral vowel is added to the chewing exercise. Complete relaxation of the laryngeal area is encouraged during phonation. When adequate progress has been made in relaxed phonation, short words and phrases are added to the chewing exercise. Finally, the chewing behavior is extinguished as more relaxed phonation is expanded into longer phrases, paragraph readings, and conversational speech.
- *Yawn-sigh approach:* Another approach for reducing laryngeal area tension is the yawn-sigh facilitating technique as first described by Boone.[24] Patients are asked to initiate the first half of a yawn behavior. The yawn serves to expand the pharynx and to stretch and then relax the extrinsic laryngeal muscles, thus lowering the larynx in the neck to a more neutral position and permitting a more forward placement of the tongue in the oral cavity. The subsequent sigh should then be more relaxed with less tension noted in the phonation of the tone. From the sigh phonation, the patient is taught

to appreciate the sensation of laryngeal relaxation. The yawn-sigh technique is then paired with vowels and then gradually expanded into words, phrases, paragraph readings, and conversational speech.

- *Biofeedback training:* The basis of biofeedback is that self-control of physiologic functions is possible with continuous, immediate information about the internal bodily state. Electromyographic biofeedback has been used successfully in the rehabilitation treatment of a wide range of neuromuscular disorders. EMG biofeedback training permits patients to monitor electrical activities of their muscles and to exert some control over these areas. This form of biofeedback training has permitted patients to view the tension of the extrinsic laryngeal muscles and to reduce or increase these tension levels utilizing auditory and visual feedback.[119,120] Stemple et al[120] demonstrated the successful use of EMG biofeedback in reducing laryngeal area tension and improving the vocal folds and voice production with a group of patients with vocal fold nodules.

Case Study 10: Ventricular Phonation

Occasionally, patients increase laryngeal area muscle tension to such an extreme that they begin phonating using the false vocal folds. This may be a functional disorder, or it may result from the patient's attempt to compensate for gross laryngeal pathology.

The patient was a 55-year-old lawyer who was referred for evaluation and treatment with the diagnosis of ventricular phonation. The problem had begun 6 weeks prior to the evaluation at about the same time that he was told he was being considered for a county judgeship. Voice quality was moderately dysphonic, characterized by harshness; however, the patient had gained a fair level of control and consistency of the voice. The major complaint was that his voice tired easily. He was not unduly concerned by the quality, which was puzzling to the voice pathologist. Results of the evaluation yielded no probable etiologic factors other than the patient's anxiety associated with the pending appointment as a judge. Laryngeal videostroboscopic observation of the vocal folds confirmed the ventricular folds as the source of voice. After further discussion, the patient recognized that he had developed the voice disorder to satisfy a psychological need. He would use the voice difficulty as an excuse if he were not appointed judge. However, the voice had habituated and needed to be changed.

Indirect therapy methods were first attempted utilizing general progressive relaxation and EMG biofeedback. The patient was readily able to reduce laryngeal tension levels, but this did not modify or reduce ventricular phonation. Direct vocal manipulation was then employed. This followed the basic treatment approach presented by Boone.[110] This approach suggests that the voice pathologist use the following 5 steps:

1. Ask the patient to inhale and exhale in a prolonged manner with a wide open mouth. He or she should not attempt to phonate at this time.
2. Repeat the same procedure with the patient phonating vowels during inhalation. This often is facilitated by the use of a higher pitch. Inhalation phonation can only be accomplished with the true vocal folds.
3. When true vocal fold inhalation phonation is achieved, ask the patient

to match this sound on exhalation phonation in the same breathing cycle. It is extremely important that the voice pathologist be persistent during this step in therapy. It is critical that patients be required to persist until they achieve appropriate target exhalation phonation.

4. When exhalation phonation is achieved, begin modifying this to a normal pitch level. This may be accomplished by singing down a musical scale in 2- to 3-note intervals on a vowel sound until the desired level is approximated.
5. Vary the vowel sounds and move on through syllables, words, phrases, and paragraphs. Stabilize the improved true vocal fold phonation during conversational speech.

It also may prove helpful to use digital manipulation of the thyroid cartilage. The position of the larynx during ventricular phonation often is high in the neck. Grasping the thyroid cartilage and holding or massaging it down during inhalation and exhalation phonation cycles may be effective.

Direct vocal manipulation proved effective in modifying this patient's voice, but only after he was appointed to the bench. Exercises to rebalance the subsystems of voice were used to return the voice to a healthy condition (see Vocal Function Exercises and Resonant Voice Therapy).

PSYCHOGENIC VOICE THERAPY

Patients who develop a disordered voice in the context of a structurally normal larynx are among the more interesting challenges in voice therapy. Several terms have been used to describe these disorders including functional dysphonia, functional aphonia, psychogenic voice disorders, conversion voice disorders, and muscle tension dysphonia (MTD). Psychological or personality disorientation often is presumed with psychogenic voice pathologies. It is more likely, however, that these voice disorders comprise a complex blend of psychological, social, and physiologic factors.[121] Beyond the controversy and confusion surrounding these disorders, is the voice pathologist's exceptional role in treating these patients. That role includes sorting through all of these factors to determine the most appropriate method of improving the voice quality.

The major types of vocal dysfunction that we will discuss under the category of psychogenic voice therapy include functional aphonia, muscle tension dysphonia, and mutational falsetto/juvenile voice. The management plans for all of these voice problems include 4 major stages:

- Stage 1 is the medical evaluation. As with all voice disorders, it is essential that the presence or absense of organic pathology be identified prior to the initiation of therapy. For the cases to be discussed here, the report of normal laryngeal structures will confirm the diagnosis of a functional disorder, in the presence of inappropriate and often unusual vocal symptoms.
- Stage 2 is the diagnostic voice evaluation. During the evaluation, the voice pathologist will develop the history of the pathology and will learn how the patient functions socially and physically within the environment. An impression of the patient's personality will evolve. The diagnostic time is also used to prepare the patient for

vocal change. This is accomplished by explaining to the patient how the vocal mechanism works and by describing what is happening physiologically within the larynx to create the present voice quality. Although no attempt is yet made to explain why this is occurring, the physiologic description provides the patient with a rationale for the vocal problem.

- Stage 3 is the direct manipulation of the voice. The type of manipulation will vary depending on the type of vocal dysfunction. Vocal manipulation most often begins during the diagnostic evaluation with the expected result being a dramatic change in the voice toward normal phonation during this first treatment session.
- Stage 4 involves probing to determine why the disorder developed. For example, in functional aphonia and MTD, the voice quality change is felt to represent a symbolic somatization of psychodynamic conflict. It may be the patient's subconscious effort to escape an unpleasant situation or the memory of the situation that promotes the reaction. Aronson[72] suggested that the most appropriate professional to deal with this type of disorder is the voice pathologist, whose complete understanding of the vocal processes and strong counseling background provides the basic skills and abilities to remediate these pathologies. Once normal voicing has been achieved, it is a natural transition to begin examining why the problem existed. By this time, the voice pathologist has gained the trust of and a positive rapport with the patient. With interview questions that are structured in a nonthreatening manner, the voice pathologist can usually determine the cause of the problem. Patients frequently volunteer the necessary information, which often opens a floodgate of emotion.

Once the cause or causes have been identified and discussed, the voice pathologist needs to determine if further professional counseling is advisable. If so, the appropriate referral should be discussed with the patient and should be made with the patient's consent. Let us now closely examine several types of functional voice problems and the voice therapy techniques for treating them.

Functional Aphonia/Dysphonia

Whispered voice or an unusual voice quality in the presence of a normal appearing vocal mechanism has been referred to as hysteric, hysterical, nervous, psychosomatic, functional, and muscle tension aphonia/dysphonia, and has been discussed in medical journals for scores of years. Many curious and unconventional treatments have been advocated in the literature. Russell[66] suggested that "hysteric aphonia" was a mental or moral ailment that required moral treatment. The method of cure was "to rouse the will, and thus rid the body of its thousand morbid things."

Ward[65] advocated the application of an astringent to the vocal folds along with simultaneous electric shock to the neck. The pain of both procedures would influence the patient to talk. Goss,[64] Ingalls,[122] and Bach[123] also utilized painful "remedies" such as bitter tonics including solutions of iron, quinine, arsenic, and strichnia.

In the early part of the 20th century, Winslow[124] and Howard[125] described

2 of the more imaginative remedies. According to Winslow:[124(pp1129,1130)]

> My method of treatment is as follows: the patient is seated before me and a careful history of the case is taken. Then with the laryngeal mirror I make a careful examination of the larynx, noting the movements of the vocal cords and the condition of the mucous membrane from the pharynx down as far as I can see. If I am satisfied that the case is one of functional aphonia, I remove the mirror. The patient is then asked to take 10 or 12 deep breaths. He is next told to raise the arms above the head 10 or 12 times. Now looking the patient directly in the eye, I say to him that there is a little piece of cartilage in his throat which is slightly out of position and as soon as I put my finger down his throat and fix it, he will be able to use his voice (this is to bring about the proper psychological attitude of the patient). Then standing to his right with my left arm under the his neck, the index finger of the left hand pushing on the cheek, between the upper and lower jaw (done to keep the patient from biting), the index finger of the right-hand is shoved down the throat beyond the epiglottis and held there until the patient makes an attempt to get away. I continue to hold my finger there until it becomes quite uncomfortable. At this stage the patient will, as a rule, make a sound like a grunt and as soon as this happens I take my finger from the throat and begin to count fairly loud from 1 to 5, at the same time urging the patient to count with me. If this does not work I repeat the count, from 1 to 5, much louder than before. It may be necessary to yell while counting before the patient begins to use his voice. When the voice is restored, I keep working for some time so that the patient will become accustomed to it. The attitude of the operator should be firm but gentle, and he must, by his demeanor, inspire the patient with the idea that he will restore the voice.

Howard[125(p104)] described his case as follows:

> Mrs. M.T., aged 51, whose nervous system had been below par since her husband had committed suicide a year-and-a-half ago, in January, 1922, contracted influenza. Prior to February 1, she enjoyed the full use of her voice, but that morning she found that she could not talk above a whisper. A diagnosis was made of functional aphonia, also known as hysterical nervous aphonia. The patient was informed that there was no paralysis of the cords; that people affected in this way always recovered, and that the voice usually came back suddenly, just as it had left. The next day, she was told that we would put her to sleep and apply medicine to the parts, and that when she woke up she could talk. She was given ether, and, while she was under the anesthetic, the region was painted with one-percent silver nitrate as a local fillip to the parts. In coming out of the anesthetic, and while only partly conscious, she mumbled something above a whisper. She was encouraged to talk louder and asked to count out loud, and she did so. She has since then been talking normally.

Although these techniques are fun to review, the problem with all of these remedies is, of course, that their practitioners were not necessarily honest with their patients. Deceit is not necessary (or ethical) in modifying the vocal condition of aphonic patients. Patients with this pathology may have an unconscious need for the voice disorder and deserve an honest professional management approach. By the time patients with functional aphonia/dysphonia are referred to a voice pathologist, they are often truly seeking relief from the disorder and are subconsciously ready for change. Often, the event that precipitated the onset of the voice disorder has passed. Some patients may continue to receive secondary gains from the disorder and resist all therapeutic modifications, but the majority of patients will respond quickly to direct voice therapy. It is extremely important to understand that these patients are not malingering. They truly believe that they have lost their normal voices and are seeking your help with the hope of voice restoration. With this orientation in mind, the following treatment strategies may be applied:

- *Nonspeech Phonatory Tasks:* Following the interview period of the diagnostic evaluation, the voice pathologist will present a physiologic description of the vocal mechanism, using simple line drawings, pictures of the vocal folds, or the patient's own laryngeal videostroboscopic examination recording. These visual displays are used to demonstrate how the adductory muscles are not pulling the vocal folds together, causing the voice to be whispered or overcontracting, causing extreme laryngeal muscle tension. In the case of aphonia, the clinician may give this type of explanation:

  > For some reason, the muscles that pull the vocal folds together are simply not pulling the way that they should. Therefore, the vocal folds are not closing all the way. When they don't close all the way, they can't vibrate and so all we can hear is a whisper. Our goal in therapy today is to manipulate the vocal muscle system in whatever manner needed to encourage the vocal folds to come together.

  With this approach, the voice pathologist has given the patient a nonthreatening, reasonable explanation as to why phonation is not occurring. No comment is yet made regarding the patient's inherent ability to phonate. In fact, the "blame" for lack of phonation has been removed from the patient and placed squarely on the faulty laryngeal mechanism.

  Traditional therapy approaches then examine the patient's ability to phonate during nonspeech phonatory behaviors such as coughing, throat clearing, laughing, crying, sighing, and gargling. When phonation is identified on one of these behaviors, it is then shaped into vowel sounds, nonsense syllables, words, and short phrases. The voice pathologist must remain patient, supportive, and persistent throughout. Most patients have not phonated for several weeks or longer. The possibility of proceeding too quickly and frightening the patient away from phonation is present. Once good, consistent phonation is established under practice conditions, the voice pathologist begins to gently insist that it be used during the therapy conversations.
- *Manual Circumlaryngeal Therapy* (Digital Massage): Aronson[72] suggested that all patients with voice disorders, regardless of etiology, should be assessed for excess laryngeal musculoskeletal tension, either as a primary or a secondary cause of the persisting dysphonia. If tension is an etiologic factor, then reducing it releases the capability of the larynx to produce normal voice. Roy et al[79] demonstrated the efficacy of manual techniques with patients with functional dysphonia including those with aphonia. A 7-step program

of digital massage for decreasing laryngeal tension was suggested by Aronson:[72(pp200,201)]

1. Encircle the hyoid bone with the thumb and middle finger, working them posteriorly until the tips of the major horns are felt.
2. Exert light pressure with the fingers in a circular motion over the tips of the hyoid bone and ask if the patient feels pain, not just pressure. It is important to watch facial expression for signs of discomfort or pain.
3. Repeat this procedure with the fingers in the thyrohyoid space, beginning from the thyroid notch and working posteriorly.
4. Find the posterior borders of the thyroid cartilage just medial to the sternocleidomastoid muscles and repeat the procedure.
5. With the fingers over the superior borders of the thyroid cartilage, begin to work the larynx gently downward, also moving it laterally at times. Check for a lower laryngeal position by estimating the increased size of the thyrohyoid space.
6. Ask the patient to prolong vowels during these procedures, noting changes in quality and pitch. Clearer voice quality and lower pitch indicate relief of tension. Because these procedures are fatiguing, rest periods should be provided.
7. Once a voice change has taken place, the patient should be allowed to experiment with the voice, repeating vowels, words, and sentences.

Aronson further stated that the rate of improvement varies depending on the cause of the tension.

With the patient with functional dysphonia, changing voice quality should be expected within the first session.

Manual techniques may also be used with other laryngeal tension disorders.[79]

■ *Falsetto Voice Technique for Functional Aphonia/Dysphonia:* Another therapy technique used for reestablishing normal voice in the functional aphonic/dysphonic patient relies on first establishing a normal falsetto voice production. This approach is based on breaking or modifying the current inappropriate laryngeal muscle posturing by substituting the falsetto voice muscle posture and then gradually lowering the voice to the normal habitual pitch. The patient again is instructed in the physiology of the laryngeal mechanism and how it relates to the vocal difficulties. The clinician explains that he or she is going to manipulate the vocal mechanism in a manner that will force the muscles to change their current posture to a different, more voice-friendly posture. The voice pathologist then produces a falsetto tone on the vowel /ai/ and tells the patient in a matter-of-fact manner that everyone can produce this tone, even those who are having vocal difficulties. The clinician again demonstrates the falsetto, and instructs the patient to produce the same sound. Some patients initially resist the falsetto production, but in our experience, with a little coaching, the majority of patients will eventually produce the tone. The falsetto is then stabilized briefly on vowels.

It is explained to the patient that we are going to use the modified laryngeal muscle posture created by the falsetto to encourage the vocal folds to vibrate normally. The patient is then given a list of 2-syllable phrases and asked to read them in the falsetto voice (see Appendix 7–A). During this exercise, the patient is constantly encouraged to read swiftly and loudly. After the voice stabilizes in a relatively strong falsetto, the patient is halted and asked to match the clinician singing down the scale about 3 to 4 notes from the original falsetto tone. The patient is then asked to continue reading the phrases at this new pitch level. The same procedure is repeated 2 or 3 more times until the patient is approximating a normal pitch level fairly closely. The patient is continually encouraged to produce these phrases louder and faster until eventually the voice "breaks" into normal phonation.

Occasionally, the patient will approximate normal phonation but then hesitate as if somewhat reluctant to produce normal voice. When this occurs, the patient is instructed to "drop way down" and produce a guttural voice quality while reading the phrases. The guttural voice is simply another method of changing the inappropriate muscle posturing. After a few minutes, the patient is taken back to the falsetto voice with the break into normal phonation usually occurring soon after.

- *Visual Biofeedback:* Providing the patient with a reasonable physiologic explanation as to why the voice is whispered or produced with too much tension is an important part of encouraging a return to normal phonation. Another technique that we have found useful is the use of direct visual feedback using laryngeal videoendoscopy. While the patient is being scoped, either with a rigid or flexible endoscope, an explanation is given related to the positioning of the vocal folds and how that positioning relates to the present vocal problem. The patient is able to monitor the video over the voice pathologist's shoulder. The patient is then instructed in various manipulations of the vocal folds such as deep breathing, light throat clearing, laughing, and attempts to produce tones of various loudness levels and pitches. We have had surprising success in the quick return of normal voicing using these procedures.

It is extremely important that the voice pathologist be patient when applying any of these therapy techniques. The normal time frame from disordered to normal voice is approximately 30 to 45 minutes (quicker with visual feedback). The voice pathologist not only must be tolerant and persistent but also must present a matter-of-fact, confident manner. Voice pathologists are not cheerleaders. They are simply confidently presenting a technique that they know will work. Why do these techniques work?

- The patient is ready for change.
- The voice pathologist has given a reasonable explanation for the present voice production.
- The voice pathologist has demonstrated confidence in the therapeutic techniques.

Following return of voice, it is necessary to explore the actual cause for the functional voice disorder. It is desirable to do this in a direct manner. For example, the voice pathologist may say:

> I'm very pleased that the muscles are all functioning well now and that

> your voice has returned to normal. It sounds very good. The thing that still puzzles me somewhat is why the muscles began posturing in the unusual manner in the first place. I can tell you quite frankly that with many other patients that we have seen with the same problem, the cause is often related to an upsetting event or some form of emotional stress. Can you think of anything that has been going on lately that might have contributed to this kind of stress?

By this time the patient has developed strong confidence in the voice pathologist and may freely provide information related to the psychosocial problems that could be related to the development of the voice disorder. In discussing these problems, the voice pathologist attempts to accomplish 2 major objectives: (1) give the patient total and final control over the laryngeal mechanism; and (2) determine the patient's general emotional state to decide the need for further professional counseling. To this point, the voice pathologist has been manipulating the voice. The patient now must understand that despite the actual cause of the aphonia/dysphonia, he or she is in total control of voice and does not need to permit the problem to recur. If it does, the patient now knows how to regain control of the voice (using whatever manipulations were used). The patient is in control. Finally, if the voice pathologist feels that the psychosocial problem has not resolved and further counseling is in order, the suggestion should be discussed with the patient, and appropriate referrals should be made.

Traditionally it has been reported in voice texts that when voice is regained through voice therapy that it is seldom lost again, and patients do not substitute other functional somatic symptoms.[126] This author could not find long-term follow-up data to support this assertion.

Functional Falsetto

Functional falsetto is the production of the preadolescent voice in the postadolescent male or female. Variously termed *mutational falsetto, persistent falsetto, puberphonia*, or, in the case of a female, *juvenile voice*, the high-pitched falsetto voice often draws unwanted attention to the postpubescent, physically mature patient. In fact, when not recognized and treated early, the unusual voice quality is often responsible for shaping the psychosocial character of the individual, with negative psychosocial consequences being greater for the male. Young males who present with this disorder have normal physical development and normal appearing larynges and vocal folds. However, the falsetto voice register is produced instead of the normal modal register. To accomplish this register, the suprahyoid muscles elevate the larynx, and the cricothyroid muscles are active while the thyroarytenoid muscles disengage. To maintain this register, respiration is usually shallow, with minimal subglottic air pressure. In fact, one of the diagnostic signs of functional falsetto is that the patient is not able to build adequate subglottic air pressure to produce a shout.

It has been suggested that functional falsetto may be the result of psychogenic factors such as failure of an adolescent male to accept an adult male role, overidentification with the mother, or social immaturity.[72] We would agree with Colton and Casper[75] who suggested that this disorder may simply result from attempts to stabilize unstable pitch and quality characteristics present in the male pubescent voice. Whatever the reason for the development of this voicing behavior, most patients are ready and willing to modify the voice with direct therapy. It has been our experience that this diagnosis is often missed in the young, postadolescent male and female. In the male, the misdiagnosis may be related to the presence of a mild dysphonia, which often accompanies the falsetto production. The dysphonia may be caused from strain placed on the laryngeal mechanism as the patient attempts to produce a more pitch-appropriate voice. The female falsetto voice most often goes unrecognized and not diagnosed unless the weak voice quality leads to negative job or social consequences.

Several therapy techniques may be used to modify functional falsetto voices. As with all functional voice disorders, the first step is to guarantee the presence of a normal laryngeal mechanism through a laryngeal examination by an otolaryngologist. The second step is to offer the patient a reasonable explanation for the vocal difficulty. Consider, for example, an explanation similar to the following:

> Often, as we grow, our many muscles grow so fast that for a while we may experience a lack of coordination or even clumsiness. I'm sure that you've known people whose legs have grown so fast in 1 year that it looks as if they are going to trip whenever they run. Well, our vocal folds are also made of muscles, and sometimes they grow so fast that we have to learn to use them correctly. That's why when voices begin to change, they crack and the voice breaks and sometimes it sounds funny.
>
> In your case, all the muscles changed and grew physically just the way they were supposed to grow, but they are not yet functioning properly. They need just a little bit of training to encourage them to work correctly. Our goal for today is to train the vocal folds to vibrate differently than they have vibrated before. I want you to do things I ask you to do with your voice and do not be surprised by some of the changes that we're going to hear.

This simple, brief explanation prepares the patient to accept the therapy procedure by providing a reasonable rationale for the problem. The third step is to utilize direct vocal manipulation. The following procedures are recommended:

- Ask the patient to produce a hard glottal attack (HGA) on a vowel. Demonstrate how the vowel should be produced with effort closure. When the glottal attack is produced correctly, the pitch will break into the normal lower register as the falsetto positioning of the intrinsic and extrinsic laryngeal muscles for the HGA cannot support initiation of this form of effort closure. If the pitch does not break, grasp the larynx with your thumb and index finger and hold it in a lowered position in the neck as the vowel is produced. If, after several trials, this fails to elicit the desired sound, depress the tongue with a tongue depressor as the patient produces the glottal attack.
- When the lower pitch is produced using the glottal attack, identify it immediately as a more appropriate voice sound. Have the patient repeat it several times using the glottal attack. Then produce several different vowel sounds while attempting to reduce and then extinguish the effort of the glottal attack. Stabilize the normal voice on vowel prolongation.

- Immediately move from vowels into words and phrases while maintaining the lower voice register. Attempt to expand the phrases through paragraph readings and into conversational speech during the initial therapy session.

Using this approach, the voice change is expected to be sudden and the progress of therapy rapid. The best way to accomplish this sudden improvement is for the voice pathologist to be aggressive with the therapy approach. It must be remembered that the voice is new to the patient. The patient's auditory feedback system does not yet identify the new voice as belonging to him or her. Initially, the voice may want to shift back into the falsetto. Positive encouragement may be necessary.

Follow-up sessions may be needed to stabilize the new voice. We often give the patient Vocal Function Exercises to build the strength and balance of the laryngeal mechanism and to balance respiration, phonation, and resonance. In addition, in our effort to aid the patient in developing total control of the voice, we often use negative practice by having the patient shift back and forth between the two voices. Interestingly, as the "new" voice is increasingly used, patients find it more difficult to produce the falsetto voice.

Most patients are somewhat excited by and proud of the new voice, but some are embarrassed by the sudden voice quality change. These patients may require a gradual desensitization program as a part of the stabilization process. A desensitization program involves establishing with the patient a personal hierarchy of communication experiences ranging from the least difficult to the most difficult speaking situations. A typical hierarchy may include:

1. talking to strangers in a fast-food restaurant or store
2. talking to family members
3. talking to selected friends
4. talking in the classroom.

One of our patients was a 17-year-old who developed normal voicing from falsetto over the Christmas holidays. The patient handled his drastic voice change in a humorous manner. He returned to school using the falsetto voice for half of the day in the classroom. During his afternoon math class, he began coughing and asked to be excused to get a drink of water. When he returned to class he exclaimed excitedly in his new normal voice, "Mr., they must have put something in the water; listen to my voice!" We also have had another experience that made the therapeutic intervention rather easy. The patient was easily able to produce the glottal attack. When it was explained to him that this was the desired voice, he replied in a normal modal voice register, "Okay, I can do that all day long if I have to." This young man had experimented with the modal voice register. He was not aware, however, that this was supposed to be his voice. As with all of these patients, we make liberal use of audio-recorded samples of the falsetto voice and the "new" voice. When this patient heard and realized the excellent quality of the modal voice, he simply began using it on a regular basis. From that experience, we have learned to first ask the patient before initiating any other therapy approaches, "Do you have any other voice?"

Our experience with female falsetto voice has been with older women who complain of a lack of power and strength in the voice. When examined stroboscopically, perceptually, and instrumentally, it becomes evident that they are producing voice in the falsetto register. In most cases, this form of voice production has been a lifelong habit and is more resistant to modification. One patient was a 68-year-old woman who had recently become a tour guide at a local museum. She complained that even using a portable amplifier, her voice was fatiguing and becoming hoarse on a daily basis. We identified the problem as a functional falsetto and began using the glottal attack to introduce her modal voice. In fact, she almost jumped out of her chair the first time she produced the loud vowel sound. She indicated that she had never been able to shout at her children. This patient was readily able to develop a strong, appropriate voice over a several week period of time and was pleased to use it as she guided people through the museum without the previous vocal fatigue and hoarseness. The problem arose when she tried to use the voice with her family. To be blunt, they hated the new voice. It simply was not their mom. Their auditory feedback systems could not accept the new voice. The patient's solution was to shift between the 2 voices depending on her vocal needs.

This juvenile-sounding female voice is not often seen in voice therapy clinics because the problem is more one of aesthetics than one that is considered a pathologic problem. An unusual high pitch with associated breathiness characterizes the voice quality of female functional dysphonia. What characterizes the juvenile voice is the "child-like" quality. Our experience has been with women who complain of laryngeal fatigue and late-in-the-day hoarseness. Like the tour guide mentioned above, the vast majority of these individuals have recently become involved in activities that require increased voice use. When these patients seek treatment, they are not aware of the functional ineffectiveness of their vocal habits. It is the role of the voice pathologist to describe the inappropriate voice components and to seek production of an improved voice.

Vocal Cord Dysfunction

As described in Chapter 4, vocal cord dysfunction (VCD) is characterized by wheezing or inspiratory stridor caused by inappropriate closure of the true vocal folds throughout the respiratory cycle. VCD is often mistaken for asthma and is treated with many pulmonary medications without relief of the symptoms.[127] During acute attacks, patients with VCD often require emergency medical treatment and in severe cases have undergone (unnecessary) tracheostomy. Treatment involves a combination of medical, psychological, and behavioral approaches.

Pharmacologic interventions including bronchodilators have been used in an attempt to relieve symptoms; however, success depends on the etiology of the disorder. Some centers use an inhalation therapy called "heliox," a mixture of helium (80%) and oxygen (20%) to relieve at least the acute symptoms and maintain symptom reduction even after cessation of the treatment.[127] Psychiatric or psychological intervention in the form of psychotherapy using methods of relaxation and supportive therapy has also been effective when emotional or psychological issues and family dynamics have been involved.[128]

Voice symptoms ranging from complete aphonia to mild hoarseness may be present in the VCD patient, but the primary role of the voice pathologist is to aid in restoring the airway. As with most disorders, educating the patient regarding the disorder is the first step. Videolaryngoscopy is an excellent tool for this purpose. It should be remembered that some patients often have been treated for an asthmatic condition for many years. It may be quite disconcerting suddenly to be told that, in fact, they have a different disorder altogether. Patients are readily able to understand the disorder when observing inappropriate movements of the vocal folds during respiration. Our normal protocol examines the vocal folds during forced inhalation and exhalation as well as during quiet breathing. We then encourage an increase in respiratory effort by having the patient walk briskly up and down steps or on a treadmill, which is in our office. This exercise often induces greater adductory movement of the vocal folds. (This is only done in a medical setting, with emergency protocol in place.) Finally, we ask the patient to simulate an "attack" while monitoring the larynx through videoendoscopy. This simulation is often very revealing. When videoendoscopy is not available, the patient may be educated with picture descriptions of inappropriate and appropriate vocal fold movements during respiration.

Because the patient now understands the disorder, direct treatment approaches may be applied. Martin et al[129] described a treatment approach that facilitates laryngeal relaxation by maintaining continuous airflow through the glottis during abdominal breathing. By focusing on self-awareness, the patient is encouraged to become aware of sensations of heightened laryngeal and respiratory tension during an episode in comparison to laryngeal sensations when voluntary control is exercised. Therapy techniques include relaxation exercises to relax the oropharyngeal and upper body musculature, using abdominal breathing without laryngeal constriction or tension, and focusing on prolonged exhalation. Martin et al[129] further recommended inhaling through the nose with the lips closed, a relaxed tongue posture, and prolonged audible exhalation through pursed lips or while producing /s/. When the patient is experiencing VCD, a quick sniff with the mouth closed may abduct the vocal folds and relieve the symptoms.

PHYSIOLOGIC VOICE THERAPY

When a voice disorder is present, we may assume that the disorder has caused a change in the functioning of the physiology responsible for voice production. These changes may be the result of a respiratory problem interrupting normal airflow or causing inappropriate subglottic air pressure responsible for driving phonation. Phonation may be affected by mass, lesion, neurologic problems, or muscle tension. Finally, functional or organic modifications of the resonators may lead to vocal dysfunction. When any one of these voice subsystems, respiration, phonation, or resonance, is affected by functional misuse or pathology, the remaining subsystems must adjust to compensate for the change. Physiologic voice therapy is a holistic therapy approach, involving all 3 subsystems, using direct physical exercise and manipulations to improve voice quality.

Case Study 11: Laryngeal Muscle Imbalance

The patient was a 35-year-old female who was referred for evaluation and treatment with a diagnosis of "voice disturbance." Voice quality during the diagnostic evaluation was normal. The patient complained, however, of laryngeal fatigue when speaking and more recently when singing; she also described ineffective use of the lower range of her singing voice. Although she could maintain a "reasonably good" singing quality if she "forced" the voice, she was sure that the forcing contributed to the fatigue. In addition, she reported feeling a "shortness of breath" as if she were "running out of air" before the end of a musical phrase. An operatic contralto, she was currently engaged to sing her first solo as a professional. She indicated that this particular aria, which she had practiced many times a day, stretched her vocal range to its lower limit.

The evaluation yielded no significant etiologic factors or voice changes except for the symptoms described by the patient. Stroboscopic evaluation of vocal function revealed grossly normal appearing vocal folds bilaterally as the folds were free of any apparent edema or other visible pathology. The mucosal waves and amplitude of vibration were normal at comfort level. Glottic closure, however, demonstrated an unusual anterior glottal chink, which became larger as the pitch was lowered. The patient was able to sustain an upper range tone for 49 seconds and a lower tone for only 21 seconds. Her measured airflow rates were consistent, with a higher airflow rate measured at low pitch.

We speculated that this voice problem reflected imbalance between cricothyroid and thyroarytenoid muscle function. It was our impression, therefore, that this laryngeal muscle imbalance, most likely caused by voice strain, contributed to the fatigue in her speaking voice and the ineffectiveness of her lower singing range. The therapy focused on strengthening and balancing the voice subsystems and was successful in remediating her symptoms. Stroboscopic observation of the vocal folds following voice therapy demonstrated the anterior chink to be gone as glottic closure was complete at all pitch levels. We speculated that this patient had spent so much time pushing her voice "to its lower limit" while practicing her aria that she altered the coordination within the laryngeal musculature.

Stemple and colleagues[130] studied voice and vocal fold changes following prolonged loud voice use in a vocally normal group of participants. Results of their investigation were consistent with the example described above in that a significant number of participants demonstrated the unusual anterior glottal chink following the voicing task. In addition, subjects experienced much difficulty in matching the lower limits of their pretest voices. These authors speculated that laryngeal muscle strain may have contributed to these results.

This 35-year-old singer demonstrated that at least 2 parts of her vocal mechanism had been negatively affected by laryngeal muscle imbalance. When the muscular system became strained and imbalanced, the respiratory system was forced to adjust and, through increased air pressure and airflow, could maintain a "reasonable" singing voice for a short period of time. For this elite vocal performer, "reasonable" was not good enough. We would speculate that had she continued to force the voice, she would have developed a back-focused tone with a combination of all the faulty subsystems leading to more serious vocal difficulty.

Case Study 12: The Postsurgical Patient

The patient, a 55-year-old insurance sales representative, was referred for evaluation and treatment following 2 surgeries for removal of bilateral vocal fold polyps. Voice quality during the evaluation was moderately dysphonic, characterized by low pitch, decreased loudness, and breathiness. He could not readily increase loudness to a shout. The patient was disturbed by the results of surgery, because it was his impression that his voice quality would be "normal" following the surgery. The voice evaluation indicated that the patient originally had a voice disorder caused by several etiologic factors. These included: (1) excessive, loud talking; (2) the use of a low-pitched telephone voice; (3) smoking 1½ packages of cigarettes per day; and (4) habitual throat clearing. Presurgical voice therapy had modified all factors except those for smoking, which was reduced but not eliminated.

The presurgical vocal mechanism had adjusted the voice subsystems to accommodate the presence of the bilateral polyps. Once the polyps were removed, the subsystems were essentially in disarray and had not automatically rebalanced to provide the expected improved voice quality. The patient had maintained the back-focused, strained voice production that had been required to produce voice prior to his surgeries. He continued producing voice with muscle tension. Direct, physiologic voice therapy was used to accomplish the task of improving the voice quality.

Case Study 13: Presbyphonia

The patient was a 74-year-old male who was referred by the otolaryngologist with the diagnosis of bowed vocal folds. He was looking forward to the voice evaluation because of the restrictions that his voice was placing on his life. Two years prior to the evaluation, the patient was widowed, and he lived alone. He was a social individual who enjoyed going to weekly lunches with his friends, attending a variety of sporting events, and until recently, singing in the church choir. He presented with a moderate dysphonia, characterized by dry, breathy hoarseness. He found it difficult to compete vocally with background noise and noticed that his voice fatigued easily with use. Recently, the patient had begun declining social invitations because it was difficult to carry on conversations with his friends. The problems with his weak voice were exacerbated by the fact that several of his close friends were hard of hearing.

The geriatric population often complains of voice weakness, fatigue, and chronic hoarseness. As described in Chapter 2, several physiologic changes occur in the aging larynx, which may account for voice quality changes. The aging larynx suffers a decrease in muscle fiber, a stiffening of the vocal fold cover, and continued calcification of the laryngeal cartilages.[131] Many geriatric patients present to otolaryngologists and voice pathologists complaining of the vocal symptoms as described above. Often, they are told that this is part of the aging process and that they would have to "live" with the problem.

Some older individuals are widowed and live alone, often with little opportunity to talk for extended periods of time. Combine the natural physiologic changes in the larynx with the lack of voice use, and these individuals develop voice problems that interfere with their communication ability when they do have the need and desire to speak. In our clinic, geriatric patients have found great success using a systematic vocal exercise program as a means of strengthening voice production by improving the relationships of the 3 subsystems of voice production: respiration, phonation, and resonance.

As previously stated, a voice pathologist must develop a large armamentarium of voice therapy treatment techniques. With experience, each clinician will choose techniques that feel comfortable, that make sense and can be easily explained to the patient, and that also work well for that clinician. Physiologic voice therapy programs integrate all of the voice subsystems into the rehabilitative effort. The following are examples of comprehensive physiologic voice therapy programs that may be applied to many patients with various pathologies of varying etiologic origins. The strength of each of these approaches is their comprehensive holistic nature. Each approach attends to all 3 subsystems of voice production. They are physiologic treatments that address respiration, phonation, and supraglottic placement of the glottal tone all at once. As seen from the previous case discussions, their applications are many including both hyperfunctional and hypofunctional disorders.

Vocal Function Exercises

The vocal function exercise (VFE) program is based on an assumption that has not been determined empirically. Nonetheless, this assumption and the clinical logic that follows has been supported through many years of clinical research,[83–87,132] experience, and observation using this exercise program. For our purposes, it is useful to consider that the laryngeal mechanism is similar to other muscle systems and may become strained and imbalanced through many etiologic factors. The analogy that we often draw with patients is a comparison of the rehabilitation of the knee to rehabilitation of the voice. Both the knee and the larynx are composed of muscle, cartilage, and connective tissue. When the knee is injured, rehabilitation includes a short period of immobilization for the purpose of reducing the effects of the acute injury. The immobilization is followed by assisted ambulation, and then the primary rehabilitation begins in the form of systematic exercise. This exercise is designed to strengthen and balance all of the supportive knee muscles for the purpose of returning the knee to as close to its normal functioning as possible.

Rehabilitation of voice may also involve a short period of voice rest following acute injury or after surgery to permit healing of the mucosa to occur. The patient then may begin conservative voice use and follow through with all of the management approaches that seem necessary. Full voice use is then resumed quickly, and the therapy program often is successful in returning the patient to normal voice production. We would suggest, however, that on many occasions patients are not fully rehabilitated because one of the important rehabilitation steps was neglected. That step is the systematic exercise program that is often necessary to decompensate maladaptive voicing behaviors by regaining the balance among airflow, to this laryngeal muscle activity, to the supraglottic placement of the tone.

Vocal function exercises first described by Barnes[133] and modified by Stemple[105] strive to balance the subsystems of voice production. The exercise program has proven successful in improving and enhancing the vocal function of speakers with normal voices,[85] opera singers,[84] teachers with voice disorders,[83] and elderly men.[134]

The program is simple to teach and, when presented appropriately, seems reasonable to patients. Many patients are enthusiastic to have a concrete program, similar in concept to physical therapy, during which they may plot the progress of their return to vocal efficiency. The program begins by describing the problem to the patient, using illustrations as needed or the patient's own stroboscopic evaluation video. The patient is then taught a series of 4 exercises to be done at home, 2 times each, twice per day, preferably morning and evening. These exercises include:

1. Sustain the /i/ vowel for as long as possible on the musical note (F) above middle (C) for females and boys, (F) below middle (C) for males. (Notes may be modified up or down to fit the needs of the patient. Seldom are they modified by more than 2 notes in either direction.) *Goal:* Based on airflow volume. In our clinic the goal is based on reaching 80 to 100 mL/s of airflow. So, if the flow volume is equal to 4000 mL, then the goal is 40 to 45 seconds. When airflow measures are not available, the goal is equal to the longest /s/ that the patient is able to sustain. Placement of the tone should be in an extreme forward focus, almost, but not quite, nasal. All exercises are produced as softly as possible, but not breathy. The voice must be "engaged." This is considered a warm-up exercise.
2. Glide from your lowest note to your highest note on the word "Knoll." *Goal:* No voice breaks. The glide requires the use of all laryngeal muscles. It stretches the vocal folds and encourages a systematic, slow engagement of the cricothyroid muscles. The word "Knoll" encourages a forward placement of the tone as well as an expanded open pharynx. The patient's lips are to be rounded and a sympathetic vibration should be felt on the lips (Figure 7–3). (The patient may also use a lip trill, tongue trill, or the word "whoop.") Voice breaks will typically occur in the transitions between low and high registers. When breaks occur, the patient is encouraged to continue the glide without hesitation. When the voice breaks at the top of the current range and the patient

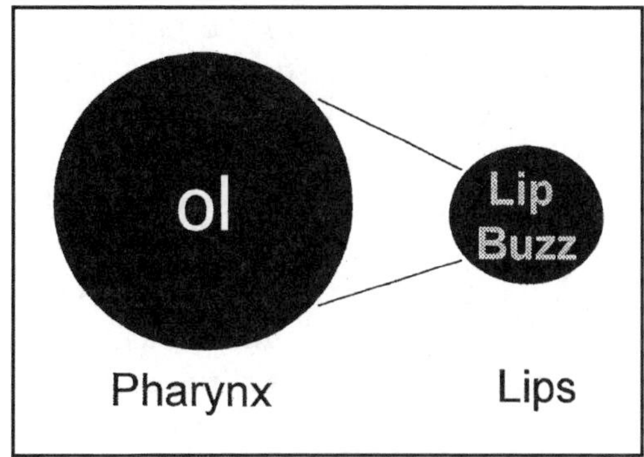

FIGURE 7–3. Open pharynx and lip buzz.

typically has more range, the glide may be continued without voice as the folds will continue to stretch. Glides improve muscular control and flexibility. This is considered a stretching exercise.

3. Glide from your highest note to your lowest note on the word "Knoll." *Goal:* No voice breaks. The patient is instructed to feel a half-yawn in the throat throughout this exercise. By keeping the pharynx open and focusing the sympathetic vibration at the lips, the downward glide encourages a slow, systematic engagement of the thyroarytenoid muscles without the presence of a back-focused growl. In fact, no growl is permitted. (The patient may also use a lip trill, tongue trill, or the word "boom.") This is considered a contracting exercise.
4. Sustain the musical notes (C-D-E-F-G) for as long as possible on the word "Knoll" minus the "Kn." (Use the middle C for females and boys and the octave below middle C for males.) *Goal:* The goal remains the same as for exercise 1. The "oll" is once again produced with an open pharynx and constricted, sympathetically vibrating lips. The shape of the pharynx to the lips is likened to an inverted megaphone. The fourth exercise may be tailored to the patient's present vocal ability. Although the basic range of middle C, an octave lower for males, is appropriate for most voices, the exercises may be customized up or down to fit the current vocal condition or a particular voice type. Seldom, however, are the exercises shifted more than 2 notes in either direction. This is considered a low-impact adductory power exercise.

Quality of the tone is also monitored for voice breaks, wavering, and breathiness. Quality improves as times increase and pathologies begin to resolve. All exercises are done as softly as possible but with good vocal fold engagement. Without engagement of the thyroarytenoid muscles, the patient will be producing a falsetto tone and air will escape between the folds at a rapid rate. Consequently, softness is a relative term as some patients, such as those with unilateral vocal fold paralysis or vocal fold bowing, may be required to be quite loud in the initial stages of therapy in order to maintain engagement. It is much more difficult to produce soft tones; therefore, the vocal subsystems will receive a better workout than if louder tones were produced. Extreme care is taken to teach the production of a forward tone that lacks tension. In addition, attention is paid to the glottal onset of the tone. The patient is asked to breathe in deeply with attention paid to training abdominal breathing, posturing the vowel momentarily, and then initiating the exercise gesture without a forceful glottal attack or an aspirate breathy attack. It is explained to the patient that maximum phonation times increase as the efficiency of the vocal fold vibration improves. Times do not increase with improved "lung capacity." Even aerobic exercise does not improve lung capacity, but rather the efficiency of oxygen exchange with the circulatory system, thus, giving the sense of more air.

The musical notes are matched to the notes produced by an inexpensive pitch pipe that the patient purchases for use at home or a CD recording of live voice doing the exercises may be given to the patient for home use. Many patients find the CD-recorded voice easier to match than the pitch pipe. In addition, many apps are now available which can be downloaded to the patient's smart phone for both pitch matching and timing by stopwatch. We have found that patients who complain of "tone deafness" often can be taught to approximate the correct notes well with practice and guidance from the voice pathologist.

Finally, patients are given a chart on which to mark their sustained times, which is a means of plotting progress (Figure 7–4). Progress is monitored over time and, because of normal daily variability, patients are encouraged not to compare today to tomorrow and so on. Rather, weekly comparisons are encouraged. Estimated time of completion for the program is 8 to 10 weeks. Some patients experience minor laryngeal aching for the first day or so of the program similar to muscle aching that

Vocal Function Exercise

Daily Record

Name__________ **Begin Date**__________

		MON	TUE	WED	THU	FRI	SAT	SUN
	Date							
	E/F	/	/	/	/	/	/	/
	C	/	/	/	/	/	/	/
AM	D	/	/	/	/	/	/	/
	E	/	/	/	/	/	/	/
	F	/	/	/	/	/	/	/
	G	/	/	/	/	/	/	/
	E/F	/	/	/	/	/	/	/
	C	/	/	/	/	/	/	/
PM	D	/	/	/	/	/	/	/
	E	/	/	/	/	/	/	/
	F	/	/	/	/	/	/	/
	G	/	/	/	/	/	/	/

		MON	TUE	WED	THU	FRI	SAT	SUN
	Date							
	E/F	/	/	/	/	/	/	/
	C	/	/	/	/	/	/	/
AM	D	/	/	/	/	/	/	/
	E	/	/	/	/	/	/	/
	F	/	/	/	/	/	/	/
	G	/	/	/	/	/	/	/
	E/F	/	/	/	/	/	/	/
	C	/	/	/	/	/	/	/
PM	D	/	/	/	/	/	/	/
	E	/	/	/	/	/	/	/
	F	/	/	/	/	/	/	/
	G	/	/	/	/	/	/	/

FIGURE 7–4. Vocal Function Exercise Daily Record.

might occur with any new muscular exercise. As this discomfort will soon subside, they are encouraged to continue the program through the discomfort should it occur.

When the patient has reached the predetermined therapy goal, and the voice quality and other vocal symptoms have improved, then a tapering maintenance program is recommended. Although some of the professional voice users choose to remain in peak vocal condition, many of our patients desire to taper the VFE program. The following systematic taper is recommended:

- Full program 2 times each, 2 times per day
- Full program 2 times each, 1 time per day (morning)
- Full program 1 time each, 1 time per day (morning)
- Exercise 4, 2 times each, 1 time per day (morning)
- Exercise 4, 1 time each, 1 time per day (morning)
- Exercise 4, 1 time each, 3 times per week (morning)
- Exercise 4, 1 time each, 1 time per week (morning)

Each taper should last 1 week. Patients should maintain 85% of their peak time, otherwise they should move up a step in the taper until the 85% criterion is met.

In short, vocal function exercises provide a holistic voice treatment program that attends to the 3 major subsystems of voice production. The respiratory, laryngeal, and resonance postures and activities inherent in these exercises demand exquisite coordination of these mechanisms leading to maximal voice output with minimal effort. The program appears to benefit patients with a wide range of voice disorders because it is reasonable in regard to time and effort. It is similar to other recognizable exercise programs; the concept of "physical therapy" for the vocal folds is understandable; progress may be easily plotted, which is inherently motivating; and it appears to balance airflow, laryngeal activity, and supraglottic placement.

Resonant Voice Therapy

Resonant voice therapy (RVT) is another holistic voice therapy program. The concept of RVT arose from performing arts trainers, especially Arthur Lessac, and speech-language pathologists from Morton Cooper in the 1970s through the current well-researched and developed Lessac-Madsen Resonant Voice Therapy of Katherine Verdolini.[135,136] Resonant voice is defined as voice production involving oral vibratory sensations, usually on the anterior alveolar ridge or higher in the face in the context of easy phonation. Resonant voice is a continuum of oral sensations and easy phonation building from basic speech gestures through conversational speech. The therapy goal is to achieve the strongest, "cleanest" possible voice with the least effort and impact between the vocal folds to minimize the likelihood of injury and maximize the likelihood of vocal health.

As with vocal function exercises, the training methodologies are experiential, focusing on the processing of sensory information. The patient is constantly asked to monitor the "feel" and to concentrate on the auditory feedback. The training model assumes similar approaches for voice restoration for voice disorders and enhancing the normal voice (excellence training). According to Verdolini,[77] the following fundamental characteristics guide RVT:

- The fundamental perceptual target is focused oral vibratory sensations in the context of easy phonation.
- The training methodology is experiential, involving an emphasis on the processing of sensory information (what the patient feels and hears).
- The singular training focus (resonance) is expected to affect multiple levels of physiology (breathing and laryngeal function).
- Large numbers of repetitions are used, in varying speech/singing and environmental contexts relevant to the learner.
- Both neuromuscular ("hardware") and cognitive ("software") shifts in voice production are expected.
- Training is strongly goal (results) driven, involving a dogged insistence on the greatest possible precision in the achievement of the perceptual tasks.

The following is a 7-step RVT program supported by outcomes research,[59] based on the work of Verdolini and developed within our own clinical voice practice.[137]

Basic Training Gesture

The patient is asked to either stand or sit with good posture; to take a comfortable breath, and to vocally sigh from a high to low pitch repeating /molm/. The pharynx is to be wide open for the /ol/, and the energy of the /m/ is to be focused in the facial bones, nose, and lips. Attempt to develop a connection between the abdominal respiratory support muscles and the face and lips. The following written instructions are provided to the patient.

Basic Training Gesture

- Holm-molm-molm-molm-molm . . . As a sigh . . .
- Extreme forward focus is required with appropriate breath support
- Make the connection from the abdominal muscles to the lips
- Patient should feel very relaxed at the end of this gesture

RVT Hierarchy Stage 1 (All Voiced)

Begin to add nonlinguistic speech contexts on repetitions of /molm-molm-molm/. You will note that all 5 exercises in this stage use voiced sounds that do not require laryngeal articulation. Choose a pitch that is slightly higher than a comfortable conversational tone for all exercises. It is helpful to match this pitch to the corresponding note on a pitch pipe and to remain consistent throughout the program.

Step 1. Repeat molm-molm-molm . . . (sustained pitch) on musical note _____.

- Vary the rate only (slow-fast-slow)
- Discover the vibrations; experiment with broad and narrow vibrations
- Eventually focus on the narrow vibration; "like a narrow beam of light"
- Increase the ease of production by reducing the effort

Step 2. Repeat molm-molm-molm . . . (sustained pitch) on musical note _____.

- Combine slow-fast-slow and soft-loud-soft

- Vary the intensity and the rate of the sustained molm-molm-molm . . .

Step 3. molm-molm-molm . . . as speech with the intonation of spoken phrases (Make up nonlinguistic phrases using only the molm-molm-molm . . .) This step helps in the transition to speech.

- Use nonlinguistic phrases; vary the rate, pitch, and loudness; constantly use abdominal breathing to support the tone production with the point of vocal tract constriction at the extreme end of the resonators. In other words, make the connection from the abdominal muscles to the lips.

Step 4. Chant the following voiced phrases on the musical note. Totally exaggerate articulation and forward resonance.

- Mary made me mad.
- My mother made marmalade.
- My merry mom made marmalade.
- My mom may marry Marv.
- My merry mom may marry Marv.
- Marv made my mother merry.

Step 5. Overinflect these same phrases as speech. Be diligent about making the connection from the abdominal breath support to the front of the face.

RVT Hierarchy Stage 2 (Voiced-Voiceless Contrasts)

You will note that the exercise difficulty has been increased with the addition of the voiceless consonant. This requires rapid laryngeal articulation, which more closely approximates the requirements of conversational voice production. As always, begin with the Basic Training Gesture and then proceed.

Step 1. mamapapa . . . vary the rate on the note _____. (comfortable conversational tone)

Step 2. mamapapa . . . combined slow-fast-slow and soft-loud-soft on the note _____.

Step 3. mamapapa . . . as speech, with the intonation of spoken phrases.

- use nonlinguistic phrases; vary the rate, pitch, and loudness; make the connection from the abdominal muscles to the lips

Step 4. Chant the following voiced/voiceless phrases on the musical note _____. (comfortable conversational tone) Totally exaggerate articulation and forward resonance

- Mom may put Paul on the moon.
- Mom told Tom to copy my manner.
- My manner made Pete and Paul mad.
- Mom may move Polly's movie to 10.
- My movie made Tim and Tom sad.

Step 5. Overinflect these same phrases as speech.

RVT Hierarchy Stage 3 (Any Phrase)

The task is now made more difficult by introducing other phrases. As usual, begin with the Basic Training Gesture.

Step 1. Chant 5- to 7-syllable phrases on the note _____. (Comfortable conversational tone)

- All the girls were laughing.

- Get there before they close.
- Did you hear what she said?
- Come in and close the door.
- Are you going tonight?
- Put everything away.
- Come whenever you can.
- We heard that yesterday.
- The player broke his leg.
- The children went swimming.

Step 2. Overinflect the same phrases with an extreme forward focus

Step 3. Repeat the same phrases in a more natural forward speech/voice production

The chanted phrase should be said in an extreme forward focus with exaggerated articulation. The overinflected phrase and the more natural production must both maintain the same forward connection and ease of phonation. It is often helpful to ask the patient to link the chanted and inflected phrases together (without taking a breath), as this will aid in maintaining appropriate respiratory support and tone focus.

RVT Hierarchy Stage 4 (Paragraph Reading)

This stage begins combining strings of phrases which expands the difficulty of the task once more. Maintain the exaggerated focus only as long as is necessary to confirm that the task has been mastered. Begin with the Basic Training Gesture. Then:

1. Read a paragraph with phrase markers; separate each phrase only by the natural inhalation of air.
2. Exaggerate focus and then repeat with a more normal speech/voice production.
3. Repeat the above with paragraphs without phrase markers (see Appendix 7–A, Paragraphs).

RVT Hierarchy Stage 5 (Controlled Conversation)

It is now time to begin carryover to conversation of the new "forward-focus" voicing behavior. Usually by this stage patients have mastered the appropriate focus and are using a more appropriate manner of voice production. This stage is confirmation of that fact. Any topic of interest is fair game for discussion from job and family to vacations and hobbies. The patient may want to establish practice times at home, such as at the dinner table, because it is difficult to concentrate on how one is talking while talking. If the foundation has been successfully established in the previous steps, however, then this challenge will be lessened:

- Practice forward speech placement in conversation
- Do not permit glottal attacks, glottal fry, and so forth

RVT Hierarchy Stage 6 (Environmental Manipulations)

Quiet conversation, as in Step 5, is an easier task than actually placing the patient in everyday situations where there is background noise and other commotion. This step encourages the patient to continue to use the new vocal habits despite ambient distractions:

- Simulate actual speaking environments consistent with the patient's needs (actual/simulated).
- Use recordings of background noise.

- Go to a noisy setting such as a cafeteria.
- Practice in a lecture environment.

RVT Hierarchy Stage 7 (Emotional Manipulations)

Challenge the use of resonant voice by animating the discussion with topics that elicit laughter, loud talking, anger, indignation, and other emotions. Use materials and topics that increasingly engage and challenge the patient based on personality, interests, work experience, and passions.

RVT Hierarchy Home Exercises

Home exercise is an essential part of RVT. In this day and age of managed care, therapy is often limited to a few actual sessions. In therapy, the patient is given the skills and tasks that must be mastered during home practice. It is evident when a patient has neglected to follow the practice recommendations.

- The critical portion of each exercise for each week is recorded by the speech-language pathologist as a home exercise example. The home program involves 5- to 10-minute sessions, twice per day, including:
  - ☐ Basic training gesture
  - ☐ Selected level of hierarchy

The patient is also encouraged to "tune" the voice with the basic training gesture several times throughout the day.

Several studies now indicate that easy, resonant voice tends to be produced with vocal folds that are barely touching or barely separated.[138,139] This posture appears to produce the strongest, clearest voice output for the least amount of vocal fold impact stress. This posture also requires the least amount of lung pressure to vibrate the vocal folds. Therefore, the postures developed in vocal function exercises and resonant voice therapy encourage a relatively strong, clear voice, which appears to provide some protection from injury and is physically easy to produce.[136] Preliminary evidence indicates that these programs provide for efficient vibration of the vocal folds and a balance among the 3 subsystems of voice production. We have found the RVT program extremely useful as a means of training a forward focus voice production. Resonant voice therapy and vocal function exercises are extremely complementary in a therapy program used for a wide variety of voice disorders including both hyperfunctional and hypofunctional disorders.

Accent Method of Voice Therapy

Another holistic treatment approach is the accent method developed by Svend Smith of Denmark and described in detail by Kotby and colleagues.[81] This voice therapy approach is designed to:

- increase pulmonary output
- reduce glottic waste
- reduce excessive muscular tension
- normalize the vibratory pattern during phonation

The technique is based on the principles of the myoelastic-aerodynamic theory of phonation. The originators state that because voice production is created by subglottal air pressure and transglottal airflow, stronger air pressures below the vocal folds result in an increased amplitude of vibration and a more stable closed phase of the vibratory cycle. The stronger closed phase improves the filtering process of the vocal tract as a result of a longer duration of the vocal fold contact within one period and a higher airflow through the glottis in the opening phase of the vibratory cycle. Together they counteract the damping effect of the resonances in the vocal tract. The expected acoustic effects of treatment are:

- increased energy of the fundamental frequency
- increased energy in the second and third formant frequencies
- reduced irregular pitch perturbations
- optimal fundamental frequency
- increased frequency range
- increased dynamic range[60]

A summary of the Accent Method procedures follows:

- Facilitate abdominal breathing: Ideally, the patient is placed in a recumbent position and normal abdominal breathing is elicited. The patient is instructed to place one hand on the stomach to monitor the abdominal movements while the clinician demonstrates abdominal breathing and upper body relaxation. A brief description of the lowering action of the diaphragm is given to demonstrate the appropriate increase in chest cavity size as air is inspired. The patient is asked to gain a consciousness over the abdominal movements for both inhalation and exhalation. Abdominal muscle control is important for achieving changes in pitch and loudness.
- The patient is then instructed to watch the clinician as fricative-like sounds are demonstrated. The sounds are first sustained individually and then with a 2-beat rhythm. The 2-beat rhythm is accented, with the first sound being weak and the second sound produced with more force. A sample of this sequenced breathing exercise would be:

  Inhale, say /s/————
  Inhale, say /sh/————
  Inhale, say /f/————

  The 2-beat accented rhythm would be:

  s-S————
  sh-SH————
  f-F————

  (The second sound is accented and sustained.)

  Throughout the accented practice, changes in body position (sitting, standing, walking, swinging the arms) are used to encourage regulation and adaptation of the breathing patterns.
- Utilize rhythmic vocal play: When the correct breathing pattern has been established, phonation is begun. Voice is initially introduced with a soft, breathy onset of the tone. Again, the clinician demonstrates the rhythm and the patient imitates the accented pattern. Each stressed sound (the second accented sound) is accompanied by a smooth abdominal contraction. Eventually, the exercises are carried out at three different speeds: largo, andante, and allegro (slow, moderate, and fast) tempos (Figure 7–5). In implementing the accent method, the clinician can utilize arm movements, tapping, or even beating on a drum to help establish the rhythm. Many vowel and consonant combinations may be used.

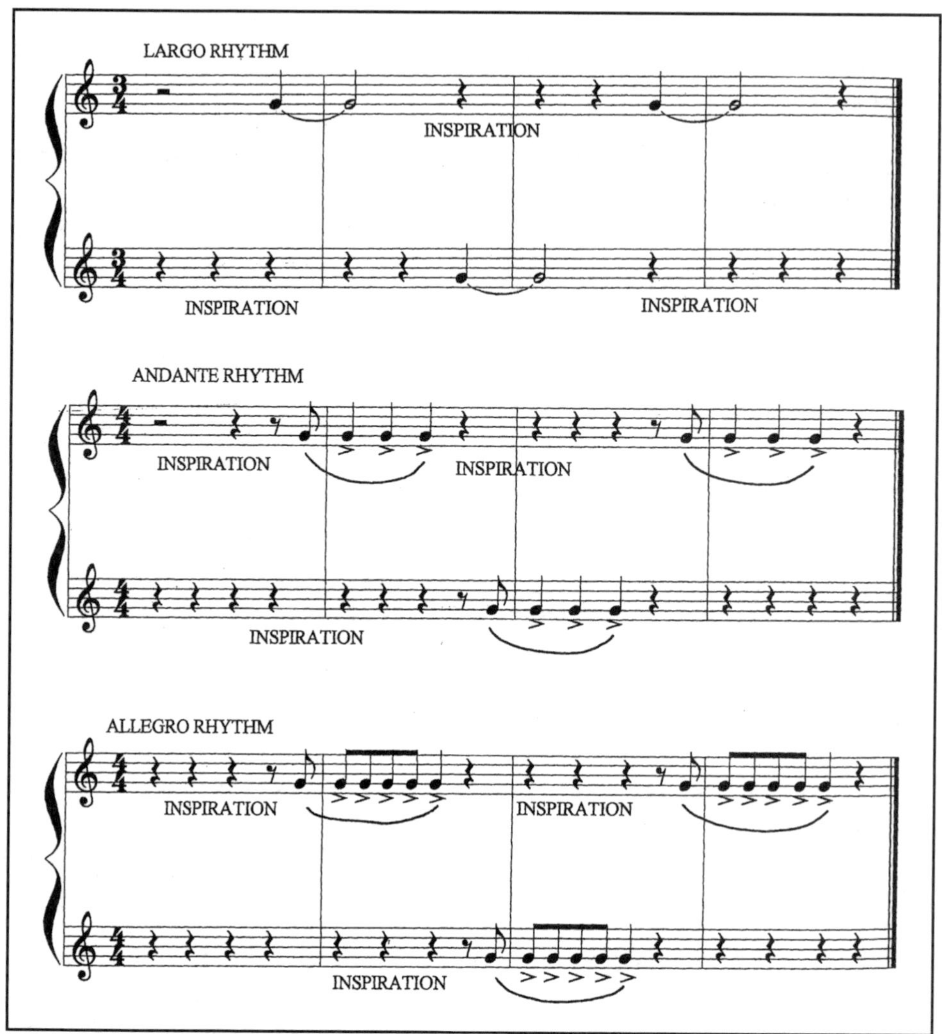

FIGURE 7–5. Largo, andante, and allegro rhythms.

The largo tempo consists of one or two main stresses in a 3-beat rhythm in which breathy phonation and consonant resistances are used at the lips and the tongue. A sample largo sequence includes:

zh-ZH

zz-ZZ-ZZ

yoi-YOI

yoi-YOI-YOI

In the andante tempo, phrases are increased in size to 3 main beats in a 4-beat rhythm, and the breathiness of the voice is eliminated. This step introduces variability in pitch, intensity, timbre, vowel shape, and time. A sample andante sequence includes:

woo-WOO-WOO-WOO

yea-YEA-YEA-YEA

yee-YEE-YEE-YEE

In the allegro tempo, the voice exercises consist of an unstressed vowel followed by 5 stressed vowels. This speed is doubled as the main beats are divided into 2 faster beats. Phrase length, intensity, and a rich variety of sounds are incorporated into the practice as well as the other tempo patterns. This step encourages more variety to the voice and approaches the natural prosody used in conversation. A sample sequence of the allegro tempo would be:

yea-YEA-YEA-YEA-YEA-YEA

ya-YA-YA-YA-YA-YA

ba-BA-BA-BA-BA-BA

no-NO-NO-NO-NO-NO

- Transfer rhythms to articulated speech: The final stage of the accent therapy involves transferring the rhythms to real speech. The transfer process includes: (1) repetitions following the clinician's model, (2) reading aloud using passages marked for phrasing and stresses, (3) monologue, and (4) conversation.
  - The accent method can be used for many different types of voice disorders. It is a therapy method that is widely used outside of the United States. There are many reasons why the method is effective in treating voice disorders. First, it is a programmed approach that follows a logical order of progression. Second, it trains new motor patterns of voice production assisted by the emphasis on steady, rhythmic body movements. Third, the Accent Method, like vocal function exercises and resonant voice therapy, at once works to improve the balance among the 3 subsystems of voice production: respiration, phonation, and resonance. Several outcome studies have demonstrated the efficiency of this approach.[78,80–82]

Lee Silverman Voice Treatment

The Lee Silverman Voice Treatment program is the most studied of all voice therapy programs. Developed by Lorraine Ramig, PhD, and her colleagues at the University of Colorado, the LSVT has been proven to significantly improve the voice quality of patients with Parkinson's disease.[140,141] LSVT is a specific, intensive treatment program that emphasizes "loud" speech. The loud voice generates improved respiratory support, articulation, and even facial expression and animation.

Five basic concepts are followed in the LSVT program. These concepts include: (1) think loud, think shout; (2) speech effort must be high; (3) treatment must be intensive; (4) patients must recalibrate their loudness level; and (5) improvements are quantified over time. Using visual feedback from a sound level meter, patients are taught the effort that is necessary to increase their loudness level. They are told to "think loud, think shout." Because most Parkinson's patients use poor breath support and talk softly, they must learn that the effort to produce adequate loudness must be high. The most efficacious way to accomplish this task is through intensive treatment. During the treatment, patients are taught to recalibrate their loudness level because the loudness that they think is normal is actually too soft. Finally, LSVT requires excellent record keeping so that the efficacy of the treatment may be demonstrated.

Efficacy studies have demonstrated that the program is most effective if therapy sessions are held daily, 4 days per week, for 4 consecutive weeks. Patients are also asked to practice therapy exercises daily at home. Voice pathologists who use LSVT must receive special training and certification in this method. An LSVT training manual is available from the National Center for Voice and Speech, and certification courses are provided nationally and internationally by Ramig and colleagues.[142–144]

TEAM MANAGEMENT OF SPECIFIC LARYNGEAL PATHOLOGIES

Voice problems arise under many conditions, and as described in Chapter 3, numerous etiologic factors may play a role. In general, however, 3 overriding categories prevail: voice use patterns and voice demands, medical or organic factors, and psychosocial or emotional contributors.[145–147] Of course, there is considerable overlap among these three groupings. Inappropriate voice behaviors or excessive vocal demands may result in organic manifestations (eg, polyps or nodules); psychological trauma or excessive emotional stress may trigger the onset of functional dysphonia. In this chapter, we have discussed the treatments that are specific to voice disorders associated with voice use patterns and voice demands and psychosocial and emotional contributors. In the remainder of this chapter, we discuss treatment alternatives for medical or organic voice disorders that often require a team approach.

With medically related voice disorders, the voice pathologist plays a supportive role by assisting in the correct diagnosis and prognosis for change based on the assessment of laryngeal anatomy, vocal fold vibratory pattern, vocal function measurement, and rehabilitative options for voice treatment. Collaboration between otolaryngologists and voice pathologists continues to expand through joint examination of the laryngeal image and vocal function; efficacious cotreatment alternatives that include medications, phonosurgery, and voice rehabilitation; and clinical delivery models that encourage a team approach to patients with voice disorders. More than ever, it is critical that the voice pathologist be aware of the medical pathologies in an otolaryngology patient population that affect voice production. Several of the medical pathologies of voice that require team treatment include vocal fold cover lesions, laryngopharyngeal reflux (LPR), vocal fold paralysis, and spasmodic dysphonia.

Vocal Fold Cover Lesions

Many benign vocal fold pathologies are the result of acute or chronic traumatic hyperfunctional voice use and respond readily to voice rehabilitation as previously described in this chapter. When standard voice therapy fails to improve voice quality, however, the otolaryngologist may recommend surgery. The term *phonosurgery* refers to laryngeal surgery that seeks to improve voice quality as the primary goal. This definition is distinct from traditional concepts of laryngeal surgery, which seeks to remove disease, with voice outcome as a secondary consideration. Advances in surgical instruments, bioimplant materials, and development of alternative surgical techniques have created phonosurgical options that are available to enhance voice quality in patients with laryngeal pathology.[148] In cases of nonmalignant mucosal lesions of the vocal folds, phonosurgery will be used to excise the lesion with a simultaneous goal of preserving the vocal fold mucosa and restoring the vocal fold edge.

Voice pathologists play a major role in treating patients who must undergo phonosurgery. First, a laryngeal videostroboscopic examination will be conducted to evaluate vocal function and determine the extent of disruption in the vibratory pattern caused by the lesion. The surgeon will study the stroboscopic image, which will help plan the surgical approach. Prior to surgery, the patient will undergo preoperative counseling with the voice pathologist. This counseling will involve vocal hygiene issues including hydration, elimination of traumatic vocal behaviors, and sometimes initiation of conservative voice use. In cases where surgery cannot be performed for several weeks, the patient will start direct voice therapy including perhaps Vocal Function Exercises and RVT. The patient is also given strict instructions for immediate postsurgical voice use. Most surgeons place patients on absolute voice rest for several days to a week following surgery. In addition, patients are encouraged to increase hydration and may be placed on a precautionary reflux regimen, including diet and medications. (Reflux precautions are described below.)

Seven to 10 days after surgery, the patient returns for a postsurgical laryngeal videostroboscopic examination. When sufficient healing is evident, postsurgical voice rehabilitation is begun. It is believed that postsurgical vocal fold condition and subsequent treatment may be significantly enhanced by the preoperative counseling and strict postoperative regimen.

Laryngopharyngeal Reflux and Gastroesophageal Reflux Disease

As described in Chapter 4, gastroesophageal reflux disease (GERD) is the reflux of gastric acid including bile, pepsin, and trypins from the stomach back into the esophagus and possibly into the pharynx. It is thought that reflux occurs normally in all individuals at some time. Reflux may cause irritation of the mucosal lining of the esophagus, pharynx, and larynx as it is released from the stomach. Gastroesophageal reflux becomes gastroesophageal reflux disease once histological changes take place within the esophagus. Symptoms of GERD may include dysphagia, odynophagia (or painful swallow), chest pain, a globus or lump in the throat sensation, onset of asthma during middle age, bloating, belching, and hiccups.[149] Long-term chronic gastroesophageal reflux may have detrimental effects on the esophagus. These include damage to the epithelial layer of the mucosal lining; the basal layer of the mucosal lining becomes thickened with extension of the papillae and loss of service cells in early inflammatory stages; stasis of the lumen, which is created with advanced inflammation; muscular atrophy; and severe gastroesophageal reflux has been implicated in gastrointestinal bleeding, Barrett's esophagus, and cancer. Individuals with GERD tend to be obese and are nocturnal refluxers. They tend to have lower esophageal dysfunction and complain of chronic heartburn.

Patients most often seen in a voice clinic by the otolaryngologist and voice pathologist experience laryngopharyngeal reflux (LPR). Most of these individuals are upright refluxers and experience upper esophageal dysfunction. Most suffer from hoarseness; globus sensation; a sense of increased mucus; and chronic throat clearing, coughing, or both. Only 18% of these patients complain of heartburn.[150] Consistent reflux into the larynx can negatively influence voice production. Beyond the obvious hoarseness, patients often complain of voice fatigue. Koufman[150] suggested that LPR might be responsible for edema, ulceration, granulation, polypoid degeneration, vocal nodules, laryngospasm, arytenoid fixation, laryngeal stenosis, and carcinoma of the larynx.

Much controversy surrounds LPR regarding its pathophysiology, diagnostic criterion, and treatment efficacy.[151,152] Evaluation of LPR by the otolaryngologist focuses on the identification of signs and symptoms of the disorder with symptoms often dictating the initiation of treatment. In an attempt to aid diagnosis of LPR, Belafsky et al developed the Reflux Finding Score (RFS) and the Reflux Symptom Index (RSI).[153,154] The RFS is an 8-item clinical severity rating scale based on the fiberoptic laryngoscopic findings. The scale includes the most common laryngeal findings related to LPR including vocal fold and infraglottic edema (pseudosulcus), erythema, and posterior commissure hypertrophy. It ranges from 0 (no abnormal findings) to a maximum of 26 (worst score possible). It has been concluded that any individual with an RES greater than 7 has LPR. On the other hand, the RSI is a 9-item self-administered outcome instrument. It has been stated that it accurately documents symptoms of patients with LPR including hoarseness, throat clearing, excess throat mucus, difficulty swallowing, coughing after eating, breathing difficulties, annoying cough, lump (globus) sensation, and heartburn. An RSI of more than 13 is considered to indicate LPR. Although both indices are widely used, there is some controversy about their sensitivity and specificity in LPR diagnosis.

Treatment of GERD and LPR incorporates three treatment levels. Level 1 involves conservative measures including dietary and lifestyle changes along with over-the-counter medications, such as antacids, H2 blockers, and protein pump inhibitors. Dietary precautions include decreasing the intake of fatty foods, spicy foods, tomato-based products, citrus fruits and fruit drinks, caffeine, carbonated beverages, alcohol, peppermint and spearmint, menthol, and onions. Lifestyle changes include decreasing or eliminating smoking, losing excess weight, wearing loose clothing that does not bind the midriff, elevating the head of the bed at night, not exercising or singing too soon after eating, and waiting 3 to 4 hours before lying down after eating.

Level 2 involves all of the dietary and lifestyle precautions mentioned in Level 1. In addition, prescription H2 blockers such as cimetidine, ranitidine, and famotidine are used to control mild to moderate GERD and LPR. H2 blockers control the acid, but the pepsin remains active. When H2 blockers prove not to be effective, then a prescription proton pump inhibitor, omeprazole, is the medication of choice. Most laryngeal manifestations of LPR can be controlled through medication and conservative measures.

Level 3 treatment is for severe reflux. Severe reflux requires the use of omeprazole, dietary and lifestyle changes, and often surgery. The most common type of surgery is a fundoplication, which essentially tightens the sphincter between the stomach and the esophagus, decreasing the regurgitation of the stomach contents into the esophagus.

Although persistent questions remain as to the actual prevalence, LPR is a common diagnosis in the voice clinic. The voice pathologist is responsible for supporting the antireflux regimen, as well as providing the most appropriate direction for voice therapy. In the acute stages of voice change, therapy may involve decreasing or eliminating throat clearing and coughing, encouraging conservative voice use, and initiating new functional voicing behaviors. We have found it useful to encourage the placement of voice into an extreme forward focus, thereby decreasing the medial impact on the arytenoid cartilages and vocal folds. Resonant voice therapy often is our treatment of choice with LPR patients.

Unilateral Vocal Fold Paralysis

Patients with unilateral vocal fold paralysis present with varied vocal symptoms, ranging from mild to severe dysphonia depending on the resting position of the paralyzed fold. When the paralyzed fold is located near the midline, voice quality is less impaired. The impairment increases when the paralyzed fold is located farther from the midline. Typically, voice is characterized by breathiness, low intensity, and diplophonia. Some patients produce an extreme vocal hyperfunction in an attempt to compensate for the lack of glottic closure; others will produce voice in a falsetto register because it becomes too much effort to maintain engagement of the thyroarytenoid muscle. Recall from Chapter 4 that this loss of vocal power and quality is due to inadequate closure of the vocal folds at midline, because the paralyzed vocal fold remains lateral to the midline and cannot meet its contralateral pair. Also, the loss of vocal fold body and tonicity result in bowing, flaccidity, and weakness of the paralyzed fold. Both factors contribute to the asymmetric, aperiodic, and incomplete vibratory closure during phonation seen in patients with unilateral vocal fold paralysis.

Treatment choices for unilateral vocal fold paralysis include voice therapy, phonosurgical management, reinnervation, or a combination of these approaches. The selection of treatment is dependent on several factors. These factors include whether the cause for the paralysis is known or unknown (idiopathic), the presence or absence of aspiration, the immediate voice needs of the patient, the distance from the time of onset of the paralysis, and the resting position of the paralyzed fold to the midline and the presence or absence of vocal fold bowing.[155]

In the case of idiopathic paralysis, a temporary vocal fold medialization (injection medialization laryngoplasty) is the treatment of choice. This is accomplished by injecting a resorbable material (such as Gelfoam paste, collagen, fat, calcium hydroxylapatite, nonanimal stabilized hyaluronic acid, or a micronized particulate form of decellularized human donor tissue, Alloderm) into the lateral aspect of the paralyzed vocal fold.[156] The injection typically is followed with behavioral voice therapy to maximize the positive effects of the medialization and to decompensate any inappropriate voice behaviors.

When the cause for the vocal fold paralysis is known, and it is determined that damage is permanent and there is no chance for return of function, then any form of management may begin immediately. Permanent dysphonia resulting from unilateral vocal fold paralysis is typically treated surgically with injection laryngoplasty, medialization thyroplasty, arytenoid adduction or arytenoidopexy, and reinnervation procedures. These treatments usually are combined with behavioral voice therapy to optimize voice production and avoid maladaptive compensatory behaviors. When the cause for the paralysis is idiopathic or there is some question as to the return of function, most surgeons will routinely observe patients for 6 to 12 months before permanent surgical intervention.[155]

The phonosurgical management alternatives for permanent unilateral paralysis may address both the midline glottic incompetence and the loss of vocal fold body and tone. The traditional surgical treatment was injection of a synthetic alloplastic, Teflon paste into the lateral margin of the paralyzed fold. The paste formed a solid mass, which displaced the paralyzed edge medially to improve midline competence. This technique was used routinely for more than 50 years with some complications reported. These complications included migration of the Teflon material into other sites of the body and granulation of tissue around the Teflon. When injected too superiorly or medially, the Teflon impaired the vibratory properties of the free edge of the paralyzed fold.[156] Teflon injection is no longer a treatment of choice.

Newer bioimplants continue to be developed and their efficacy explored as injectable alternatives to Teflon. These include expanded polytetrafluoroethylene and polyacrylamide hydrogels, which not only attend to improving the glottic gap but reportedly enhance the vibratory properties in both paralyzed and scarred vocal folds.[157–159]

Another surgical approach to medialization of the paralyzed vocal fold is laryngeal framework surgery. Laryngeal framework surgery is manipulation of the cartilagenous framework that houses the vocal folds. The procedure offers certain advantages over injection methods for the treatment of unilateral paralysis. First, it is completely noninvasive of the vocal fold body and mucosa; second, it is potentially reversible, barring excessive scarring of the surgical site. The Type 1 thyroplasty[160] utilizes a surgical implant (Silastic block) that is inserted and locked into a small window of the lamina of the thyroid cartilage. The Silastic implant will actively "push" the paralyzed fold toward the glottal midline to improve glottic closure. The exact size and placement of the implant are critical; if positioned too high or low, a vertical level mismatch will result, and voice quality will be suboptimal. In our practice, the voice pathologist is involved in monitoring the position of the vocal folds and the quality of the voice during surgery. The patient is under a local anesthesia during the surgery. The voice pathologist or surgeon places a flexible laryngeal videoendoscope and monitors the relative position of the vocal folds as the paralyzed fold is medialized. The patient's voice quality is also monitored perceptually. The combination of visual and auditory perceptual monitoring often leads to excellent postsurgical voice quality.

Isshiki and his colleagues introduced the concept of laryngeal framework surgery over 40 years ago.[161] Multiple types of framework surgery that manipulate the cartilage to alter the vocal fold configuration and restore voice in patients with unilateral paralysis, vocal fold bowing, and pitch disorders have been developed.[162–164] Laryngeal framework surgery is also being explored now for use in managing pediatric laryngeal disorders.[165]

Along with a fold medialization, surgeons often enhance the adduction of the paralyzed vocal fold through a procedure known as arytenoid adduction. In this procedure, the vocal process of the arytenoid is manually adducted toward the midline of the glottis. Once positioned appropriately, it is sutured in place, thus improving the posterior closure of the vocal folds.[166]

Injection techniques and laryngeal framework surgery address the deficit of midline closure in their approaches to management of unilateral vocal fold paralysis. To address the loss of vocal fold body and tonicity posed by atrophy and weakness of the denervated vocal fold, reinnervation techniques have been developed. These techniques include nerve muscle pedicle[164] and nerve anastomosis.[167] The principles behind neuromuscular reinnervation techniques include transplanting muscle blocks that can provide innervation to the paralyzed muscle, and the contraction characteristics of the donor muscle or nerve will be imparted to the paralyzed muscle. Thus, selection of an appropriate donor nerve or muscle (ie, one that is compatible with the contraction properties of the original) is important. Neuromuscular pedicle reinnervation is limited to a single muscle, usually the lateral cricoarytenoid (LCA) or thyroarytenoid (TA), which are both vocal fold adductors.

An alternative to the nerve-to-muscle reinnervation is nerve-to-nerve reinnervation. Recurrent laryngeal nerve (RLN)-to-RLN reinnervation is not consistently successful and does not always provide functional return of adductor and abductor activity. Furthermore, RLN-to-RLN anastomosis may result in dysphonia because of jerky movements and excessive synkinesis of adductor and abductor muscles simultaneously. Crumley[167] has developed a nerve anastomosis procedure using the ansa cervicalis as a donor to the recurrent laryngeal nerve. Because the ansa nerve delivers a slower firing rate, no jerky movements or paradoxical vocal fold bulging result. Instead, a quiet tonicity of the vocal fold body is achieved (synkinesis), providing a better vibratory source for voice production.

Although reinnervation techniques increase the likelihood of vocal fold tonicity, they do not restore vocal fold mobility, and subsequent medialization procedures may still be necessary for an optimal result. Both surgical treatments can be used in combination with laryngeal framework surgery, and some otolaryngologists have advocated this combination approach to decrease the glottal gap and improve the tonicity of the vocal fold body.[164] Laryngeal electromyography (LEMG) is a valuable diagnostic and prognostic test for patients with vocal fold paralysis. LEMG is effective in localizing the neural site of lesions, which aids in determining the cause and the prognosis of the paralysis. With LEMG, the nature and stage of the neuropathy as well as the prognosis for recovery may be determined. The presence of spontaneous neural activity, for example, indicates ongoing degeneration, and the finding of severely decreased recruitment indicates a poor prognosis for complete recovery.[168] Use of this diagnostic test might preclude much of the waiting that is inherent in the treatment of unilateral vocal fold paralysis.

Voice therapy for unilateral vocal fold paralysis often can be very effective. The goal of therapy is to improve glottic closure without causing supraglottic hyperfunction. Historically, descriptions of voice therapy for this population have discussed the process of strengthening the nonparalyzed vocal fold for the purpose of crossing the glottal midline for better approximation of the folds. There is question as to whether a strengthening process actually occurs. Nonetheless, by whatever process is operational, improvement in voice quality will occur when glottic closure is improved.

In an attempt to compensate for a lack of glottic closure, some patients with unilateral vocal fold paralysis develop a vocal and laryngeal hyperfunction. This hyperfunction actually decreases the efficiency of vocal function and usually impairs voice quality to a greater level than what might be expected from the paralysis alone. The task of voice therapy with these cases is to decrease this hyperfunctional behavior.

Several therapy techniques have been suggested for use with unilateral vocal fold paralysis patients. They include:

- hard glottal attack exercises
- pushing exercises
- lateral digital pressure
- head tilt method
- half-swallow boom technique
- vocal function exercises

We have been known to try all of these techniques with an individual patient in an attempt to find a strategy that works.

Because of the potential for developing vocal hyperfunction, the hard glottal attack and pushing exercises have fallen out of favor with voice pathologists. These exercises continue to be useful with patients with vocal fold paralysis who also use the falsetto register for voice production, however. Because of the effort to produce voice caused by the lack of glottic closure, some patients default to the high-pitch, breathy voice of the falsetto. When this is the case, we might attempt to engage the thyroarytenoid muscle of the nonparalyzed fold using the hard glottal attack. The technique used is similar to that described for the adolescent male with functional falsetto. To produce a hard glottal attack the patient is instructed to:

- breathe in
- build air pressure without letting your air out; posture the vowel in your mouth at the same time
- release the vowel

In the first week, the patient is given the list of vowels and vowel-consonant combinations to practice the glottal attack twice per day for 1 week:

- Say each vowel 2 times using a hard glottal attack:

  a, e, i, o, oo

- Say each word 2 times using a hard glottal attack:

  eat, it, ate, etch, at, ooze, oats, ought, out, up, I'm

When the patient returns 1 week later, the glottal attack exercise is reviewed. If progress has been adequate, the exercise is made more challenging by asking the patient to again produce the glottal attack with the addition of stretching the vowel while gliding down to a lower pitch. Gliding down in pitch encourages contraction of the working thyroarytenoid muscle, whereas sustaining the tone for a longer period of time encourages low-impact adduction. The patient is instructed to practice this modified hard glottal attack exercise, using the above vowels and words, 2 times each, 2 times per day for 1 week.

When the patient returns for the third therapy session, the glottal attack exercise with the stretched vowel and the glide to lower pitch is reviewed. If progress has been adequate, the same exercise is made more challenging by asking the patient to incorporate an isometric push. The isometric push may be accomplished by pressing the hands together in front of the body or pulling up on the arms of a chair at exactly the same time that the air pressure is being built and the vowel is being postured. The isometric push is then released when the vowel is released.

It has been our experience that if patients are able to extinguish use of the falsetto voice, improvement will most likely occur within a 3-week period of time. Continuing with glottal attack and isometric pushing exercises beyond this time frame may risk increased vocal hyperfunction. Remember, the purpose of introducing this exercise program is to develop use of the modal register for patients who are using the falsetto register as compensation for the unilateral vocal fold paralysis. It is important to monitor patient performance during this therapy to ensure against inadvertent supraglottic hyperfunction.

Lateral digital pressure, sometimes known as manual compression of the thyroid cartilage, has proven to be beneficial for improving the voice quality of some patients with unilateral vocal fold paralysis.[169] While the patient is sitting in an upright position, looking straight forward, and producing a vowel sound, the therapist uses his or her thumb and forefinger to apply pressure to one side of the thyroid cartilage. Different amounts of pressure are applied while the therapist explores any change that may occur in voice quality. Both sides of the thyroid cartilage receive pressure during the exploration. When improved voice quality is identified, the exercise will progress through words and phrases. The patient is taught to use his or her own digital pressure for practice at home. The ultimate goal of this approach is to improve voice quality while extinguishing the digital pressure.

The head-turn approach uses the natural repositioning of the vocal folds by simply turning the head to one side or the other. Again, the patient is instructed to sit in an upright position. While turning the head slowly to one side, he or she is asked to phonate. The therapist will monitor any change in voice quality while the head is being turned. When a head-turn position is found that improves voice quality, the exercise will progress through words and phrases. The position of the head is stabilized in therapy so that the patient may be able to practice using this same position at home. The ultimate goal of this approach is to improve voice quality while extinguishing the turning of the head.[169]

McFarlane et al[169] also suggested the use of what they termed the half-swallow boom technique. It is suggested that this technique is another means of repositioning the vocal folds for the purpose of exploring improved voice quality in the unilateral vocal fold paralysis patient. The patient is asked to take a breath and go through the motions of initiating the first part of a swallow. Apparently, the pharyngeal and laryngeal muscle movements that occur during the half-swallow improve glottic closure. At the peak of the half-swallow, the patient is asked to forcefully say "boom." When this technique is successful, the boom will demonstrate a louder and clearer voice quality. The muscle manipulations created by the half-swallow are stabilized on the boom and then expanded to other words and phrases.

The effect of these exercises is variable and often depends on the degree of vocal fold gap. We must emphasize that outcome studies are lacking for all of the above approaches and encourage the reader to consider participating in such studies. To a certain extent, the prognosis for success of rehabilitative therapy can be predicted following the results of the videostroboscopic image. When light "touch" closure is achieved in glottic waveform, despite the position of the paralyzed fold, the likelihood of discrete benefits from behavioral therapy is greater than for vibratory patterns that display no touch closure whatsoever. When touch closure is present, we have found that low-impact Vocal Function Exercises are extremely effective in improving the vocal function and voice quality of patients with unilateral vocal fold paralysis.

It is important to note that many patients with idiopathic etiologies for unilateral vocal fold paralysis have spontaneous return of function within 1 year of onset. For this reason, timing of surgical management is typically delayed at least 6 months to 1 year postonset. Voice therapy often combined with injection laryngoplasty of a temporary absorbable material may facilitate recovery of serviceable voice during the waiting. Rehabilitation also can prevent the patient from adopting maladaptive compensatory strategies. Finally, the effects of vocal fold paralysis may have a strong emotional impact on patients, and therapy may serve as a time to monitor progress and support the patient's need to adjust communicative demands at home, work, and in social settings to accommodate the disorder. Occasionally, referral to mental health professionals for additional support may be appropriate.

Case Study 14: Unilateral Vocal Fold Paralysis

The patient was a 65-year-old, recently retired high school teacher. One month prior to the voice evaluation, he underwent an anterior approach to a cervical fusion. Upon recovering from the anesthesia, he noticed a severe hoarseness. He was not alarmed at that time, because it was his impression that the hoarseness was a temporary condition caused by intubation. When the hoarseness persisted for 2 weeks following the surgery, however, he sought the opinion of an otolaryngologist. Results of the laryngeal examination confirmed the presence of a right true vocal fold paralysis. The patient was then referred to the voice center for evaluation treatment.

The patient presented with a moderate-to-severe dysphonia characterized by a weak, high-pitched breathy voice. Results of the laryngeal videostroboscopic evaluation demonstrated the posterior aspect of the paralyzed fold to be near the midline but, because of a significant bowing of the right fold, a large glottal gap was present, accounting for his poor voice quality.

Therapy was immediately employed involving the hard glottal attack exercises protocol described above. Once again, this exercise was used only for the purpose of establishing engagement of the normal thyroarytenoid muscle. No improvement was made in voice production over a 3-week period of time. Other therapy methods, such as digital pressure, head tilt, and the half-swallow boom, were attempted without success. It was determined that the size of the glottal gap caused by the vocal fold bowing precluded improvement through behavioral therapy.

Because of the potential for spontaneous recovery of the right recurrent laryngeal nerve, permanent surgical intervention was not yet possible. This patient was extremely debilitated as a result of his poor voice quality. The weak voice interfered with many of his family and social activities. It was suggested in consultation with the laryngologist that this patient might benefit from a temporary Gelfoam injection of the paralyzed fold. Accomplished as an outpatient procedure, the Gelfoam was injected into the lateral aspect of the paralyzed fold. Stroboscopic observation of vocal fold vibration following injection demonstrated significantly improved glottic closure. The patient's voice quality was also improved to a mild-to-moderate dysphonia characterized by a breathy hoarseness. In addition, the falsetto was replaced by his modal register.

The patient was extremely pleased with the improvement of voice quality. Gelfoam, however, provides only a temporary improvement because of absorption, which occurs within 2 to 3 months. The improvement resulting from this procedure gave the voice pathologist the opportunity to try other therapy approaches that might have provided a more permanent vocal change; Vocal Function Exercises were immediately employed. The patient practiced the exercise program for 9 weeks, making steady improvement in his maximum phonation times. His voice quality also steadily improved, so much so that there was speculation that the function of the right true vocal fold had returned. Subsequent stroboscopic evaluation, however, demonstrated that the vocal fold remained paralyzed. Even though the Gelfoam had resorbed, glottic closure remained improved and the voice quality was adequate for the patient's daily voicing activities.

This was a case where the team approach was successful. Voice therapy was not effective as long as the large glottal gap was present. A more permanent medialization procedure was not possible. The combination of a temporary improvement in glottic closure and direct voice therapy led to a significantly improved voice quality. As it turned out, this patient's right true vocal fold paralysis was permanent. He did not choose to undergo a more permanent surgical procedure as his voice quality was acceptable to him.

Spasmodic Dysphonia

Spasmodic dysphonia (SD) is a rare, chronic, disabling voice disorder that typically begins gradually in the fifth decade of life. It tends to occur more frequently in women than men, and can be a progressive condition that worsens with time, and fails to plateau in one-third of cases.[170] As described in Chapter 4, SD is a focal dystonia of the central motor system. As with other focal dystonias, SD is characterized by abnormal involuntary movements that are action induced and task specific. Perceptually, the voice symptoms are classified into 2 primary groups—adductor and abductor SD; however, a mixed variant has also been described. Approximately 25% to 30% of patients with SD will have a coexisting voice tremor.[170,171] Adductor spasmodic dysphonia, which appears to be the most common variant, is characterized by strained, strangled phonation with occasional intermittent stoppages of voice. The severity may range from very mild, intermittent symptoms to a very severe, persistent struggle to produce phonation. The abductor type is characterized by abductor vocal fold spasms causing sudden, intermittent explosions or breathy air escape. Abductor spasms appear to occur most frequently on voiceless consonants.

Currently, the diagnosis of SD is based almost exclusively on auditory-perceptual features.[172] However another voice disorder, muscle tension dysphonia (MTD), can mimic the voice characteristics of the subtypes of SD, thus leading to diagnostic confusion.[173–175] Unlike SD, MTD is considered a "functional" voice disorder wherein hyperfunctional laryngeal and extralaryngeal muscle activity is offered as the proximal cause of the dysphonia (see Chapter 4).[176] In clinical practice, a validated set of diagnostic criteria do not exist to distinguish SD and MTD; thus, the differential diagnosis can be extremely difficult, even for experienced clinicians.

Researchers have begun to compare characteristics of SD and MTD to determine if there are features that reliably distinguish the 2 disorders and lead to improved differential diagnosis. Distinguishing the adductor form of spasmodic dysphonia (ADSD) from MTD has received the most attention. As mentioned previously, ADSD has been described as a "task-specific" or "task-dependent" dystonia, implying that certain vocal tasks may increase or decrease the likelihood of provoking spasmodic overclosure of the vocal folds.[177] In ADSD, it has been asserted that vocal tasks such as singing, crying, laughing, whispering, shouting, or speaking in falsetto are relatively free of voice breaks and the strained, strangled vocal quality perceived during connected speech produced at normal pitch and loudness.[173] Descriptions of task dependency in ADSD have been expanded to include variable voice symptoms on the basis of phonetic content or context. For instance, it has recently been shown that voice produced during sustained vowels in ADSD is often (ie, in 50% of cases) less severely affected (ie, fewer voice breaks, less strain) as compared to voice produced during contextual speech.[178] In contrast to ADSD, MTD appears not to be as task dependent. That is, all vocal tasks regardless of phonetic context (ie, sustained vowels and connected speech) are believed to be equally difficult for patients with MTD, seemingly due to the constant hyperfunction of the intrinsic and extrinsic laryngeal musculature during phonation.[179,180] Researchers have reported additional speech/voice tasks that influence dysphonia severity in patients with ADSD, and perhaps speak to its task-dependent nature. For instance, increasing severity of phonatory signs on the basis of the relative loading of voiced versus voiceless consonants has also been cited as evidence of task-dependency in SD.[171,173,181] Roy and colleagues confirmed that voice signs (based on listener ratings) increase or lessen in connected speech of many patients with ADSD on the basis of the proportion of the voiced or voiceless consonants. Sentences loaded with voiced consonants provoked more frequent and severe spasms/voice breaks in contrast to sentences loaded with voiceless consonants. Again, however, only half of the patients with ADSD behaved in the stereotypic manner (ie, the all-voiced sentence was perceived as worse than the voiceless-laden sentence) suggesting that absence of task-dependency does not necessarily rule out ADSD as a possible diagnosis. But, because only 10% of patients with MTD displayed differential performance on the basis of phonetic loading, the authors advised that strong evidence of differential performance on the basis of task should raise substantially the suspicion for ADSD.[181]

In summary, although perceptual voice evaluation remains the standard for diagnosis of ADSD, knowledge of factors that influence the severity of voice symptoms seems critical to successful differential diagnosis. Consequently, during clinical assessment, voice clinicians who use generic stimulus materials that do not control for specific phonetic content may miss critical phenomenological features of the types of SD. Rather, observing a patient's performance on stimulus materials that maximally provoke voice symptoms in ADSD (ie, all-voiced phonemes), as compared to more facilitative phonetic environments (ie, predominantly voiceless phonemes, or sustained vowels), can help to accentuate differences between ADSD and MTD and lessen the likelihood of misdiagnosis. Similarly, observing the opposite pattern wherein there is worsening of voice symptoms associated with voiceless-laden sentences as compared to all voiced contexts should raise suspicion of abductor SD (ABSD) over ADSD. Further research is necessary to determine the diagnostic worth of differential performance observed during falsetto, singing, whispering, shouting, laughing, and crying as a means to distinguish ADSD from MTD. Although a diagnostic algorithm has been recently proposed which highlights reduced dysphonia during these particular vocal behaviors in SD, the diagnostic precision of this algorithm (and its individual components) awaits experimental assessment.[182]

Due to the relative rarity of SD and the challenges associated with differential diagnosis, regrettably we still see patients who have sought treatments from many laryngologists, speech pathologists, psychologists and psychiatrists, and chiropractors. They have been prescribed various drugs and holistic remedies and have gone through relaxation training, EMG and thermal biofeedback, hypnosis, acupuncture, acupressure, and faith healing hoping to find help for their voice disorder. The history and effectiveness of various treatments for SD are reviewed in the section that follows.

Herbert Dedo,[183] a San Francisco otolaryngologist, innovated the use of unilateral recurrent laryngeal nerve section for the treatment of adductor spasmodic dysphonia. Creation of the unilateral vocal fold paralysis decreased the opportunity for the vocal folds to spasm at the midline. This treatment enjoyed early favorable results.[184] However, long-term success has been debated due to relapse of symptoms within a few years of treatment, and the approach has fallen out of favor.[145,185]

Botulinum toxin (BOTOX) injections for the treatment of spasmodic dysphonia have become the primary management option.[186–188] For adductor spasmodic dysphonia, a small amount of BOTOX is injected into the vocalis muscle, resulting in decreased spasm activity for a period of 3 to 6 months. Individual responses vary, but the overall success of this treatment method in the management of adductor spasmodic dysphonia has been positive.[186,189]

When used as a therapy for abductor spasmodic dysphonia, BOTOX is injected into the posterior cricoarytenoid muscle on the side of the larynx. This injection decreases the ability of the vocal folds to spasm in the abducted position. Bilateral injections of the posterior cricoarytenoid muscles are avoided due to potential compromise of the airway. BOTOX injections for abductor spasmodic dysphonia yield less predictable success.[190–192]

Physicians use 2 techniques to inject BOTOX in the vocal folds for adductor spasmodic dysphonia. An intraoral technique using a long, curved syringe[193] permits the otolaryngologist to visualize the vocal folds during the injection. Topical anesthesia is used to decrease the gag reflex. While the patient holds his or her tongue, the otolaryngologist visualizes the vocal folds with a laryngeal mirror in one hand and injects the folds with the syringe in the other hand. This procedure has the advantage of visual inspection of the injection site, ensuring correct placement of the toxin in the vocalis muscle. It requires excellent patient compliance to tolerate the curved syringe placement (Figures 7–6 and 7–7).

The most common method of injection, which can be used for both adductor and abductor spasmodic dysphonia uses percutaneous electromyography to discern correct locations in the intrinsic muscles (vocalis for ADSD and posterior cricoarytenoid for ABSD). After palpating the laryngeal cartilage landmarks, the otolaryngologist inserts the needles and injects the toxin. This method usually requires the collaboration of the otolaryngologist with a neurologist. The neurologist assists in the setup and

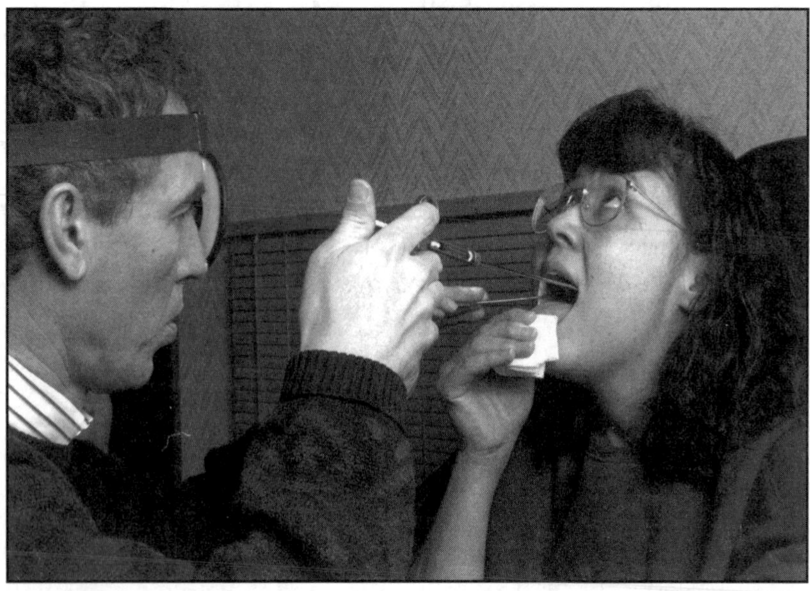

FIGURE 7–6. Botox injection with curved syringe in a transoral approach.

interpretation of the electromyographic feedback (Figure 7–8). Placement of the EMG electrode in the correct muscle is verified using speech tasks designed to discriminate intrinsic laryngeal muscle activity. Both the timing and the quality of the sound of muscle activity recording indicate when the needle edge is located in the appropriate muscle body.

The efficacy of rehabilitative voice therapy with spasmodic dysphonia is controversial, but many voice pathologists have reported success in decreasing compensatory vocal behaviors with patients who are experiencing early or mild symptoms of SD or who used therapy in conjunction with BOTOX. Techniques for reducing compensatory symptoms of adductor spasmodic dysphonia include the use of increased pitch, increased breathy quality, use of /h/ onset in phonation, and relaxation training.

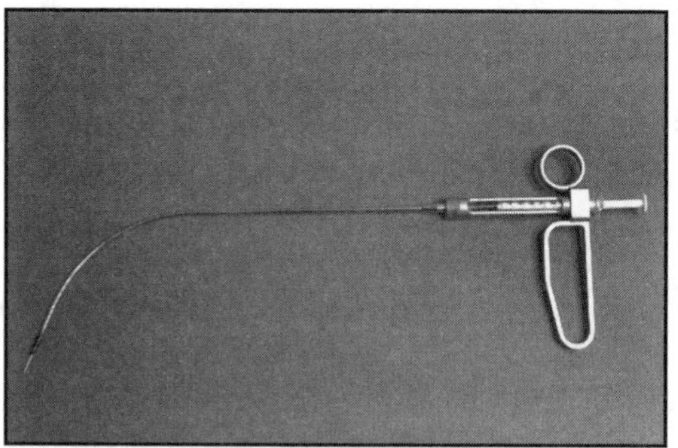

FIGURE 7–7. The curved syringe designed to inject the vocal folds through a transoral approach.

Most patients with adductor spasmodic dysphonia demonstrate a decrease in the frequency and severity of spasms when using a slightly elevated pitch. Using an increased breathy quality decreases the force of glottal impact, thus decreasing the potential for spasm. The same logic is used to justify the use of the consonant /h/ at the onset of phonation. Because many patients with spasmodic dysphonia develop an extreme hyperfunctional posture in an attempt to "push" the voice through the spasms, relaxation training often helps overcome

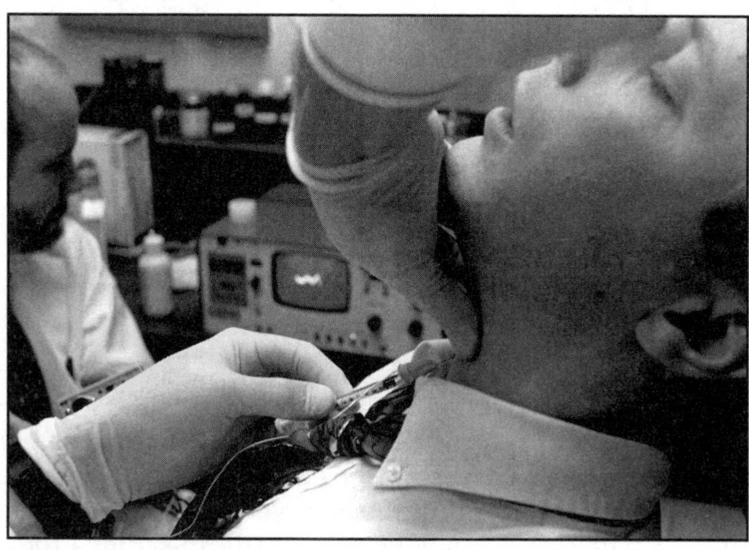

FIGURE 7–8. Botox injection using a percutaneous technique with EMG guidance.

this habit. Murry and Woodson[194] demonstrated that patients who follow up BOTOX injections with voice therapy often extend the effectiveness of the injections for a longer period of time than patients who do not have voice therapy.

In addition to the direct therapies mentioned above, the voice pathologist is responsible for educating the patient with spasmodic dysphonia about the disorder. SD is an insidious disorder that often causes emotional upheaval. It can lead to depression, reclusive behavior, and, at the extreme, thoughts of suicide. The disorder has been known to challenge careers, friendships, and marriages. We believe that patients must be well educated regarding their disorder. Knowledge is power. Knowledge permits the patient to put a face on the disorder and to better plan ways of coping with it. Much written information regarding spasmodic dysphonia is shared with the patient. The patient is introduced to the National Spasmodic Dysphonia Association, which publishes information pamphlets, sponsors support groups, supports research, and holds a national convention for patients with spasmodic dysphonia. In addition, much supportive information regarding this disorder may be found on the association's Web page (http://www.dysphonia.org/).

SUCCESSFUL VOICE THERAPY

This chapter provided the reader with a discussion of several orientations of voice therapy. One of the joys in providing therapy for patients with voice disorders is that many, if not most, improve. It is important to understand that the clinician and the patient share equally in the success or failure of voice therapy. The voice pathologist must be well grounded in anatomy, physiology, etiologic correlates, laryngeal pathology, and the psychodynamics of voice production. He or she must also possess outstanding skills in human interaction. These human interaction skills include the ability to talk to people, to skillfully and systematically divine the important aspects of the voice disorder, and then to counsel appropriately.

The clinician must also understand all aspects of voice disorders, including the less obvious nuances of various pathologic conditions. By understanding voice disorders, realistic expectations of therapy will result and can be shared with the patient. The successful voice pathologist also will apply the management techniques appropriately. Every patient is an individual with different problems and individual needs. Patients with similar voice disorders will not necessarily respond to the same management approaches. Successful voice therapy is dependent on the clinician's awareness and use of all management techniques that seem appropriate. Misapplied techniques often result in failure.

Successful voice therapy also can be enhanced through patient education. For patients to be motivated to change vocal behaviors, they must understand why change is required. Without a full understanding of the problem, the total management burden remains on the clinician. The clinician must use education to shift the burden for improvement to the patient. The patient must become an equal partner in the process of voice improvement.

Finally, the criteria for termination of therapy must be understood and agreed upon by both the voice pathologist and the patient. Documentation of the baseline voice production is essential to this process. Throughout the therapy program, it is necessary to subjectively and objectively plot progress for the purpose of accountability and to support the decision to continue or terminate therapy. It must be remembered that the patient lives with his or her voice on a daily basis. The patient may not appreciate the gradual, sometimes subtle changes that occur over time. Documentation of progress throughout the therapy program may demonstrate to the patient changes that he or she would not otherwise appreciate. These demonstrations are inherently motivating.

Assuming adequate preparation of the voice pathologist, the success of voice therapy may also be related to the patient. Successful voice therapy is dependent on the patient agreeing that a problem exists and having the motivation necessary to follow through and comply with the management suggestions. Patients also must be willing to share information. Information gathered during the patient interview is only valuable if it is complete and accurate. Even the most skilled clinician has experienced situations in which, after several sessions of therapy, the patient finally shares information critical to management decisions. Successful voice therapy is dependent on an open and honest relationship between patient and clinician. Ultimately, the patient has final control over the information he or she is willing to share.

Vocal image has a strong psychological influence on many people. Patients often find it difficult to modify even moderate-to-severe vocal disturbances because of the effect this change may have on their image. Voice therapy is composed of a series of choices that both the clinician and the patient make. One choice that must be made by the patient is to shed the vocal image by following the management suggestions of the clinician. Successful voice therapy is dependent on the patient recognizing negative vocal behaviors and choosing the need to modify these behaviors.

Successful voice therapy, therefore, is a negotiation. The clinician's goal should always be the development of the best voice possible. This goal must be made clear to the patient. The patient's goal, however, may be beyond reasonable expectations or may be somewhat less than the best voice possible. It is the responsibility of the voice pathologist to negotiate the definition of each patient's successful voice therapy.

Some people are totally dependent on their voices for their livelihood. In one respect, these individuals are often a joy to work with in therapy because of their inherent motivation for improvement. On the other hand, their special needs and concerns require additional knowledge and understanding. Chapter 8 will introduce you to these individuals and provide you with a framework for successfully treating their voice disorders.

REFERENCES

1. Stemple J. *Voice Therapy: Clinical Studies.* St. Louis, MO: Mosby Year Book; 1993.
2. Thomas L, Stemple J. Voice therapy: does science support the art? *Comm Dis Rev.* 2007;1:51–79.
3. Andrews ML. *Voice Treatment for Children and Adolescents.* 2nd ed. San Diego, CA: Singular; 2002.

4. Bloch C, Gould W. Voice therapy in lieu of surgery for contact granuloma: a case report. *J Speech Hear Dis.* 1974;39: 478–485.
5. Holmberg E, Hillman R, Hammarberg B, Sodersten M, Doyle P. Efficacy of a behaviorally based voice therapy protocol for vocal nodules. *J Voice.* 2001;15: 395–412.
6. Roy N, Gray, S, Simon M, Dove H, Corbin-Lewis K, Stemple J. An evaluation of the effects of two treatment approaches for teachers with voice disorders: a prospective randomized clinical trial. *J Speech Lang Hear Res.* 2001;44:286–296.
7. Roy N, Weinrich B, Gray S, et al. Voice amplification verses vocal hygiene instruction for teachers with voice disorders: a treatment outcomes study. *J Speech Lang Hear Res.* 2002;45:623–638.
8. Schneider P. Tracking changes in dysphonia: a case study. *J Voice.* 1993;7: 179–188.
9. Verdolini-Marston K, Burke M, Lessac A, Glaze L, Caldwell E. Preliminary study of two methods of treatment for laryngeal nodules. *J Voice.* 1995;9:74–85.
10. Aaron V. A vocal hygiene program for high school cheerleaders. *Lang Speech Hear Serv Sch.* 1991;22:287–290.
11. Broaddus-Lawrence P, Treole K, McCabe R, Allen R, Toppin L. The effects of preventative vocal hygiene education on the vocal hygiene habits and perceptual voice characteristics of training singers. *J Voice.* 2000;14:58–71.
12. Chan R. Does the voice improve with vocal hygiene education? A study of some instrumental voice measures in a group of kindergarten teachers. *J Voice.* 1994;8:279–291.
13. Nilson H, Schneiderman C. Classroom program for the prevention of vocal abuse and hoarseness in elementary school children. *Lang Speech Hear Serv Sch.* 1983;14:114–120.
14. Timmermans B, De Bodt M, Wuyts F, Van de Heyning P. Training outcome in future professional voice users after 18 months of voice training. *Folia Phoniatr Logopae.* 2004;56:120–129.
15. Timmermans B, De Bodt M, Wuyts F, Van de Heyning P. Analysis and evaluation of a voice-training program in future professional voice users. *J Voice.* 2005;19:202–210.
16. Punt N. Lubrication of the vocal mechanism. *Folia Phoniatr.* 1974;36:287–288.
17. Solomon N, DiMattia M. Effects of a vocally fatiguing task and systemic hydration on phonation threshold pressure. *J Voice.* 2000;14:341–362.
18. Verdolini K, Titze I, Fennell A. Dependence of phonatory effort on hydration level. *J Speech Hear Res.* 1994;37: 1001–1007.
19. Verdolini-Marston K, Titze I, Druker D. Changes in phonation threshold pressure with induced conditions of hydration. *J Voice.* 1990;4:142–151.
20. Verdolini-Marston K, Sandage M, Titze I. Effect of hydration treatments on laryngeal nodules and polyps and related voice measures. *J Voice.* 1994;8:30–47.
21. Deem J, Miller L. *Manual of Voice Therapy.* 2nd ed. Austin, TX: Pro-Ed; 2000.
22. McFarlane S. Treatment of benign laryngeal disorders with traditional methods and techniques of voice therapy. *Ear Nose Throat J.* 1988;67:425–435.
23. Zwitman D, Calcaterra T. The "silent cough" method for vocal hyperfunction. *J Speech Hear Disord.* 1973;38: 119–125.
24. Boone D. *The Voice and Voice Therapy.* Englewood Cliffs, NJ: Prentice-Hall; 1971.
25. Hicks D, Bless D. Principles of treatment. In: Brown BV, Crary M, eds. *Organic Voice Disorders: Assessment and Treatment.* San Diego, CA: Singular Publishing Group; 2000:171–191.
26. Koufman J, Blalock P. Is voice rest never indicated? *J Voice.* 1989;3:87–91.
27. Myerson M. Vocal rest in laryngeal disease. *Ann Otorhinolaryngol.* 1958;67: 491–495.

28. Prater R. Voice therapy: techniques and applications. *Otolaryngol Clin North Am.* 1991;24:1075–1092.
29. Sataloff R. The professional voice: part III. Common diagnoses and treatments. *J Voice.* 1997;1:283–292.
30. van der Merwe A. The Voice Use Reduction Program. *Am J Speech Lang Pathol.* 2004;13:1208–1218.
31. Myerson MC. Vocal rest in laryngeal disease. *Ann Otorhinolaryngol.* 1958;67: 491–495.
32. Yiu EM, Chan RM. Effect of hydration and vocal rest on the vocal fatigue in amateur karaoke singers. *J Voice.* 2003; 17(2):216–227.
33. Froeschels E, Kastein S, Weiss DA. A method of therapy for paralytic conditions of the mechanisms of phonation, respiration and glutination. *J Speech Hear Disord.* 1955;20(4):365–370.
34. Yamaguchi H, Yotsukura Y, Sata H, et al. Pushing exercise program to correct glottal incompetence. *J Voice.* 1993;7(3): 250–256.
35. Yiu EM, Ho EYY. Short-term effect of humming on vocal quality. *Asia Pac J Speech Lang Hear.* 2002;7:123–137.
36. Brodnitz FS, Froeschels E. Treatment of nodules of vocal cords by chewing method. *AMA Arch Otolaryngol.* 1954; 59(5):560–565.
37. Froeschels E. Hygiene of the voice. *Arch Otolaryngol.* 1943;38:122–130.
38. Froeschels E. Chewing method as therapy. *Arch Otolaryngol.* 1952;56:427–434.
39. Brewer DW, McCall G. Visible laryngeal changes during voice therapy: fiberoptic study. *Ann Otol Rhinol Laryngol.* 1974;83(4):423–427.
40. McFarlane SC. Treatment of benign laryngeal disorders with traditional methods and techniques of voice therapy. *Ear Nose Throat J.* 1988;67(6):425–428, 430–432, 434–435.
41. Boone DR, McFarlane SC. A critical view of the yawn-sigh as a voice therapy technique. *J Voice.* 1993;7(1): 75–80.
42. Xu JH, Ikeda Y, Komiyama S. Biofeedback and the yawning breath pattern in voice therapy: a clinical trial. *Auris Nasus Larynx.* 1991;18(1):67–77.
43. Andrews S, Warner J, Stewart R. EMG biofeedback and relaxation in the treatment of hyperfunctional dysphonia. *Br J Disord Commun.* 1986;21(3):353–369.
44. Prosek RA, Montgomery AA, Walden BE, Schwartz DM. EMG biofeedback in the treatment of hyperfunctional voice disorders. *J Speech Hear Disord.* 1978; 43(3):282–294.
45. Stemple JC, Weiler E, Whitehead W, Komray R. Electromyographic biofeedback training with patients exhibiting a hyperfunctional voice disorder. *Laryngoscope.* 1980;90(3):471–476.
46. Yiu EM, Verdolini K, Chow LP. Electromyographic study of motor learning for a voice production task. *J Speech Lang Hear Res.* 2005;48(6):1254–1268.
47. Yamaguchi H, Yotsukura Y, Kondo R, et al. Nonsurgical therapy for vocal nodules. *Folia Phoniatr.* 1986;38:372–373.
48. Laukkanen AM, Syrja T, Laitala M, Leino T. Effects of two-month vocal exercising with and without spectral biofeedback on student actors' speaking voice. *Logoped Phoniatr Vocol.* 2004; 29(2):66–76.
49. D'Antonio L, Lotz W, Chait D, Netsell R. Perceptual-physiologic approach to evaluation and treatment of dysphonia. *Ann Otol Rhinol Laryngol.* 1987;96 (2, pt 1):187–190.
50. Rattenbury HJ, Carding PN, Finn P. Evaluating the effectiveness and efficiency of voice therapy using transnasal flexible laryngoscopy: a randomized controlled trial. *J Voice.* 2004;18(4): 522–533.
51. Holbrook A, Rolnick MI, Bailey CW. Treatment of vocal abuse disorders using a vocal intensity controller. *J Speech Hear Disord.* 1974;39(3):298–303.
52. Lodge JM, Yarnall GD. A case study of vocal volume reduction. *J Speech Hear Disord.* 1981;46(3):317–320.

53. Roy N, Weinrich B, Gray SD, et al. Voice amplification versus vocal hygiene instruction for teachers with voice disorders: a treatment outcomes study. *J Speech Lang Hear Res.* 2002;45(4):625–638.
54. Boone DR. Treatment of functional aphonia in a child and in an adult. *J Speech Hear Disord.* 1966;31:69–74.
55. Maryn Y, DeBodt M, Van Cauwenberge P. Ventricular dysphonia: clinical aspects and therapeutic options. *Laryngoscope.* 2003;113:859–866.
56. Gray B, England G, Mahoney J. Treatment of benign vocal nodules by reciprocal inhibition. *Behav Res Therapy.* 1986;3:187–191.
57. Blood G. Efficacy of a computer-assisted voice treatment protocol. *Am J Speech Lang Pathol.* 1994;3:57–66.
58. Fisher HB, Logemann JA. Objective evaluation of therapy for vocal nodules: a case report. *J Speech Hear Disord.* 1970;35(3):277–285.
59. Roy N, Weinrich B, Gray SD, Tanner K, Stemple JC, Sapienza CM. Three treatments for teachers with voice disorders: a randomized clinical trial. *J Speech Lang Hear Res.* 2003;46(3):670–688.
60. Bloch CS, Gould WJ. Voice therapy in lieu of surgery for contact granuloma. *J Speech Hear Disord.* 1974;39:478–485.
61. Drudge MK, Philips BJ. Shaping behavior in voice therapy. *J Speech Hear Disord.* 1976;41(3):398–411.
62. McCrory E. Voice therapy outcomes in vocal fold nodules: a retrospective audit. *Int J Lang Commun Disord.* 2001 (36 suppl):19–24.
63. Murry T, Woodson GE. A comparison of three methods for the management of vocal fold nodules. *J Voice.* 1992;6:271–276.
64. Goss F. Hysterical aphonia. *Boston Med Surg J.* 1878;99:215–222.
65. Ward W. Hysterical aphonia. *Chicago Med J Examiner.* 1877;34:495–505.
66. Russell J. A case of hysterical aphonia. *Br Med J.* 1864;8:619–621.
67. West R, Kennedy L, Carr A. *The Rehabilitation of Speech.* New York, NY: Harper & Brothers; 1937.
68. Van Riper C. *Speech Correction Principles and Methods.* Englewood Cliffs, NJ: Prentice-Hall; 1939.
69. Murphy A. *Functional Voice Disorders.* Englewood Cliffs, NJ: Prentice-Hall; 1964.
70. Brodnitz F. *Vocal Rehabilitation.* 4th ed. Rochester, NY: American Academy of Ophthalmology and Otolaryngology; 1971.
71. Andrews M. *Voice Therapy for Children.* San Diego, CA: Singular Publishing Group; 1991.
72. Aronson A. *Clinical Voice Disorders: An Interdisciplinary Approach.* New York, NY: Brian C. Decker; 1980.
73. Aronson AE. *Clinical Voice Disorders.* 3rd ed. New York, NY: Thieme; 1990.
74. Case J. *Clinical Management of Voice Disorders.* 3rd ed. Austin, TX: Pro-Ed; 1996.
75. Colton R, Casper J. *Understanding Voice Problems: A Physiological Perspective for Diagnosis and Treatment.* Baltimore, MD: Williams & Wilkins; 1996.
76. Stemple JC. A holistic approach to voice therapy. *Semin Speech Lang.* 2005; 26:131–137.
77. Verdolini K. *Resonant Voice Therapy.* In: Stemple JC, ed. *Voice Therapy: Clinical Studies.* 2nd ed. San Diego, CA: Singular Publishing; 2000:46–62.
78. Smith S, Thyme K. Statistic research on changes in speech due to pedagogic treatment (the accent method). *Folia Phoniatr (Basel).* 1976;28(2):98–103.
79. Roy N, Bless DM, Heisey D, Ford CN. Manual circumlaryngeal therapy for functional dysphonia: an evaluation of short and long-term treatment outcomes. *J Voice.* 1997;11(3):321–331.
80. Fex B, Fex S, Shiromoto O, Hirano M. Acoustic analysis of functional dysphonia: before and after voice therapy (Accent Method). *J Voice.* 1994;8(2):163–167.

81. Kotby MN, Shiromoto O, Hirano M. The accent method of voice therapy: effect of accentuations on FO, SPL, and airflow. *J Voice.* 1993;7(4):319–325.
82. Bassiouny S. Efficacy of the accent method of voice therapy. *Folia Phoniatr Logopaed.* 1998;50:146–164.
83. Roy N, Gray SD, Simon M, Dove H, Corbin-Lewis K, Stemple JC. An evaluation of the effects of two treatment approaches for teachers with voice disorders: a prospective randomized clinical trial. *J Speech Lang Hear Res.* 2001;44(2):286–296.
84. Sabol JW, Lee L, Stemple JC. The value of vocal function exercises in the practice regimen of singers. *J Voice.* 1995; 9(1):27–36.
85. Stemple JC, Lee L, D'Amico B, Pickup B. Efficacy of vocal function exercises as a method of improving voice production. *J Voice.* 1994;8(3):271–278.
86. Gillivan-Murphy P, Drinnan M, O'Dwyer T, Ridha H, Carding P. The effectiveness of a voice treatment approach for teachers with self-reported voice problems. *J Voice.* 2006;20(3): 423–431.
87. Bell S, Kidd B, Leemkuil C, Smith A, McCrae C. Vocal function exercises (VFE) versus resonant voice therapy (RVT) in the treatment of hyperfunctional voice disorders. American Speech-Language-Hearing Association Annual Convention. Boston, MA; November 2007.
88. Chen SH, Huang J, Chang W. The efficacy of resonance method to hyperfunctional dysphonia from physiological, acoustic and aerodynamic aspects: the preliminary study. *Asia Pacif J Speech Lang Hear.* 2003;8:200–203.
89. Verdolini-Marston K, Burke MK, Lessac A, Glaze L, Caldwell E. Preliminary study of two methods of treatment for laryngeal nodules. *J Voice.* 1995;9(1): 74–85.
90. Roy N, Leeper HA. Effects of the manual laryngeal musculoskeletal tension reduction technique as a treatment for functional voice disorders: perceptual and acoustic measures. *J Voice.* 1993; 7(3):242–249.
91. Van Lierde KM, De Ley S, Clement G, De Bodt M, Van Cauwenberge P. Outcome of laryngeal manual therapy in four Dutch adults with persistent moderate-to-severe vocal hyperfunction: a pilot study. *J Voice.* 2004;18(4): 467–474.
92. Herrington-Hall BL, Lee L, Stemple JC, Niemi KR, McHone MM. Description of laryngeal pathologies by age, sex, and occupation in a treatment-seeking sample. *J Speech Hear Disord.* 1988;53(1):57–64.
93. Coyle SM, Weinrich BD, Stemple JC. Shifts in relative prevalence of laryngeal pathology in a treatment-seeking population. *J Voice.* 2001;15(3):424–440.
94. Dejonckere PH, Pepin F. [Study of the Lombard effect by measuring equivalent sound level]. *Folia Phoniatr (Basel).* 1983;35(6):310–315.
95. Dobres R, Lee L, Stemple JC, Kummer AW, Kretschmer LW. Description of laryngeal pathologies in children evaluated by otolaryngologists. *J Speech Hear Disord.* 1990;55(3):526–532.
96. Wilson D. *Voice Problems of Children.* 2nd ed. Baltimore, MD: Williams and Wilkins; 1979.
97. Andrews M. Psychosocial aspects of children's behavior. In: Stemple J, ed. *Voice Therapy: Clinical Studies.* St. Louis, MO: Mosby Year Book; 1993:26–32.
98. Zwitman DH, Calcaterra TC. The "silent cough" method for vocal hyperfunction. *J Speech Hear Disord.* 1973; 38(1):119–125.
99. Solomon NP, DiMattia MS. Effects of a vocally fatiguing task and systemic hydration on phonation threshold pressure. *J Voice.* 2000;14(3):341–362.
100. Verdolini K, Titze IR, Fennell A. Dependence of phonatory effort on hydration level. *J Speech Hear Res.* 1994;37(5): 1001–1007.

101. Verdolini-Marston K, Titze IR, Druker DG. Changes in phonation threshold pressure with induced conditions of hydration. *J Voice.* 1990;4:142–151.
102. Ainsworth S. *Speech Correction Methods: A Manual of Speech Therapy and Public School Procedures.* New York, NY: Prentice-Hall; 1948.
103. Cooper M. *Modern Techniques of Vocal Rehabilitation.* Springfield, IL: Charles C Thomas; 1973.
104. Fairbanks G. *Voice and Articulation Drill Book.* 2nd ed. New York, NY: Harper and Brothers; 1960.
105. Stemple J. *Clinical Voice Pathology: Theory and Management.* Columbus, OH: Charles E. Merrill; 1984.
106. Travis G. *Speech Pathology.* New York, NY: D Appleton and Company; 1931.
107. Hollien H, Moore P, Wendahl RW, Michel JF. On the nature of vocal fry. *J Speech Hear Res.* 1966;9(2):245–247.
108. Arnold GE. Physiology and pathology of the cricothyroid muscle. *Laryngoscope.* 1961;71:687–753.
109. McWilliams B. Some factors in the intelligibility of cleft palate speech. *J Speech Hear Disord.* 1954;19:524–527.
110. Boone D. *The Voice and Voice Therapy.* 2nd ed. Englewood Cliffs, NJ: Prentice-Hall; 1977.
111. Lee L. Refocusing laryngeal tone. In: Stemple J, ed. *Voice Therapy: Clinical Studies.* St. Louis, MO: Mosby Year Book; 1993:49–53.
112. Coleman R. A comparison of the contributions of two voice quality characteristics to the perception of maleness and femaleness in the voice. *J Speech Hear Res.* 1976;19:168–180.
113. Nittrouer S, McGowan R, Milenkovic P, Beehler D. Acoustic measurement of men's and women's voices: a study of context effects and covariations. *J Speech Hear Res.* 1976;33:761–775.
114. Spencer L. Speech characteristics of male-to-female transsexuals: a perceptual and acoustic study. *Folia Phoniatri Logopae.* 1988;40:31–42.
115. Terrango I. Pitch and duration characteristics of the oral reading of males on a masculinity-femininity dimension. *J Speech Hear Res.* 1966;9:590–595.
116. Wolfe V, Ratusnik D, Smith H, Northrup G. Intonation and fundamental frequency in male to female transsexuals. *J Speech Hearing Disord.* 1990;55:43–50.
117. Jacobson E. *Progressive Relaxation.* 2nd ed. Chicago, IL: University of Chicago Press; 1938.
118. Froeschel E. Chewing method as therapy. *Arch Otolaryngol.* 1952;56:427–434.
119. Prosek R, Montgomery A, Walden B, Schwartz D. EMG biofeedback in the treatment of hyperfunctional voice disorders. *J Speech Hearing Disord.* 1978;43:282–294.
120. Stemple J, Weiler E, Whitehead W, Komray R. Electromyographic biofeedback training with patients exhibiting a hyperfunctional voice disorder. *Laryngoscope.* 1980;90:471–475.
121. Rammage L, Nichol H, Morrison M. The psychopathology of voice disorders. *Hum Comm Can.* 1987;11:21–25.
122. Ingalls E. Hysterical aphonia, or paralysis of the lateral cricoarytenoid muscles. *JAMA.* 1890;15:92–95.
123. Bach J. Hysterical aphonia. *Med News Philadelphia.* 1890;57:263–264.
124. Winslow P. Functional aphonia. *N Y Med J.* 1919;109:1129–1130.
125. Howard C. Report of a case of functional aphonia cured under general anesthetic. *JAMA.* 1923;80:104.
126. Stevens H. Conversion hysteria: A neurologic emergency. *Mayo Clin Proc.* 1968;43:54–64.
127. Christopher KL, Wood RP, 2nd, Eckert RC, Blager FB, Raney RA, Souhrada JF. Vocal-cord dysfunction presenting as asthma. *N Engl J Med.* 1983;308(26):1566–1570.
128. Selner JC, Staudenmayer H, Koepke JW, Harvey R, Christopher K. Vocal cord dysfunction: the importance of psychologic factors and provocation

challenge testing. *J Allergy Clin Immunol.* 1987;79(5):726–733.

129. Martin R, Blager F, Gay M, Wood R. Paradoxic vocal cord motion in presumed asthmatics. *Semin Respir Med.* 1987;8:332–337.
130. Stemple JC, Stanley J, Lee L. Objective measures of voice production in normal subjects following prolonged voice use. *J Voice.* 1995;9(2):127–133.
131. Linville SE. *Vocal Aging.* San Diego, CA: Singular Publishing; 2001.
132. Pasa G, Oates J, Dacakis G. The relative effectiveness of vocal hygiene training and vocal function exercises in preventing voice disorders in primary school teachers. *Logoped Phoniatr Vocol.* 2007;32(3):128–140.
133. Barnes J. *Voice therapy.* Meeting of the Southwestern Ohio Speech and Hearing Association. Cincinnati, OH; 1977.
134. Gorman S. Senile laryngis. In: Stemple JC, ed. *Voice Therapy: Clinical Studies.* 2nd ed. San Diego, CA: Singular Publishing; 2000:182–188.
135. Lessac A. *The Use and Training of the Human Voice: A Biodynamic Approach to Vocal Life.* Mountain View, CA: Mayfield Publishing; 1997.
136. Verdolini K. *Resonant Voice Therapy.* Iowa City, IA: National Center for Voice and Speech; 1998.
137. Stemple JC, ed. *Voice Therapy: Clinical Studies.* 2nd ed. San Diego, CA: Singular Publishing; 2000.
138. Berry DA, Verdolini K, Montequin DW, Hess MM, Chan RW, Titze IR. A quantitative output-cost ratio in voice production. *J Speech Lang Hear Res.* Feb 2001;44(1):29–37.
139. Verdolini K, Druker DG, Palmer PM, Samawi H. Laryngeal adduction in resonant voice. *J Voice.* 1998;12(3):315–327.
140. Ramig L, Bonitati C, Lemke J, Horii Y. Voice treatment for patients with Parkinson disease: development of an approach and preliminary efficacy data. *J Med Speech Lang Pathol.* 1994;2: 191–209.
141. Ramig L, Mead C, Scherer R, Horii Y, Larson K, Kohler D. *Voice therapy and Parkinson's disease: a longitudinal study of efficacy.* The Clinical Dysarthria Conference. San Diego, CA; 1988.
142. Countryman S, Hicks J, Ramig L, Smith M. Supraglottal hyperadduction in an individual with Parkinson disease: a clinical treatment note. *Am J Speech Lang Pathol.* 1997;6:74–84.
143. Ramig L, Pawlas A, Countryman S. *The Lee Silverman Voice Treatment: A Practical Guide for Treating the Voice and Speech Disorders in Parkinson Disease.* Iowa City, IA: National Center for Voice and Speech; 1995.
144. Ramig LO, Countryman S, Thompson LL, Horii Y. Comparison of two forms of intensive speech treatment for Parkinson disease. *J Speech Hear Res.* 1995; 38(6):1232–1251.
145. Aronson A. *Clinical Voice Disorders: An Interdisciplinary Approach.* 2nd ed. New York, NY: Brian C. Decker; 1985.
146. Damste P. Diagnostic behavior patterns with communicative abilities. In: Bless D, Abbs J, eds. *Vocal Fold Physiology.* San Diego, CA: College-Hill Press; 1987:435–444.
147. Rubin W. Allergic, dietary, chemical, stress, and hormonal influences in voice abnormalities. *J Voice.* 1987;1:378–385.
148. Ford C, Bless D. Introduction. In: Ford C, Bless D, eds. *Phonosurgery.* New York, NY: Raven Press; 1991:1–3.
149. Redmond E, Wetscher G. Introduction. In: Hinder R, ed. *Medical Intelligence Unit: Gastroesophageal Reflux Disease.* Austin, TX: RG Landes Company; 1993:1–6.
150. Koufman J. Gastroesophageal reflux and voice disorders. In: Rubin J, ed. *Diagnosis and Treatment of Voice Disorders.* New York, NY: Igaku-Shoin; 1995:161–175.
151. Hicks DM, Ours TM, Abelson TI, Vaezi MF, Richter JE. The prevalence of hypopharynx findings associated with gastroesophageal reflux in normal volunteers. *J Voice.* 2002;16(4):564–579.

152. Milstein CF, Charbel S, Hicks DM, Abelson TI, Richter JE, Vaezi MF. Prevalence of laryngeal irritation signs associated with reflux in asymptomatic volunteers: impact of endoscopic technique (rigid vs. flexible laryngoscope). *Laryngoscope.*2005;115(12):2256–2261.
153. Belafsky PC, Postma GN, Koufman JA. The validity and reliability of the Reflux Finding Score (RFS). *Laryngoscope.* 2001;111(8):1313–1317.
154. Belafsky PC, Postma GN, Koufman JA. Validity and reliability of the Reflux Symptom Index (RSI). *J Voice.* 2002;16(2):274–277.
155. Kendall K. Evaluation and management of unilateral vocal fold paralysis: a survey, part II. *Phonoscope.* 1998;1: 141–147.
156. Ford C. Laryngeal injection techniques. In: Ford C, Bless D, eds. *Phonosurgery.* New York, NY: Raven Press; 1991: 123–141.
157. Rosen CA, Gartner-Schmidt J, Casiano R, et al. Vocal fold augmentation with calcium hydroxylapatite (CaHA). *Otolaryngol Head Neck Surg.* 2007;136(2): 198–204.
158. Kwon TK, Rosen CA, Gartner-Schmidt J. Preliminary results of a new temporary vocal fold injection material. *J Voice.* 2005;19(4):668–673.
159. Coskun HH, Rosen CA. Gelfoam injection as a treatment for temporary vocal fold paralysis. *Ear Nose Throat J.* 2003; 82(5):352–353.
160. Isshiki N, Okamura H, Ishikawa T. Thyroplasty type I (lateral compression) for dysphonia due to vocal cord paralysis or atrophy. *Acta Otolaryngol.* 1975;80(5–6):465–473.
161. Isshiki N, Morita H, Okamura H, Hiramoto M. Thyroplasty as a new phonosurgical technique. *Acta Otolaryngol (Stockholm).* 1974;78:451–457.
162. Blaugrund S. Laryngeal framework surgery. In: Ford C, Bless D, eds. *Phonosurgery.* New York, NY: Raven Press; 1991:183–200.
163. Isshiki N. Laryngeal framework surgery. *Adv Otolaryngol Head Neck Surg.* 1991;6:37–56.
164. Koufman J. Thyroplasty for vocal fold medialization: an alternative to Teflon injection. *Laryngoscope.* 1986;96: 726–731.
165. Smith M, Gray S. Laryngeal framework surgery in children. In: Titze I, ed. *Progress Report 5.* Iowa City, IA: National Center for Voice and Speech; 1994:91–98.
166. Isshiki N, Tanabe M, Sawada M. Arytenoid adduction for unilateral vocal cord paralysis. *Arch Otolaryngol.* 1978; 104(10):555–558.
167. Crumley R. Laryngeal reinnervation techniques. In: Ford C, Bless D, eds. *Phonosurgery.* New York, NY: Raven Press; 1991:201–212.
168. Koufman J, Walker F. Laryngeal electromyography in clinical practice: indications, techniques, and interpretation. *Phonoscope.* 1998;1:57–70.
169. McFarlane S, Watterson T, Lewis K, Boone D. Effect of voice therapy facilitation techniques on airflow in unilateral paralysis patients. *Phonoscope.* 1998;1:187–191.
170. Tanner K, Roy N, Merrill R, Sauder C, Houtz D, Smith M. Spasmodic dysphonia: onset, course, socioemotional effects and treatment response. *Ann Otol, Rhinol, Laryngol.* 2011;120(7): 465–473.
171. Barkmeier JM, Case JL, Ludlow CL. Identification of symptoms for spasmodic dysphonia and vocal tremor: a comparison of expert and non-expert judges. *J Commun Disord.* 2001;34:21–37.
172. Chetri DK, Merati AL, Blumin JH, Sulica L, Damrose EJ, Tsai VW. Reliability of the perceptual evaluation of adductor spasmodic dysphonia. *Ann Otol Rhinol Laryngol.* 2008;117:159–165.
173. Ludlow CL. Management of the spasmodic dysphonias. In: Rubin JS, Sataloff RT, Korovin G, Gould WJ, eds. *Diagnosis and Treatment of Voice Disor-*

ders. New York, NY: Igaku-Shoin; 1995: 436–454.

174. Higgins MB, Chait DH, Shulte L. Phonatory air flow characteristics of adductor spasmodic dysphonia and muscle tension dysphonia. *J Speech Lang Hear Res*. 1999;42:101–111.
175. Roy N, Ford CN, Bless DM. Muscle tension dysphonia and spasmodic dysphonia: the role of manual laryngeal tension reduction in diagnosis and management. *Ann Otol Rhinol Laryngol*. 1996;105:851–856.
176. Roy N. Functional dysphonia. *Curr Opin Otolaryngol Head Neck Surg*. 2003; 11:144–148.
177. Finitzo T, Freeman F. Spasmodic dysphonia, whether and where: results of seven years of research. *J Speech Hear Res*. 1989;32:541–555.
178. Roy N, Gouse M, Mauszycki SC, Merrill RM, Smith ME. Task specificity in adductor spasmodic dysphonia versus muscle tension dysphonia. *Laryngoscope*. 2005;115:311–313.
179. Leonard R, Kendall K. Differentiation of spasmodic and psychogenic dysphonias with phonoscopic evaluation. *Laryngoscope*. 1999;109:295–300.
180. Sapienza CM, Walton S, Murry T. Adductor spasmodic dysphonia and muscular tension dysphonia: acoustic analysis of sustained phonation and reading. *J Voice* 2000;14:502–520.
181. Roy N, Mauszycki SC, Merrill RM, Gouse M, Smith ME. Toward improved differential diagnosis of adductor spasmodic dysphonia and muscle tension dysphonia. *Folia Phon Logo*. 2007;59: 83–90.
182. Ludlow CL, Adler CH, Berke GS, et al. Research priorities in spasmodic dysphonia. *Otolaryngol-Head Neck Surg*. 2008;139:495–505.
183. Dedo H. Recurrent nerve section for spastic dysphonia. *Ann Otol Rhinol Laryngol*. 1976;85:451–459.
184. Dedo H, Izdebski K. Intermediate results of 306 recurrent laryngeal nerve sections for spastic dysphonia. *Laryngoscope*. 1983;93:9–16.
185. Aronson A, DeSanto G. Adductor spasmodic dysphonia: three years after recurrent laryngeal nerve resection. *Laryngoscope*. 1983;93:1–8.
186. Blitzer A, Brin M. Laryngeal dystonia: a series with botulinum toxin therapy. *Ann Otol Rhinol Laryngol*. 1991;100:85–90.
187. Blitzer A, Brin M, Fahn S, Lovelace R. Localized injections of botulinum toxin for the treatment of focal laryngeal dystonia. *Laryngoscope*. 1988;98:193–197.
188. Ludlow C, Naunton R, Sedory S, Schulz G, Hallett M. Effects of botulinum toxin injections on speech in adductor spasmodic dysphonia. *Neurology*. 1988;38:1220–1225.
189. Blitzer A. Botulinum toxin A and B: a comparative dosing study for spasmodic dysphonia. *Otolaryngol Head Neck Surg*. 2005;133(6):836–838.
190. Klein AM, Stong BC, Wise J, Delgaudio JM, Hapner ER, Johns MM 3rd. Vocal outcome measures after bilateral posterior cricoarytenoid muscle botulinum toxin injections for abductor spasmodic dysphonia. *Otolaryngol Head Neck Surg*. 2008;139(3):421–423.
191. Woodson G, Hochstetler H, Murry T. Botulinum toxin therapy for abductor spasmodic dysphonia. *J Voice*. 2006; 20(1):137–143.
192. Bielamowicz S, Squire S, Bidus K, Ludlow CL. Assessment of posterior cricoarytenoid botulinum toxin injections in patients with abductor spasmodic dysphonia. *Ann Otol Rhinol Laryngol*. 2001;110(5, pt 1):406–412.
193. Ford C, Bless D, Lowery D. Indirect laryngoscopic approach for injection of botulinum toxin in spasmodic dysphonia. *Otolaryngol Head Neck Surg*. 1990; 103:752–758.
194. Murry T, Woodson G. Combined-modality treatment of adductor spasmodic dysphonia with botulinum toxin and voice therapy. *J Voice*. 1995;9: 460–465.

Appendix 7–A
Phrases and Sentences Graduated in Length

Two-Syllable Sentences and Phrases

I am.	I will.	You can.	all right	Get up.
You are.	Oh no.	I'm fine.	King me.	black eye
He is.	Do it.	Look out.	Call me.	Cast off.
We are.	Don't go.	They're gone.	lost time	down here
You are.	What time?	Try it.	My, my.	eat out
They are.	I'll try.	Why not?	No good.	free up
Come in.	Stop it.	no time	Oh my.	gee whiz
Get out.	Catch up.	too bad	part time	hot time
Keep out.	Watch out.	Get lost.	Guess what?	I'm fine.
Get up.	Thank you.	tee time	right now	last night
So long.	Go home.	Buy now.	Start up.	My mom.
Stand up.	Strike out.	Come back.	too much	next time
Sit down.	Turn right.	Don't go	used up	on top
Jump up.	first base	end run	Vote now.	post card
How much?	home plate	fast food	Where to?	rest stop
Push it.	Wake up.	great big	uptown	run down
Why not?	You bet.	grown up	Yes sir.	Step down.
Help me.	Good night.	Have some.	Yes ma'am	Sew up.
Prove it.	Goodbye.	I was.	Act now.	Where to?
Tell me.	too much	just so	Be good.	May I?

Three-Syllable Sentences and Phrases

Pick it up.	Is that so?	Put that back.	See you soon.
Put it down.	Bake a pie.	Make salad.	Catch the ball.
Bring it here.	Ride the horse.	Fly away.	I said no.
I don't know.	Close the door.	Wear a tie.	more or less
Why not go?	Sweep the floor.	Go downtown.	Clean the tub.

Come over.
Go away.
Here we are.
Good morning.
Can you go?
Do it now.
How are you?
Help me please.
Is a time?
I'm on time.
Am I late?
I told you.
over there
What about?
Should we go?

Start the game.
Set the clock.
That's all right.
Go downtown.
not so fast
Hit the ball.
Sleep all night.
Ring the bell.
Don't do it.
That's not true.
Come back here.
Start a fire.
Mop the floor.
Go to school.
Write a check.

Race the car.
down the road
back by 5
I found it.
Run it down.
Hurry up.
Come back soon.
It's snowing.
like old times
pretty eyes
far away
Go to sleep.
Call me soon.
You look good.
I feel fine.

Wash dishes.
Fly the kite.
Build a house.
Light the lamp.
Wind your watch.
Don't touch it.
There she is.
I'm sorry.
Don't buy that.
Write a book.
buy and sell
Look around.
Share the toy.
Push and pull.
a red light

Four-Syllable Sentences and Phrases

It's very hot.
Fry the bacon.
Am I on time?
Are you ready?
I didn't know
Pick the apples.
a baby boy
Feed the kitten.
Don't wait for me.
Can we go now?
I don't know why.
How are you now?
Bring some money.

What could I do?
Will you be there?
You should say so.
Am I early?
Where do you sit?
I told you so.
That's not my fault.
How do you feel?
Show it to me.
Let's wait for them.
What time is it?
What have you done?
They are so slow.

Give it to me.
Please say something.
Is that enough?
Write a letter.
Answer the phone.
When do we go?
Was I correct?
Do it again.
They all have jobs.
Open your eyes.
We must go now.
Did you know that?
How do you do?

over the top
I like ice cream.
Open the door.
Bake apple pie.
I don't like that.
Should we go now?
Is that your car?
Where do you live?
Turn to the left.
Fill the bird bath.
Turn on the light.
Walk down the hall.
Let's go swimming.
Play volleyball.
Tell me the truth.
Did you hear me?
Keep on trying.
Put it away.
It stopped snowing.
Type the letter.
Let's go downtown.

Five-Syllable Sentences

Give it to me now.
You are a good dog.
Come back when you can
He has a nice car.
How much do you want.
There's not enough room.
The wind blew all day
Do it before noon.
Do you want to go?
Go to the bookstore.
I want some pizza.
Do you have a dime?
I'll come back today.
Have you talked to them?
Don't give it to me.
It's not all my fault.
I don't want to talk.
They are very nice.
You shouldn't do that.
They played in the sand.
The rain was welcome.
We designed our house.
She burst the balloon.
Speak clearly to them.
He is very shy.
There's not enough time.
They've sold their horses.
The crowd was pushed back.
He planted sweet corn.
The weather was cold.
Who pulled the alarm?
Bring a stronger rope.
The dogs were barking.
We picked the berries.
Let's watch some TV.
We rode the rapids.
That's a better one.
Is she your sister?
We went to the bank.
Please open the door.
I wouldn't do that.
Did he say maybe?
Stop, look, and listen.
Bring a keg of beer.
Answer the question.
I'm moving forward.
Use a safety pin.
Are you running now?
How did the race go?
The light bulb burned out.
Why don't you like it?
You made a mistake.
Where did you grow up?
Can you believe it?
Open the window.
Keep on working hard.
I missed the last class.
Let's play basketball.
The room was noisy.
I was so nervous.

Six-Syllable Sentences

Mike was cutting the grass.
The player broke his arm.
All the girls were laughing.
Get there before they close.
Did you hear what she said?
Come in and close the door.
Are you going tonight?
Put everything away.
Come whenever you can.
We heard that yesterday.
The player broke his leg.
The children went swimming.
It's time to go to class.
Please open window.
Hit the ball to shortstop.
Don't wait till it's too late.
Meet me at the courthouse.
Feed the dog his supper.
What's on TV tonight?
What's not right must be wrong.
Go to the store with me.
The fields were very dry.
Did you find your notebook?
Let's go skiing today.
Do you like your new job?
Promise that you won't tell.
May I borrow that too?
How are you this morning?
Beth was washing her clothes.
The flags blew in the wind.
He slept under the tree.
We don't want it to rain.
He couldn't start the fire.
Do you think he's happy?
When should we come around?
Let's go to a movie.
How much rent do you pay?
Who's on the telephone?

Seven- and Eight-Syllable Sentences

What movie would you like to see?
There's plenty of room in my house.
Sometimes I think you're very wrong.
Would you come by about 7?
May I have another piece?
I was raised in the Midwest.
Were you able to hear him speak?
The fisherman caught a large fish.
Please make sure your hands are clean.
The snow was a welcome sight.
All the fences were jumped with ease.
What's your favorite music?
I need to go to the bank.
Let's not take too much time here.
Why are there only 7?
The clock stopped at 4:39.

We grew roses on the back fence.

Show me how it should be done.

Yesterday he bought a new car.

I have too much to do today.

What do you want on your pie?

We ran a match race yesterday.

Come over this afternoon.

Put it back where you found it.

The boy found it by the cooler.

We went skiing on the lake.

I eat breakfast every day.

Do you think we should start that now?

The trip was exciting.

Make sure you turn off your printer.

Nine- and Ten-Syllable Sentences

We need to go to the grocery store.

I scored 100% on the test.

She has 5 brothers and 4 sisters.

Two of the brothers are in college.

That was the best time I ever ran.

Let's go to the ballgame on Saturday.

I couldn't believe how many were there.

She went to Florida during spring break.

Would you hold the door open for me?

I'm very happy that you could come.

He ordered a hamburger for lunch.

The snow melted before we could ride sleds.

We went fishing on Lake Superior.

I'm tired of cafeteria food.

What good movies have you seen lately?

Let's go scuba diving this summer.

She had an interview this afternoon.

I studied all night long for this test.

The marching band practiced before the game.

I'm going home for the holidays.

Do you have to work after class today?

There wasn't one parking space to be found.

Sometimes it's hard to keep up with the news.

You look absolutely marvelous.

What time do you think we should leave today?

The party was over by 1:30.

I should be finished in time to leave then.

Why don't you take a 15-minute break?

Who was it that called on the telephone?

It's your turn to wash the dishes tonight.

Eleven- to Fifteen-Syllable Sentences

The instructor was rigid in his opinion.

There were 800 people in the psychology class.

With any luck, this course shouldn't be too difficult.

My pen ran out of ink in the middle of the test.

American history is my favorite class.

I would have helped you with that problem if you had only asked.

I want to jog for an hour before I begin to study.

My parents are coming to visit for the weekend.

How many more tests do you have this semester?

It's important that you listen closely in his class.

I wrote for so long that my hand began to cramp.

What was in the package you received this afternoon?

Most people wouldn't even consider doing that.

We stood in line for 2 hours to buy the tickets.

I just can't seem to get this program to run.

Most of this information can be found in the library.

Were you able to finish your project on time?

I was happy when classes were canceled because of the snow.

Everyone was shocked when he announced the surprise test.

The professor wouldn't start before she had had her coffee.

Two students from Taiwan were in my physics class.

We are going on a picnic if it doesn't rain.

My audio recorder could not pick up his voice.

What time do you want to leave the basketball game?

Our dormitory had a false alarm last night.

I can't wait until the Christmas holidays.

I swam 10 laps this morning before eight o'clock.

Someone left his coat in the biology lab.

Make sure that you have all the facts and then proceed.

The library was so quiet, you could hear your heartbeat.

Sixteen- to Twenty-Syllable Sentences

The proposal was opposed by everyone who was eligible to vote.

How many times must we listen to the same thing over and over again?

I had steak, fried potatoes, and a tossed salad for dinner last night.

We knew as soon as we entered the room that someone had been there before us.

He posed the most important question that we would have to consider.

If I can raise the money, I'm going to fly to California.

Though we had been there only for a week, it seemed more like a month.

Let me know if there's anything I can do to help you get ready.

Since the building did not have air conditioning, the class was unbearable.

Nobody noticed when we entered the room a half-hour late.

Did you hear the plans to renovate the stadium for next year?

How many people do you think it will take to permit us to break even?

The runner developed the blister on his foot halfway through the race.

Students were caught painting victory signs on the railroad overpass.

How many months do you think it will take for us to finish this project?

We should be able to afford it if 6 of us rent the apartment.

He commuted to the university every day for 5 years.

She had already learned many of the skills in her co-op job.

I had 18 more hours to complete for graduation.

The referee had obviously made a serious error in judgment.

The smoke was so thick in the lab that the sprinkler suddenly came on.

We carefully placed the project on the table for the instructor's inspection.

Someone threw an aerosol can in the fire, causing a loud explosion.

Would you rather take a written or an oral examination?

If you wait too long then you're going to miss a great opportunity.

I've been invited to go on vacation with my best friend's family.

It's impossible to measure the knowledge gained from this seminar.

Most people would not have the imagination to create such a thing.

Stop at the store on your way home and pick up a gallon of milk.

We can't decide whether or not to participate in formal graduation.

PARAGRAPH READINGS

Passage 1

For the most wild yet the most homely narrative which I am about to pen,/ I neither expect nor solicit belief./ Mad indeed would I be to expect it,/ in a case where my very senses reject their own evidence./ Yet, mad am I not—/and very surely do I not dream./ But tomorrow I die, and today I would unburden my soul./ My immediate purpose is to place before the world,/ plainly, succinctly, and without comment,/ a series of mere household events./ In their consequences, these events have terrified—/have tortured—have destroyed me./ Yet I will not attempt to expound them./ To me, they have presented little but horror—/to many they will seem less terrible than baroque./ Hereafter, perhaps, some intellect may be found which will reduce my phantasm to the commonplace—/some intellect more calm, more logical, and far less excitable than my own,/ which will perceive, in the circumstances I detail with awe,/ nothing more than an ordinary succession of very natural causes and effects.

—Edgar Allen Poe, from *The Black Cat*

Passage 2

Mr. President and Gentlemen of the Convention:/ If we could first know where we are, and whither we are tending,/ we could better judge what to do, and how to do it./ We are now far into the fifth year since a policy was initiated/ with the avowed object, and confident promise, of putting an end to slavery agitation./ Under the operation of that policy, that agitation not only has not ceased,/ but has constantly augmented./ In my opinion,/ it will not cease until a crisis shall have been reached and passed./ "A house divided against itself cannot stand."/ I believe this government cannot endure permanently, half slave and half free./ I do not expect the Union to be dissolved;/ I do not expect the house to fall;/ But I do expect that it will cease to be divided./ It will become all one thing or all the other./

Either the opponents of slavery will arrest the further spread of it,/ and place it where the public mind shall rest in the belief that it is in the course of ultimate extinction;/ or its advocates will push it forward till it shall become alike lawful in all the States,/ old as well as new,/ North as well as South. . . .

—Abraham Lincoln

Passage 3

The wrath of God is like great waters that are dammed for the present;/ they increase more and more, and rise higher and higher, till an outlet is given;/ and the longer the stream is stopped, the more rapid and mighty is its course,/ when once it is let loose./ 'Tis true, that judgment against your evil work has not been executed hitherto;/ the floods of God's vengeance have been withheld;/ but your guilt in the meantime is constantly increasing,/ and you are every day treasuring up more wrath;/ the waters are continually rising, and waxing more and more mighty;/ and there is nothing but the mere pleasure of God that holds the waters back,/ that are unwilling to be stopped, and press hard to go forward./

If God should only withdraw his hand from the floodgate, it would immediately fly open,/ and the fiery floods and the fierceness and the wrath of God would rush forth with inconceivable fury/ and would come upon you with omnipotent power;/ and if your strength were ten thousand times greater than it is,/ yea, ten thousand times greater than the strength of the stoutest, sturdiest devil in hell,/ it would be nothing to withstand or endure it./

The bow of God's wrath is bent, and the arrow made ready on the string,/ and justice bends the arrow at your heart, and strains the bow,/ and it is nothing but the mere pleasure of God,/ and that of an angry God, without any promise or obligation at all,/ that keeps the arrow one moment from being made drunk by your blood.

—Jonathan Edwards

Passage 4

In the long history of the world,/ only a few generations have been granted the role in defending freedom in its hour of maximum danger./ I do not shrink from this responsibility;/ I welcome it./ I do not believe that any of us would exchange places with any other people or any other generation./ The energy, the faith, the devotion which we bring to this endeavor/ will light our country and all that serve it,/ and the glow from that fire can truly light the world./

And so, my fellow Americans,/ ask not what your country can do for you;/ ask what you can do for your country./

My fellow citizens of the world,/ ask not what America will do for you,/ but what together we can do for the freedom of man.

Finally, whether you are citizens of America or citizens of the world,/ ask of us here the same high standards of strength and sacrifice which we ask of you./ With a good conscience our only sure reward,/ with history the final judge of our deeds,/ let us go forth to lead the land we love,/ asking His blessing and His help,/ but knowing that here on earth God's work must truly be our own.

—John F. Kennedy

Passage 5

While I was in San Francisco, I enjoyed my first earthquake. It was one which was long called the "great" earthquake, and is doubtless so distinguished till this day. It was just afternoon, on a bright October day. I was coming down Third Street. The only objects in motion anywhere in sight in the thickly built and populous quarter, were a man in a buggy behind me, and a streetcar wending slowly up a cross street. Otherwise, all was solitude and a Sabbath stillness. As I turned the corner, around a frame house, there was a great rattle and jar, and it occurred to me that here was an item!—no doubt fight in that house. Before I could turn and seek the door, there came a really terrific shock; the ground seemed to roll under me in waves, interrupted by violent joggling up-and-down, and there was a heavy grinding noise as of brick houses rubbing together. I fell up against the frame house and hurt my elbow. I knew what it was, now, and from mere reportorial instinct, nothing else, took out my watch and noted the time of day; at that moment a third and still severer shock came, and as I reeled about on the pavement trying to keep my footing, I saw a sight! The entire front of a tall four-story brick building in Third Street sprung outward like a door and fell sprawling across the street, raising a dust like a great volume of smoke! And here came the buggy—overboard went the man, and in less time than I can tell it the vehicle was distributed in small fragments along three hundred yards of the street. One could have fancied that someone had fired a charge of chair-rounds and rags down the thoroughfare. The streetcar had stopped, the horses were rearing and plunging, the passengers were pouring out of both ends, and one fat man had crashed halfway through a glass window on one side of the car, got wedged fast and was squirming and screaming like an impaled madman. Every door or of every house, as far as the eye could reach, was vomiting a stream of human beings; and almost before one could execute a wink and begin another, there was a massed multitude of people stretching in endless procession down every street my position commanded. Never was solemn solitude turned into teeming life quicker.

—Mark Twain, from *The San Francisco Earthquake*

Passage 6

They tell us, sir, that we are weak; unable to cope with so formidable an adversary. But when shall we be stronger? Will it be the next week, or the next year? Will it be when we are totally disarmed, and when a British guard shall be stationed in every house? Shall we gather strength by irresolution and inaction? Shall we acquire the means of effectual resistance, by lying supinely on our backs, and hugging the delusive phantom of hope, until our enemies should have bound us hand and foot? Sir we are not weak, if we make proper use of the means which the God of nature hath placed in our power. Three millions of people, armed in the holy cause of liberty, and in such a country as that which we possess, are invincible by any force which our enemy can send against us.

Besides, sir, we shall not fight our battles alone. There is a just God who presides over the destinies of nations; and who will raise up friends to fight our battles for us. The battle, sir, is not to the strong alone; it is to the vigilant, the active, the brave. Besides, sire, we have no election. If we were base enough to desire it, it is now too late to retire from the contest. There is no retreat, but in submission and slavery! Our chains are forged! Their clanking may be heard on the plains of Boston! The war is inevitable and let it come! I repeat it, sir, let it come!

It is in vain, sir, to extenuate the matter. Gentlemen may cry peace, peace but there is no peace. The war is actually begun! The next gale that sweeps from the north will bring to our ears the clash of resounding arms! Our brethren are already in the field! Why stand we here idle? What is it that gentlemen wish? What would they have? Is life so dear, or peace so sweet, as to be purchased at the price of chains and slavery? Forbid it, Almighty God! I know not what course others may take; but as for me, give me liberty, or give me death!

—Patrick Henry

Passage 7

Friends and fellow-citizens: I stand before you tonight under the indictment for the alleged crime of having voted at the last Presidential election, without having the lawful right to vote. It shall be my work this evening to prove to you that in thus voting, I not only committed no crime, but, instead, simply citizen's rights, guaranteed to me and all United States citizens by Constitution, beyond the power of any State to deny.

The preamble of the Federal Constitution says:

"We, the people of the United States, in order to form a more perfect union, establish justice, insure domestic tranquility, provide for the common defense, promote the general welfare, and secure the blessings of liberty to ourselves and our posterity, do ordain and establish this Constitution for the United States of America."

It was we, the people; not we, the white male citizens; nor yet we, the male citizens; but we, the whole people, who formed the Union. And we formed it, not to give the blessings of liberty, but to secure them; not to the half of ourselves and the half of our posterity, but to the whole people women as well as men. And it is a downright mockery to talk to women of their enjoyment of the blessings of liberty while they are denied the use of their only means of securing them provided by this democratic-republican government the ballot.

For any State to make a sex qualification that must ever result in the disfranchisement of one entire half of the people is to pass a bill of attainder, or an ex post facto law, and is therefore a violation of the supreme law of the land. By it the blessings of liberty are forever withheld from women and their female posterity. To them this government has no just powers derived from the consent of the governed. To them this government is not a democracy. It is not a republic. It is an odious aristocracy; a hateful oligarchy of sex; the most hateful aristocracy ever established on the face of the globe; an oligarchy of wealth, where the rich govern the poor. An oligarchy of learning, where the educated govern the ignorant, or even an oligarchy of race, where the Saxon rules the African, might be endured; but this oligarchy of sex, which makes fathers, brothers, husbands, sons, the oligarchs over the mothers and sisters, the wives and daughters of every household which ordains all men sovereigns, all women subjects, carries dissension, discord and rebellion into every home of the nation.

Webster, Worcester, and Bouvier all define a citizen to be a person in the United States, entitled to vote and hold office. The only question to be settled now is: Are women persons? And I hardly believe any of our opponents will have the hardihood to say they are not. Being persons, then, women are citizens; and no State has a right to make any law, or to enforce any old law, that shall abridge their privileges or immunities. Hence, every discrimination against women in the constitutions and laws of the several States is today null and void, precisely as is every one against Negroes.

—Susan B. Anthony

Passage 8

It chanced on Sunday, when Mr. Utterson was on his usual walk with Mr. Enfield, that their way lay once again through the by-street; and that when they came in front of the door, both stopped to gaze on it.

"Well," said Enfield, "that story's at an end at least. We shall never see more of Mr. Hyde."

"I hope not," said Utterson, "Did I ever tell you that I once saw him, and shared your feeling of repulsion?"

"It was impossible to do the one without the other," returned Enfield. "And by the way, what an ass you must have thought me, not to know that this was a back way to Dr. Jekyll! It was partly your own fault that I found it out, even when I did."

"So you found it out, did you?" said Utterson. "But if that be so, we may step into the court and take a look at the windows. To tell you the truth, I am uneasy, about poor Jekyll; and even outside, I feel as if the presence of a friend might do him good."

The court was very cool and a little damp, and full of premature twilight, although the sky, high up overhead, was still bright with sunset. The middle one of the three windows was half-way open, and sitting close beside it, taking the air with an infinite sadness of mind, like some deconsolate prisoner, Utterson saw Dr. Jekyll.

"What! Jekyll!" he cried. "I trust you are better."

"I am very low, Utterson," replied the doctor drearily, "very low. It will not last long, thank God."

"You stay too much indoors," said the lawyer. "You should be out, whipping up the circulation like Mr. Enfield and me. (This is my cousin—Mr. Enfield—Dr. Jekyll.) Come now; get your hat and take a quick turn with us."

"You are very good," sighed the other. "I should like to very much; but no, no, no, it is quite impossible; I dare not. But indeed, Utterson, I am very glad to see you; this is really a great pleasure; I would ask you and Mr. Enfield up, but the place is really not fit."

"Why then," said the lawyer, good-naturedly, "the best thing we can do is to stay down here and speak with you from where we are."

"That is just what I was about to venture to propose," returned the doctor with a smile. But the words were hardly uttered, before the smile was struck out of his face and succeeded by an expression of such abject terror and froze the very blood of the two gentlemen below. They saw it but for a glimpse for the window was instantly thrust down and they turned and left the court without word. In silence, too, they traversed the bystreet; and it was not until they had come into a neighboring thoroughfare, where even upon a Sunday there were still some stirrings of life, that Mr. Utterson at last turned and looked at his companion. They were both pale; and there was an answering horror in their eyes.

"God forgive us, God forgive us," said Mr. Utterson.

But Mr. Enfield only nodded his head very seriously, and walked on once more in silence.

—Robert Louis Stevenson, from *Dr. Jekyll and Mr. Hyde*

POETRY READINGS

Passage 1

Annabel Lee

It was many and many a year ago,
In a kingdom by the sea,
That a maiden there lived whom you may know
By the name of Annabel Lee;
And this maiden she lived with no other thought
Than to love and be loved by me.
She was a child and I was a child,

In this kingdom by the sea,
But we loved with a love that was more than love
I and my Annabel Lee
With a love that the winged seraphs of Heaven
Coveted her and me.
And this was the reason that, long ago,
In this kingdom by the sea,
A wind blew out of a cloud, by night
Chilling my Annabel Lee;
So that her highborn kinsmen came
And bore her away from me,
To shut her up in a sepulcher
In this kingdom by the sea.
The angels, not half so happy in Heaven,
Went envying her and me;
Yes! That was the reason (as all men know,
In this kingdom by the sea)
That the wind came out of the cloud,
chilling and killing my Annabel Lee.
But our love it was stronger by far than the love
Of those who were older than we
Of many far wiser than we
And neither the angels in Heaven above
Nor the demons down under the sea,
Can ever dissever my soul from the soul
Of the beautiful Annabel Lee;
For the moon never beams without bringing me dreams
Of the beautiful Annabel Lee;
And the stars never rise but I see the bright eyes
Of the beautiful Annabel Lee;
And so, all the night-tide, I lie down by the side
Of my darling, my darling, my life and my bride,
In her epulcher there by the sea
In her tomb by the sounding sea.

—Edgar Allen Poe

Passage 2

Bonny Barbara Allan

In Scarlet town, where I was born,
There was a fair maid dwelling,
Made every youth cry Well-a-away!
Her name was Barbara Allan.
All in the merry month of May,

When green buds they were swelling,
Young Jemmy Grove on his death-bed lay,
For love of Barbara Allan.
O slowly, slowly rose she up,
To the place where he was lying,
And when she drew the curtain by,
"Young man, I think you're dying."
O 'tis I'm sick, and very, very, very sick,
And 'tis a' for Barbara Allan";
"O the better for me ye's never be,
Tho your heart's blood were spilling,
"O dinna ye mind, young man," said she,
"When ye was in the tavern drinking,
That ye made the healths go round and round,
And slighted Barbara Allan?"
He turned his face unto the wall,
And death was with him dealing:
"Adieu, Adieu, my dear friends all,
And be kind to Barbara Allan."
And slowly, slowly rose she up,
And slowly, slowly left him,
And sighing said she could not stay,
Since death of life had left him.
She had not gane a mile but twa,
When she heard the dead-bell knelling,
And every jow that the dead-bell gave
Cried, "Woe to Barbara Allan!"
"O mother, mother, make my bed!
O make it soft and narrow!
Since my love died for me today,
I'll die for him tomorrow."

—Unknown

Passage 3

The Old Cloak

This winter's weather it waxeth cold,
And frost it freezeth on every hill,
And Boreas blows his blast so bold
That all our cattle are like to spill.
Bell, my wife, she loves no strife;
She said unto me quietly,
"Rise up, and save cow Crumbock's life!"
Man, put thine old cloak about thee!"

HE

O Bell my wife, why dost thou flyte?
Thou kens my cloak is very thin.
It is so bare and over wom,
A cricket cannot creep therein.
Then I'll no longer borrow nor lend;
For once I'll new apparell'd be;
Tomorow I'll to town and spend;
For I'll have a new cloak about me.

SHE

Cow Crumbock is a very good cow:
She has been always true to the pail;
She has help'd us to butter and cheese, I trow
And other things she will not fail.
I would be loth to see her pine.
Good husband, counsel take of me:
It is not for us to go so fine
Man, take thine old cloak about thee!

HE

My cloak it was a very good cloak,
It hath been always true to the wear;
But now it is not worth a groat:
I have had it four and forty year.
sometime it was of cloth in grain:
'Tis now but a sieve, as you may see:
It will neither hold out wind nor rain;
And I'll have a new cloak about me.

SHE

It is four and forty years ago
Since the one of us the other did ken;
And we have had, betwixt us two,
Of children either nine or ten:
We have brought them up to women and men:
In the fear of God I trow they be
And why wilt thou thyself misken?
Man, take thine old cloak about thee!

HE

O Bell my wife, why dost thou flyte?
Now is now, and then was then:
Seek now all the world throughout,
Thou kens not clowns from gentlemen:
They are clad in black, green, yellow, and blue,

So far above their own degree.
Once in my fife I'll take a view;
For I'll have a new cloak about me.

SHE

King Stephen was a worthy peer;
His breeches cost him but a crown;
He held them sixpence all too dear,
Therefore he called the tailor 'lown.'
He was a king and wore the crown,
And thou'se but of a low degree:
It's pride that puts this country down:
Man, take thine old cloak about thee!

HE

Bell my wife, she loves not strife,
Yet she will lead me, if she can:
And to maintain an easy life
I oft must yield, though I'm good-man.
It's not for a man with a woman to threap,
Unless he first give o'er the plea:
As we began, so will we keep,
And I'll take my old cloak about me.

—Unknown

Passage 4

By-low, My Babe

By-low, my babe, lie still and sleep;
It grieves me sore to see thee weep.
If thou wert quiet I'd be glad;
Thou mourning makes my sorrow sad.
By-low, my boy, thy mother's joy,
Thy father breeds me great annoy
By-low, lie low.
When he began to court my love,
And me with sugared words to move,
His feignings false and flattering cheer
To me that time did not appear.
But now I see most cruelly
He cares not for my babe nor me
By-low, lie low.
Lie still, my darling, sleep awhile,
And when thou wak'st thou'llt sweetly smile;

But smile not as thy father did,
To cozen maids—nay, God forbid!
But yet I fear thou wilt grow near
Thy father's heart and face to bear
By-low, lie low.
I cannot choose, but ever will
Be loving to thy father still;
Where'er he stay, where'er he ride
My love with him doth still abide.
In weal or woe, where'er he go,
My heart shall not forsake him; so
By-low, lie low.

—Unknown

8

The Professional Voice

The voice so sweet, the words so fair,
As some soft chime had stroked the air;
And though the sound were parted thence,
Still left an echo in the sense.
Eupheme-Samuel Johnson

OVERVIEW

We have described the laryngeal mechanism in terms of its physical structure and function and have discussed many etiologic factors that may lead to the development of various laryngeal pathologies. We then presented management strategies designed to help patients return the laryngeal mechanism to as near a normal state as possible, yielding improved or normal voice qualities. A large group of individuals are, by the very nature of their occupations, at a greater risk of developing voice problems and laryngeal pathologies. These individuals are directly dependent on vocal communication for their livelihood. They are classified as users of "professional" voice.

The impact of a voice disorder on this population is twofold. It not only causes vocal symptoms that are characteristic of the disorder, it also carries with it a high level of emotional strain and anxiety. This anxiety may be caused by the disorder's potential impact on the person's reputation, the ability to meet professional commitments, or simply the ability to perform his or her job. These concerns and anxieties add to the actual causes of the voice disorder and must also be addressed in a positive manner within the vocal management program.

The management approach must go beyond the manipulation of inappropriate vocal properties and must involve all aspects of vocal hygiene counseling. Rehabilitation will often require the involvement of a team of professionals. The team may comprise the professional voice user, otolaryngologist, voice pathologist, and professional voice user's teacher of singing, vocal coach, producer, and manager. Successful voice rehabilitation may depend on the abilities of these disciplines to compromise and work together with the patient's long-term vocal health as the primary consideration. Ideally, the professional voice user will ultimately become responsible for the well-being of his or her vocal health.

THE PROFESSIONAL VOICE USER

We are all dependent on vocal communication in our everyday lives. Most people view the loss of voice for even a brief time as a major inconvenience. Those who rely directly on their voices for their livelihoods in a public forum are likely to experience more than an inconvenience with the development of a voice disorder. Voice disorders, whether they are acute or chronic, may threaten, shorten, change, or even end some careers. For example, the singer who develops acute laryngitis on opening night may suffer poor reviews. The stage actor who develops intermittent periods of dysphonia caused by vocal misuse may develop a reputation of unreliability. The effectiveness of a political campaign may be diminished when the politician becomes dysphonic and is unable to project the desired image.

This chapter focuses primarily on the elite vocal performer (singers and actors) for whom a slight alteration in vocal quality can have a devastating effect. Twenty-five to thirty-five percent of the national U.S. workforce is a professional voice user.[1] The elite performer is equivalent of the vocal athlete whose voice must perform optimally for his or her livelihood. There are other professionals including educators, ministers, lawyers, salespeople, auctioneers, lecturers, and health care providers, to name a few, who fall into the category of professional voice users such that when vocal quality is affected, job performance is also affected.[2,3] Many less "public" professionals are also "at risk" for the development of laryngeal disorders with the same level of social, emotional, and job-threatening anxieties present. Individuals who depend on their voices to function successfully in their occupations, may be considered professional voice users. For many, the care and proper use of the voice may never become an issue. For others, a voice disorder may create real or imagined personal threats. A voice disorder may have an impact on the person's quality of life.[4] The psychodynamics of vocal management may dictate the success or failure these professionals experience within their professions.

HISTORY

The 20th century benefited from the visionary efforts of G Paul Moore, PhD, Hans von Leden, MD, and Wilber J Gould, MD, in their advancement of the treatment of the professional voice. Their fundamental foundation of building a multidisciplined treatment approach, combining professionals from art and science, continues to generate national and international collaborative research in the area of voice. From this collaborative effort, professional conferences on voice are held both nationally and internationally.

These conferences bring together otolaryngologists/phoniatricians, speech-language pathologists/logopedists, vocologists, voice scientists, biomechanical engineers, physicists, singing teachers, voice coaches, singers, actors, performers, acting teachers, acousticians, and other professionals interested in the area of voice. They provide information on the most recent advancements in the areas of technology, science, and clinical applications regarding the study of voice. In 1971, New York's Juilliard School of Music hosted the first Voice Foundation Symposium on the Care of the Professional Voice (http://www.voicefoundation.org) under the direction of W J Gould, MD. This symposium, currently held in Philadelphia under the chairmanship of Robert T Sataloff, MD, presented its 42nd conference in 2013. This conference is the oldest organization dedicated to voice medicine, science, and education. Its mission is to enhance knowledge, care, and training of the voice through educational programs and publications for voice care professionals, the public, and professional voice users, and through supporting and funding research. An annual symposium is held each year on the care of the professional voice focusing on new research on vocal production and techniques for the treatment of voice disorders. The Voice Foundation supports a bimonthly peer-reviewed journal, the *Journal of Voice* (http://www.jvoice.org), which publishes the transcripts from the symposium as well as articles on voice medicine and clinical and laboratory research. Other national and international conferences are held yearly or every several years focusing on the professional voice. In 1980, researchers in the fields of voice science and laryngology presented biennially at the Vocal Fold Physiology conferences. This conference continues to be held; however, the name has changed to International Conferences on Voice Physiology & Biomechanics and the 8th conference was held in 2012. The International Association of Logopedics and Phoniatrics (IALP) (http://www.ialp.info), started in 1924 by Emil Froeschels in Vienna, Austria, brought about the collaboration of professionals and scientists interested in speech and voice worldwide. It is the oldest international organization with members from more than 57 countries and 58 worldwide affiliated societies. This organization has consultative status with the World Health Organization of the United Nations and works in association with the UN Department of Public Information. The IALP meets every 3 years, and the 29th IALP World Congress is scheduled to be held in Torino, Italy, in 2013. Another interdisciplinary conference for voice professionals is the Pan-European Voice Conference (PEVOC) (http://www.pevoc.org) established in 1995. Their meetings are held biennially with the 10th conference being held in Prague, Czech Republic, in 2013. A global interest in voice care to promote laryngeal research brought about the first World Voice Congress held in 1995 in Oporto, Portugal.

April 16 is World Voice Day. This date was initiated in Brazil in 1999 as the Brazilian National Voice Day and has become an international event ever since its conception. The goal of World Voice Day is to heighten public awareness regarding the importance of the voice and vocal problems. It is also a day of "celebration of interdisciplinary and interaction between arts and science."[5] In 2002, the American Academy of Otolaryngology-Head and Neck Surgery officially recognized this day in the United States (http://www.entnet.org). Various cities in the United States celebrate World Voice Day by providing voice screenings, sponsoring concerts/vocal performances, conducting media interviews, and providing educational material on maintaining good vocal health as well as other events.

Throughout the United States, and in some other countries, otolaryngology offices have adopted the team approach in the treatment of voice disorders. Otolaryngological centers throughout the United States pride themselves on being providers of voice care excellence. In addition to the otolaryngologist and voice pathologist, a teacher of singing is often on staff. The voice pathologist is licensed to provide voice therapy for the injured voice, and the teacher of singing provides instructions pertaining to singing and vocal technique. Dual specialization exists where teachers of singing are also certified speech-language pathologists. The American Speech-Language-Hearing Association (ASHA) and National Association of Teachers of Singing (NATS) published a joint statement on voice therapy for singers.[6] In this statement, any member of NATS who has taken the recommended coursework outlined is qualified to work with an otolaryngologist and a speech-language pathologist as a team in remediating diagnosed voice disorders. This professional is precluded from doing voice therapy unless he or she is also licensed and certified as a speech-language pathologist. Likewise, the voice pathologist who works with singers needs to receive instructions in vocal pedagogy and voice performance and should not provide singing instruction unless the voice pathologist is an experienced teacher of singing and has met the requirements of NATS.

The National Association of Teachers of Singing (NATS) (http://www.nats.org) was founded in 1944 by the American Academy of Teachers of Singing, the New York Singing Teachers Association, and the Chicago Singing Teachers Guild.[7] This organization strives to promote the highest standards of singing through teaching and research. The association's periodical, *Journal of Singing*, is the only professional journal in the United States devoted to singing and the teaching of singing.[8] This journal publishes articles 5 times yearly on the art of singing, vocal function, vocal literature, care of the professional voice, voice science, diction, voice medicine, and voice pedagogy. NATS provides workshops, intern programs, master classes, and conferences at chapter levels and at the national level.

Another organization that serves the professional voice user is the Voice and Speech Trainers Association (VASTA) (http://www.vasta.org). Founded in 1986, this organization is dedicated to voice and speech training for the professional voice user in acting and the performing arts. The mission of VASTA is to advance the needs of voice and speech specialists, teachers, and students in training and in practice and advance the art, research, and visibility of the voice and speech. The association publishes a *VASTA eNewsletter*. Annual conferences and workshops are also published on the website.

Both NATS and VASTA extend an affiliation membership to professionals or groups in related fields interested in the professional voice. Many voice pathologists and otolaryngologists have memberships in both organizations and receive publications and attend conferences to learn current research and training directions in the performing arts.

Internationally, the British Voice Association (BVA) began in the 1980s as a study group for individuals interested in learning more about the voice. It was initially established as the Voice Research Society, and in 1991 the name was changed to the British Voice Association (http://www.britishvoiceassociation.org.uk). The BVA has over 600 multidisciplinary professionals working to promote the field of voice through symposiums, conferences, workshops, training courses, and interactive study days.

Because voice pathologists, teachers of singing, and theater trainers all work with the performer and because some of the techniques used are similar, a word of caution is in order. It is critical that we maintain focus within our scope of practice and respect other's professional boundaries. Treating voice and speech disorders has legal implications and requires a master's degree in speech pathology, as well as a license and certification. Similarly, voice pathologists are not trained to teach singing or acting; therefore, it is necessary to work together to achieve the professional goals in vocally rehabilitating the performer. Our collaborative efforts will bring about impressive results and provide the best possible care for performers to use their instrument optimally in speech and singing and maintain a healthy laryngeal mechanism. Table 8–1 lists the websites of our collaborative partners.

Table 8–1. Websites of Our Collaborative Partners in Voice Care

WEBSITES
American Academy of Otolaryngology-Head and Neck Surgery http://www.entnet.org
Pan-European Voice Conference http://www.pevoc.org
The British Voice Association http://www.britishvoiceassociation.org.uk
The International Association of Logopedics and Phoniatrics http://www.ialp.info
Journal of Voice http://www.jvoice.org
The National Association of Teachers of Singing http://www.nats.org
The Voice Foundation http://www.voicefoundation.org
Voice and Speech Trainers Association http://www.vasta.org

THE "AT-RISK" STATUS

Individuals who use their voices professionally are subject to the development of laryngeal pathologies due to any of the etiologic factors mentioned in previous chapters. As voice pathologists, we must be acutely aware of the influences of phonotrauma and vocal misuse on the laryngeal system. We cannot assume the professional voice user understands the relationship of these at-risk behaviors and how these behaviors correlate with changes in vocal performance. We find only a few professional voice owners who have even a vague awareness of the anatomy and physiology of the vocal mechanism. Also, although many people possess "trained" voices for acting, singing, and public speaking and excellent techniques for these functions, other vocal misuses and abuses are often present as primary causes of their vocal difficulties.

Similarities between singers and actors and individuals who are athletes are quite parallel. Athletes, because of the physical nature of their work, are at greater risk than most people for developing muscular and joint injuries. Likewise, because actors and singers are dependent on their voices and, as a rule, demand more from them than the average speaker, they are at greater risk for developing laryngeal pathologies.[9] Despite these similarities, a major difference exists between the management approaches of athletes and professional voice users. The prized athlete generally rests the injury long enough for it to heal and for the possibility of permanent damage to be eliminated. Singers and actors, however, usually minimize the disability to avoid canceling an engagement and continue to use the voice, often risking permanent damage. After all, "The show must go on!"

The less "public" professional voice users behave in the same manner as singers and actors. Educators continue to teach, speech-language pathologists continue to practice, teachers of singing continue to teach, vocal coaches continue to teach acting, salespeople continue to sell, preachers/ministers continue to preach, and receptionists continue to perform their vocal duties, rather than risk loss of income or damage to their professional reputation.

PROFESSIONAL ROLES

Successful treatment of voice disorders in the professional voice user relies on a multidisciplinary team to attend to the various vocal needs and to the individual's professional and social needs to assist in the prevention, care, and training of all types of voice problems. Each member of the team should have a keen understanding of the pathophysiology of the individual's voice disorder. The key members of the voice care team include the otolaryngologist, voice pathologist, and primary care physician. Other specialists may include the singing teacher, drama coach, music educators, vocal coaches, psychologist, psychiatrist, allergist, neurologist, gastroenterologist, pulmonologist, and occasionally other medical specialties. The composition of the voice care team may differ from individual to individual, depending on the patient's level of vocal usage and demand to return to normal performance. Each individual may react differently to the same type of voice disorder, some willing to accept immediate treatment and others electing to go at a slower pace in remediating the problem(s).

The voice care team members treating the professional voice user will depend on the patient's profession and level of vocal usage. The otolaryngologist, voice pathologist, and primary care physician most often provide support for the nonperformance professional. The otolaryngologist evaluates the laryngeal condition and then treats the condition with rest, medication, surgery, or referral. The voice pathologist evaluates the causes of the laryngeal pathology and then establishes a program for the modification or elimination of these behaviors. The primary care physician continues to treat the patient for other health-related problems that may or may not contribute to the voice disorder.

Professionals who use the voice for stage and singing performances are often subjected to demands of other individuals in addition to the otolaryngologist and voice pathologist. These individuals may include the producer of the event, the director, the agent and/or manager of the performer, the stage manager, and possibly the vocal teacher or coach. Let us examine the roles of each.

The Otolaryngologist

The major role of the otolaryngologist in the treatment of the professional voice is in the physical diagnosis of the laryngeal mechanism to determine the condition and the function of the mechanism at that moment. When presented with a laryngeal pathology in a professional voice user, the otolaryngologist is often asked to "get me through this performance!" When faced with an important performance, such as a one-time audition, opening night, or a one-night stand, it is often possible for the otolaryngologist to administer anti-inflammatory steroid hormones (prednisone-like drugs) and vasoconstrictors that may make it possible for the patient to perform. In making the decision to help a patient make it through the single important performance, however, it is extremely important to balance the risk of further or more permanent damage against the need to perform. The performer must understand that a "quick fix" is possible but not the long-term solution. Administering drugs in these cases is much like doping a racehorse or an athlete. A short period of voice rest is often recommended after such performances. Caution to the performer in seeking out a physician who readily prescribes these medications because they usually mask the symptoms and may cause further damage and longer recovery periods. For chronic vocal disorders there may be a necessity for daily medication, such as those precipitated by laryngopharyngeal reflux[10–13] or allergies, to maintain a balance. Administration of medication(s) depends on the etiology of the dysphonia. Input from the voice pathologist is paramount to the successful recovery of the performer's voice. Depending on the etiology of the vocal problem, surgery is usually withheld as a last resort and performed when the patient has complied with all presurgical conditioning procedures in voice therapy.

When phonosurgery is performed, great care is taken to preserve the free vibratory vocal fold edge preserving the mucosal wave. As previously mentioned, voice is dependent on respiration, phonation, and resonance. Surgery that alters any one of these components can affect the voice quality of the vocal performer. The surgeon should discuss possible subtle changes with the patient prior to surgery.[14] Postsurgical guidelines, reviewed prior to surgery, must be strictly followed to assure proper healing and recovery. Minimal recommendations following laryngeal surgery include 7 days of complete vocal rest, consuming 2 L of water daily, and the elimination of all caffeinated beverages.

The Voice Pathologist

The voice pathologist evaluates all aspects of voice use and production including breath support, phonation, and resonance or (placement) of the voice to determine the causes of the voice disorder. When working with the professional voice user, nonstage voicing habits and the performer's technique need to be assessed separately to determine the etiologic factors that contribute to the voice disorder. These voicing habits may not be apparent during the office evaluation and case history interview. It is useful to obtain tape recordings of the speaker's voice in various settings, set up role-play scenarios, and whenever possible, observe live performances. This need is especially critical with teachers, salespeople, ministers, preachers, politicians, and lecturers. It is essential when working with performers. Inappropriate vocal components that are not heard during the quiet conversational voice used throughout the diagnostic evaluation are often quite evident during public presentations. The voice pathologist "must become familiar with the full range of vocal stressors that may be found in the performance environment."[15]

Once the causes for the disorder have been identified, however subtle, the impact these causes have on the vocal mechanism must be described in detail to the patient. The voice pathologist must compile all the data collected from patient history, observation, acoustic and aerodynamic testing, videostroboscopy, as well as the patient's perceptual and physiological sensations to develop a hypothesis of the cause as it relates to respiration, phonation, and resonance. Using pictures, diagrams, and models to describe the laryngeal mechanism and the pathology is extremely helpful for patient understanding. If a copy of the videolaryngostroboscopic evaluation is available, the educational benefits are enormous. Many people who use voice for their livelihoods have very little knowledge of the normal structure and function of the laryngeal mechanism. Providing this information is an important role of the voice pathologist. Issues regarding general vocal hygiene should be discussed as they relate to the patient's specific voice disorder. A management plan is then tailored to the patient and is designed to modify or eliminate the causes of the voice disorder.

If pathology is present and begins to resolve, efforts are made to rebuild the patient's vocal confidence. The public voice is gradually reintroduced and tested by the patient for effectiveness. When the laryngeal mechanism is healthy and the patient's confidence has been renewed, the patient is discharged from therapy with periodic recheck times established.

At times, the diagnostic evaluation of a singer will yield no etiologic factors responsible for the development of the voice disorder. When this occurs, a competent vocal coach should be found who would evaluate the present singing techniques and modify them as needed to attain a healthy mechanism.

The final goal of voice therapy is not only the return of normal laryngeal structure and function, but also the development of an understanding that the ultimate responsibility for the well-being of the laryngeal mechanism rests with the professional voice user and not the otolaryngologist, voice pathologist, producer, agent, manager, or coach. In spite of the pressures to perform in the presence of vocal difficulties, the owner of the voice must take charge. Decisions regarding whether or not to perform may be made by honestly answering a single question: "Will I compromise the rest of my career by performing tonight?"

When working with performers, it is important for the voice pathologist to understand specific vocabulary with which the performer is familiar and how the vocal problem may result in a physical alteration or limitation of a desired effect. Examples of terms (see glossary of singing terms at the end of this chapter) include *messa di voce, vibrato, passaggio, leggiero,* and *tessitura,* to name a few. Voice pathologists are directed to study the science behind the performance in an attempt to understand the working mechanics of each integral part as it relates to the whole system.[16–19] Performers understand imagery and visualization terms (such as focus, lift, placement, mask, dark color, bright color, ring, and buzz) that are used to describe specific artistic outcome of a tone. These terms are difficult to define scientifically but take on an interpretation and meaning within the individual and between the performer and singing or acting teacher. It may be beneficial for the voice pathologist to learn the "feel" of these terms by taking classes or observing a master instructor in the performing arts.

The Producer

The producer of a public event has the major responsibility of guaranteeing that the money invested in the performance is secure. The producer is responsible for overseeing the operations of the event and for reacting quickly and positively to any situations that could threaten the event's success. These situations include dealing with the physical and emotional problems and needs of the performers. Keeping in mind that the producer's main concern is the financial success of the event, it is not difficult to understand that this pressure would possibly make the producer less than sympathetic of a performer's vocal problems. The inability to perform is a threat not only to the event's success, but ultimately to the producer's reputation, which is responsible for securing investors for future events. The producer may, therefore, apply great pressure on the performer or the performer's manager or agent to guarantee that the "show must go on."

The Agent or Manager

The agent or manager is responsible for the overall career development of the professional voice user. Career development involves selling the performer's services to producers, developing public relations strategies, deciding appropriate jobs to accept or reject, scheduling performances, and often handling business affairs.

There is huge competition among a great number of performers for a very limited number of parts. Professionals who are good enough or lucky enough to find steady work in the performing arts are usually associated with top managers. These performers often sustain themselves as attractive employees through their own professional reliability. It is the manager's or agent's responsibility to guarantee that his or her clients remain as attractive as possible to those in the hiring positions. The success and the financial gain of the manager or agent are totally dependent on his or her ability to keep clients working. The more clients work, the more attractive is the manager to other potential clients. Producers will not hire performers who have developed reputations for unreliability. This reputation may be developed quickly, especially by performers in the nonstar category. Therefore, we may understand the pressure that the manager or agent may place on a client to perform even in the presence of vocal difficulties. This pressure to perform is not an indictment of producers, managers, or agents, but is simply a statement of the reality of competing interests.

CLINICAL PATHWAYS

A number of disciplines are involved with the voice care team. How can all the disciplines work together, and who should address what problems when the professional has a vocal problem? There is no set protocol for providing care for the professional voice user. Nonetheless, the key personnel providing care for the professional voice user include the otolaryngologist, voice pathologist, and vocal pedagogue. Let us look at some possibilities.

Otolaryngology-Voice Pathology-Voice Pedagogy

Referrals to the otolaryngologist come from many sources. There are self-referrals, but more often, referrals come from primary care physicians. The chief complaint is dysphonia with hoarseness. Additionally, the individual may be referred for complaints of a "lump" sensation in the throat, dysphagia, sinus drainage, allergies, ear problems, throat discomfort, cough, airway problems, or possible neurological involvement. Other medical disciplines also refer directly to the otolaryngologist. The otolaryngologist diagnoses the etiology of the voice problem after taking a thorough medical history and examining the larynx via a mirror examination or using a flexible endoscope or videostroboscopy.[20] The individual is treated medically if warranted. The otolaryngologist refers to the voice pathologist for evaluation. The voice pathologist works to:

- re-educate the individual on vocal hygiene
- provide vocal exercises designed to balance the subsystems of voice production
- provide vocal exercises to promote an open front focus using diaphragmatic breath support
- provide exercises to reduce muscular tension
- design regimens to eliminate all phonotrauma behaviors and vocal misuses
- provide continued support in counseling the patient regarding reflux precautions if needed.

Voice therapy is recommended prior to removal of any mass lesion(s) that may have been created from improper or phonotraumatic vocal techniques. If therapy does not occur prior to surgical removal of a lesion(s) and the patient is unaware of the possible etiology of the dysphonia, the likelihood of recurrence is much greater.[21,22] During vocal rehabilitation with the voice pathologist, it is advisable that the performer work with the voice teacher or vocal coach. Often the individual has altered vocal technique in response to the dysphonia. It is necessary for the performer to learn or relearn to use a healthy technique that will reduce or eliminate the chances of future vocal problems. It is important for the professional voice user to follow suggestions to stay vocally healthy. Table 8–2 lists tips for staying vocally healthy.

Voice Pedagogy-Otolaryngologist-Voice Pathology

When working closely with the professional voice user, the teacher of singing or vocal coach may detect subtle perceptual changes or possible limitations

Table 8–2. Tips for Staying Vocally Healthy

Seek medical attention if the following occur, and never ignore warning signs like hoarseness; chronic coughing; throat clearing; change in vocal quality; loss of voice; change in the range of the singing voice; sore, burning, or achy throat; throat pain; or problems swallowing. **Voice disorders can be caused by infections, misuse and phonotraumatic behaviors, benign and malignant growths, neuromuscular diseases, and psychogenic causes.**
• Drink plenty of water, "pee pale"—systemic hydration is important for a healthy voice and to keep secretions thin. • Avoid caffeinated beverages (tea, coffee, or soft drinks) as they are drying agents. • Avoid recreational drug use and/or excessive alcohol use. • Avoid breathing chemicals, dust, or other harmful inhalants or irritants. • Do not smoke, and avoid smoky rooms. • Take "vocal naps" throughout the day to rest the voice, especially if vocally active • Rest the voice regularly, especially if singing aggressively. Take 1 day off for every 3 days of performing or 2 days off for every 5 days of performing. • Avoid talking too loudly, especially in a noisy environment. • Do not talk above loud noise, and reduce ambient noise or turn off the television, radio, machinery, vacuum cleaner, blowers, etc, before talking in person or on the phone. • Avoid yelling or screaming at sporting events—use nonverbal expressions such as clapping or blowing a whistle to show enthusiasm. • Hold face-to-face conversations. • Move closer to the person(s) engaged in conversation or move into a quieter location to talk without yelling or straining the voice. • Use amplification when speaking to large groups or speaking in a large room. • Avoid overuse of the speaking and singing voice—rest the voice when the voice is tired or fatigued. • Avoid throat clearing by substituting a hard swallow, taking a sip of water and swallowing, or using a nonvocalized clear and swallow. • Try to cough quietly. If there is a need to cough, take a deep breath and support from the diaphragm instead of using the throat to cough up secretions. May use a "huff" cough support with a deep breath. • Do not sing higher or lower than is comfortable. • Do not sing if it hurts, or if it hurts to swallow. • Check with your physician or pharmacist on medications (over the counter or prescription) that may have adverse drying effects on the tissue of the larynx. • Use a facial steam inhaler for direct moisturization of the tissue of the larynx and vocal folds to help with excessive dryness or thick secretions in the throat. • Use good posture and support the voice with a deep breath (diaphragmatic breathing) to prevent vocal strain or tension. • Get plenty of rest, especially the night before a vocally demanding day or performance. • Do not whisper.

in the voice. The performer may have acute or chronic vocal problems. Symptoms may include increased effort to initiate voicing, difficulty sustaining voice (especially on softer tones), increase in recovery time, loss of vocal range, vocal fatigue or pain after performance, and more notable, *passaggio*. The referral to the otolaryngologist may come directly from the teacher of singing or vocal coach. Once assessed by the otolaryngologist, the individual is then referred to the voice pathologist to interpret and describe stroboscopic findings. Findings may indicate a muscle tension dysphonia. Voice therapy would then be recommended to focus on a return to healthy laryngeal function in both speech and singing.

Voice Pedagogy-Voice Pathology-Otolaryngology

Over the last 30 years, teachers of singing and vocal coaches have worked closely with trained speech-language pathologists who have specialized in the area of voice, particularly if a voice lab is within the same city or nearby. Some voice labs offer stroboscopic screenings for freshman vocal or theatrical majors to serve as a baseline. In most voice labs throughout the United States, the voice pathologist performs videolaryngostroboscopic examinations, interprets laryngeal function, and reviews these results with the otolaryngologist. By establishing these close professional working relationships, the teacher of singing or vocal coach may refer directly to the voice pathologist when the performer is having vocal problems. Often the individuals have not seen an otolaryngologist; therefore, medical referral would then come from the voice pathologist.

Otolaryngology-Voice Pedagogy

The performer may be on the road, traveling to different cities when a vocal problem develops. An otolaryngologist may see the performer and treat the problem medically if needed. The performer's problem may be with vocal technique or style. Performers generally study or have studied with a teacher of singing or vocal coach. It would be appropriate for the otolaryngologist to refer back to the vocal pedagogue to address issues of technique; address changes in style, repertoire, or environmental conditions; and evaluate preexisting conditions that are or have been troublesome for the individual. The vocal pedagogue can offer suggestions on vocal rehearsals, vocal use, and vocal warm-ups.

Voice Pathologist-Voice Pedagogy

The performer may have worked or is currently working with a voice pathologist for vocal rehabilitation and wants to return to performing. Once the underlying condition that caused or contributed to the dysphonia improves, it is appropriate for the voice pathologist to refer to the voice pedagogue for assessment of the singing or acting voice. This is recommended to prevent future injury to the voice during performance.

Vocal Types and Vocal Range

It is beneficial for the voice pathologist to understand vocal types and vocal range of professional singers. Vocal types and vocal range of singers can be confusing. These terms are often used interchangeably and are thus misleading. When evaluating a nonclassical singer or a person who sings for the enjoyment of singing and ask what the person's range is, the reply is, "I am an alto or soprano." Vocal type refers to the kind of voice classified using terms such as *tessituras*, vocal timbre or tone, register transition points, etc. There are 6 operatic vocal types—bass, baritone, tenor, contralto/alto, mezzo-soprano, and soprano; however, within each of the vocal types there are subtypes such as a bass-baritone or a dramatic coloratura soprano. In choral music, music sung by a choir, there are 4 vocal types including soprano, tenor, alto, and bass.

Vocal range refers to the full spectrum of notes that each singer is able to produce, from the lowest to the highest pitch. A well-trained singer who has learned how to utilize the vocal instrument optimally will have a more extensive range than an untrained singer. Table 8–3 demonstrates vocal type according to gender and estimated vocal range.[23]

The soprano voice type has a bright tone with usually a strong head voice, and this female voice type is often the lead singer in operas or performances. In contrast, the mezzo soprano has a stronger middle voice and is considered a darker or deeper tone. The contralto voice type has a darker and richer tone compared to the mezzo soprano. The

Table 8–3. Vocal Type by Gender and Range

Gender	Voice Types	Vocal Range (Estimate Notes)	Description of Voice Type
Female	Soprano	A3 to F6 or G6	Highest of the adult female voices
	Soprano (head voice)	E4 to F5	
	Mezzo Soprano	G3 to C6	Most common adult female voice
	Mezzo Soprano (head voice)	E4 to E5	
	Contralto/Alto	E3 to G5	Lowest of the adult female voices
	Contralto/Alto (head voice)	G4 to D5	
Male	Falsetto, Countertenor	G3 to F5	Highest adult male voice and with projection
	Tenor	C3 to G5	Typical highest of the adult male voice
	Baritone	F2 to E4	Most common of the adult male voice
	Bass	F2 to E4	Lowest of the adult male voice

countertenor is the highest of the adult male voice types and is similar to the range of the female contralto voice. The most comfortable range for this type of singer lies above the tenor male voice. The countertenor's head voice is bright in tone and may be confused with a female voice. The typical high adult male voice is the tenor whose voice is bright and strong in the head voice. The baritone vocal type is the most common adult male voice, and the strength of that vocal type lies in the middle of the range. A deep, dark resonating vocal type is that of the bass adult male which is the lowest of the range. The most comfortable range for this type is below the baritone level.

In the operatic world, vocal types can be subdivided into categories based on vocal agility. These 5 categories are light, lyric, full, dramatic, and coloratura. Light refers to a voice that is bright and youthful as well as sweet and lightweight. This type of voice would be youthful, flirty, and fun. A lyric voice refers to a medium-size voice with warm color, and the singer would need to sing long and even phrases. A lyric voice would be cast for a romantic or sympathetic role and must be loud enough to be heard over the orchestra. The full voice is louder and heavier as well as being strong. A dramatic voice is powerful and louder than a full voice and considered big, heavier, and with increased strength to sing over a large orchestra. The coloratura voice is considered flexible, and the vocalist must be able to move quickly through fast singing lines easily. These 5 classical descriptors can be used in combination with a lyric coloratura soprano. This singer must have warmth and be able to move through lines quickly verses a dramatic coloratura soprano requiring a powerful voice, yet be able to have the rapid flexibility in singing the lines fast and with ease.

CATEGORIES OF SINGERS

Bunch and Chapman[24] systematically categorized the performance abilities of singers. They described 18 types of singers (opera to street singers) and 9 categories based on performance achievement (superstar to child). Using these categories in research, the authors offer a definitive way of evaluating singers solely on accomplishment and achievement in performance and compare types of singing within the same category and at different levels among categories.

VOCAL REGISTERS

The term *vocal register* can be used for both the speaking and singing voice. Vocal registers refer to the different ranges of vocal fundamental frequencies and vocal fold edge patterns and are classified as modal, pulse/glottal fry, and falsetto/loft. The lowest register is referred to as the pulse/glottal fry, with the modal being the middle register, and the falsetto the highest register. Conversational speech falls in the modal range of frequencies; however, individuals may speak toward the lower range and drop to the pulse register at the end of a sentence.[25,26]

Hollien[27] described the registers can be differentiated and identified on perceptual vocal quality, the physiological length or thickness, and vibratory patterns of the vocal folds and the aerodynamic characteristics related to subglottal pressure, airflow, glottal resistance, and vocal intensity.

The pulse register or glottal fry is characterized by decreased vocal fold stiffness,[28] decreased lung pressure and airflow,[29] and decreased length and thickness of the vocal folds.[30] Chen et al[31] reported the speed quotient of glottal fry was increased during electroglottographic results compared to modal phonation. This was most likely due to the decrease in lung pressure resulting in a longer duration of the open phase. Glottal fry is the production of a low fundamental frequency with a range of 35 to 50 Hz which is the same for males and females.[32]

The modal register is also referred to as the chest or speech register that includes the range of frequencies used in speaking. For men, the range of fundamental frequencies is around 75 to 450 Hz and for females around 130 to 520 Hz.[33] Blomgren et al[34] reported the average modal speaking frequency for adult females is 211 Hz (range 175–266 Hz) and 117 Hz (range 86–170 Hz) for adult men.

The falsetto register (highest) occurs with the contraction of the cricothyroid muscles. The true vocal folds elongate and mass decreases, resulting in increased tension on the vocal folds and stiffness. Reduction of amplitude of vibration and mucosal wave and decreased glottal closure and higher open quotient during the vibratory cycle have been observed in high-speed films[35,36] and stroboscopy.[37] The falsetto voice has frequencies occurring above modal register and is recognizable in the adult male voice with a speaking pitch of 300 to 600 Hz.[38]

COMMON ETIOLOGIC FACTORS

Personality Factors

Intense, volatile, excitable, emotional, neurotic, anxious, temperamental, moody, intemperate, vain, and unstable are all terms Punt used when describing the personalities of professional actors and singers.[39] Although these personality attributes have also been described as necessary for the successful artist, a person's emotional or mental state will have an effect on vocal production. Weiner supported this view when he stated the human voice is one of the most accurate and sensitive indicators of the state of a personality; it tends to mirror what is happening in a person's life.[40]

Punt further indicated the direct relationship between emotions and voice quality by observing that in times of extreme stress, even the trained voice user will project emotional problems into the voice.[39] The vocal mechanism may even be perfectly healthy and free of visible pathology, but its precision of movement may be adversely affected by the state of mind and the emotions of the owner of the voice.

Many of these personality factors are also present in many "unartistic" professional voice users. For example, salespeople are often described as driven, intense, and fast talking. Ministers may be subjected to great emotional strain due to the personal needs and problems of congregational members. Physicians may be under stress due to demands of patients and their families. Educators and lecturers struggle with anxiety regarding teaching responsibilities.

They may also worry about receiving good evaluations or securing jobs or promotions. In short, inherent personality characteristics, which are to some extent demanded of professional voice users, along with the anxieties and stresses created by the various professional challenges, may all contribute to the development of a voice disorder.

Phonotrauma

Individuals who use their voices professionally are subject to the same vocal misuses and phonotraumatic behaviors as those found in the general speaking public. However, the overall effect that phonotraumatic behaviors have on the livelihood of the professional voice user is more detrimental. For example, the laryngeal changes associated with shouting at a football or basketball game would not be the same for the professional and nonprofessional voice users. Let us speculate that mild edema and erythema developed resulting in a mild to moderate dysphonia. The nonprofessional voice user would be able to return to work the next day with no ill effect on job performance, whereas the professional voice user may suffer the consequences of a missed performance, a lost sale, an inadequate public appeal, and so forth.

Another factor associated with phonotrauma and professional voice users is the unique, itinerant lifestyle they live. Inherent in the lifestyles of many public "performers" are periods of socializing and other extraneous activities that may contribute to vocal hyperfunction. These activities may include talking over noise in the hustle and bustle of the backstage area following a performance; loud talking during post performance dinners and parties; or unusual vocal demands created by frequent public appearances that take place in noisy public forums for promotional purposes.

Phonotrauma and vocal misuse behaviors may also occur during performances. Many singers and actors have highly trained voices, but others may be guilty of using inappropriate vocal techniques. These inappropriate uses of vocal components may be present while singing musical roles not suited to the artist's voice, while using inappropriate respiratory support for a particular role, or while singing or speaking with an improper tone focus. Although loud singing and stage shouting need not be vocally abusive, they often create vocal problems in the untrained voice. When these activities do cause vocal problems, the difficulties usually are the result of a lack of abdominal/diaphragmatic breath support, the use of hard glottal attacks, and a general constriction of the upper vocal tract. Training to promote an open front focus using abdominal/diaphragmatic breath support in the speaking voice is beneficial for the singer, actor, and nonprofessional voice user.

By the nature of their acting roles, actors often work in less than optimal conditions on stage. Some theaters are designed with appropriate acoustics, whereas others place more demands on the human voice. Volatile or emotional character portrayals can be potentially harmful even to the trained "vocal athlete." Many are requested to scream, cry, shriek, cough, gasp, and so forth, in addition to competing with various accompanying background music, noises, and sounds. Costumes and makeup may place added restrictions, creating limited mobility and requiring more demand on the voice.[41]

Assessment of vocal technique by a trained acting-voice trainer on body alignment, body tension, breath support, relaxation, and isolation of the articulators, forward placement, and presentation style is essential to develop and maintain a healthy acting voice. The actor must be aware and note areas of body tension, such as locked knees, clenched jaw, relaxed abdominal breathing, and proper alignment of the head being balanced over a lengthened and relaxed neck and spine. A projected voice should be produced with relaxed articulators and a forward resonating focus, connecting the breath through the vocal tract without muscular tension.[42]

Another potential form of phonotrauma in the singer is the use of a singing technique known as belting. Belting is often used in theatrical shows for projection of the voice. The belted singing voice is produced at a high intensity level with strong vocal fold adduction. As long as the respiratory effort is adequate to support the voice and the supraglottic structures are not constricted, belting is not abusive. Vocal problems occur when the respiratory effort is inadequate for the high intensity level, causing constriction of the entire upper airway. Numerous popular singers have constructed successful careers using this form of singing, but many others have suffered harsh vocal consequences as a result of this form of laryngeal hyperfunction.

After a big performance, voice rest or vocal naps (short periods of no talking throughout the day) over a 2- or 3-day period is recommended to allow for healing. Longevity of the voice may depend on the need to incorporate a vocal recovery period and take time for tissue regeneration.[43]

Phonotrauma may also be related to environmental conditions in which the performer works. For example, the classical singer may be forced to compete with an overly enthusiastic and loud orchestra in a hall with limited or poor acoustics and a musty backstage area. Rock singers often compete with the high intensity levels of their own heavily amplified electronic instruments. Other entertainers sing or perform in small clubs with dense ambient smoke and must compete with noisy patrons and poor amplification. Actors compete with various special effects, such as smoke and background noises. Considering the environments in which many professionals are asked to perform, it is surprising that more voice disorders do not occur.

Other less "public" professional voice users have their own forms of vocal abuse. The following are examples:

- Teachers who shout during playground, cafeteria, or bus duty
- Salespeople who often hold business meetings or make sales presentations over lunch in noisy restaurants
- Ministers who give sermons at the top of their loudness range without the aid of a amplification
- Politicians who present frequently in various surroundings without use of amplification.

Many salespeople use a pseudoauthoritative voice with greater vocal effort. Continued use of this hyperfunctional voice will often lead to laryngeal pathology. A demanding vocal load, particularly under conditions of speaking in increased levels of background noise, poor environmental acoustics, and poor atmospheric humidity are factors that may contribute to vocal difficulties.[44]

In concluding this section on phonotrauma and the professional voice user, it is strongly suggested that the voice pathologist consider the obvious when evaluating these patients. These may include common vocal behaviors such as shouting at children, pets, or during sporting events; talking loudly to a hard-of-hearing relative; constantly clearing the throat, having a persistent cough, grunting during exercise such as weight lifting, engaging in prolonged talking, using abusive laughter, and shouting in anger. All of these behaviors are just as likely to occur in the professional as in the nonprofessional voice user.

Drugs

Many medications can contribute to laryngeal side effects and become detrimental to the professional voice user.[45] Many factors (such as age, gender, body composition, metabolism, and concurrent administration of other medications) can influence a person's response to a medication(s). Some individuals are very sensitive to minimum dosing levels; therefore, finding the correct dosage for the performer is critical to prevent or reduce possible side effects that may affect the voice.[46,47] There are a number of prescription medicines and over-the-counter agents that can adversely affect the voice.[48,49]

Recreational drugs such as alcohol, cigarettes, marijuana, and cocaine have significant adverse effects on voice production. All of these agents are irritating to the respiratory tract and larynx and may contribute to the development of voice disorders. Some of the reasons given by professional voice users for using these abusive agents include the following:

- stress and pressures of auditions and subsequent rejection
- stress of giving performances that will always please the audiences
- tight schedules that yield minimal time for relaxation
- difficult personal relationships
- individual emotional conflicts.

In addition to these reasons, it is fair to say that our culture has influenced the use of alcohol and "recreational" drugs not only in this population, but also in the general population.

Alcohol is abusive both as a local oral and laryngeal irritant and as a vasodilator of the mucosal lining of the larynx. The effect of vasodilatation is drying of the mucous membrane that increases the likelihood of vocal fold hemorrhage during phonation. Excessive consumption of alcohol may lead to a chronic dysphonia, which has been commonly described as a "gin" or "whiskey" voice.[50] Caffeine is also a vasodilator and has a dehydrating effect on the mucosal membrane. It is found in products such as coffee, tea, soda, chocolate, and prescription and nonprescription drugs. Excessive caffeine intake can lead to thick, sticky mucus that accumulates on the true vocal fold surface. Thick mucus on the vocal folds can lead to chronic habitual throat clearing or coughing. Cigarette and marijuana smoke are both irritants of the respiratory tract and larynx. Both types of smoke dry out the mucosal lining of the larynx causing mild edema and erythema. This laryngeal condition causes an increased sensitivity that often creates excessive coughing, which is also vocally abusive. Cocaine is also a local irritant that produces changes in the nasal, pharyngeal, and laryngeal mucosal linings.

Hydration

Hydration is extremely important for optimal mucosal wave vibration and performance of the entire laryngeal system. Systemic tissue hydration is necessary for the 3 subsystems of voice to work efficiently without effort to produce voice. The body functions optimally when it is adequately hydrated. Dehydration causes depletion of moisture content at the cellular level, and systemic dehydration can augment the problem. We can use the late Dr Van Lawrence's axiom, "sing wet and pee pale" as a rule of thumb in monitoring one's degree of internal systemic hydration. For adults, 2 L of water is recommended for adequate daily consumption.

Verdolini-Marston et al[51] manipulated conditions of hydration (no-treatment, hydrated, and slightly dehydrated) and found phonation threshold pressure, especially for higher pitches, decreased in the hydrated condition. Highest phonation threshold pressures were found for the dry condition, especially at low pitches. Hydration is also an important ingredient for treatment of nodules and polyps during therapy with greater improvement seen following hydration.[52] The inverse relation between phonatory effort and hydration levels, especially for high pitches, was observed in a double-blind, placebo-controlled study.[52] Increased perturbation measures were recorded following inhalation of dry air.[53,54] These studies support the clinical finding of a relationship between hydration and vocal performance and relative humidity and vocal performance.

COMMON PATHOLOGIES

The professional voice user may be susceptible to the development of all types of laryngeal pathologies, but functional pathologies are most likely to occur because of improper or excessive use of voice. These common pathologies include acute and chronic noninfectious laryngitis, vocal nodules, vocal fold polyps, contact ulcers or granulomas, gastroesophageal reflux disease, laryngeal fatigue, vocal fold cysts, and vascular pathologies.

Acute and Chronic Noninfectious Laryngitis

On examining the causes of all laryngeal pathologies in the professional voice user, it is most important to determine whether the cause is long-standing and frequently occurring or whether or simply an acute occurrence. Acute noninfectious laryngitis is usually the result of an unusual, short-term period of vocal misuse. It may result from shouting, vocal enthusiasm at a sporting event, singing out of the optimum range, or consuming an unusual amount of alcohol, caffeine, or cigarettes in a short period of time.

During acute laryngitis, the vocal folds usually have a dull pink color or a thickened, sticky mucus lining. The major symptoms may vary from mild to a severe dysphonia characterized by hoarseness, lowered pitch, and impairment in the vocal range. Singers with acute laryngitis demonstrate difficulty in achieving the upper parts of their ranges, especially at low-intensity levels.

Treatments for acute laryngitis include elimination or modification of the causes, steam inhalation, and short-term voice rest when possible. Voice rest permits the laryngeal muscles and the mucosal lining to rebound from the acute abuse. Continued speaking or singing in the presence of the pathology may lead to more serious pathologies such as submucosal hemorrhages or nodules.

Chronic abuse or misuse of the laryngeal mechanism may lead to the development of chronic, noninfectious laryngitis. A chronic vocal problem is one lasting longer than several weeks. This laryngeal pathology is usually indicative of a long history of vocal difficulties. The etiology of chronic dysphonia may be the result of chronic coughing, throat clearing, laryngopharyngeal reflux, smoking, and yelling or a combination of several abusive behaviors. The vocal characteristics of the chronic condition are similar to acute laryngitis; the dysphonic quality is more permanent and resistant to change. Long-term voice misuse causes drying of the mucous membrane and a more persistent voice fatigue than does the acute condition.

Typical treatment for both acute and chronic laryngitis involves a short period of vocal rest or incorporation of vocal "naps" throughout the day, followed by identification and modification of the causative factors. When a performance or presentation cannot be postponed, it is possible for the otolaryngologist to prepare the patient for the performance with the use of laryngeal spray solutions or corticosteroids that diminish laryngeal sensitivity and reduce congestion and edema. This treatment is usually considered if a period of vocal rest is available after the performance.[39] Because of the high risk of more serious laryngeal damage, this treatment is only used when it is absolutely necessary that the patient perform.

The effects of a dysphonic voice quality caused by noninfectious, chronic laryngitis may have serious implications on the livelihoods of some individuals. Others, however, have used their voice disorders to their advantage by developing distinctive vocal characteristics. More often, the long-term vocal effects of chronic laryngitis lead to the premature end of a performance career or a reduction in earning capabilities.

Vocal Nodules

To the professional voice user, one of the most frightening of all laryngeal pathologies, and the bane of all professional singers, is vocal nodules. We suspect that this fear is present mainly because nodules are one of the most common and most discussed pathologies even among people with a relative naiveté regarding voice disorders. It is not unusual for even the most trained professional singer to develop small bilateral nodules during particularly forceful singing.

The voice symptoms of vocal nodules are extremely variable depending on their size, duration of existence, and mechanical effects on phonation. Efforts to produce normal phonation in the presence of nodules leads to forceful methods of phonation causing voice fatigue and often an inappropriate constriction of the supraglottic structures. Higher tones are most adversely affected, especially when produced at lower intensity levels. Glottal closure is generally hourglass in shape causing airflow leak. Phonation breaks, breathiness, decreased frequency range, and decreased maximum sustained phonation usually occur when nodules are of moderate size or larger. Fibrous nodules create greater stiffness in vibration with decreased amplitude of vibration and mucosal wave.

The treatment of vocal nodules again involves identification and modification of their causes. Along with traditional vocal hygiene counseling, much emphasis is placed on patient education and counseling regarding the impact of nodules on the patient's career. Often, the anxiety level expressed by the patient as a result of the pathology is much higher than the pathology warrants. With the patient's complete cooperation, nodules may often be resolved quickly and effectively with minimal career interruption. Frankly, it is often much easier to modify the causes of vocal nodules than to reverse the long-standing causes of chronic laryngitis.

The voice diagnostic examination may occasionally fail to identify any possible causes for the development of vocal nodules, especially in singers. When causes cannot be identified, evaluation of the singing technique by a competent vocal coach is appropriate. It is not the voice pathologist's role to evaluate artistic techniques or abilities. If the vocal coach or singing teacher finds the technique faulty, then voice lessons designed to improve vocal technique are advised.

Vocal nodules occur more often in the untrained singing voice than in the classically trained voice. Some pop and rock singers have capitalized on dysphonic voice qualities; others agonize over their inability to produce adequate phonation. Resolution of the nodules through traditional voice therapy coupled with vocal training become essential for many untrained singers who wish to continue their careers. Although voice therapy is not long term (approximately 3 months or less), the patient must often sacrifice some performance time in order to restore voice quality. However, it is better to spend time in concentrated voice training to resolve the problem than to continue the vocal struggles. A little time taken now may help to ensure a long career. The alternative may be no career at all.

Peppard et al[55] compared singers and nonsingers with vocal fold nodules to control groups of singers and nonsingers, and found the trained singers without nodules to perform superiorly in all tasks. The singers with nodules were found to have smaller nodules with less impairment of vibratory function and less severe vocal symptoms than their nonsinging counterparts. The singers with nodules also performed better on frequency range and maximum phonation time tasks, in comparison to the nonsingers with nodules, but not as well as normal singers. Singers with vocal problems probably tend to seek evaluation sooner because their vocal demands would show a diminution in performance.

Surgery is occasionally recommended for the excision of vocal nodules, but as a rule of thumb, surgery should be avoided on professionals' vocal folds, if at all possible. Although the physical risks of the surgery may be minimal, the psychological effects could be most damaging. Some patients are reluctant to return to full vocal use for fear of redeveloping the laryngeal pathology. Their fear is often so strong that even though the laryngeal mechanisms are normal, the patients will not use full voice. Of course, this fear jeopardizes their careers. Vocal fold surgery performed without strong counseling from the surgeon or voice pathologist is not advised. Even when surgery is performed, the causes of the pathology must be modified to reduce the possibility of recurrence, and the patient must also follow a plan for successful return to normal phonation.

Contact Ulcers and Granulomas

Contact ulcers occur most commonly in male public speakers, teachers, sales representatives, politicians, and actors. Contact ulcers can result from a grinding, hammering action of the vocal processes of the arytenoid cartilages. These actions occur during the repeated use of a loud, low-pitched, pseudo-authoritative voice, which is often used to project a desired masculine or authority image. The mild to moderate dysphonia that is a result of slowly developing ulcerations is characterized by a low-pitch, husky voice quality. Other factors also associated with the development of contact ulcers involve cigarette smoking, excessive alcohol and caffeine consumption, and reflux of stomach acids into the posterior laryngeal area. Contact ulcers are most effectively treated through retraining the appropriate use of the vocal components of pitch and loudness. Reduction or elimination of alcohol, caffeine, and smoking is also strongly advised. If reflux is the cause of contact ulcers and granulomas, an antireflux regimen is recommended. These patients will need to be monitored closely until the resolution of the pathology.

Gastroesophageal Reflux Disease/ Laryngopharyngeal Reflux

Probably the most underdiagnosed and most common gastrointestinal problem that affects professional voice users is gastroesophageal reflux disease (GERD). Incidence of 7% to 10% of the population has been reported in the literature.[56] Professional and nonprofessional voice users are prone to many of the precipitating factors that promote reflux. See the listed symptoms and precipitating factors in Chapter 4. Many singers or actors prefer to eat a minimal amount of food prior to a performance. They may then eat a larger meal after the performance, late in the evening. Some individuals may overeat and go to bed with a full stomach. When in a reclined body position, the larynx, esophagus, and stomach are on the same plane, and the gastric contents from the stomach may reflux all the way to the posterior laryngeal area.[57] Foods that reportedly promote reflux include coffee (caffeinated or decaffeinated), sodas, chocolate, high-fat foods, citrus beverages, tomato products, spicy foods, and alcohol. Smoking and weight gain have also been shown to increase reflux. Other contributing factors include stress and poor sleep habits.

Possible physiological etiologies of gastroesophageal reflux include a hiatal hernia, lower esophageal sphincter dysfunction, and esophageal dysmotility. Individuals diagnosed with GERD complain of heartburn and acid regurgitation with the report of a burning or bitter taste in the throat. Some patients will report a sensation of a "lump" in the throat feeling or present with symptoms of chronic cough (nonproductive), hoarseness, chronic throat clearing with little mucus production, and chest pain or discomfort. Singers report any of the above symptoms but may also experience difficulty singing notes in the upper range. Others may report a history of chronic laryngitis. It is also noted that prevalence of acid reflux has been implicated in the pathogenesis of vocal fold nodules[58] as well as posterior laryngitis,[59,60] subglottic stenosis,[61] and contact ulcer[62] and granuloma.[63]

Physical examination of the larynx may show erythematous arytenoids,[64] small contact ulcerations or granuloma in the vocal process area. The most commonly observed changes involve a thickening or mounding of tissue (pachydermia), opalescence coloration of the tissue in the interarytenoid space, or both. A cobblestone appearance of the tissue in the posterior laryngeal area may be seen directly superior to the esophageal inlet. The true vocal folds may appear edematous and erythematous. The amplitude of vibration and mucosal wave can range from mildly to severely decreased.

Treatment includes dietary restrictions (avoiding foods that are acidic or are irritants) and behavioral lifestyle changes. Lifestyle changes involve weight reduction (if necessary), avoidance of overeating or eating late at night (not within 3 to 4 hours of bedtime), smoking cessation, elevating the head of the bed or using a wedge-shaped pillow, and taking an antacid between meals and before bedtime. Patients are strongly advised to follow these restrictions in addition to taking their prescribed medicine as directed by the physician. If a conservative approach is not effective in treatment (approximate 3-month trial), additional medical tests may be ordered. These may include ambulatory 24-hour double-probe pH monitoring to measure frequency and duration of gastric reflux into the esophagus, barium esophagram with fluoroscopy, or direct endoscopy. A gastroenterological workup may be necessary if patients report pain in the substernal area (region of the lower esophageal sphincter).

The combination of medical, dietary, and lifestyle changes in conjunction with voice therapy is highly successful in the treatment of laryngopharyngeal reflux.[65] Voice therapy is beneficial to ensure easy onset of phonation when speaking. Retraining singing habits to eliminate initial hard onsets during singing may also need to be addressed. Recommending the use of an amplification device is also helpful to increase vocal volume and avoid overadduction of the vocal folds.

Voice Fatigue

As reported in Chapter 4, it is possible that pathological conditions of the larynx, voice misuse, or voice overuse will lead to laryngeal fatigue. The singer or actor with laryngeal fatigue will complain about a lack of consistency in the quality of the vocal output, decreased endurance, loss of frequency and intensity control, and complaints of effortful, unstable, and ineffective voice production. In both the speaker and the singer, discomfort and muscular aching in the laryngeal area are often present.

Theories about the existence of laryngeal muscle fatigue have been reported for many years, giving rise to the term *laryngeal myasthenia*. This term reflects the sensations of tiredness that the patient reports following vocalization. Punt[39] attempted to categorize what he described as a muscular disorder of the larynx into 3 groups: acute, subacute, and chronic myasthenia.

Acute myasthenia was described as being caused by a brief period of severe vocal misuse and abuse. Edema and erythema of the mucosal lining of the vocal folds may also accompany the myasthenia. Subacute myasthenia was described as having many causes. Punt[39] suggested these causes include long-term vocal misuse, emotional difficulties, coughing, throat clearing, and overwork of the voice. He also suggested that the lack of preseason vocal training could lead to subacute myasthenia. This would be comparable to the football player who puts on the pads and equipment and takes part in a full-scale scrimmage the first day of training camp. More than likely the player would experience muscle strain, soreness, or even a pulled leg muscle. Because the larynx is also a muscular system, Punt hypothesized that attempting to sing or act without proper conditioning after an extended layoff would cause a subacute weakness. Chronic myasthenia was described as having the same causes as the subacute type. The difference was in the length of time that the causes were present. In chronic myasthenia, the voice user continues the same improper vocal habits over many years, creating the possibility of a more permanent laryngeal muscle weakness, which is also more resistant to change.

Discussion of laryngeal pathologies typically focuses on what the eye can see. The presence or absence of mucosal change or growths is described. The discussion of laryngeal fatigue attempts to describe the changes in the balance of the 3 subsystems of voice production: respiration, phonation, and resonance. Evaluation of this disorder is therefore limited to the patient's history as well as laryngeal videostroboscopy. Vibratory patterns of the vocal folds as observed through stroboscopy will often demonstrate underlying vocal incoordination through the observance of out-of-phase vibrations and incomplete glottic closure,[66] as well as high airflow rates and decreased maximum phonation times.[67] In the case of laryngeal fatigue, the underlying causes of the disorder (ie, imbalance of the voice subsystems), not the apparent vocal symptoms, must be treated. The voice user must understand that the voice mechanism requires daily care. It must be trained, warmed up, cooled down, and kept in shape, in much the same manner as the legs of a dancer or the arm of a baseball pitcher.

Treatment of voice fatigue in the professional voice user involves identification of the underlying causes and then modification or elimination of those causes. The voice pathologist may choose to initiate Vocal Function Exercises for balancing the 3 subsystems of voice production, or Resonant Voice Therapy, or both to promote an open frontal focus (see Chapter 7). When significant progress has been made in improving voice production, the patient may be reintroduced to professional voice use.

Vocal Fold Hemorrhage and Vascular Pathologies

Vocal fold hemorrhages result from a rupture of a blood vessel within the vocal fold. Hemorrhages can be caused by internal or external laryngeal trauma. A sudden vocal quality change is the most common symptom; however, a more permanent dysphonia may result if submucosal scarring develops following resolution of the hematoma.[68] Professional singers may observe immediate changes with a reduction in pitch range or a development of an "edge" to the voice. As the blood disperses into the submucosal tissue, it creates a mass effect, causing a decrease in amplitude and mucosal wave. Unilateral and bilateral hemorrhages can result.[69] Other professional voice users may note progressive hoarseness, vocal fatigue, or both over a period of days.

Professional voice users may be more susceptible to vocal injury secondary to vocal demand and strain placed on the voice. They may also seek medical treatment immediately because they feel and hear even a slight aberrant vocal change that may not be apparent to others. Hemorrhages result from harsh coughing, throat clearing, sneezing, yelling, forceful singing, shearing effect from an existing mass lesion such as a cyst, or vascular insults; inflammatory changes; and blunt external injury to the larynx. Increased risks are greater in individuals who use aspirin, ibuprofen, or other medications that alter blood clotting abilities.[68] Other risk factors that have been associated with vocal fold hemorrhage involve hormonal influences. Hormonal imbalances among women including abnormal menstrual cycles, use of estrogen supplements, gynecological surgery, and use of birth control pills,[70] as well anecdotal reported premenstrual and early menstrual hormonal changes, have influenced the development of vocal fold hemorrhages.

Treatment for recovery from a vocal fold hemorrhage is complete vocal rest for 1 to 2 weeks. Singers are advised to significantly reduce voice use and seek medical advice if a sudden vocal quality change occurs during a performance. Individuals can often return to their prehemorrhagic vocal quality if early diagnosis is made and the person is compliant with absolute voice rest. Limited use of the speaking voice may resume 1 to 2 weeks following complete voice rest. Routine voice therapy and singing lessons are recommended following resolution of the hemorrhage to address the phonotraumatic behaviors that caused the problem and to address maladaptive compensatory behaviors that may be present secondary to the injury. For full recovery, singers may be restricted from singing for 6 weeks.[68,71] Hemorrhages that result from the presence of a mass lesion take longer to heal and recover. Although rare, sometimes a hemorrhage needs evacuation of the hematoma, especially when enlarged vessels are involved.[72]

Several vascular lesions other than vocal fold hemorrhages (Plate 30) can present problems for professional voice users. These include the following:

- Vascular dilatation arising from a thickened capillary located on the vibratory edge or on the superior surface of the true vocal folds (Plate 31)
- Capillary ectasia, which is a varicose dilation of the capillaries of the vocal fold (Plate 32).
- Hemangioma presenting as a purplish red, firm mass that can be either sessile or pedunculated.

Singers may not have any vocal problems if small capillary ectasia exists on the superior surface of the true focal folds away from the vibrating free edge; however, larger capillary ectasia and hemangioma may have significant effects on vocal quality. Videostroboscopy is an essential tool for distinguishing vascular lesion(s) and is necessary for developing a plan of treatment. Abitbol[72] reported that most patients treated with capillary ectasia were female professional singers who reported they were experiencing increased strain and hormonal problems.

A 22-year-old singer had been experiencing vocal difficulties for several months. Her chief complaints were inability to consistently sing the high notes in her range and increased breathiness when singing in her upper range. She complained of not being able to hold the higher notes as long in duration as compared to the lower notes. Her range was becoming narrower. Longer warm-ups were needed, and she was having difficulty singing softly and initiating a tone. She complained of a feeling of increased mucus and vocal fatigue with use. A videostroboscopic examination revealed a questionable right intracordal cyst with accompanying capillary ectasia. Increased edema and erythema were observed bilaterally with contralateral nodular tissue thickening. Mucus started to accumulate on the vocal fold surface after sustained phonation. A posterior glottal chink was observed for sustained lower pitches, whereas an hourglass glottal closure was observed for sustained higher pitches. Under simulated slow motion stroboscopy, the amplitude of vibration was moderately decreased on the right and mildly to moderately decreased on the left. Mucosal wave was moderately to severely decreased on the right and mildly to moderately decreased on the left. An open phase predominated during the vibratory cycle, and the symmetry of vibration was irregular during the initiation and ending of phonation, as well as during changes in pitch and loudness.

Because of the increased edema and erythema and uncertainty of a possible underlying cyst, the otolaryngologist and voice pathologist recommended a 4- to 5-week period of trial voice therapy with a repeat videostroboscopy in 5 weeks. The individual was enrolled in voice therapy with therapy consisting of a hydration program, vocal hygiene counseling including no singing, Resonant Vocal Therapy, and Vocal Function Exercises. A repeat videostrobe was performed the fifth week following the initiation of therapy. Results showed that with no edema and erythema present, an intracordal cyst was evident with prominent capillary ectasia and a feeder vessel to the area of the cyst. The contralateral nodular thickness was significantly reduced in size. The individual was taken into surgery for a microlaryngoscopy to remove the right true vocal fold cyst and for superficial laser vaporization of the dilated vessel. Great care was taken not to disrupt the vibrating free edge of the vocal fold.

The individual was placed on 7 days of complete voice rest following surgery with a strict hydration program of drinking at least 2 L of water daily. Voice therapy resumed 1 week following surgery with light humming and Resonant Voice Therapy. Conservative voice use was recommended for the second week following surgery. The individual was reintroduced to the Vocal Function Exercises the second week following surgery. She started vocal lessons the fourth week following surgery. This was in addition to seeing the voice pathologist. She resumed singing 6 weeks following surgery.

CLINICAL ASSESSMENT OF THE VOCAL PERFORMER

As part of a multidisciplinary team in assessing vocal performers, various instrumentation and assessment tools may be used across the disciplines which are warranted to help diagnose and evaluate the vocal condition of the individual. The otolaryngologist's objective is to visualize the larynx and provide a medical diagnosis of the presence or absence of laryngeal pathology and to recommend the appropriate management strategies. Visualization of the larynx via laryngoscopy, a comprehensive clinical history, and a physical examination are the minimum recommendations for a person with dysphonia, as set forth by the American Academy of Otolaryngology-Head and Neck Surgery.[73] The SLP's objective is to assess vocal function objectively and subjectively. Although a standard assessment protocol for functional assessment of voice is lacking in the United States, there is evidence outlined by Roy and colleagues for selected acoustic, auditory-perceptual, functional, and aerodynamic measures to be used in the clinical voice evaluation protocol.[74]

The SLP has a number of assessment tools used to evaluate how the voice functions from day to day as well as how these measures are affected by the underlying physiological function of the larynx. These tools help the SLP determine the individual's prognosis for improvement as well as support recommendations suggested by the multidisciplinary team. Assessment of the professional singer necessitates attention to detail outlined by Sataloff which includes a thorough knowledge of the performer's environment on and off stage as it relates to vocal use and vocal performance.[75] A tool to assess a performer's perception of singing difficulties and vocal health is the Singer's Voice Handicap Index (SVHI).[76] The SVHI is scored on a 0 to 100 scale with a higher score indicating more voice handicap. The Ambulatory Phonation Monitor (KayPENTAX, Lincoln Park, NJ), designed to objectively document key phonatory behaviors over a period of time, has been effective in quantifying real-time total phonation time, fundamental frequency, and vocal intensity. This instrument was created to measure vocal dose, which is defined as vocal fold tissue exposure to vibration over time.[77,78] The reliability of the Ambulatory Phonation Monitor has been verified measuring phonation data in real time in a number of studies.[78–81] This instrument's use has shown a significant higher vocal load for music teachers compared with elementary classroom teachers[82] as well as a case study documenting voice use and vocal efficiency of 2 graduate students' voice use before, during, and after an intense week of opera rehearsals.[83] The area of vocal dose among singers is certainly needed to establish valid baseline data for both healthy singers and those singers experiencing dysphonia. The individual phonetogram or voice range profile (VRP) is often used to assess the laryngeal possibilities of vocal intensities and fundamental frequencies when evaluating the professional singer.[84,85] The VRP has been used to study students in vocal training, soloists, amateur singers, and female professional opera soloists.[86–90] This tool can be valuable for pre- and postmeasures for individuals undergoing voice therapy secondary to dysphonia.[91]

SUPPORTIVE TRAINING AND TECHNIQUES

Throughout the years, a number of philosophical techniques have been written about and presented to focus on effective and efficient use of coordinated movements. These include the following:

- Alexander Technique
- The Linklater Method
- The Feldenkrais Method
- The Lessac System
- Estill Voice Training

Trained instructors have continued to pass these techniques down to others throughout the decades. Many vocal teachers and vocal coaches as well as performers have been trained in these techniques. The underlying philosophical concept of these techniques is based on establishing a balance and integration between the mind and body that permits physiologic freedom of movement during performance. The term *movement* is used in a generic sense and encompasses everything people do. These techniques incorporate auditory, visual, and kinesthetic awareness to attain self-discovery of freedom of movement. Increasing one's awareness of what facilitates beneficial and natural movement on a conscious level is paramount to influence changes at all levels. Only after a conscious level of self-discovery of ease of total function can one achieve a state of unconscious acts of repetition that will allow for effortless performance. In a performer it is the coordinated and integrated movement of the emotional, physical, and artistic demands on the voice in synchrony that must be met. Professionals have refined movements that appear effortless and natural to their audiences. The following are general descriptions of these techniques.

Alexander Technique

Frederick Matthias Alexander (1869–1955), from Australia, was a professional Shakespearean actor. During his career, he repeatedly developed laryngitis while performing. He wrote of "gasping" and "sucking in air," and his breathing became audible during his recitations. Despite medical treatment as well as vocal training, nothing helped. He sought out to self-analyze his technique of delivery. While practicing in front of a mirror, he discovered that increased muscular tension contributed to his vocal problems. Throughout the years he discovered that proper alignment of the head, neck, and torso was critical in every body activity. From his work, he developed a hands-on teaching method that promoted balance, support, and coordination through freedom of movement. He began teaching his method to singers and actors in London in the 1890s. This technique has helped instrumentalists, dancers, singers, actors, and athletes. It can be incorporated into all facets of one's life.[92]

The Alexander Technique focuses on developing awareness and consciously controlling body movements to allow for integration and coordination of the mind and body to perform activities without effort and muscular tension. Alexander believed that habituated maladaptive habits limited and impaired coordinated movement and postural patterns and even impeded learning. These unconscious habits alter sensory feedback and change perceptions and feelings, which affect people both physically and mentally in everything they do. Alexander's "respiratory re-education" focuses on proper body alignment and coordination of breathing with ease of vocalizing. For additional reading on the development of the technique and Alexander's self-discoveries, the reader is directed to the text *Technique: The Essential Writings of F. Matthias Alexander.*[93]

One learns the mind-body integration of whole patterns of coordinated movement and body alignment through the guidance of certified instructors.

Hands-on guidance helps the individual experience the freedom of a more natural movement without the interference of maladaptive habituated patterning, thus allowing for sensory internalization of ease of coordinated movement. The Alexander Technique has benefited athletes, singers, dancers, and musicians through the coordination of improving respiratory support, vocal production, and speed and accuracy of movement, and to achieve greater conscious control of reactions.

Certified instructors of the Alexander Technique in the United States can be located through 2 professional organizations: North American Society for the Teachers of the Alexander Technique (http://www.amsatonline.org) or Alexander Technique International (http://alexandertechniqueworldwide.com).

The Linklater Method

Actress Kristin Linklater trained and studied under Iris Warren at the London Academy of Music and Dramatic Art in England. In 1963, she came to the United States and has trained numerous teachers, actors, directors, and public speakers. Liberating our "natural" voices minus tension and habituated patterns is the basic premise of her designed approach. It is assumed that all individuals have a voice capable of performance through a 2- to 4-octave natural pitch range. It is also assumed that as humans, we have physiological tensions and psychological inhibitory responses that impair the ability of the natural voice to perform.

Emphasis on mind-body unity through physical awareness and relaxation unravels the habitual patterns that impede the natural voice. Linklater states, "breath and sound must always be connected to thought and feeling so that the two processes work simultaneously to activate and release inner impulses and to dissolve physical blocks."[94(p2)] Her method incorporates combining imagery and imagination to achieve a sound that is produced freely under any conditions. Emphasis is placed on awareness of postural alignment, breath support, relaxation of the articulators, resonance to enhance vocal range, and bridging the voice to acting "speaking the text."[94] For information on training, one can visit the website at (http://kristinlinklater.com).

The Feldenkrais Method

Moshe Feldenkrais (1904–1984), born in Russia, held mechanical and electrical engineering degrees, as well as a doctor of science in physics from Sorbonne in Paris. He had an interest in athletics and earned a black belt in judo. Suffering from serious knee injuries, which led him to study human anatomy, psychology, and physiology, he developed a method of awareness coordinated mind-body exercises. A type of supportive therapy, the individual becomes aware of his or her own movement and functioning, including habituated tensions and rigidity, and learns new ways of coordinated patterning that enhances overall efficiency and improves muscular function with greater effectiveness. One aims to achieve movement with minimal effort and maximum efficiency.

There are 2 modalities to learning in the Feldenkrais Method: Functional Integration and Awareness Through Movement.[95–97] Functional Integration involves noninvasive, hands-on body manipulations performed while sitting, standing, or lying down. These body manipulations help the individual learn and feel appropriate movements through tactile and kinesthetic input that are inhibitory and increase overall bodily functioning. Once internalized, the individual can focus attention to habituated tense movement and cognitively change positioning to the newly acquired neuromuscular patterning that is free of tension and rigidity.

Awareness Through Movement involves verbal instruction of sequential movements in basic body positions of sitting, standing, or lying on the floor. The instructor focuses on self-awareness through sensations and how to achieve improved motor functioning with comfort and ease and abandon habitual patterns. The goal is to improve flexibility and coordination in all movement. For the professional singer, this method teaches to a balance of mind-body actions and release tension and muscle strain to achieve optimal performance. Information on training and workshops can be found at the Feldenkrais Institute (http://www.feldenkraistinstitute.org).

The Lessac System

Arthur Lessac studied at the Eastman School of Music in Rochester, New York, and is a professor emeritus of Theatre, State University of New York at Binghamton. Renowned both as an actor and as a singer, his method strives to cultivate awareness or attention in coordinating mind and body. The performer must "physically experience the feeling while at the very same time behaviorally feel the experience."[98(p1)] The focus of this method is on kinesthetic awareness where the performer is requested to physically feel and cognitively process their vocal sounds to replace habituated behaviors.

According to Lessac,[98] there are 4 concepts that are essential for the performer. These include: (1) body esthetics, (2) inner harmonic sensing, (3) organic instructions, and (4) the "familiar event" principle. Body esthetics focuses on sensations and expanding awareness such as bodily feelings or sounds of being open, flowing, and rhythmic versus closed, turbulent, or rigid. Internal bodily processing provided with integration from the 5 senses of hearing, feeling, tasting, seeing, and smelling, creates an intrinsic harmonious feeling. It is through inner harmonic sensing (like a sixth sense) that performers develop intrasensitivity when engaged in a bodily activity. Organic instructions refer to the performer being in conscious control of the body and mind as to not inhibit freedom of movement. The last step is finding a number of familiar events that are pleasing and can be imaged to evoke a body action that is performed naturally without effort.

Lessac's method in producing voice requires awareness of the anatomy and the ability to produce a natural forward vowel without facial, oral, and neck tension. Tonal production relies on an awareness of a buzz or ring vibration felt on the alveolar ridge, in the nasal area, and forehead with effortless projection of the tone. Consonants are viewed as musical instruments. Playing the consonant, one should feel its vibrations and range. Finally, one adds meaning to each consonant and then applies that meaning to speech with emotional feelings. One can obtain information on training workshops at http://lessacinstitute.com/.

Estill Voice Training

Jo Estill, a classically trained singer, founded Estill Voice Training (originally called Estill Voice Craft) and the Figures for Voice (originally known as Compulsory Figures for Voice) in 1988.

Although classically trained, she was best known for her work with "belting"[99] that can be heard in musical theater singing. The Figures for Voice is a series of vocal exercises learned to control laryngeal structures independently and in combination to create different vocal qualities.[100–104]

The Estill method is taught through a series of workshops held by certified course instructors and can be located on the Internet (http://www.estillvoice.com/). Participants in the courses learn 13 compulsory figures that focus on vocal onset and offset, laryngeal height, and laryngeal sphincter control. The figures are then incorporated in combination for shaping the vocal tract in 6 vocal qualities: speech, falsetto, sob, twang, opera, and belting. The 13 Figures for Voice are True Vocal Folds: Onset/Offset Control, False Vocal Folds Control, True Vocal Folds: Body-Cover Control, Thyroid Cartilage Control, Cricoid Cartilage Control, Larynx Control, Velum Control, Tongue Control, Aryepiglottic Spincter Control, Jaw Control, Lips Control, Head and Neck Control, and Torso Control.

SUMMARY

This chapter serves as an overview of the professional voice user and is not meant to be all-inclusive. In the last 25 years, we have witnessed a strong interest in interdisciplinary research and training at the institutions that combine medicine, science, and the arts. As a result of the collaborative efforts among these disciplines, a plethora of research articles, books, CDs, and YouTube videos are available resources for us all to use. A multidisciplinary team is essential in providing the best care possible for the individual with vocal problems.

GLOSSARY OF TERMS USED IN SINGING

A cappella: solo or group singing without instrumental sound

Allegro: quick, fast

Alto (or contralto): the lowest female singing voice

Aria: a lyric song for solo voice with orchestral accompaniment, generally expressing intense emotion; found in opera, cantata, and oratorio

Baritone: a type of male voice in the middle range between bass and tenor

Bass: a type of male singing voice; the lowest vocal range of all voice

Cantata: a vocal composition sung with an instrumental accompaniment, in several self-contained parts, and often involving a choir

Chest voice: resonance of pitches is felt in the chest or throat. It is the speaking voice of individuals and generally the most comfortable way of singing for most singers.

Coloratura: (coloring) refers to runs, trills, and florid decorations in vocal music. A high soprano with vocal ability to produce notes above high C (C6) and possess a tessitura ranging from A4 to A5 or higher

Countertenor: a type of male singing voice whose vocal range goes into falsetto
Crescendo: gradually increasing in volume
Decrescendo: reduction in volume
Diminuendo: lessening the tone from loud to soft
Falsetto: a type of vocal phonation above the normal range and is characteristically breathy, and flute-like
Fortissimo: as loud as possible
Glissando: "gliding" to include all possible pitches between the initial and final pitch sounded
Head voice: resonance of pitches is felt vibrating in the head or nasal area of the singer
Legato: smooth and connected quality, with no noticeable interruption between the notes
Leggiero: light and delicate
Messa di voce: gradual swelling and diminishing of the voice (crescendo and diminuendo on a sustained tone)
Mezza voce: "half voice"; singing softly with breath support
Mezzo forte: moderately loud
Octave: interval of 8 diatonic or full notes of a musical scale. Can refer to 8 notes above or below another note.
Overtone: partial higher than the fundamental
Passaggio: break between vocal registers: males is generally E–F♯ above middle C4 and for females A♭–B♭ above middle C
Pianissimo: very soft
Portamento: a continuous gliding from one note to another including all intervening tones
Singer's formant: a high-spectrum peak occurring between 2.3 and 3.5 kHz; a "ring" that is heard in a voice
Soprano: a type of female singing voice; the highest vocal range of all types
Staccato: opposite of legato. Each note is separate from the one before and after.
Tenor: highest range for the male singing voice
Tessitura: the general range of pitch found in a melody or vocal part to be most comfortable
Timbre: sound quality or tone quality
Trill: rapid alteration of 2 pitches
Vibrato: regular fluctuation in pitch, timbre, intensity, or a combination of the 3
Vocalises: vocal exercises to develop flexibility and control of pitch and tone

REFERENCES

1. Koufman J, Isaccson G. The spectrum of vocal dysfunction. In: Koufman J, Isaccson G. eds. *The Otolaryngologic Clinics of North America: Voice Disorders.* Philadelphia, PA: WB Saunders; 1991: 985–988.
2. Titze I, Lemke J, Montequin D. Population in the U.S. workforce who rely on voice as a primary tool of trade: a preliminary report. *J Voice.* 1997;11: 254–259.
3. Fritzell B. Voice disorders and occupations. *Logoped Phoniatr Vocol.* 1996;21: 7–12.
4. Krischke S, Weigelt S, Hoppe U, et al. Quality of life in dysphonic patients. *J Voice.* 2005;19:132–137.
5. Svec, JG, Behlau, M. April 16th:World Voice Day. *Folia Phoniatr Logop.* 2007;59: 53–54.
6. American Speech-Language-Hearing Association. The role of the speech-language pathologist and teacher of singing in remediation of singers with voice disorders. *ASHA.* 1993;35:63.

7. Westerman JG. What's in a name? *J Singing*. 1996;53:1–2.
8. McKinney J. Something old—something new. *J Singing*. 1997;53:1–2.
9. Khambato A. Laryngeal disorders in singers and other voice users. In: Ballantyne J, Groves J, eds. *Scott Brown's Diseases of the Ear, Nose, and Throat*. 4th ed. London, UK: Butterworths; 1979.
10. Tutuian R, Castell DO. Diagnosis of laryngopharyngeal reflux. *Curr Opin Otolaryngol Head Neck Surg*. 2004;12: 174–179.
11. Ford C. Evaluation and management of laryngopharyngeal reflux. *JAMA*. 2005;294:1534–1540.
12. Hawkshaw MJ, Pebdani P, Robert T. Sataloff RT. Reflux laryngitis: an update, 2009–2012. *J Voice*. 2013;27:486–494.
13. Garrett CG, Cohen SM. Otolaryngological perspective on patients with throat symptoms and laryngeal irritation. *Curr Gastroenterol Rep*. 2008;10:195–199.
14. Irving RM, Epstein R, Harries MLL. Care of the professional voice. *Clin Otolaryngol*. 1997;22:202–205.
15. Wilder CN. Speech-language pathology and the professional voice user: an overview. In: Sataloff RT, ed. *Professional Voice: The Science and Art of Clinical Care*. Vol. 1. 3rd ed. San Diego, CA: Plural Publishing; 2005: 957–960.
16. Sundberg J. *The Science of the Singing Voice*. Dekalb, IL: Northern University Press; 1987.
17. DeJonckere PH, Hirano M, Sundberg J. *Vibrato*. San Diego, CA: Singular Publishing Group; 1995.
18. Titze I. *Principles of Voice Production*. Englewood Cliffs, NJ: Prentice-Hall; 1994.
19. Vennard W. *Singing: The Mechanism and the Technic*. New York, NY: Carl Fischer; 1968.
20. Cohen SM, Pitman MJ, Noordzij JP, Courey M. Evaluation of dysphonic patients by general otolaryngologists. *J Voice*. 2012;26:772–778.
21. Lancer M, Syder D, Jones AS, Le Bortillier A. The outcome of different management patterns for vocal cord nodules. *J Laryngol Otol*. 1988;102:423–427.
22. Murry T, Woodson GE. A comparison of three methods for the management of vocal fold nodules. *J Voice*. 1992;6:271–276.
23. Hirano M. *Clinical Examination of Voice*. New York: Springer-Verlag; 1981.
24. Bunch M, Chapman J. Taxonomy of singers used as subjects in scientific research. *J Voice*. 2000;14:363–369.
25. Wolk L, Abdelli-Beruh NB, Slavin, D. Excessive use of glottal fry when speaking is considered potentially harmful to the true vocal fold mucosa. *J Voice*. 2012;26:111–116.
26. Ylitalo R, Hammarberg B. Voice characteristics, effects of voice therapy, and long-term follow-up of contact granuloma patients. *J Voice*. 2000;14: 557–566.
27. Hollien H. On vocal registers. *J Phonetics*. 1974;2:125–143.
28. Whitehead R, Metz D, Whitehead G. Vibratory patterns for the vocal folds during pulse register phonation. *J Acoust Soc Am*. 1984;75:1293–1297.
29. McGlone R, Shipp T. Some physiologic correlates of vocal fry phonation. *J Speech Hear Res*. 1971;14:769–775.
30. Hollien H, Girard G, Coleman R. Vocal fold vibratory patterns of pulse register phonation. *Folia Phoniatrica*. 1977;29:200–205.
31. Chen Y, Robb MP, Gilbert HR, Electroglottographic evaluation of gender and vowel effects during modal and vocal fry phonation. *J Speech Hear Res*. 2002; 45:821–829.
32. Sorensen D, Horii Y. Frequency characteristics of male and female speakers in the pulse register. *J Comm Dis*. 1984; 7:65–73.
33. Baken RJ. An overview of laryngeal function of voice production. In: Sataloff RT, ed. *Voice Science*. San Diego, CA: Plural Publishing; 2005:147–165.

34. Blomgren M, Chen Y, Ng ML, Gilbert HR. Acoustic, aerodynamic, physiologic, and perceptual properties of modal and vocal fry registers. *J Acoust Soc Am.* 1998;103:2649–2658.
35. Farnsworth DW. High-speed motion pictures of the human vocal cords. *Bell Lab Record.* 1940;18:203–206.
36. Echternach M, Dippold S, Sundberg J, Arndt S, Zander MF, Richter B. High-speed imaging and electroglottography measurements of the open quotient in untrained male voices' register transitions. *J Voice.* 2010;24:644–650.
37. Timcke R, von Leden H, and Moore P. Laryngeal vibrations: measurements of the glottic wave, part 2: physiologic vibrations. *Arch Otolaryngol.* 1959;69: 438–444.
38. Boone DR, McFarlane SC, VonBerg SL, Zraick RI. *The Voice and Voice Therapy.* 9th ed. Boston, MA: Pearson Education; 2014:52–53.
39. Punt N. *The Singer's and Actor's Throat: The Vocal Mechanism of the Professional Voice User and Its Care and Health in Disease.* 3rd ed. London, UK: William Heinemann Medical Books; 1979.
40. Weiner H. Medical problems and treatment: panel discussion. In: Lawrence V, ed. *Transcripts of the 7th Symposium on Care of the Professional Voice Part III: Medical/Surgical Therapy.* New York, NY: The Voice Foundation; 1978.
41. Raphael BN. Special considerations relating to members of the acting profession. In: Sataloff RT, ed. *Professional Voice: The Science and Art of Clinical Care.* 3rd ed. San Diego, CA: Plural Publishing; 2005:339–341.
42. Freed SL, Raphael BN, Sataloff RT. The role of the acting-voice trainer in medical care of professional voice users. In: Sataloff RT, ed. *Professional Voice: The Science and Art of Clinical Care.* Vol. 1. 3rd ed. San Diego, CA: Plural Publishing; 2005:1051–1060.
43. Titze I. A few thoughts about longevity in singing. *NATS J.* 1994;50:36–38.
44. Wingate JM, Brown WS, Shrivastav R, Davenport P, Sapienza, CM. Treatment outcomes for professional voice users. *J Voice.* 2007;21:433–449.
45. Watts CR, Early S. Cortocosteroids: effects on voice. *Curr Opin Otolaryngol Head Neck Surg.* 2002;10:168–172.
46. Martin FG. Drugs and vocal function. *J Voice.* 1988;2:338–344.
47. Sataloff RT, Lawrence VL, Hawkshaw M, Rosen DC. Medications and their effects on the voice. In: Benninger MS, Jacobson BH, Johnson AF, eds. *Vocal Arts Medicine: The Care and Prevention of Professional Voice Disorders.* New York, NY: Thieme Medical Publishers; 1994: 216–225.
48. Sataloff RT, Hawkshaw M, Anticaglia J. Medications and the voice. In: Sataloff RT, ed. *Professional Voice: The Science and Art of Clinical Care.* Vol 1. 3rd ed. San Diego, CA: Plural Publishing; 2005:905–924.
49. Nair G, Sataloff RT. Vocal pharmacology: introducing the subject at Drew University. *J Singing.* 1999;55:53–63.
50. Sataloff R. *Professional Voice: The Science and Art of Clinical Care.* New York, NY: Raven Press; 1991:chap 5.
51. Verdolini-Marston K, Titze IR, Druker DG. Changes in phonation threshold pressure with induced conditions of hydration. *J Voice.* 1990;4:142–151.
52. Verdolini-Marston K, Sandage M, Titze I. Effect of hydration treatments on laryngeal nodules and polyps and related voice measures. *J Voice.* 1994;8: 30–47.
53. Verdolini K, Titze IR, Fennell A. Dependence of phonatory effort on hydration level. *J Speech Hear Res.* 1994;37: 1001–1007.
54. Hemler RJB, Wieneke GH, Dejonckere PH. The effect of relative humidity of inhaled air on acoustic parameters of voice in normal subjects. *J Voice.* 1997;11:295–300.
55. Peppard RC, Bless DM, Milenkovic P. Comparison of young adult singers

and nonsingers with vocal nodules. *J Voice*. 1988;2:250–260.

56. Nebel L, Forbes M, Castell D. Symptomatic gastroesophageal reflux: incidence and precipitating factors. *Am J Dig Dis*. 1976;21:953–956.
57. Koufman JA, Aviv JE, Casiano RR, Shaw GY. Larngopharyngeal reflux: position statement of the committee on speech, voice, and swallowing disorders of the American Academy of Otolaryngology-Head and Neck Surgery. *Otolaryngol Head Neck Surg*. 2002; 127:32–45.
58. Kuhn J, Toohill RJ, Ulualp SO, et al. Pharyngeal acid reflux events in patients with vocal cord nodules. *Laryngoscope*. 1998;108:1146–1149.
59. Shaker R, Milbrath M, Ren J, et al. Esophagopharyngeal distribution of refluxed gastric acid in patients with reflux laryngitis. *Gastroenterology*. 1995; 109:1575–1582.
60. Koufman JA. The otolaryngologic manifestations of gastroesophageal reflux disease GERD: a clinical investigation of 225 patients using ambulatory 24-hour pH monitoring and an experimental investigation of the role of acid and pepsin in the development of laryngeal injury. *Laryngoscope*. 1991;101(suppl 53):1–78.
61. Jacob P, Kahrilas PJ, Herzon G. Proximal esophageal pH-metry in patients with reflux laryngitis. *Gastroenterology*. 1991;100:305–310.
62. Toohill RJ, Jindal JR. Gastroesophageal reflux as a cause of idiopathic subglottic stenosis. *Oper Tech Otolaryngol Head Neck Surg*. 1997;8:149–152.
63. Ohman L, Olfsson J, Tibbling I, Ericsson G. Esophageal dysfunction in patients with contact ulcer of the larynx. *Ann Otol Rhinol Laryngol*. 1983;92:228–230.
64. Lumpkin SMM, Bishop S, Katz P. Chronic dysphonia secondary to gastroesophageal reflux disease GERD: diagnosis using simultaneous dual-probe prolonged pH monitoring. *J Voice*. 1989;3:351–355.
65. Ross J, Noordzji JP, Woo P. Voice disorders in patients with suspected laryngo-pharyngeal reflux disease. *J Voice*. 1988;12:84–88.
66. Stemple JC, Stanley J, Lee L. Objective measures of voice production in normal subjects following prolonged voice use. *J Voice*. 1995;9:127–133.
67. Eustace CS, Stemple JC, Lee L. Objective measures of voice production in patients complaining of laryngeal fatigue. *J Voice*. 1996;10:146–154.
68. Spiegel JR, Sataloff RT, Hawkshaw M, Caputo RD. Vocal fold hemorrhage. In: Sataloff RT, ed. *Professional Voice: The Science and Art of Clinical Care*. 2nd ed. San Diego, CA: Singular Publishing; 2005:541–554.
69. Abitbol J. Vocal cord hemorrhages. *J Voice*. 1988;2:261–266.
70. Lin PT, Stern JC, Gould WJ. Risk factors and management of vocal cord hemorrhages: an experience with 44 cases. *J Voice*. 1991;5:74–77.
71. Sataloff RT. Vocal fold hemorrhage: diagnosis and treatment. *NATS J*. 1995; 51:45–48.
72. Abitbol J. *Atlas of Laser Voice Surgery*. San Diego, CA: Plural Publishing; 1995.
73. Schwartz SR, Cohn SM, Dailey SH, et al. Clinical practice guideline: hoarseness (dysphonia). *Otolaryngol Head Neck Surg*. 2009;141:S1–S31.
74. Roy N, Barkmeier-Kraemer J, Eadie T, et al. Evidence-based clinical voice assessment: a systematic review. *Am J Speech Lang Pathol*. 2013;22:212–226.
75. Sataloff RT. *Vocal Health and Pedagogy: Advanced Assessment and Treatment*. 2nd ed. San Diego, CA: Plural Publishing; 2006.
76. Cohen SM, Jacobson BH, Garrett CG, et al. Creation and validation of the Singing Voice Handicap Index. *Ann Otol Rhinol Laryngol*. 2007;116:402–406.
77. Titze I, Svec J, Popolo P. Vocal dose measures: quantifying accumulated vibration exposure in vocal fold tissues. *J Speech Lang Hear Res*. 2003;46:919–932.

78. Cheyne HA, Hanson H, Genereux R, Stevens K, Hillman R. Development and testing of a portable vocal accumulator. *J Speech Lang Hear Res*. 2003; 46:1457–1567.
79. Hillman RE, Heaton JT, Maski A, Zeitels S, Cheyne H. Ambulatory monitoring of disordered voices. *Ann Otol Rhinol Laryngol*. 2006;115:795–801.
80. Popolo PS, Svec JG, Titze IR. Adaptation of a pocket PC for use as a wearable voice dosimeter. *J Speech Lang Hear Res*. 2005;48:780–791.
81. Szabo A, Hammarberg B, Granqvist S, Sodersten M. Methods to study preschool teachers' voice at work: simultaneous recordings with a voice accumulator and a DAT recorder. *Logoped Phoniatr Vocol*. 2003;28:29–39.
82. Morrow S, Conner NP. Comparison of voice-use profiles between elementary classroom and music teachers. *J Voice*. 2009;25:367–372.
83. Scholoneger MJ. Graduate student voice use and vocal efficiency in an opera rehearsal week: a case study. *J Voice*. 2010;25:e265–e273.
84. Damsté H. The phonetogram. *Pract Otorhinolaryngol*. 1970;32:185–187.
85. Schutte H, Seidner W. Recommendations by Union of European Phoniatricians (UEP): standardizing voice area measurement/phonetography. *Folia Phoniatr*. 1983;35:286–288.
86. LeBorgne WD, Weinrich BD. Phonetogram changes for trained singers over a nine-month period of vocal training. *J Voice*. 2002;6:37–43.
87. Awan S. Phonetographic profiles and F0-SPL characteristics of untrained versus trained vocal groups. *J Voice*. 1991;5:41–50.
88. Siupsinskiene N, Lycke H. Effects of vocal training on singing and speaking voice characteristics in vocally healthy adults and children based on choral and nonchoral data. *J Voice*. 2011;25: e177–e189.
89. Hunter EJ, Svec JG, Titze IR. Comparison of the produced and perceived voice range profiles in untrained and trained classical singers. *J Voice*. 2006; 20:513–526.
90. Lamarche A, Ternstro S, Pabon P. The singer's voice range profile: female professional opera soloists. *J Voice*. 2010;24:410–426.
91. Speyer R, Wieneke GH, van Wijck-Warnaar I, Dejonckere PH. Effects of voice therapy on the voice range profiles of dysphonic patients. *J Voice*. 2003;17:544–556.
92. Conable B, Conable W. *How to Learn the Alexander Technique: A Manual for Students*. Columbus, OH: Andover Press; 1995.
93. Alexander FM. *Alexander Technique: The Essential Writings of F Matthias Alexander*. New York, NY; Carol Publishing Group; 1995.
94. Linklater K. *Freeing the Natural Voice*. New York, NY: Drama Book Publishers; 1976.
95. Rywerant Y. *The Feldenkrais Method: Teaching by Handling*. New Canaan, CT: Keats Publishing; 1983.
96. Feldenkrais M. *Body and Mature Behavior*. New York, NY: International Universities Press; 1970.
97. Feldenkrais M. *Awareness through Movement*. New York, NY: Harper & Row; 1972.
98. Lessac A. *The Use and Training of the Human Voice: A Bio-Dynamic Approach to Vocal Life*. Mountain View, CA: Mayfied Publishing; 1997.
99. Estill, J. Belting and classic voice quality: some physiological differences. *Med Probl Perform Ar*.1988;3:37–43.
100. Yanagisawa E, Kmucha, ST, Estill J. The role of the soft palate in laryngeal function and in selected voice qualities. *Ann Otol Rhinol Laryngol*. 1990;99:18–28.
101. Yanagisawa E, Estill J. The contribution of aryepiglottic constriction to "ringing" voice quality. *J Voice*. 1989;3:342–350.

102. Yanagisawa E, Kmucha ST, Estill J. Endolaryngeal changes during high intensity phonation: video laryngoscopic observations. *J Voice.* 1990;4:346–354.
103. Yanagisawa E, Mambino L, Estill J, Talkin D. Supraglottic contributions to pitch raising. *Ann Otol Rhinol Laryn.* 100:19–30.
104. Yanagisawa E, Citardi M, Estill J. Videoendoscopic analysis of laryngeal function during laughter. *Ann Otol Rhinol Laryn.* 1996;105:545–549.

9

Rehabilitation of the Laryngectomized Patient

OVERVIEW

Total rehabilitation of the laryngectomized patient involves interaction of a number of specialists from a multidisciplinary team. The diagnosis of laryngeal cancer has a significant impact on the individual's emotional and physical health. Multimodality treatment including chemotherapy, radiation, surgery, and rehabilitation involves various health professionals participating in the individual's progression of care. A primary participant on the team is the voice pathologist. The voice pathologist's role goes beyond basic speech retraining approaches to include both patient and family counseling. This chapter will discuss:

- etiology and symptoms of laryngeal cancer
- staging and treatment of the disease
- methods of voice restoration for the laryngectomized patient
- identifying risk factors for laryngeal cancer
- physical changes following surgery
- emotional needs of the patient and significant others
- social adjustments that must also be considered for total rehabilitation.

INCIDENCE OF LARYNGEAL CANCER

Head and neck cancer describes a range of cancers that arise in the head and neck region that includes oral cavity, pharynx, larynx, nasal cavity, paranasal sinuses, thyroid, and salivary glands. The incidence of head and neck cancer worldwide exceeds half a million cases annually, ranking it as the fifth most common cancer,[1] with oral cancer being the most common site and laryngeal cancer the second most common site within the head and neck region.[2] Each year the American Cancer Society estimates the number of new cancer cases and deaths expected in the United States and reports cancer incidence, mortality, and survival rates based on incidence data from the National Cancer Institute, Centers for Disease Control and Prevention, and the North American Association of Central Cancer Registries and mortality data from the National Center for Health Statistics. Cancer statistics are published yearly in the journal *CA: A Cancer Journal of Clinicians,* and the estimated number of new cases of laryngeal cancer in the United States in 2013 is 12,260 (9,680 for males and 2,580 for females). The total number of estimated deaths in the United States from laryngeal cancer is 3630 (2860 males and 770 females).[3]

Laryngeal cancer accounts for approximately 1.7% of all new cancers diagnosed annually worldwide, with around 182,000 new laryngeal cancers yearly.[4] Laryngeal cancers make up less than 1% of all cancers and nearly 6% of all cancers of the respiratory system. According to the American Cancer Society (http://www.cancer.org), the rate of laryngeal cancer is decreasing by 2% to 3% a year. Squamous cell carcinomas comprise 90% of head and neck cancers. Fifty-six percent of squamous cell carcinomas of the larynx most often occur in the glottal region which is made up of the true vocal folds, anterior commissure, and posterior commissures, with 31% in the supraglottic larynx, which comprises any five subsites of the supraglottic part of the larynx (ventricular folds, arytenoids, suprahyoid epiglottis, infrahyoid epiglottis, laryngeal aspect of the aryepiglottic folds), and approximately 1% in the subglottic larynx, which starts 0.5 cm below the free edge of the true vocal fold and ends at the level of the inferior border of the cricoids.[5] Approximately 60% of patients present with advanced disease (stages III and IV), and prognosis is poor for these individuals.[6]

The 5-year survival rate of patients with laryngeal cancer has varied little in the last 20 years. Shah et al[5] looked at 16,213 patients with laryngeal cancer and found a 5-year survival rate of 75%. Advanced laryngeal disease (stages III or IV) among these patients demonstrated less than 40% survival.

ETIOLOGY

The primary carcinogens for laryngeal cancer appear to be inhaled cigarette, pipe, and cigar smoke. The sites at greatest risk for developing cancer from smoking are anatomical areas that have direct exposure to irritants. Risks of developing laryngeal carcinoma will vary depending on daily consumption, type, and manner of tobacco use.[7] A synergistic effect between tobacco use and large amounts of alcohol consumption has been reported. Alcohol appears to potentiate the cancer-causing effect of tobacco smoke, creating a significantly higher risk than if each were used alone.[8] An individual who has more than 40-pack-year history of smoking and consumes 5 alcoholic drinks per day has a 40-fold increased risk of developing head and neck cancer.[9]

Alcohol and tobacco have been consistently implicated as being carcinogenic, but laryngeal cancer may certainly develop in their absence. The human papillomavirus (HPV) is a risk factor for development of head and neck cancers.[10,11] Although more than 118 HPVs have been described,[12] HPV 16 and 18 are known as the most carcinogenic types[13] associated with head and neck cancers.[14] An estimated 14,000 cases per year of oral cavity and pharynx, larynx, and esophageal tumors can be attributed to HPV.[15,16] Gastroesophageal reflux can also be a factor that may contribute to the development of laryngopharyngeal cancers. Studies have suggested that gastric acids refluxed at the level of the larynx may influence the development of laryngeal and pharyngeal cancers.[17–20]

SYMPTOMS OF LARYNGEAL CANCER

Cancer is the uncontrolled, rapid growth of malignant cells. As cancer cells grow and divide, they accumulate and form tumors, destroying and invading normal tissue. Cancer is a pathological diagnosis and is classified by the body part in which it develops. Cancer cells can also spread to other parts of the body traveling through the bloodstream or lymphatic system. Metastasis is the spread of cancer from a primary tumor to a new site. For example, if laryngeal cancer spreads to the lymph glands in the neck, the primary site is still the larynx, with metastasis to the neck. Early identification of laryngeal carcinoma increases the chance that malignancy will remain localized with successful optimal treatment results.

The larynx can be divided into three regions: supraglottis, glottis, and subglottis. The supraglottis is composed of the lingual and laryngeal area of the epiglottis, laryngeal aspect of the aryepiglottic folds, arytenoids, and the ventricular folds. The supraglottis is distinct from the glottis and subglottis. Embryologically the supraglottis is derived from the buccopharyngeal anlage (brachial arches III and IV). The glottis is composed of the superior and inferior surfaces of the true vocal folds, which includes the anterior and posterior commissures and is derived from the laryngotracheal anlage (brachial arches V and VI).[21] Work by Pressman and colleagues[21] indicates fascial compartmentalization and lymphatic drainage is distinct for the supraglottis and glottis and is the basis for the supraglottic horizontal laryngectomy. Dye studies have also confirmed the larynx is divided into right and left compartments. The subglottis is composed of the inferior region of the glottis extending to the lower margin of the cricoid cartilage. The area surrounding the larynx is referred to as the hypopharynx and includes the pharyngoesophageal junction, right and left pyriform sinuses, lateral and posterior hypopharyngeal walls, and the postcricoid region.

Cancer can arise in any of these three anatomical regions, but symptoms vary depending on the origin of cancer development. Laryngeal cancers that form on the vocal folds (glottis) are often detected early due to the mass effect that interrupts the vibration of the vocal folds. Hoarseness is the most common symptom when lesions involve the true vocal folds. Vocal fold lesions can cause a change in vocal pitch, increased effort to produce voicing and, if large enough, breathing problems (dyspnea) and audible breathing (stridor). Persistent hoarseness may motivate an individual to see a physician because of a fear of "throat" cancer. However, the fear of cancer may also elicit the opposite reaction—refusal to seek medical evaluation. As hoarseness is one of the seven warning signals of possible cancer as listed by the American Cancer Society,[22] individuals should seek a medical evaluation if hoarseness extends beyond a 2-week period.

Cancers that originate in the supraglottis, subglottis, or hypopharyngeal areas are usually discovered at later stages because the symptoms may be vague. When the vocal folds are not involved, the lesion may present with many symptoms including:

- lump in the throat sensation
- persistent throat clearing
- mass or lump in the head and neck area
- persistent coughing
- sense of discomfort in the throat
- persistent sore throat
- difficulty breathing/airway obstruction (dyspnea)
- burning sensation when swallowing
- difficulty swallowing or pain when swallowing (odynophagia)
- referred pain from the larynx to the ear (otalgia)
- unexplained weight loss
- hemoptysis
- halitosis or foul odor

In the later stages of cancer, malignancy will cause difficulty swallowing[23,24] and breathing with the eventual appearance of hoarseness.[25] Supraglottic tumors present with more symptoms in comparison to glottic tumors with higher occurrence of dysphagia, otalgia, globus sensation, shortness of breath and neck masses.[26] If the malignancy progresses beyond the confines of the larynx, it is likely to metastasize to the lymphatic system and appear as a lump on the neck. Pain is rarely reported until the later stages of the disease.

MEDICAL EVALUATION

An individual who is suspected of having cancer is referred to an otolaryngologist usually by his or her primary care physician. Background information is taken regarding current symptoms, medical history of the patient, and family history. All possible risk factors are assessed. An indirect mirror laryngoscopy performed by the otolaryngologist is the first step in evaluating the presence of laryngeal cancer. The otolaryngologist assesses the laryngeal structures, vocal fold mobility, tissue coloration, and presence of pathology. Elicitation of the gag reflex or the inability to sustain the vowel /i/ for a given period of time may create an abbreviated view of the laryngeal structures when using mirror laryngoscopy; therefore, a flexible fiberoptic endoscope may be used to give the examiner longer imaging capabilities. When the endoscopy instrumentation is coupled with a video camera, computer, and monitor, a complete visual examination can be documented and reviewed. Endoscopy examinations can be performed with either a flexible or rigid scope. A flexible nasendoscopy is performed by passing the endoscope through one of the patient's nares. With the flexible scope, the nasopharynx, pharynx, and larynx can all be assessed. Once the scope is positioned to view the true vocal folds, the patient is requested to perform a number of various speech tasks including abductory and adductory phonatory tasks to assess vocal fold mobility.

Rigid endoscopy with stroboscopy is performed with the endoscope positioned in the mouth as far back as the oropharynx. The true vocal folds and laryngeal structures are magnified, thus allowing for visualization of any tissue change. Stroboscopic images showing changes in the true vocal fold mucosal lining may indicate precancerous lesions or carcinoma in situ. Nonvibratory segments may indicate a more invasive lesion. Arytenoid movement is assessed to rule out true vocal fold paresis or paralysis, which can be either unilateral or bilateral.

Noninvasive imaging techniques that include computed tomography (CT) scanning that creates a cross-sectional 3-dimensional image of the inside structures, or magnetic resonance imaging (MRI) producing detailed images of soft tissue, are performed to view the laryngeal structures to delineate morphological features of the tumor, tissue, and organ and to determine the exact location and size of the lesion, presence or absence of regional lymph node metastasis, and/or presence or absence of distant metastases. A positron emission tomography (PET) scan may be preferred, which uses a form of sugar that contains a radioactive atom to view cancer that has spread to the lymph nodes or to other organs in the body. Cancer cells absorb glucose and tumors are then illuminated. PET scans pinpoint the exact location of the tumor(s) and are useful in the initial staging and restaging after treatment.[27,28] Imaging for detection of nodal metastases is higher for both sensitivity and specificity with PET as compared with high-resolution CT studies.[29]

If a malignant lesion is suspected based on the laryngeal examination and positive scans, a panendoscopy or direct view under a microscope in the operating room with the patient asleep (under general anesthesia) is performed to biopsy the lesion(s). A biopsy involves excising small samples of tissue under suspicion and evaluating them microscopically to determine the cell type. The most common type of laryngeal cancer is squamous cell. The otolaryngologist will also note the location and extent of the lesion. A modified barium swallow examination may be performed if there is a complaint of dysphagia. During this examination, barium coats the inside of the throat to assess for penetration or aspiration of liquids or solid food. All microscopic, visual, and x-ray information is analyzed, and the appropriate treatments are planned. Treatment may include radiation therapy, chemotherapy, surgery, or combination of these.

STAGING AND TUMOR-NODE-METASTASIS CLASSIFICATION

Laryngeal cancer is classified using the American Joint Commission on Cancer (AJCC) tumor-node-metastasis (TNM) and the presence or absence of metastasis staging system (Table 9–1).[30] The clinical staging of cancer was developed with the underlying premise that cancers of similar histology or site of origin share similar patterns of growth and metastasis. TNM staging is a clinical decision made by the physician after gathering information from different tests.

Table 9–1. The TNM Classification System

Primary Tumor (T)	
TX	Primary tumor cannot be assessed
TO	No evidence of primary tumor
Tis	Carcinoma in situ
Supraglottis	
T1	Tumor is limited to one subsite of the supraglottis with normal vocal cord mobility
T2	Tumor invades the mucosa of more than one adjacent subsite of the supraglottis or glottis or region outside the supraglottis (eg, mucosa of base of tongue, vallecula, and medial wall of pyriform sinus) without fixation of the larynx
T3	Tumor limited to the larynx with vocal cord fixation and/or invades any of the following: postcricoid area, pre-epiglottic space, paraglottic space, and/or inner cortex of the thyroid cartilage
T4a	Moderately advanced local disease Tumor invades through thyroid cartilage and/or invades tissues beyond the larynx (eg, trachea, soft tissues of neck including deep extrinsic muscle of the tongue, strap muscles, thyroid, or esophagus)
T4b	Very advanced local disease Tumor invades prevertebral space, encases carotid artery, or invades mediastinal structures
Glottis	
T1	Tumor is limited to the vocal cord(s) (may involve anterior or posterior commissure) with normal vocal cord mobility
T1a	Tumor is limited to one vocal cord
T1b	Tumor involves both vocal cords
T2	Tumor extends to the supraglottis and/or subglottis, and/or with impaired vocal cord mobility
T3	Tumor limited to larynx with vocal cord fixation and/or invasion of paraglottic space, and/or inner cortex of the thyroid cartilage
T4a	Moderately advanced local disease Tumor invades through the outer cortex of the thyroid cartilage and/or invades tissues beyond the larynx (eg, trachea, soft tissues of neck, including deep extrinsic muscles of the tongue, strap muscles, thyroid, or esophagus)
T4b	Very advanced local disease Tumor invades prevertebral space, encases carotid artery or invades mediastinal structures
Subglottis	
T1	Tumor limited to the subglottis
T2	Tumor extends to the vocal cord(s) with normal or impaired mobility
T3	Tumor limited to the larynx with vocal cord fixation

Table 9–1. *continued*

Subglottis *continued*	
T4a	Moderately advanced local disease Tumor invades cricoid or thyroid cartilage and/or invades tissues beyond the larynx (eg, trachea, soft tissues of neck including deep extrinsic muscles of the tongue, strap muscles, thyroid, or esophagus)
T4b	Very advanced local disease Tumor invades prevertebral space, encases carotid artery, or involves mediastinal structures
Regional Lymph Nodes (N)*	
NX	Regional lymph nodes cannot be assessed N0; no regional lymph node metastasis
N1	Metastasis in a single ipsilateral lymph node, 3 cm or less in greatest dimension
N2	Metastasis in a single ipsilateral lymph node, more than 3 cm but not more than 6 cm in greatest dimension, or in multiple ipsilateral lymph nodes, none more than 6 cm in greatest dimension; or in bilateral or contralateral lymph nodes, none more than 6 cm in greatest dimension
N2a	Metastasis in a single ipsilateral lymph node more than 3 cm but not more than 6 cm in greatest dimension
N2b	Metastasis in multiple ipsilateral lymph nodes, none more than 6 cm in greatest dimension
N2c	Metastasis in bilateral or contralateral lymph nodes, none more than 6 cm in greatest dimension
N3	Metastasis in a lymph node more than 6 cm in greatest dimension
Distant Metastasis (M)	
M0	No distant metastasis
M1	Distant metastasis

Stage Grouping	***T Stage***	***N Stage***	***M Stage***
Stage 0	Tis	N0	M0
Stage I	T1	N0	M0
Stage II	T2	N0	M0
Stage III	T3	N0	M0
	T1	N1	M0
	T2	N1	M0
	T3	N1	M0

continues

Table 9–1. *continued*

Stage Grouping	*T Stage*	*N Stage*	*M Stage*
Stage IVA	T4a	N0	M0
	T4a	N1	M0
	T1	N2	M0
	T2	N2	M0
	T3	N2	M0
	T4a	N2	M0
Stage IVB	T4b	Any N	M0
	Any T	N3	M0
Stage IVC	Any T	Any N	M1

*Note: Metastases at level VII are considered regional lymph node metastases.

These include a physical examination which may determine nodal location and spread of the disease upon palpation and endoscopic examination[31] as well as imaging examinations such as x-rays, CT scans, MRI, or PET scans to show the location, size, and extent of metastases if the cancer has spread. In addition, laboratory tests, surgical exploration, and biopsy of tissue are used for accurate staging.[8,30] Cancer is a diagnosis of pathology, and the sample tissue removed from the site in question confirms the diagnosis and cell type. The TNM staging system has been revised throughout the years since the first edition in 1968 for 47 body sites. Revisions of the staging system are based on improved understanding of the natural history of the tumor and technological advancements to better assess the extent of tumors. The TNM staging system revisions of head and neck tumors are based on expert opinions and published articles, as well as advances in technology to assess the extent of tumor and treatment strategies.[30] In describing the anatomic extent of the lesion, "T" refers to features of tumor size (expressed in centimeters of diameter), location, and extent of spread into surrounding tissues. "N" identifies the absence or presence and extent of the regional lymph node metastasis, and "M" refers to the absence or presence of distant metastasis. The numbers assigned to the TNM classification system refer to the extent of the tumor. Laryngeal cancer is described using a stage grouping that gives information about the tumor, lymph nodes, and metastasis. The stage is described using Roman numerals from I to IV. The higher numbers indicate more metastasis to the surrounding neck tissue and are associated with more advanced disease. There are 4 different types of staging: (1) clinical staging—based on the physical examination, imaging tests, and biopsies; (2) pathologic staging—used when individuals have had surgery to remove or explore the extent of cancer and is used in conjunction with the results from the clinical staging; (3) posttherapy or post-neoadjuvant therapy—determines the amount of cancer remaining after treatment with chemotherapy and/or radiation therapy prior to surgery or when surgery is no longer needed and uses the clinical and/or pathologic staging guidelines; and (4) restaging—used if cancer has recurred after treatment and determines the best treatment options for return of cancer.[30] A patient with a clinical classification of Stage IV, T4 N1 M0 has a large tumor with metastasis to the lymph nodes but no distant spread of the disease.

This clinical classification system assists the physicians in planning treatment, serves as a prognostic indicator, facilitates communication within and among treatment centers, and serves as a baseline to compare the results of treatment. The staging system also serves for improving stratification of individuals for inclusion in clinical trials.[32]

LYMPH NODE DISTRIBUTION

The lymph nodes of the neck area are divided into 6 different levels within defined anatomic triangles (Figure 9–1).

The cervical lymphatic drainage system is important to understand for neck metastases from the primary tumor and helps to understand neck dissections. Level I includes all nodes above the level of the lower body of the hyoid bone and is subdivided into 2 sublevels. Level IA or the submental area includes nodes that lie between the medial margins of the anterior bellies of the digastric muscles, above the lower body of the hyoid bone, and below the mylohyoid muscle. These nodes are at risk for metastatic disease from cancers in the floor of the mouth, anterior oral tongue, anterior mandibular alveolar ridge, and lower lip. Level IB or the submandibular area, consists of nodes between the anterior belly of the digastric muscle medially, the stylohyoid muscle, and the body of the mandibular bone laterally. This area also includes the preglandular and the postglandular nodes as well as the prevascular and postvascular nodes. The nodes in this area are at greatest risk for harboring metastases arising from the oral cavity, anterior nasal cavity, soft tissue structures of midface, and submandibular gland. When surgery is performed in this area, the submandibular gland is removed.

The Level II or upper jugular (cervical) group of lymph nodes extends from the skull base around the upper third of the internal jugular vein and adjacent spinal accessory nerve to the inferior border of the hyoid bone, and the nodes are laterally covered by the body of the sternocleidomastoid muscle. There are two sublevels with IIA nodes located anterior to the vertical plane defined by the spinal accessory nerve and IIB nodes located posterior to the vertical plane defined by the spinal accessory nerve. The upper jugular nodes are at greatest risk for metastases from cancers coming from the oral cavity, nasal cavity, nasopharynx, oropharynx, hypopharynx, larynx, and parotid gland.

Level III or middle jugular nodes are located around the middle third of the internal jugular vein extending from the inferior border of the hyoid bone to the inferior border of the cricoid cartilage. These nodes are at risk for metastatic disease from the oral cavity, nasopharynx, oropharynx, hypopharynx, and larynx.

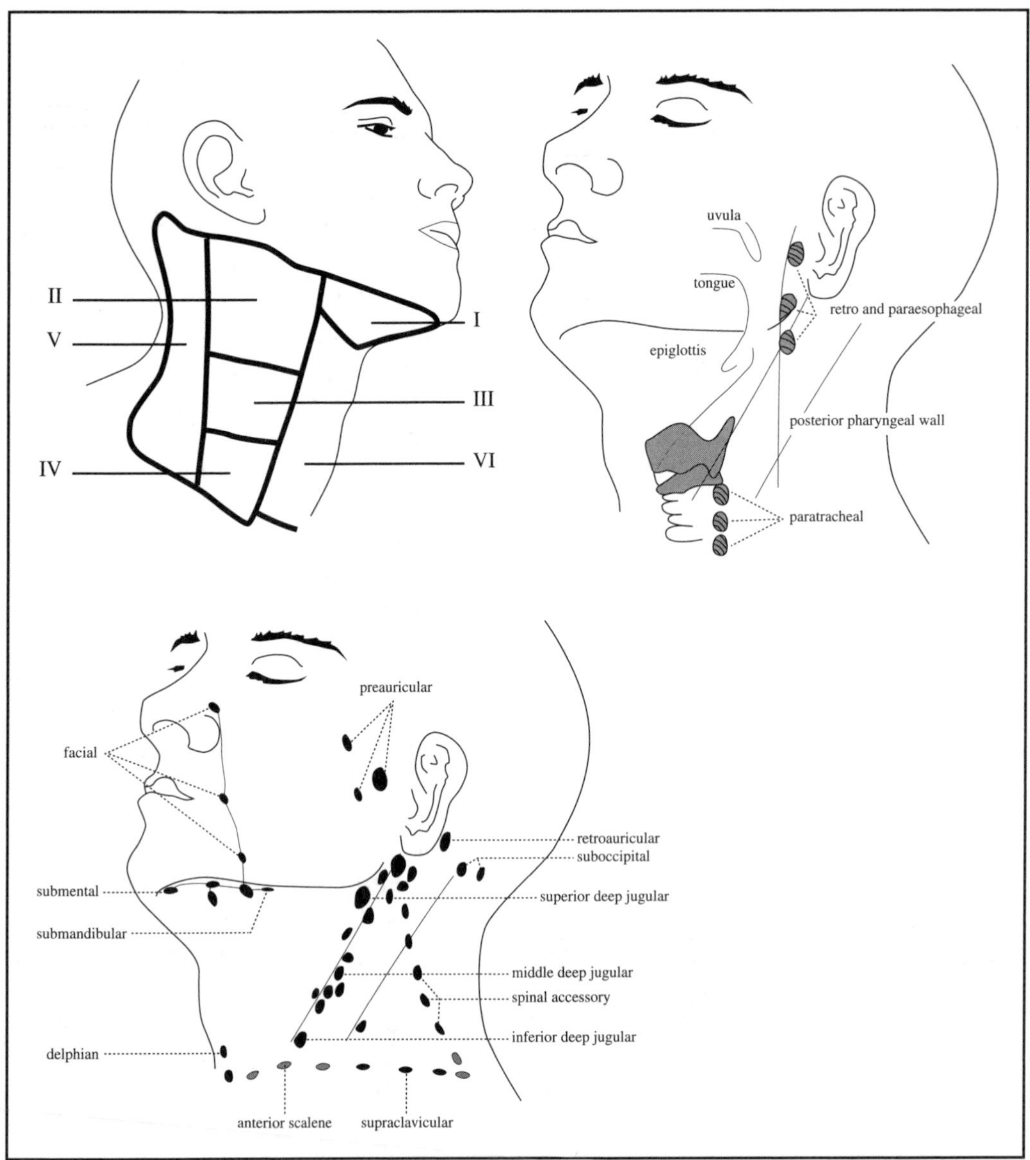

FIGURE 9–1. Lymph node distribution of the head and neck area. I = submental and submandibular nodes; II = upper jugulodigastric group; III = middle jugular nodes draining the nasopharynx and oropharynx, oral cavity, hypopharynx, and larynx; IV = inferior jugular nodes draining the hypopharynx, subglottic larynx, thyroid, and esophagus; V = posterior triangle group; VI = anterior compartment group.

Level IV lymph nodes are located around the lower third of the internal jugular vein extending from the inferior border of the cricoid cartilage to the clavicle inferiorly. The sentinel or Virchow's node, which is located under the clavicle, is included at this level. Nodes in this area are susceptible to metastases arising from the hypopharynx, thyroid, cervical esophagus, and larynx.

Level V lymph nodes comprise the posterior triangle group. These nodes are located along the lower half of the spinal accessory nerve and the transverse cervical artery. This triangular area includes nodes from the anterior boarder of the trapezius muscle posteriorly, the posterior border of the sternocleidomastoid muscle anteriorly, and the clavicle caudally. There are 2 sublevels with VA containing nodes in the superior area including the spinal accessory nodes, and inferiorly VB includes nodes following the transverse cervical vessels and the supraclavicular nodes located directly above the clavicle. The sublevels VA and VB are separated by a horizontal plane through the inferior border of the anterior cricoid arch.

Level VI lymph nodes lie in the anterior compartment that surrounds the midline visceral structures extending from the level of the hyoid bone above to the suprasternal notch below with the lateral borders being the common carotid arteries. This area includes the pretracheal and paratracheal nodes, precricoid (Delphian) node, and the perithyroidal nodes including the lymph nodes along the recurrent laryngeal nerves. The nodes in this area are at risk for metastases from cancers coming from the thyroid gland, glottis and subglottic larynx, apex of the pyriform sinus, and cervical esophagus.[33]

The spread of cancer in the larynx is dependent on the site of origin and T classification of the primary tumor.[30] The true vocal folds are devoid of lymphatic capillaries, and when glottal carcinoma is diagnosed early, treatment outcome is very favorable. Nodal spread from glottal carcinoma occurs when tumor extends into the supraglottic or subglottic areas and may involve nodes at the upper, middle, and lower jugular regions. The supraglottis has an extensive lymphatic network, and drainage from these nodes passes through the thyrohyoid membrane and drains into the upper jugular, mid jugular, and lower jugular nodes of the jugular chain. In the subglottic area, the lymphatic system is less developed but forms 3 lymphatic channels of 1 anterior and 2 posterolateral.[34] Primary tumors occurring in the subglottic area spread to surrounding tissue and then to the mid and lower jugular nodes with contralateral spread of the disease.[30]

TREATMENT OPTIONS

Conservation

Attempts to establish a curative treatment for laryngeal carcinoma date back to the latter 1800s. In 1876, Billroth performed the first total laryngectomy in the treatment of laryngeal carcinoma. Surgery thus remained the treatment modality until the advent of fractionated external beam radiation in the early 1920s. Histological refinements permitted better understanding of the lymphatic system and metastases in the larynx, which brought about conservation treatments. For many years, surgery and radiation therapy were mainstays of treatment in managing head and neck cancers. In 1991, a landmark clinical trial conducted by the Department of Veterans Affairs Laryngeal Cancer Study[35] changed clinical practice by introducing an organ preservation protocol by comparing induction chemotherapy followed by radiation therapy to surgery followed by radiation therapy for individuals with resectable stage III or IV laryngeal cancer. This study revealed no significant difference in survival rate after more than 10 years of follow-up and laryngeal preservation in almost two-thirds of the survivors. Since this study, investigation research on organ preservation of the larynx in advanced laryngeal cancers has looked at combining chemotherapy and radiation therapy.[36,37] The goal in treatment of laryngeal carcinoma is to maximize the cure rate while preserving voice and swallowing function through refined surgical techniques, advancement in the delivery of radiation therapy, and the combination of various chemotherapy agents with radiation therapy.

Combined Treatments

Chemotherapy is the use of drugs that are either administered orally or intravenously and are designed to kill cancer cells. This treatment is a systemic therapy to work on cancer cells that are actively reproducing. Chemotherapy can be administered either neoadjuvant (before) or adjuvant (after) surgery, radiation therapy, or both. In recent years, systemic chemotherapy used with radiotherapy has improved the survival rates of organ preservation.[38–41] Chemotherapy is also used as a palliative treatment if there is recurrent or metastatic disease and the patient does not qualify for any other treatment modalities. There are different types of chemotherapy drugs which can be found on http://www.cancer.org.

Some of the side effects of chemotherapy include:

- nausea
- fatigue
- loss of appetite as a result of change in taste
- weakened immune system
- mucositis or sores in the mouth
- xerostomia
- vomiting
- bowel changes (diarrhea/constipation)
- hair changes/loss
- chemo brain
- hearing loss
- low blood counts
- depression

Radiation Therapy

When a lesion is isolated in a specific location and is in the early stages of laryngeal cancer, radiation therapy (also referred to as radiotherapy) is the most definitive treatment. In more advanced stages of laryngeal carcinoma, radiation therapy can be used for either definitive or adjuvant (additional) treatment.

Radiation therapy involves the use of high-energy x-rays or particles directed to a marked treatment field targeting the tumor site and surrounding tissue. Generally, radiotherapy treatments to the head and neck area are administered in the form of an external beam rather than interstitially (within tissues). Radiotherapy affects all cells, both normal and cancerous, within the area being radiated. The objective of radiation therapy is to administer the maximum dosage (fractions) allowable for destruction of the tumor without irreversibly damaging surrounding healthy structures and tissue. The radiation beam is usually generated by a machine called a linear accelerator. A limiting factor in dosage administration of radiation is normal tissue reaction to the radiation. Conventional accelerated radiotherapy involves approximately

6000 cGY in 25 to 30 fractions of radiation administered daily over a 6- to 7-week period to a specified field[42] that is defined by the radiation oncologist. Some radiotherapy procedures, such as hyperfractionated acceleration, are administered twice a day.

Schemes of administering radiation have changed with advancement of newer technology and 3-dimensional reconstruction of the tumor site. Three-dimensional conformal radiotherapy (3D CRT) combines multiple radiation treatment fields delivered in specific doses to the tumor area. Intensity-modulated radiation therapy (IMRT), a form of 3D-CRT, occurs when high-precision computer-guided treatment generates small radiation pencil beams that conform to the tumor, minimizing toxicity to nearby normal tissues. Because tumors come in different shapes and sizes, 3D CRT uses computers and special imaging techniques to define the tumor. CT, MRI, or PET scans are used to create the detail of the tumor as well as the surrounding tissue. Higher doses of radiation can be tailored to the gross tumor volume with sharp dose gradients delivered to the surrounding tissue. To ensure complete accuracy of the beam directed to the tumor, a custom fabricated mask is individually customized to the patient to maintain complete immobilization of the head, neck, and shoulders during treatment.[43] Intensity-modulated radiation therapy delivers higher doses of radiation than conventional dosing to the tumor site, with less radiation administered to the adjacent surrounding normal tissues, thus preserving function. Less damage to surrounding tissue is advantageous to a patient. For example, with conventional accelerated radiotherapy a patient may have permanent xerostoma (dry mouth) due to destruction of the parotid gland. With intensity-modulated radiotherapy, the parotids are preserved, thus maintaining a better quality of life without laryngeal dryness and quicker healing time.[42]

Radiation therapy may also be administered as an adjuvant treatment before or after surgery or in combination with chemotherapy. When surgery is required to excise a malignant lesion, the surgeon may choose to "shrink" the lesion with radiation therapy prior to surgery. Following surgery, radiation may be used to kill any cancerous cells that were not detected and removed at the time of surgery. Generally, individuals who have radical neck dissections to remove metastatic lymph nodes at the time of a total laryngectomy will undergo radiation treatments following surgery. Patients obtain the best results with postoperative radiation therapy if treatments begin within 6 weeks following surgery and end within 100 days of surgery.[44,45] Radiation therapy can also be used to palliate symptoms such as pain caused by metastases.

Most patients experience various side effects as a result of radiation therapy. If an individual receives radiation to the neck area without surgery, the treatments may also cause increased hoarseness. All of these side effects may progressively worsen as the treatments progress and gradually subside when they are completed. The healing process following surgery appears to progress more rapidly when the patient has not undergone radiation therapy prior to surgery. Radiation therapy may cause some of the following side effects:

- Difficulty swallowing (dysphagia) or pain when swallowing (odynophagia)
- Diminished taste/loss of appetite

- Skin irritation or redness of the radiated area
- Tissue swelling
- Tissue hardening (fibrosis)
- Fatigue
- Possible breathing problems secondary to increased edema
- Decreased salivary flow
- Dry mouth (xerostomia)
- Sore throat
- Nausea
- Hoarseness or change in vocal quality
- Fluid in middle ear creating a hearing loss
- Dryness in the ear canal creating buildup of earwax
- Mucositis
- Hypothyroidism
- Hair loss of the area in the field of radiation
- Damage to dentition
- Tissue necrosis
- Osteoradionecrosis (bone death)
- Lymphedema

Surgery

Total laryngectomy involves the surgical excision of the entire cartilaginous larynx including the epiglottis, its inferior and superior muscular and membranous attachments, the hyoid bone, and the extrinsic strap muscles, and may include the upper 2 or 3 tracheal rings. If the cancer cells have metastasized to the cervical lymph nodes, surgery will include a neck dissection(s). Robbins et al[33] describes 4 neck dissection classifications:

1. Radical neck dissection is the standard procedure for cervical lymphadenectomy, and subsequent procedures are variants of this procedure. During a radical neck dissection the cervical lymph nodes removed extend from the inferior border of the mandible to the clavicle, from the lateral boarder of the sternohyoid muscle, hyoid bone, and contralateral anterior belly of the digastric muscle medially, to the anterior border of the trapezius muscle. This includes all lymph nodes from levels I to V as well as the internal jugular vein, sternocleidomastoid muscle, and spinal accessory nerve. A radical neck dissection may be performed on the right, left, or both sides of the neck.
2. Modified radical neck dissection involves all lymph nodes from levels I to V with preservation of 1 or more nonlymphatic structures (internal jugular vein, sternocleidomastoid muscle, and spinal accessory nerve), for example, modified neck dissection with preservation of the spinal accessory nerve.
3. Selective neck dissection refers to preservation of 1 or more of the lymph node groups from levels I to V that are routinely removed for a radical neck dissection. Selective neck dissection is based on the predictable patterns of metastases according to the site of the cancer. The lymph nodes that are at the greatest risk for oral cancer are located in levels I, II, and III. For oropharyngeal, hypopharyngeal, and laryngeal cancers, nodes in the levels of II, III, and IV are at risk, whereas for thyroid cancer, level VI nodes are at risk for metastases.
4. Extended neck dissection refers to the removal of additional lymph node groups or nonlymphatic structures relative to the radical neck dissection (eg, lymph nodes groups that would include parapharyngeal, superior mediastinal, perifacial, and paratracheal or nonlymphatic

structures such as the carotid artery, hypoglossal nerve, vagus nerve, and paraspinal muscles).

The biological function of the larynx is to serve as a valve to protect the trachea and lungs from aspiration of swallowed liquids and solids (Figure 9–2).

After laryngeal excision, the original pulmonary airway cannot be protected or maintained. Thus, the trachea is redirected and sutured to the external neck area just above the notch of the sternum. This opening in the neck is called a stoma. The stoma serves as the point of air exchange with the atmosphere. There no longer remains a connection between the trachea and the pharynx, nose, and mouth (Figure 9–3).

The esophagus remains intact during the total laryngectomy. Because of the previous attachment of the larynx and the pharynx, the anterior pharyngeal walls must be joined and sutured together with the hypopharynx and then sutured to the upper esophagus. When the pharynx is sutured to the base of the tongue, the oral-pharyngeal-esophageal track is completed. The passage of liquids and foods remains the same as before the surgery.

Concurrent Chemoradiotherapy

Careful diagnosis, advancement of technology, precise staging of cancers, novel chemotherapy agents, and dosing schedules have contributed to changes in the treatment of laryngeal cancer. Combining 2 or 3 types of treatment may be the most effective in treatment of the size and stage (extent) and location of the tumor. The rationale in support of the use of chemotherapy concurrently administered with radiation is threefold: (1) organ preservation, (2) the action of chemotherapy as a radiosensitizer by improving the probability of local control and survival secondary to the destruction of radioresistant cells, and (3) the possibility that treatment may systemically and potentially eradicate distant micrometastases.[46] A surgeon, radiation oncologist, and medical oncologist make up the team of cancer specialists when combined therapies are used to treat the patient.

Chemotherapy is the administration of anticancer drugs intravenously or by mouth. The cytotoxic drugs are systemically delivered via the circulatory system to the individual cells, killing or changing the cancerous cells and inhibiting tumor growth. The 2 most common cytotoxic drugs used in the treatment of head and neck carcinomas are cisplatin (alkylating agent) and 5-fluorouracil (5-FU) (antimetabolites). Alkylating agents are drugs that react chemically and damage the DNA in the cell nucleus preventing the cell from dividing and growing. Antimetabolites damage cells by interfering with the production of DNA, preventing essential nutrients to the cells' normal growth process.[47] Cisplatin is the only evidence-based drug that has been extensively studied in head and neck[48,49] in combination with chemoradiotherapy and is a widely used standard therapy administered with a 100 mg/m^2 every 3 weeks regimen in combination with ~70 Gy radiation delivered in 1.8 to 2.0 Gy daily fractions.[49,50] Other single chemotherapy agents studied have been: carboplatin, 5-fluorouracil, taxane, hydroxyurea, tirapazamine, cetuximab, and methotrexate. Multiagent-based chemoradiotherapy of combining several drugs are being studied and offers improved radiosensitization of tumor cells with increased systemic benefits.[51–55]

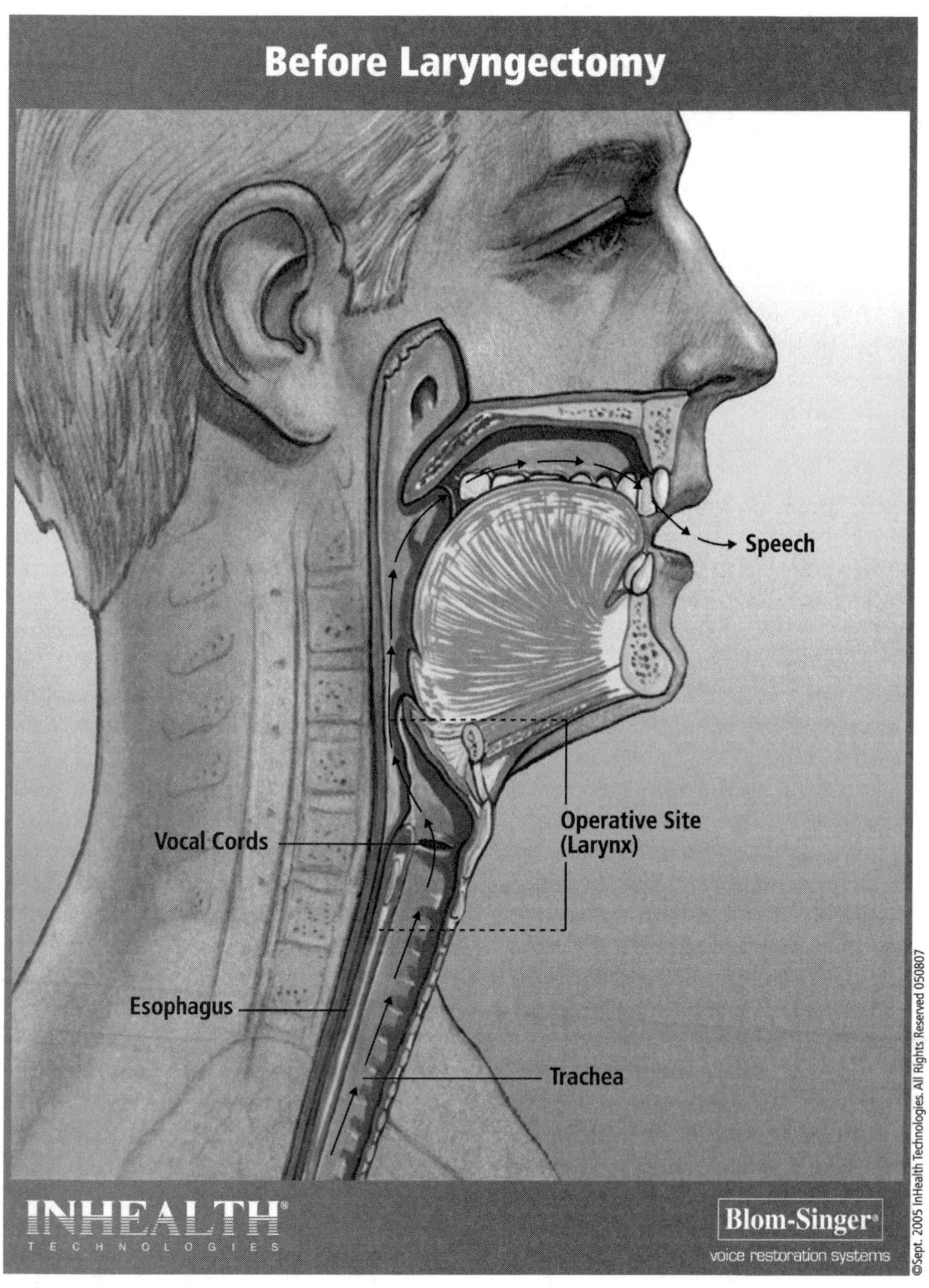

FIGURE 9–2. Larynx before laryngectomy. (Photo courtesy of InHealth Technologies, http://www.inhealth.com)

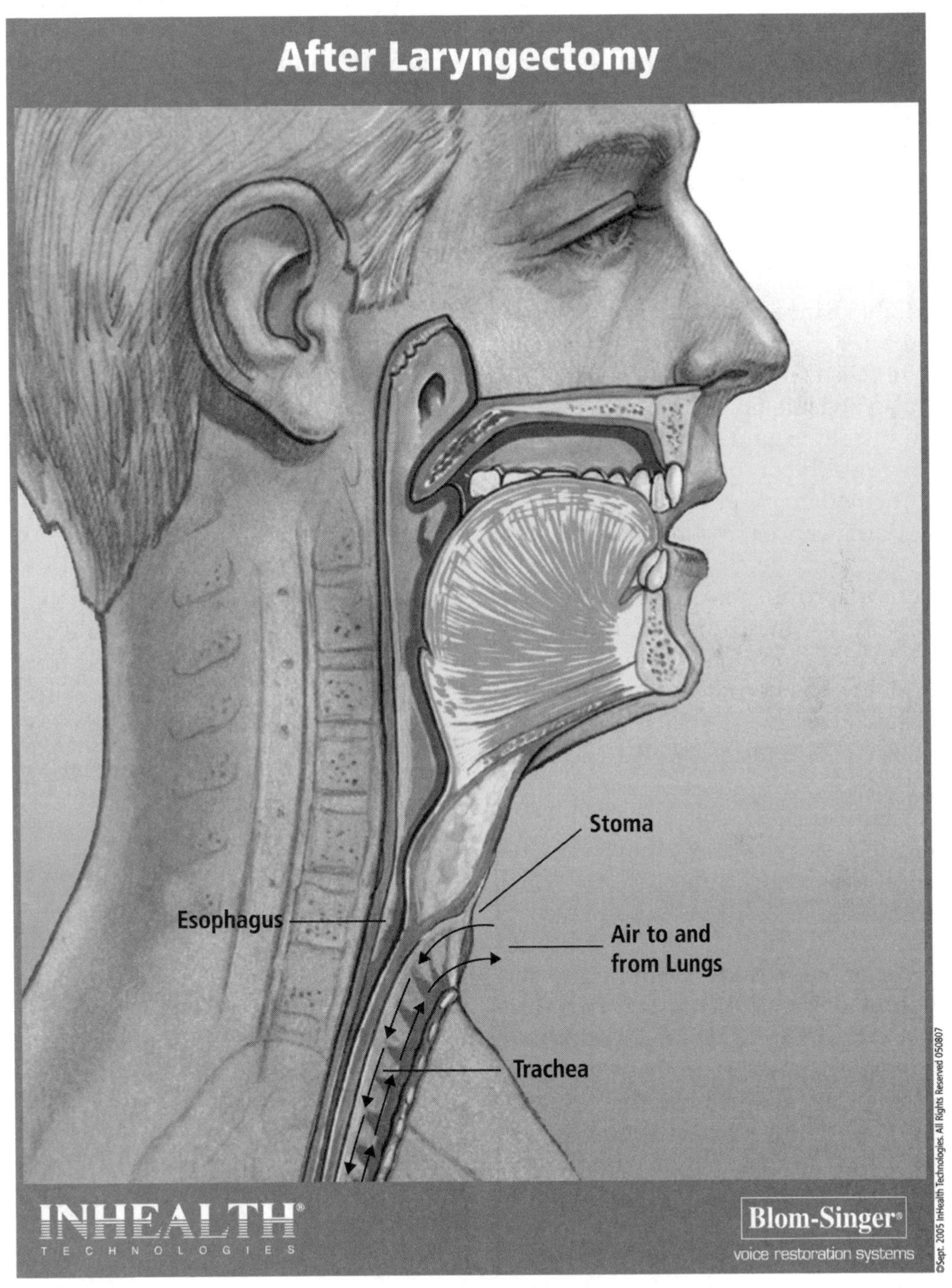

FIGURE 9–3. After laryngectomy. (Photo courtesy of InHealth Technologies, http://www.inhealth.com)

Research has shown trends that chemotherapy concurrent with radiation therapy has promising long-term effects; however, clinical trials are currently being conducted to determine the best regimens (single-agent or multiagent chemoradiotherapy) for treatment of patients with advanced carcinoma in the head and neck. Chemotherapy is also used for palliative measures in unresectable cancers of individuals where radiation treatments and/or surgery have failed to control tumor growth. It is also a viable option for patients who are unable to undergo surgery due to other health concerns. A meta-analysis of chemotherapy in patients with head and neck cancer has shown a survival benefit with concurrent chemoradiotherapy for the management of locoregionally advanced disease in comparison to radiation alone.[56] This treatment modality has become widely accepted and is now the standard of care for intermediate and advanced-stage laryngeal cancer.[57]

Side effects from chemotherapy may include nausea, vomiting, fatigue, hair loss, sores in the mouth (mucositis), dermatitis, loss of appetite secondary to a change in sense of taste, dry mouth (xerostomia), weakened immunity system, bleeding, bruising, allergic reactions, diarrhea and/or constipation, as well as possible damage to other internal organs including the kidneys, heart, lungs, liver, and nervous system. Individuals undergoing chemotherapy must have frequent blood tests to monitor blood counts. With the advancement of antinausea medications, most individuals can tolerate chemotherapy. During treatment it is advised that patients do not smoke, eat frequent small meals, hydrate with water, and avoid alcoholic and caffeinated beverages, aspirin, and exposure to known infections and viruses. It is important to note that not all individuals experience side effects from chemotherapy. Side effects are usually dependent on the type of drug administered, the amount given, and the duration of the treatment. Most side effects resolve after treatment is completed.

METHODS OF RECONSTRUCTION

When cancer involves other structures such as the pharynx, hypopharynx, or esophagus, in addition to the larynx, additional surgical reconstruction techniques are used to help restore function while retaining socially acceptable cosmesis. Because tissue is removed from the cancerous site, muscle tissue or sections of the alimentary tract can be used to reconstruct the defect. This gives support and protection to the head and neck area where the tissue was resected. The factors that account for the success of tissue transfer are pre- or postradiation treatments, revascularization, and nutritional status of the individual. Reattachment of the microvessels of the flap to the remaining tissue is important to prevent necrosis. Radiation and poor nutritional intake are negative indicators for tissue transfer. The type of reconstruction is dependent on the location and extent of tissue resection and presents a challenge in restoring the physiologic requirements for the swallowing and voice production. Each reconstruction technique has merit as well as disadvantages for voice restoration.[58] The following is a discussion of some of the methods of reconstruction.

- Myocutaneous flaps
  The pectoralis major (taken from the chest) myocutaneous flap has been used to reconstruct the pharynx and provide protection of the carotid following radical neck dissection.[59,60] Because it is highly vascularized and easily accessible for reconstruction, the pectoralis muscle is commonly used as a regional flap for reconstruction. Voice production is generally functional but not equal to tracheoesophageal voice (use of voice prosthesis) production following a total laryngectomy. These patients are also subject to changes that may occur from wound healing and radiation treatments.
- Free flaps
  A free flap is tissue removed from a donor site and placed into the recipient site using microvascular anastomosis (connecting the vessels). A donor site that is often used for pharyngoesophageal reconstruction is the radial forearm.[61] The radial forearm flap is much thinner with less bulk compared to the pectoralis muscle flap. It has excellent vascularity and is not adversely affected by postoperative radiation. Although radial forearm flaps used in reconstruction of the laryngopharynx tend to be stiffer in comparison to pharyngeal mucosa, patients can achieve acceptable and functional voicing with a voice prosthesis.[58]
- Jejunal free flap
  A portion of the jejunum (second portion of the small intestine) can be used to replace a laryngopharyngectomy defect. Due to discoordination of the intrinsic jejunal peristalsis and increased mucus production, individuals may develop swallowing problems.[62] Voicing is characterized by a wet, gurgly, hypotonic, soft quality with decreased intensity and generally poor quality. Sustained voicing is decreased secondary to the hypotonicity of the tissue.
- Gastric pull-up
  When removing the entire esophagus, a gastric pull-up can be performed that involves the transposition of the entire stomach.[58] Usually, patients need to eat smaller meals and more frequently. Voice restoration can be performed as a secondary procedure; however, the resulting voice is characterized by a wet quality with decreased volume.

Patients undergoing flap reconstruction surgery may experience difficulty swallowing. A videofluoroscopy study can be very informative in assessing the patency of the reconstructed area during swallowing and for voicing. If the reconstructed area is narrowed, the patient may undergo dilation of the lumen. When an individual with reconstruction has a voice prosthesis for communication purposes but is not able to produce voice after a reasonable amount of training, the voice pathologist needs to investigate and introduce other methods of communication to provide the patient with functional speech.

NEED FOR FOLLOW-UP TREATMENT

Individuals treated for laryngeal cancer are at risk for developing recurrences or new cancers in the head and neck area. These individuals must be closely followed after treatment. Recurrent cancers are likely to return within the first 2 years after initial treatment. It is important for the otolaryngologist to follow the patient on a monthly basis during the first year, bimonthly visits the second year, quarterly visits the third year, and 6-month follow-up the fourth and fifth years. If a patient remains free of cancer after 5 years from the initial date of being diagnosed, yearly visits are generally recommended.

Following treatment, the patient is advised to immediately report any new symptoms to the otolaryngologist to rule out possible recurrences. The voice pathologist must also be keenly aware of any physical changes or patient-reported symptoms that may be signs of recurrences or metastatic disease. These changes should be shared immediately with the otolaryngologist. The following case illustrates the importance of this medical follow-up.

An 83-year-old gentleman who communicated using tracheoesophageal speech came to the clinic with difficulty talking. A new, small, raised, and irritated area was visible on the left of the patient's stoma. Also, he reported a recent weight loss. Both the weight loss and the unusual appearing tissue were suspicious. The physician was notified and a biopsy was performed. The result of the biopsy was recurrent squamous cell carcinoma and the patient underwent chemotherapy. Several months following chemotherapy, the site of the lesion remained free of disease.

Multidisciplinary Rehabilitation Team

Rehabilitation of the total laryngectomized individual involves many different professionals. A multidisciplinary team approach is essential to serve the medical, psychological, communication, and social needs of the patient and family. In medical settings where a large number of total laryngectomees are treated each year, it is possible to form such a team from existing professional personnel. The interaction of the multidisciplinary team involves evaluating treatment options and the total needs of the patient and the family. These needs may include treatment modalities, preconsultation and preparing the individual for surgery and/or combined modality of chemoradiation therapy, providing support and educational training through the hospital stay and treatments, planning for discharge support, and planning actions to meet future needs. The primary goal is to return the patient to as normal a lifestyle and quality of life as possible. The type of cancer determines what specialists may be seen. Individuals serving on a multidisciplinary team include the follow professionals:

- Head and Neck Surgeon
  The surgeon serves as the primary case manager and is responsible for diagnosis of the disease, treatment planning, and the entire medical management of the patient. The surgeon informs the patient of the medical condition and details the implications of the surgery and subsequent medical treatments. She or he makes referrals to other medical team members regarding treatment options. Referrals to other medical personnel are important to help the patient obtain all necessary information regarding the various treatment modalities. When necessary, the surgeon also makes referrals to other appropriate team members.

- Plastic and Reconstructive Surgeon
  A plastic and reconstructive surgeon may also join the surgical team. In some settings when surgery involves removal of structures such as the pharynx, hypopharynx, or esophagus in addition to a total laryngectomy, the plastic and reconstructive surgeon uses microvascular surgery to repair these defects by removing healthy muscle or skin from other parts of the body to reconstruct the tissue.

- Radiation Oncologist
  The radiation oncologist studies the stage of the tumor and the involvement of surrounding tissue as well as uninvolved critical structures to determine if radiation therapy would be an acceptable definitive treatment option for the patient. If radiotherapy is selected, the radiation oncologist plans the type, chooses the treatment schema, and calculates optimal dosage levels that will irradiate the tumor and slow spread of the disease while preserving function.

- Medical Oncologist
  The oncologist specializes in the treatment of cancer through the administration of chemotherapy. The oncologist reviews the tumor type and selects a chemotherapeutic regimen including the chemical agents, dosage levels, and treatment schedules. If a patient qualifies to be in a clinical research trial, the oncologist manages the protocol to be followed. The oncologist works closely with the radiation oncologist when combined modality treatment of chemotherapy and radiotherapy is pursued.

- Speech-Language Pathologist
  The speech-language pathologist (SLP) is directly responsible for evaluating and providing for the patient's short-term and long-term communication needs as well as management of swallowing if needed. Intervention occurs throughout the individual's treatment of the disease including pretreatment consultation. The initial speech pathology consultation with the patient may include family members and or close friends. It is an informational-educational session discussing issues related to changes in speech and alternate forms of communication (should the patient undergo surgical removal of the larynx). Management of swallowing problems is also discussed as needed in the course of treatment, and the patient is assured of intervention if needed. It is important that the patient be seen prior to radiation or chemoradiation treatment and followed during radiation as voice and swallowing can be affected as a result of edema. For alaryngeal speech therapy, the patient is seen postoperatively by the speech-language pathologist to address communication needs, swallowing issues, and voice restoration. Management of lymphedema of the head and neck which is common following radiation therapy can be addressed by the SLP.[63] (A complete description of the speech-language pathologist's role follows in the section entitled The Role of Speech Pathology.

- Oncology Nurse
  The oncology nurse is an essential member of the multidisciplinary team in the rehabilitation of the laryngectomized patient during the patient's hospitalization. Beyond the day-to-day care and moral support provided by the nurse, the nurse is responsible

for teaching the patient and family the skills necessary for independent stoma care including use of a suctioning machine. The nurse helps the patient understand and accept the new experience of breathing through the stoma and often uncomfortable experience of coughing and sneezing from the stoma. Stoma hygiene is important, and the tasks of caring for the respiratory system must be learned prior to hospital discharge. The patient is educated and trained to care for a stoma vent or possible tracheostomy tube, as needed. The nurse also serves in a supportive role for the hospitalized patient undergoing chemotherapy for the treatment of laryngeal carcinoma.

- Dietitian
  Patients respond better to surgery and heal more rapidly when they are in good nutritional health. The dietitian is responsible for evaluating the nutritional needs of each patient and correcting nutritional imbalances. Because of the social habits of some patients and presurgical swallowing problems experienced by others, many patients who undergo a total laryngectomy do not maintain adequate nutritional health. Occasionally, surgery is not scheduled until the patient's nutritional level can be improved. This improvement may involve supplementing food intake with high levels of nutrients that may be taken orally or in an intravenous solution. Following surgery, the dietitian monitors caloric intake and determines the nutritional requirements necessary for the patient to gain and maintain an adequate weight. The patient and family are also advised of the proper eating habits necessary upon discharge. If the patient receives radiation and/or chemotherapy, the dietitian also monitors the patient's weight and nutritional intake.

- Radiologist
  The radiologist interprets the results of the chest x-ray, computerized tomography (CT) scan, magnetic resonance imaging (MRI), or positive emission test (PET) and aids the surgeon in planning the most appropriate treatment approach.

- Histopathologist
  A histopathologist is a physician who makes diagnoses from tissue samples.

- Physical Therapist
  Patients who undergo total laryngectomy with radical neck dissection and those who undergo radiation therapy to the neck may require the services of a physical therapist. Surgical trauma and excision of neck and shoulder muscles and the spinal accessory nerve will often limit the patient's ability to freely move the arm, shoulder, and neck of the dissected side. Radiation may stiffen the muscle fibers and limit mobility in the neck area. The physical therapist designs and implements therapy programs based on the physical disabilities created by the surgery.

- Dentist and/or Prosthodontist
  Radiation-induced oral mucosal tissue changes may include stomatitis, xerostomia, tissue necrosis, hypogeusia (taste change), and trismus. These conditions affect the patient's oral sensations as well as function. A pretreatment dental examination with prophylaxis for patients receiving radiation therapy is recommended.

The dentist evaluates the condition of the mouth and teeth, documenting baseline conditions and possible risk factors prior to treatment. If extensive decay or poor dentition is present, dental extraction or repair is recommended to prevent further complications secondary to radiation. If the teeth are in good condition, the dentist will recommend a preventive program. Preradiation dental cleaning is recommended to reduce bacterial infections. To reduce any radiation-induced oral problems, the dentist may prescribe daily fluoride treatments and instructions on proper brushing and flossing. Checkups are recommended during radiation treatments if problems arise, 2 months following treatment and then every 6 months.

A prosthodontic evaluation prior to radiation treatment assures proper fitting or adjustment to dentures and or prosthetic devices. Devices may need adjustments to prevent sliding or friction against tissue to alleviate possible irritation. Dentures and appliances are removed during treatments. Following completion of radiation therapy and when appropriate, patients who have undergone dental extractions can be fitted for dentures or prosthetic appliances to help with chewing and speech.

- Clinical Social Worker
  The social worker helps patients, families, and friends cope with the diagnosis of cancer and helps with obtaining the necessary services in the community to address psychological or social barriers to treatment. The social worker assists the patient and family to identify the appropriate resources needed which may include transportation to and from treatment, home health care, rehabilitative or skilled care, community support programs, lodging and housing, financial support programs, crisis intervention, counseling, advance directives, and hospice care.

- Psychologist
  The psychologist provides extended patient and family counseling as needed. The laryngectomized patient is required to make many emotional and social adjustments. The psychologist helps the patient deal with such issues as potential death, serious illness, disfigurement, anger, postoperative depression, changing family roles, self-image, fears of recurrence, and sexuality. A review of the literature by Humphris emphasizes the importance of this team member in providing psychosocial support.[64]

- Audiologist
  Hearing acuity and presbycusis may need to be addressed in this population. Hearing sensitivity may change following a laryngectomy.[65] It is also possible that normal eustachian tube functioning may be impaired by surgery or subsequent radiation therapy, or both, causing middle ear dysfunction. The audiologist is responsible for evaluating the auditory condition of the laryngectomized patient and recommending amplification when appropriate. Hearing loss may impede the patient's speech monitoring during the rehabilitation process.[66,67]

  In addition to testing the patient, audiological evaluation of the spouse or companion is strongly recommended.[68] Successful rehabilitation may be limited if the spouse is unable to hear the patient's speech efforts adequately.

- The Laryngectomized Visitor
  An important team member is the nonprofessional who has experienced the patient's situation and has adjusted well. The laryngectomized visitor who has learned to speak well may lift the patient's spirits and provide motivation for successful recovery and rehabilitation. It is also recommended that the visitor's spouse meet with the patient's spouse. Spouse-to-spouse support is often just as valuable as patient-to-patient support.

SPECIAL CONCERNS OF THE LARYNGECTOMIZED PATIENT

The ultimate goal of a total laryngectomy is to "cure" the patient of cancer through surgical excision of the malignancy. Because of the ability to isolate and excise the cancer through laryngeal excision, cancer of the larynx is one of the most curable forms of cancer when the disease is identified early. The results of the surgery leave the patient with the major problem of reestablishing oral communication. The patient must also address several other physical, psychological, and social concerns. If the patient is to live a quality life, the ability to make the appropriate adjustments is just as important as reestablishing speech. Let us consider some of these concerns.

Communication

The only vital or essential part of oral communication missing following a total laryngectomy is a sound generator. The patient's language and cognitive abilities as well as the ability to articulate remain intact. Although implications of the loss of voice have been explained well to the patient, the impact is often not fully realized until the patient awakens from the anesthesia and automatically tries to speak. The realization is even more dramatic later when the patient attempts to express his or her feelings and needs and is constrained by cumbersome writing or unintelligible articulation and mouthing of words and phrases. Most of us take our ability to speak for granted, because speaking is an automatic act. If the speaking ability is withdrawn or impaired, we quickly realize the profound loss of this expressive communication modality.

The laryngectomized individual is soon confronted with communication deprivation. There is a distinct difference in communicating to make one's needs known (such as hunger, thirst, yes, no, bathroom, etc) and communicating complex thoughts, feelings, and actions. The initial forms of communication for the laryngectomized patient are usually writing and mouthing words. Writing is slow and laborious for both the patient and the reader, and, of course, not all patients can write. Mouthing words is effective only if the patient's articulation is excellent and if the listener has the ability to understand speech without sound. Patients often have many thoughts that they would like to express, but because of the effort required to communicate, do not try. If this situation continues, the patient will soon become isolated.

Therefore, it is in the patient's best interest to reestablish some form of oral communication as soon as possible. This goal may be accomplished soon after surgery, while still hospitalized, with the use of an artificial larynx. A long-standing negative bias against early use of an artificial larynx prevailed for years based on the worry that the patient would develop a dependency on the device and would therefore not be as likely to develop other forms of alaryngeal speech. Currently, clinicians understand that early oral communication is essential, and that withholding an available means of communication is more likely to disrupt the rehabilitation process.

The early days following surgery are usually quite traumatic for the patient and the family. Providing an effective means of communication will ease this trauma. Other forms of communication can be explored as soon as the patient is medically and physically healed and released by the physician.

Physical Concerns

Respiration

Another concern of the laryngectomized patient is adjustment to breathing through the stoma. Prior to surgery, normal respiratory exchange had the advantages of the nose. The nose is essentially an air treatment center. Before reaching the lungs, the air is filtered by the hairs in the nose, humidified by the mucous membrane of the nose and pharynx, and warmed along the entire upper respiratory tract. The laryngectomized patient no longer has advantages of a natural filtering, moistening, and warming air treatment system. Without a substitute, untreated air is inhaled directly into the trachea and lungs. The laryngectomee is subjected to the atmospheric conditions whether the air is dry or humidified. Dry air causes increased mucous buildup with thicker secretions and decreased ciliary function.

Passive heat and moisture exchange (HME) stoma air-filtering systems are available for the laryngectomee. These specially designed filters are placed over the stoma by peristomal adhesion and serve to compensate for the loss of upper airway function.[69–72] Air is exchanged through the filter which filters out unwanted particles from entering the trachea. Inhaled air is filtered and humidified by the natural moisture in the material created by the condensation from the exhalations, and warmed by the warmth of the material. This warm, filtered, moist air exchange reduces the amount of mucus and the likelihood for mucus to become encrusted and build up in the bronchial pathway, thus decreasing coughing. The HME system partially restores breathing resistance and improves lung function. Commercially available heat and moisture exchangers include:

- InHealth Blom-Singer Easy Touch Speech Button and MucusShield Occluder (Figure 9–4)

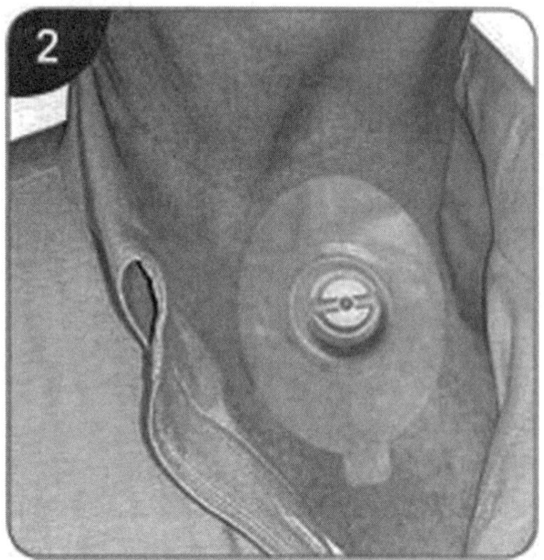

FIGURE 9–4. Patient wearing Blom-Singer Easy Touch HME System with adhesive housing. (Photo courtesy of InHealth Technologies, http://www.inhealth.com)

- Provox HME System and Provox Micron HME and Filter (Figure 9–5A)
- Provox HME System with Provox LaryTube and Adhesive Housing (Figure 9–5B)

Selection of an HME may be dependent on daily cost as well as fixation of the device to the stoma.[73]

Other stoma covers (Figure 9–6) can be worn directly over the stoma and are made of porous material, either cloth or foam.

Stoma covers provide a protective function as well as improve the cosmetic appearance of the neck. The exchange of air through the material of the stoma cover aids to warm the air and add moisture when breathing. Stoma covers protect the airway by filtering out dust, fumes, insects, and other foreign matter. Hygienically, stoma covers help to block mucus when expelled from a cough or sneeze. The laryngectomized patient should also consider wearing stoma covers for cosmetic reasons. The general population is often uncomfortable around laryngectomized patients with an uncovered stoma in full view. This accommodation is part of the patient's social adjustment and acceptance. Stoma covers are health benefits as well. Covering the stoma is especially beneficial in cold weather and when the air is very dry. It is recommended the patient use a room humidifier following

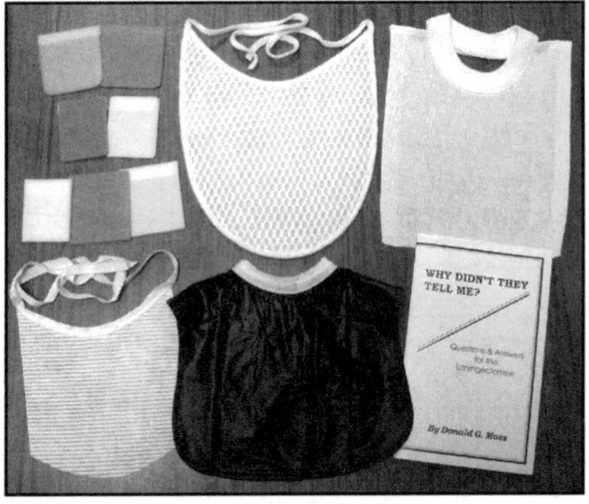

FIGURE 9–6. Stoma cover starter kit (Photo courtesy of Luminaud, http://www.luminaud.com)

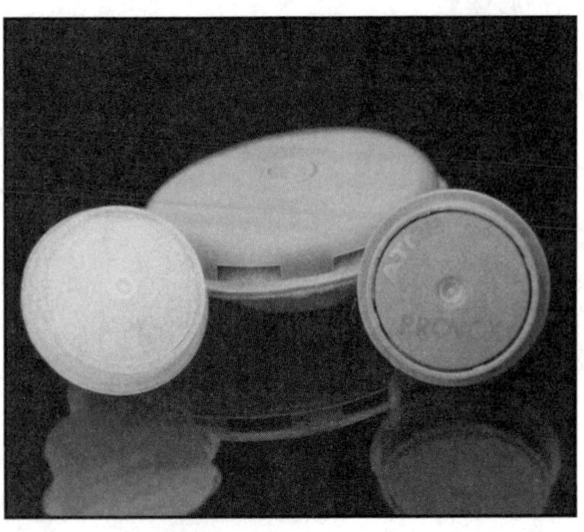

A

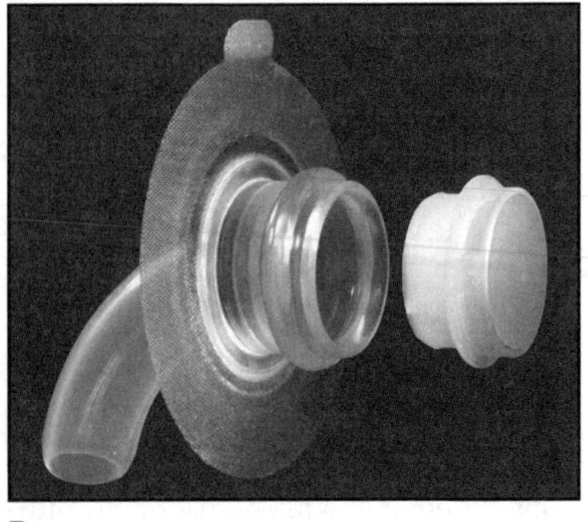

B

FIGURE 9–5. A. Provox HME, Provox Micron and Provox HME. **B.** Provox HME system with Provox LaryTube and Adhesive Housing. (Photos courtesy of Atos Medical, http://www.atosmedical.com)

surgery to limit drying and irritation of the lining of the trachea.[74]

Recent research has investigated speech breathing behaviors in tracheoesophageal speakers in varied speech tasks.[75,76] Given pulmonary air is used to produce tracheoesophageal speech, Bohnenkamp[75] noted that tracheoesophageal speakers used higher lung volumes with increased rib cage and abdominal excursion at the onset of speech in reading and spontaneous speech as compared to laryngeal speakers. Tracheoesophageal speakers also terminated speech below their resting expiratory level.

Coughing and Sneezing

Breathing is only one of the respiratory functions of the stoma. Laryngectomized patients also cough and sneeze through the stoma. Patients need to be reminded to cover the stoma instead of the mouth when coughing; otherwise, the discharged mucus is expelled into the air or on others. Another concern is the "runny" nose. Posterior drainage and swallowing remain intact. However, because the respiratory connection between the nose and the lungs no longer exists, drainage from the nose cannot be prevented. The laryngectomized patient must either wipe or use the small amount of intraoral pressure to blow the nose free of mucus. A tissue or handkerchief should be available at all times.

Tracheal Tubes and Tracheostoma Vents

Concerns regarding the stoma also include the use and care of the tracheal tubes and tracheostoma vents (Figures 9–7A and 9–7B).

At the time of surgery, a tracheal tube may be inserted in the stoma as a means of keeping it open and maintaining the air passage. As the tissue shrinks

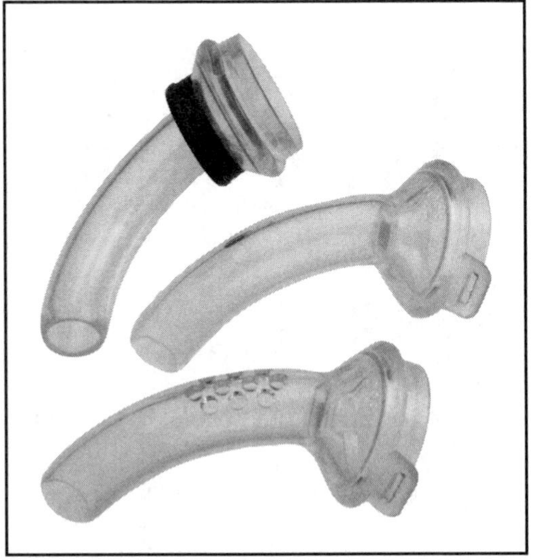

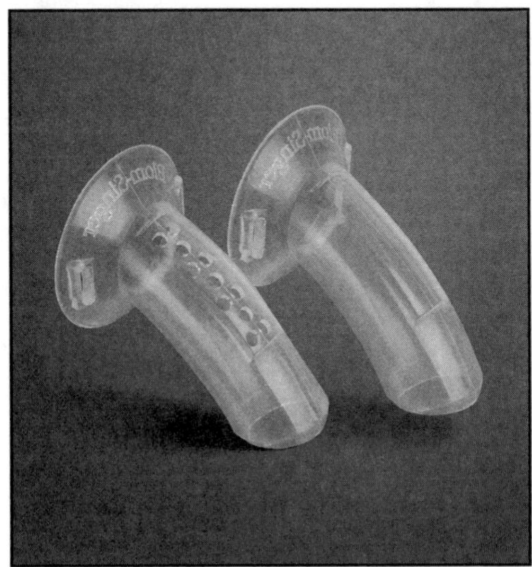

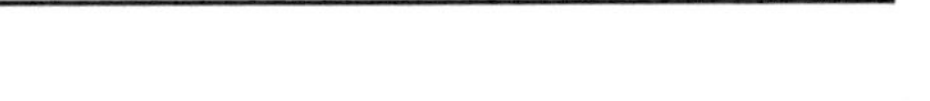

A B

FIGURE 9–7. A. Provox LaryTubes. **B.** Blom-Singer laryngectomy tubes. (Photos courtesy of InHealth Technologies, http://www.inhealth.com)

during the healing process, the tube maintains the integrity of the stoma, preventing a reduction in its size. Generally the patient does not need a tracheal tube; however, if after several days the stoma starts to shrink, the physician may insert a tracheostoma vent to prevent further stenosis. Tracheostoma vents are manufactured in various diameter sizes and lengths. A variety of devices can be used to maintain stoma patency (Figures 9–8A and 9–8B). A trained clinician will assess and prescribe the best device for the given patient's needs.

As mentioned previously, it is important for the patient to assume independent care of the stoma, which includes cleaning the tracheal tube or vent. Following surgery, most patients secrete and cough thick mucus plugs. These plugs hinder air exchange, making breathing difficult. Care of the stoma and tracheal tube involves removing the inner tube (cannula) for washing, removing dried mucus from the stoma with a long-handle tweezers, and suctioning accumulated mucous secretions from the trachea with a suction machine.[77] Mild soap and water can be used to clean the tracheostoma vent. Patients are taught to inhale a small amount of commercially prepared saline solution into the stoma to thin out thick secretions, making it easier to suction or expel mucus. Regular stoma care maintains an open airway and prevents irritating mucus crusts from forming on the skin around the stoma.

As healing progresses, most patients are able to reduce gradually and eventually eliminate the use of a tracheal tube or stoma vent. Some patients are required to wear a tracheostoma vent 24 hours per day to prevent stoma stenosis, whereas others maintain an adequate stoma size by wearing a vent only several hours per day. The tracheostoma vent can be fenestrated (opened) to accommodate the voice prosthesis for tracheoesophageal speech. There are several types of silicone laryngectomy tubes, stoma buttons, or tracheostoma vents that can

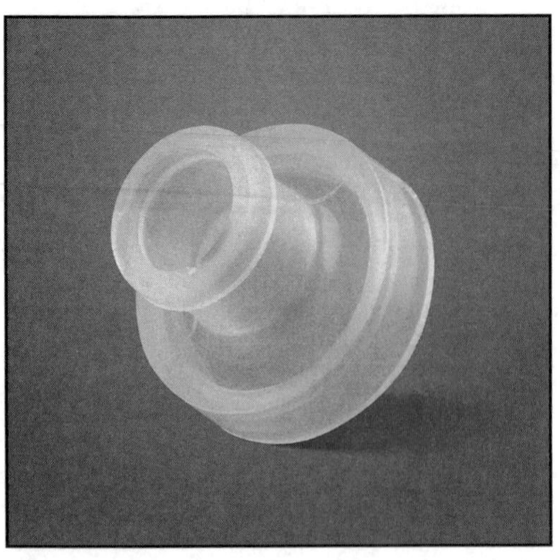

A

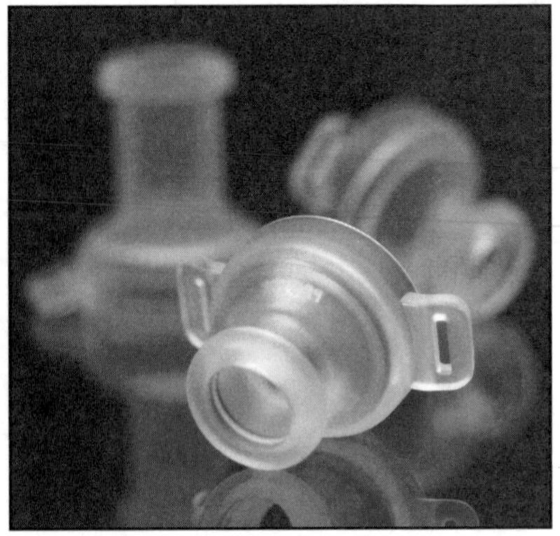

B

FIGURE 9–8. **A.** Barton-Mayo tracheostoma button. **B.** Provox LaryButtons. (Photos courtesy of Atos Medical, http://www.atosmedical.com)

be used to maintain stoma patency. The Provox LaryTube, Barton-Mayo Tracheostoma Button, Provox LaryButton, and Andres Fahl Laryngotec Blom-Singer Laryngectomy tube can all be used with a heat and moisture exchanger.

Swallowing

If possible, a presurgical clinical swallowing assessment should be performed to assess oral-motor function regarding range of motion, strength, dentition, and ability to manipulate and propel material from the oral cavity.[78] Prior to surgery, swallowing difficulties may be associated with size and location of the tumor, which can affect bolus flow and clearance in the oropharyngeal phase of swallowing. Manofluorography studies revealed postoperative swallowing changes with prolonged pharyngeal transit times in postlaryngectomy patients with and without tongue impairment. However, longer transit times were noted for individuals with tongue impairment secondary to decreased lingual propulsion.[79] Dysphagia ranges from 10% to 60% following a total laryngectomy[80] as a result of a number of causes which include surgery,[81] gastroesophageal reflux, radiotherapy,[82] postoperative complications such as pharyngocutaneous fistulae,[83] and anatomical variations such as anterior pharyngeal pouches or pseudodiverticulum.[79]

If a tracheoesophageal puncture (TEP) is performed as part of the primary procedure, the patient is fed through the catheter that is directed down the esophagus via the TEP. Usually, the patient is permitted by the otolaryngologist to begin drinking clear liquids orally on the seventh day following surgery. This assumes normal healing has taken place. Sometimes, patients develop fistulas that delay oral feeds. A bedside swallowing evaluation by the speech-language pathologist assesses labial, lingual, and palatal range of movement and makes recommendations regarding the consistency of food intake. A modified barium swallow examination is performed to assess the oral, pharyngeal, and esophageal phase of swallowing should a patient develop swallowing problems. Some patients develop esophageal narrowing secondary to wound healing and/or radiation therapy, which create a feeling of food sticking in the throat. Esophageal dilatations improve swallowing for these patients.

Smell and Taste

Smell and taste are related physical changes that are affected in the laryngectomized patient. Because the patient has lost the ability to inhale air through the nose, the ability to smell is impaired even though there is no impairment in the olfactory organ itself. The odor is simply not able to reach the organ to be sensed. Deterioration of olfaction after a total laryngectomy can be profound in the inability to detect smoke or leaking gas and create safety problems as fumes directly enter the lungs without the person being aware of it.[84]

The chemical sense of smell can occur through orthonasal olfaction or retronasal olfaction. Orthonasal refers to the flow of air through the nose or by sniffing which sends the odor to the olfactory epithelium, which excites the olfactory nerve, CN I. Airflow also enters the nasal passages posteriorly when breathing out the nose, or chewing or swallowing, which is thus referred to as retronasal olfaction.[85] Although the olfactory nerve, CN I, is the primary pathway for smell, certain odorants such as ammonia may stimulate the trigeminal nerve, CN V, located in the oral mucosa of the mouth and nose. Sensations of an irritation, tickling, burning, warming, cooling, and stinging may be perceived through chemoreceptors in the mouth.[86] Although methodology testing was different in 2 olfactory studies with total laryngectomees, hyposmia or reduced olfactory acuity ranged from 68%[87] to 100%.[88]

Van Dam noted approximately one-third of the laryngectomized patients were able to smell by moving jaw and/or facial muscles and floor of mouth and mastication versus those who were non-smellers. From the observation of this study and comments from the patients, the nasal airflow-inducing maneuver (NAIM) was developed. The NAIM was described by Hilgers et al[89] as the "polite yawning" technique or yawning with the lips closed. This technique is designed to create negative pressure in the oral cavity and oropharynx to permit orthonasal airflow to allow for odor molecules to reach the olfactory epithelium. With closed lips, the oral cavity is enlarged by lowering the jaw, floor of mouth, tongue, base of tongue, and soft palate in a downward relaxed rapid movement as in a "polite yawn." The yawning movement is repeated in quick rapid succession to enable the air to reach the olfactory area. Long-term results of the polite yawning technique can rehabilitate the olfactory acuity in approximately 50% of individuals who have undergone a total laryngecotmy.[90,91] Daily practice of the technique is necessary to optimize long-term benefits.

Laryngectomized patients should prevent odor-related disasters by placing smoke detectors in every room that might have a fire (such as a living room with a fireplace) or where people sleep. Carbon monoxide detectors placed in the home are highly recommended as carbon monoxide is an odorless gas. Electric stoves are preferred over gas unless the gas stove is equipped with an automatic pilot light. There are other detectors for propane, natural gas, and gasoline that are available through the gas company, marine electronics stores, or recreational vehicle dealers. Caution is also given to check expiration dates on food or to date leftovers and to throw out food if there is any doubt of spoilage.

Diedrich and Youngstrom[66] reported that 31% of the laryngectomized patients they studied reported a diminished ability to taste. As taste is greatly influenced by the ability to smell,[92] the act of eating may often be reduced to simply a necessity. Some patients report that this may be attributed to their adjustment to the loss of smell, as this sense is related to taste. Although smell and taste are impaired, maintaining good nutritional intake is paramount. Taste can improve by keeping the lips together, chewing intensively, and moving the food back and forth to optimize the retronasal and some orthonasal olfaction.[89] Rehabilitation of the laryngectomy should address the loss of smell and taste and incorporate the teaching of olfactory rehabilitation using the NAIM.

Safety

Safety issues related to breathing through the stoma are real concerns of the laryngectomized patient and family. In the event of accident or illness, emergency medical personnel must be alerted that the patient is a neck breather so appropriate medical aid may be administered. This may include mouth-to-stoma resuscitation or administration of oxygen via the stoma. *First Aid for (Neck-Breathers) Laryngectomees* is a helpful pamphlet that provides explicit instructions for resuscitation. It is available from the International Association of Laryngectomees.[93] Patients are strongly advised to wear medical alert bracelets (Figure 9–9), carry an emergency identification card, and place emergency identification cards on the windshields of their cars and in obvious locations in their homes (Figures 9–10A and 9–10B).

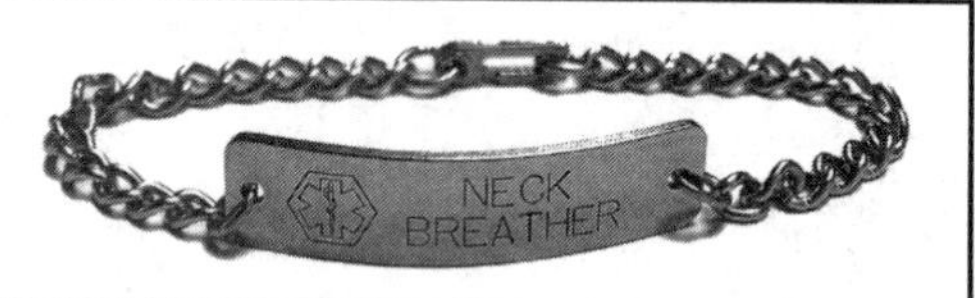

FIGURE 9–9. Neck breather bracelet. (Photo courtesy of Luminaud, http://www.luminaud.com)

The laryngectomized patient should inform the medical emergency personnel who service the area in which they live of their surgical alterations including first aid procedures for neck breathers. The local fire or emergency medical station will record the information in the computer to alert personnel should an emergency call come from the specified residence.

EMERGENCY!!

LARYNGECTOMEE

***Total Neck Breather** – no vocal cords*

I breathe ONLY through an opening in my neck, NOT through my nose or mouth.

If I have stopped breathing:

1. Remove anything that covers the opening in my neck. Expose my entire neck.
2. Keep neck opening clear and protected from liquids.
3. RESUSCITATE WITH AIR OR OXYGEN TO NECK OPENING, OR USE MOUTH-TO-NECK BREATHING.

BE PROMPT—SECONDS COUNT

I NEED AIR NOW!

(See Other Side)

Medical Problems
☐ Epilepsy ☐ Glaucoma
☐ Diabetes ☐ Peptic Ulcer
☐ Other________________________

Medicines Taken Regularly
☐ Anticoagulants ☐ Cortisone or ACTH
☐ Heart Drugs
(Name & Dose)____________________
☐ Other ________________________

Dangerous Allergies
☐ Drugs (Name)_________________
☐ Penicillin
☐ Other________________________

Other Information
☐ Hard of Hearing ☐ Speak no English
☐ Wear contact lenses
☐ Other ________________________

My Name ________________________

Address ________________________

____

____
Physician's Name Phone

____
Relative's Name Phone

____
Other

A

FIGURE 9–10. A. Emergency card front and back. *continues*

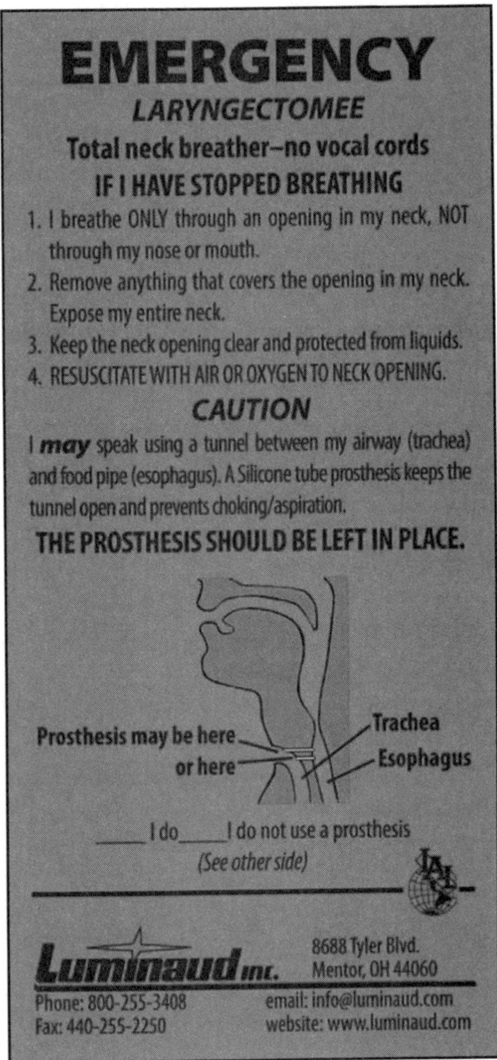

EMERGENCY

LARYNGECTOMEE

Total neck breather–no vocal cords

IF I HAVE STOPPED BREATHING

1. I breathe ONLY through an opening in my neck, NOT through my nose or mouth.
2. Remove anything that covers the opening in my neck. Expose my entire neck.
3. Keep the neck opening clear and protected from liquids.
4. RESUSCITATE WITH AIR OR OXYGEN TO NECK OPENING.

CAUTION

I ***may*** speak using a tunnel between my airway (trachea) and food pipe (esophagus). A Silicone tube prosthesis keeps the tunnel open and prevents choking/aspiration.

THE PROSTHESIS SHOULD BE LEFT IN PLACE.

Prosthesis may be here
or here
Trachea
Esophagus

____ I do ____ I do not use a prosthesis

(See other side)

Luminaud inc.
8688 Tyler Blvd.
Mentor, OH 44060
Phone: 800-255-3408
Fax: 440-255-2250
email: info@luminaud.com
website: www.luminaud.com

FIGURE 9–10. *continued* **B.** Emergency card showing voice prosthesis placement. (Photos courtesy of Luminaud, http://www.luminaud.com)

Activities related to water, such as bathing, fishing, and swimming, are important to discuss with the patient. Safety around water is of the utmost importance. Bathing and showering may, therefore, present special problems for the patient. A special rubber shower collar (Figure 9–11) is available as a safety aid for this purpose.

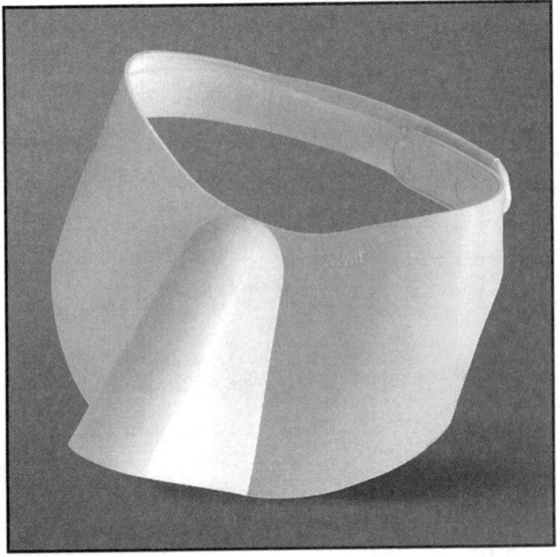

FIGURE 9–11. Shower collar. (Photo courtesy of InHealth Technologies, http://www.inhealth.com)

The collar fits tightly around the neck to deflect water from entering the stoma. Holes on the underside of the collar permit safe air exchange. This device is recommended for patients who prefer to take showers.[79] Shower guards (Figures 9–12A and 9–12B) are also available, which are used with the peristomal adhesives. These devices are shaped at a right angle that deflects the water away from the stoma.

Water sports require their own forms of caution and safety. Those who want to continue swimming as a hobby are advised to seek special training.[74] A Larkel (modified snorkel) is a device that allows the laryngectomee to swim safely. Special training is essential in learning to use this device. This activity is extremely dangerous for the patient and is not advisable. Fishing from the bank or dock requires caution. The patient should fish only where there is easy access to the water and where footing is stable. Boating may also be hazardous, and the laryngectomized patient

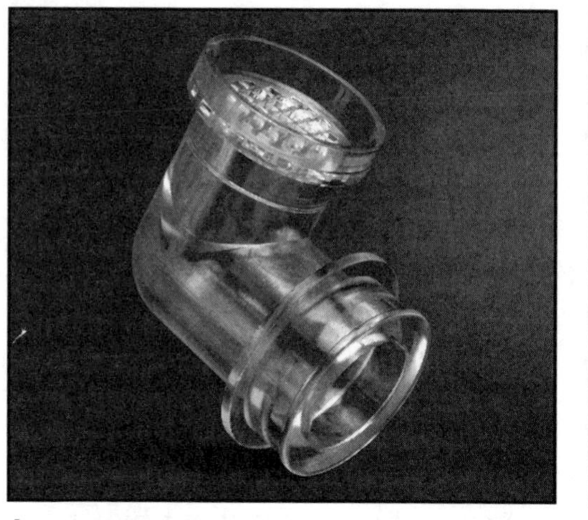

A

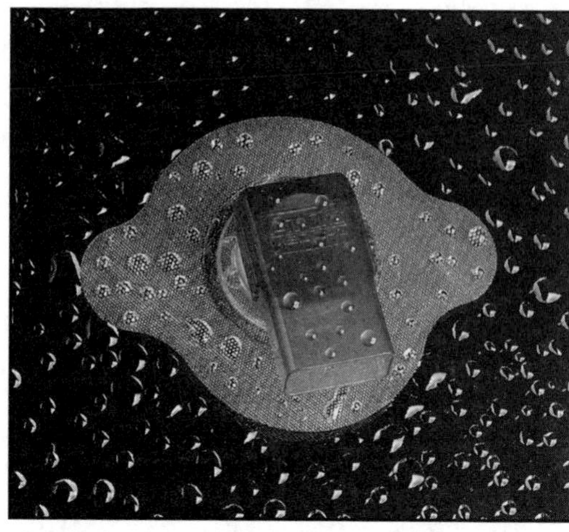

B

FIGURE 9–12. A. Blom-Singer shower guard. **B.** Provox ShowerAid. (Photos courtesy of Atos Medical, http://www.atosmedical.com)

is cautioned to limit boating activities to stable crafts. A superior quality life vest should be worn, and extreme caution should be maintained at all times.

Lifting

One of the biological functions of the larynx is to allow pulmonary air to be trapped within the lungs when the vocal folds are held in complete adduction making it easier to lift objects. The laryngectomized patient can no longer regulate the larynx to build thoracic air pressure. Theoretically, lifting should be difficult for the laryngectomee. In Diedrich and Youngstrom's survey of patients, they found that 45% of their patients reported no difficulty lifting, 42% reported some difficulty, and 13% reported great difficulty.[66] The majority of the surveyed patients did not experience problems with lifting. Laryngectomees who usually have problems have undergone radical neck dissection and experience related neck, shoulder, and arm movement problems.

Psychosocial Concerns

The laryngectomized patient may have many psychological adjustments to make.[94] In an excellent review of the basic psychological stages of patients, Gardner described adjustments that were made preoperatively, immediately postoperatively, and upon reentering the familiar environment.[77] These adjustments focused on the patient's reaction to the disease, the physical changes as a result of the surgery, self-concept based on the feeling of adequacy and appearance, and emotional reactions related to the physical and psychological changes.

When told they have cancer of the larynx, it is not unusual for patients to be more concerned about the disease than about the ramifications of surgery. To many individuals, cancer is synonymous with death.[95] On hearing that they have cancer, patients often do not hear the complete explanation of the disease and its treatment as provided by the physician. Reality must eventually be dealt with and the patient must move forward toward understanding the surgery and its consequences.

The Laryngectomized Speaker's Source Book, published by the International Association of Laryngectomees (IAL), provides an excellent description of the fears and concerns of the patient.[96] (The IAL is an international teaching and support group composed of and operated by laryngectomized individuals.) It describes fears related to the operation such as taking the anesthetic, fear of pain following surgery, fear of mutilation, and fear of not being able to speak.

The immediate postoperative period may be a time of considerable frustration. Many patients experience acute physical stress; worries about health, families, and finances; and uncertainties about the future. The concept of being a "whole" person may also arise. The reaction of some patients is to resign themselves to being cared for by others, to become dependent. Those who make the appropriate adjustments work through these difficulties and maintain their presurgical independence. All of these concerns and frustrations are compounded by the inability to communicate feelings adequately because of limited nonverbal means.

As the patient returns to a normal environment, many family and social issues must be resolved. It is quite possible, especially in the typical age group, that temporary role reversals occur during the hospitalization and rehabilitation period. Husbands may take over the domestic roles of their wives, or wives may assume the traditional male roles of the family. When role reversals take place, it is necessary for the family to evaluate relationships and either maintain new role distributions or return to previous roles.

Personal and sexual relationships may also be affected by the laryngectomy. Individuals with strong interpersonal relationships and positive self-images will seldom experience difficulties or sexual disorientation. Following surgery, however, some patients experience less than adequate self-images and often need psychological counseling to work through these problems.

Blood and Blood[97] found that the laryngectomized patient who spoke openly and candidly about his or her disability and rehabilitation process was more socially accepted than the patient who was reticent or acted embarrassed about the situation. Therefore, the well-adjusted patient may find more success in attempting to return to the previous work setting. Many patients, even those who require skilled oral communication such as managers, businesspeople, and salespeople, have successfully returned to their jobs and careers. When patients are not able to meet previous job requirements because of physical or communication deficits, job retraining or employment changes may be required. The various state rehabilitation commissions may be helpful in training patients for new employment opportunities. Some patients choose early retirement following laryngectomy surgery.

SPEECH REHABILITATION

The goal of the speech rehabilitation program following total laryngectomy is to achieve the most effective speech possible for the individual speaker in terms of age, gender, and dialect. As we have discussed, there are three options available to the total laryngectomy patient:

- artificial larynx
- esophageal speech
- surgical prosthetics

No categorical statements concerning the "best" approach can be made. Each option must be weighed and evaluated against each patient's own set of circumstances. The deciding factor is based on which method is the most effective for the individual patient. Watterson and McFarlane advocate learning two modes of communication, one to serve as the primary mode of speaking and the other to use as a backup if needed.[98]

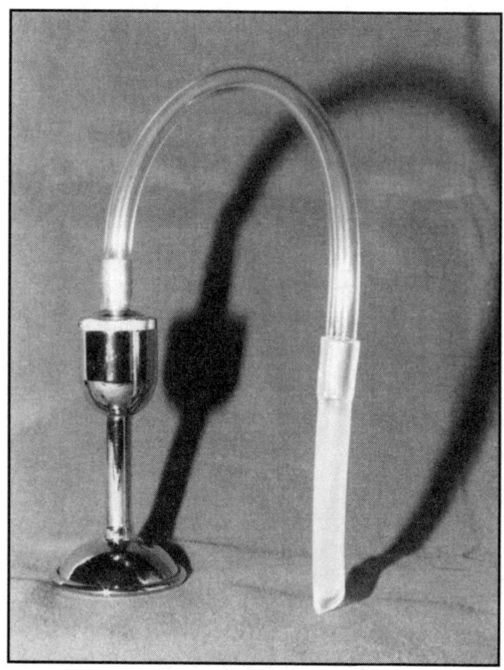

FIGURE 9–13. Tokyo artificial larynx. (Photo courtesy of Limco Solutions, http://www.limcosolutions.com)

Artificial Larynges

Pneumatic Artificial Larynx

Historically, the development of artificial larynges dates back to 1859.[99] Throughout the years, two major types of artificial larynges have emerged, pneumatic and electronic, with the electronic being the most widely used of the 2 types. Although seldom used in the United States, the Tokyo pneumatic artificial larynges (Figure 9–13) is still available for purchase.[100]

This device is more commonly used in South and East Asia where languages such as Mandarin, Cantonese, and Taiwanese are spoken, as these languages have linguistic markers of pitch and intonation which are important for intelligibility and expression.[101] The pneumatic larynx utilizes pulmonary air as its power source. A cuff that contains a reed or a membrane fits over the stoma. As the patient expels air for speech, a flexible rubber or plastic tube placed into the patient's mouth transmits the vibration from the membrane. The patient articulates as the sound is produced. Loudness variations occur as the air pressure levels change during breathing for speech. Sound quality from the pneumatic larynges may be more pleasing than the electromechanical device because there is no electronic noise or buzzing sound with this device. The major disadvantage of the pneumatic instruments is the presence of the tube in the mouth, which may interfere with articulation and eventually collect saliva or moisture condensation within the tube or on the diaphragm. The cuff, as well, may become clogged with mucus. This device requires the use of one hand for placement of the cuff over the stoma.

Electronic Artificial Larynges

There are three types of electronic artificial larynges, neck-type devices (Figure 9–14), oral devices (Figure 9–15), and intraoral devices (Figure 9–16).

All electronic larynges are battery-powered sound generators. Some of the devices operate using 9-volt alkaline batteries, and others use rechargeable batteries. These devices may differ in size, weight, quality of sound, ability to control pitch and volume, appearance, types of batteries needed, and durability. There are a number of battery-operated electronic artificial larynges that are commercially available for purchase.

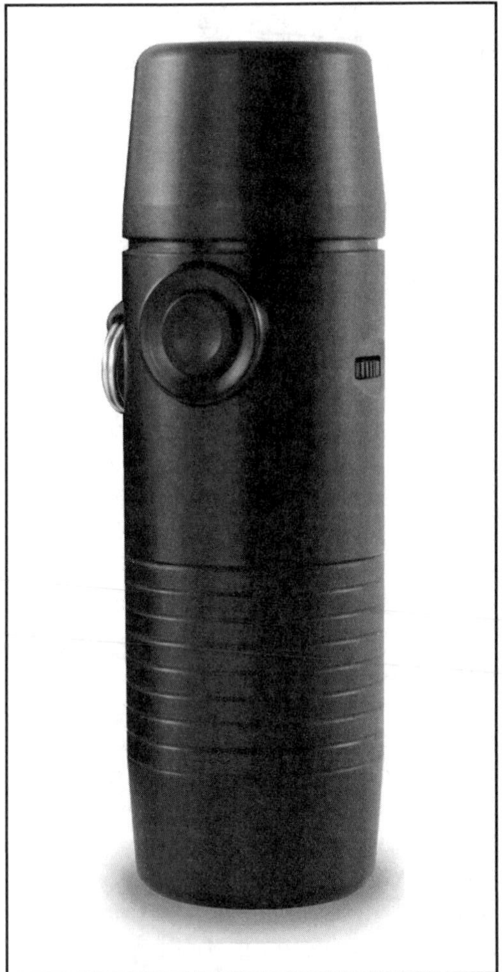

FIGURE 9–14. TruTone. (Photo courtesy of Griffin Laboratories, http://www.griffinlab.com)

Neck-Type Devices. The neck-type artificial larynges are the most popular of the alaryngeal devices. The sound source is a diaphragm in the head of the instrument that is set into vibration when the speaker activates the device by depressing the on/off button. The speaker operates the neck-type artificial larynges by placing the head of the device firmly on the side of the neck, under the chin, or on the cheek allowing for the sound to be transmitted through the tissues and into the oropharynx (Figure 9–17) and articulates normally. Artificial larynges range in cost and relative quality from around $200 to $600. The electronic devices permit variations in volume and pitch through manipulation of switch controls.

Oral Devices. An oral artificial larynx, such as a Cooper-Rand, is a device that can be used for patients who cannot achieve adequate sound transfer on the skin. The device generates sound in a small transducer and transmits the sound through a plastic sound conduction tube. The speaker places the plastic tube, which is attached to the tone generator, approximately 1 to 1½ inches in the mouth on top of the tongue. The plastic tube can either enter the mouth at midline or from the corner of the mouth with the tube entering at a diagonal. The speaker is instructed to coordinate the activation of the sound generator and speech simultaneously. Practice should incorporate the use of natural pauses and reducing rate of speech to improve intelligibility.

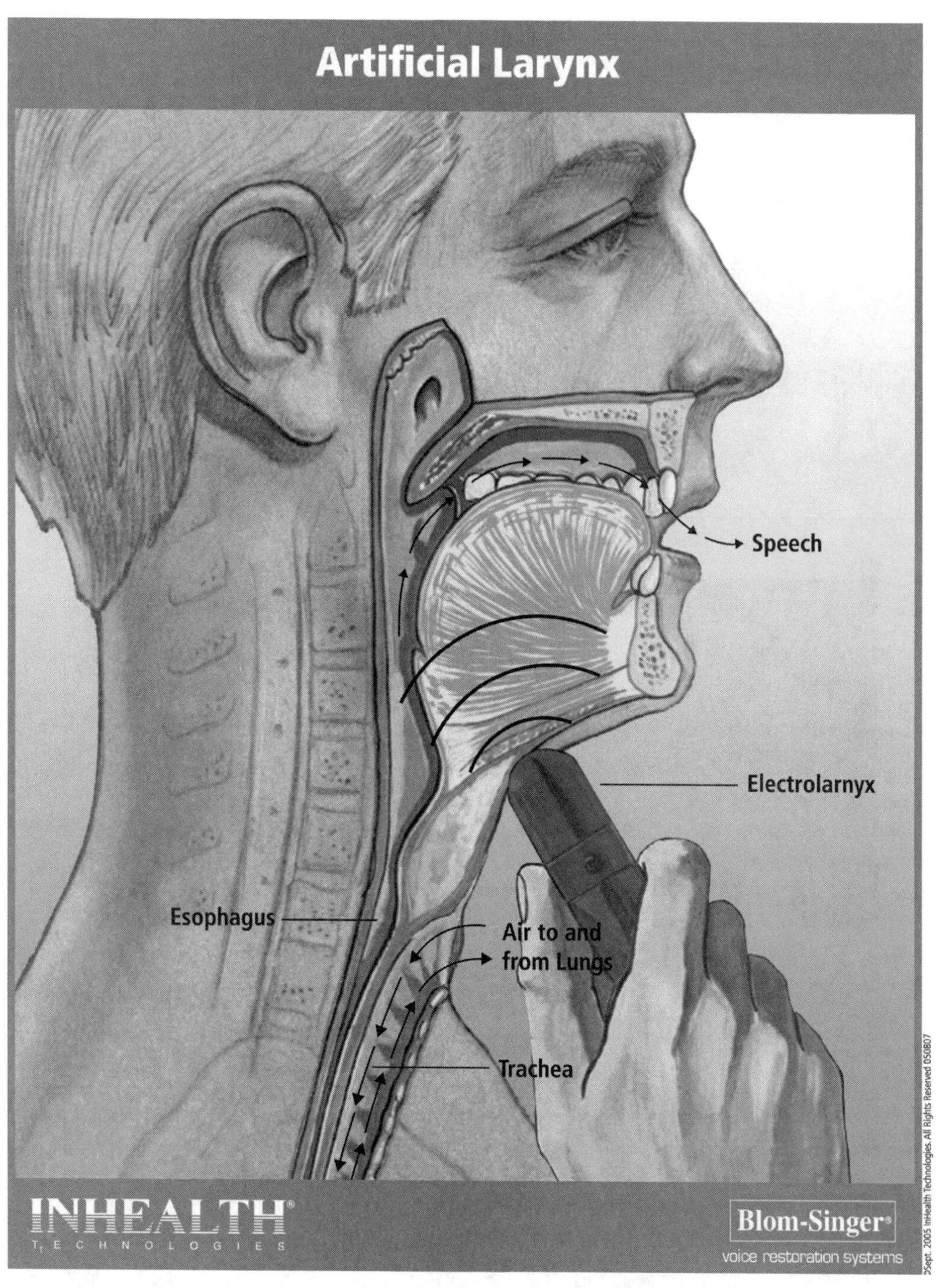

FIGURE 9–15. Cooper-Rand artificial larynx. (Photo courtesy of Luminaud, http://www.luminaud.com)

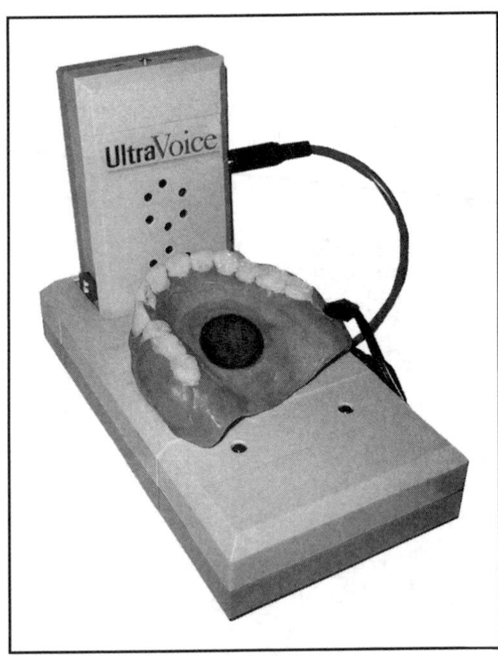

FIGURE 9–16. Ultra Voice Plus II with charger. (Photo courtesy of UltraVoice, http://www.ultravoice.com)

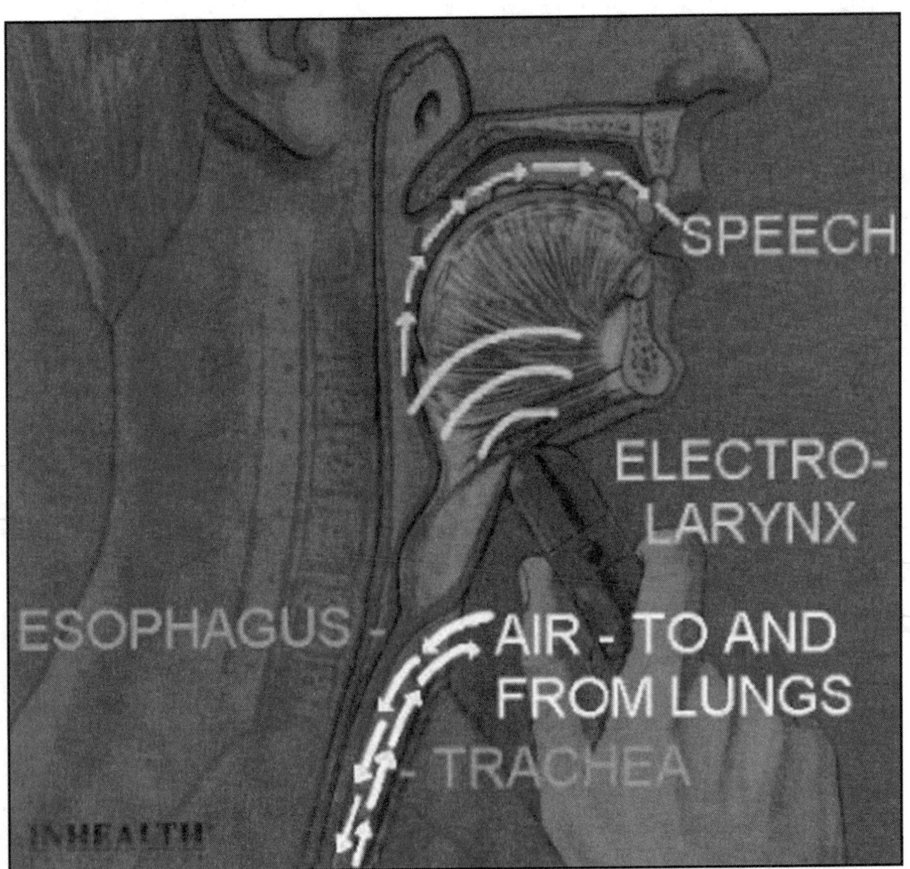

FIGURE 9–17. Representation of speech being produced with a neck-type artificial larynx. (Photo courtesy of InHealth Technologies, http://www.inhealth.com)

Most neck-type devices can be converted into an oral device by affixing a rubber or plastic adapter onto the head of the electrolarynx. The plastic conduction tube is then inserted into the center of the adapter for sound to be transmitted through it. An oral artificial device is ideal for patients who experience extensive scar tissue or edema of the neck preventing adequate transfer of sound through the tissues when using a neck-type electrolarynx. This type of device can be effectively used immediately following surgery to communicate with the hospital staff and family members. As with the pneumatic device, the disadvantage involves the oral tube's interference with articulation and collection of saliva within the tube.

Intraoral Devices. The Ultravoice Plus II (see Figure 9–16) is an intraoral device that can be custom mounted into an upper denture or an orthodontic retainer.

There is a built-in loudspeaker and amplifier that have a flexible membrane cover to protect it from saliva, food, or liquids. It consists of a lightweight oral unit mounted into the acrylic denture, a high-speed signal processor control unit, and a charging unit that charges the batteries in both the oral unit and control unit simultaneously. The individual has the ability to control loudness. The pitch is controlled by a high-speed digital signal processor, which works in real time. This means that the prosody more closely mimics the natural voice. This device is individually customized, as maxillary impressions must be taken to fit the patient properly. This device is costly; however, it may be the only device that some patients can use. Training involves slowing the rate of speech and coordinating loudness levels and pitch for improved tonal quality during conversational speech.

A 66-year-old gentleman was evaluated by the otolaryngologist following a several month history of persistent hoarseness. He did not complain of any hemoptysis, shortness of breath, or dysphagia. He quit smoking 2 years prior to the evaluation and had a history of smoking 2 packs of cigarettes per day for 40 years.

Videolaryngostroboscopic examination revealed the presence of a whitish granular lesion involving the anterior aspect of the right true vocal fold. Vocal fold mobility was normal bilaterally. The otolaryngologist revealed no evidence of lymphadenopathy. A microlaryngoscopy with biopsy confirmed squamous cell carcinoma and was staged a T1a lesion. The patient was evaluated by the radiation oncologist and elected to receive radiation therapy. He received 67.6 Gy over a 2-month period with resolution of the malignancy.

Fourteen months after receiving radiation treatments, an enlarged left cervical mass appeared. Biopsy revealed metastatic squamous cell carcinoma. All available options were presented to this patient including a total laryngectomy, radiation and chemotherapy, and a combination of surgery and radiation therapy. The patient did not want to lose his larynx and opted for the radical neck dissection and partial laryngectomy with follow-up radiation therapy. The patient underwent a right anterolateral partial laryngectomy with a left radical neck dissection and an additional 90 Gy of radiation therapy. After completion of radiation therapy, this patient presented with significant radiation mucositis involving the oral cavity, pharynx, and hypopharynx. He also experienced difficulty swallowing accompanied with pain. Secondary to radionecrosis of the larynx 7 months following the second series of radiation treatments, the patient underwent a total laryngectomy with a tracheoesophageal puncture and reconstruction of pectoralis major myocutaneous flap.

The patient was seen for his initial voice prosthesis fitting 7 weeks following his surgery. This patient experienced a slow course of healing secondary to the previous radiation treatments. The patient was initially fitted with a 3.0-cm voice prosthesis. He achieved short bursts of voicing on vowels. The patient was also fitted with a tracheostoma vent secondary to stoma stenosis. Due to the inability to produce voicing 2 months following his second round of radiation treatments, an insufflation test was administered. Voicing was weak and inconsistent with ability to sustain vowels for approximately 1 second. Alternative methods of voicing were initiated. A neck-type electrolarynx failed because of poor sound transfer into the oral cavity secondary to the neck tissue hardening from the radiation treatments. An oral adapter was placed onto the head of the electrolarynx. The patient was trained using the oral device; however, intelligibility was minimal at best. Three esophagrams over a 7-month period revealed gradual narrowing and finally stenosis of the cervical esophagus. Esophageal dilatations were performed to dilate the esophagus for swallowing. Secondary to poor healing, the otolaryngologist did not advise performing a myotomy. Although the patient was trained to use the oral adapter to speak, it was not adequate for communication purposes. Since the patient was edentulous, and had to get a new set of dentures made, it was recommended that he try the UltraVoice speaking device. Although all modes of alaryngeal speech were tried with this individual, the intraoral device was the most effective and provided the best intelligibility for this individual given his complicated recovery period. This patient has remained cancer free 5 years following his total laryngectomy.

Treatment Considerations—Artificial Larynges

The following are suggestions when instructing the patient to use an artificial larynx for communication. Some patients will quickly master the art of using the device, while others may require several sessions of speech therapy as well as follow through on structured home exercises. The following is a discussion of various factors that affect speech intelligibility using artificial larynges.

Articulation. Instruct the patient to slightly overarticulate words without overexaggerating oral movements. Patients who articulate with little oral movement are difficult to understand when using an artificial larynx. Teaching patients to overarticulate slightly will help open the vocal tract to improve resonance of the sound. Teach patients to enhance articulation by instructing them to use intraoral air for the articulation of voiceless consonants. If a patient has dentures, encourage the individual to wear them as this adds in intelligibility when articulating. It is important to teach the individual to coordinate the on-off switch of the device for onset and offset of voice. The device will continue to transmit sound during voiceless consonants if the device is activated; therefore, training is necessary to work on the contrast of voiced and voiceless consonants.[102]

Placement. The speech-language pathologist should experiment with various placements of the device around the neck area for the best possible sound transfer into the oral cavity. While the patient is asked to count, the speech-language pathologist moves the electrolarynx around the neck area, finding the place on the neck that transmits the clearest and loudest sound into the oral cavity. All patients have a particular site that serves to transmit the sound with the optimal amount of energy into the oral cavity. This is referred to as the "sweet spot" and is the placement of best sound transfer to minimize the electronic buzz of the device and where the sound is perceived coming from the oral cavity.[103] The difference in sound between this placement and other placement sites should be demonstrated. The best placement site is usually under the mandible and slightly off midline of the neck. The vibrating head of the artificial larynx should be directed toward the oral cavity to enhance vocal tract resonance. The patient's cheek may be the best placement, especially if the neck tissue is dense or hardened from radiation treatments.

Larynx to Skin Seal. Instruct the patient to place the head of the artificial larynx against the palm of the hand to demonstrate acquiring a seal without sound leakage. This technique will help the patient to understand how to manipulate the sound generator control. Success in using the neck device electrolarynx rests on proper placement of the vibrating head, and it must be sealed firmly against the skin to prevent noise leakage from the device. Speech intelligibility is markedly affected if the device is not flush to the skin. In individuals who have undergone radiation to the neck, find the most soft and supple area of the neck to facilitate the optimal transfer of sound.

Developing Conversational Speech. Once the "sweet spot" is found for the best sound transfer, request the patient practice finding this area quickly and precisely with consistency. Using the mirror as well as marking the site with a piece of tape will help the patient locate the area on the neck. Counting, reading short phrases and sentences, and responding to questions can serve as practice material both in therapy and practicing at home.

Expand quickly into conversational speech. As the patient becomes consistent with placement and appropriate sound generation when reading phrases and sentences, advance to conversational level. Patients will have a tendency to talk in a monotonous, robot-like speech. Demonstrate and insist on the use of normal phrasing, with appropriate cessation of sound for natural pauses, and with normal rate. The initiation and ending of speech must be coordinated with the activation and deactivation of the sound generator, respectively.

Coordination of Movements. Teach the patient to remove the artificial larynx from the neck when not speaking. Patients are likely to fall into the habit of leaving the device positioned on or near the neck during conversational speech. The flow of conversation will be greatly enhanced if the patient places the artificial larynx on the neck only when she or he wants to talk. This serves as a natural signal to other speakers, much as when we take a deep breath prior to speaking during conversation, that the patient has something to say.

Stoma Noise. Following surgery, the laryngectomized patient breathes through the stoma. If air is forced through the stoma, either during inhalation or exhalation, a noise can be heard which is referred to as "stoma noise" This stoma noise can interfere with the patient's intelligibility of speech and become annoying for the listener. Rapid muscular contraction of the thoracic or abdominal muscles may result in increased air turbulence at the level of the stoma. If you ask the patient to whisper or speak with increased loudness, much stoma noise will be produced. To help eliminate or reduce the amount of stoma noise, teach the patient to mouth, not whisper, the words. The patient should practice reading phrases by just mouthing the words, and at the same time, monitor the amount of stoma noise being heard. The patient who has mastered these steps should be encouraged to discontinue whatever nonoral means of communication used previously. Usually, patients agree to this transition with little argument because oral communication is much more flexible and expansive. The patient will continue to improve simply by using the artificial larynx in all speaking situations. As a final means of demonstrating its effectiveness, the voice pathologist should consider talking to the patient on the telephone during a therapy session to assess telephone intelligibility. The 60 to 80 Hz tone generated by the artificial larynx is carried well over the telephone. Using the artificial larynx on the telephone reopens another avenue of communication for the patient.

Esophageal Speech

An artificial larynx provides the patient with a new, external source of sound vibration. Esophageal voice utilizes the patient's remaining anatomical structures to provide a new, internal source for sound generation. These vibrating structures are the cricopharyngeus muscle of the upper esophagus and the middle and inferior pharyngeal constrictor muscles. When used for sound generation, these structures collectively are termed the pharyngo-esophageal (PE) segment. The PE segment lies approximately at the level of C-5 (Figure 9–18).

To generate sound, the PE segment needs a power source. Because the patient can no longer inhale air into the nose and mouth, another air source must be found. This source is simply the atmospheric air that is always present in the oral and nasal cavities. With training, patients can be taught to place this ambient air into the upper esophagus, which serves as an air reservoir, and then expel this air while vibrating the PE segment and surrounding tissues.[104] When the patient articulates using this sound for voice, esophageal speech is produced. Fluent esophageal speech depends on the rapid intake and release of air form the esophagus.

A number of factors seem to influence the success of learning esophageal speech including physiological and psychological factors.[100] Proficient esophageal speakers appear to possess the anatomical structure necessary to produce esophageal vibration and display a high degree of individual motivation to focus on dedicated daily practice, accept small incremental improvement throughout the learning process, as well as setbacks, and remain positive and relaxed throughout therapy.

The first step in developing esophageal speech is learning how to place air into the upper esophagus. The two major methods of air intake are the

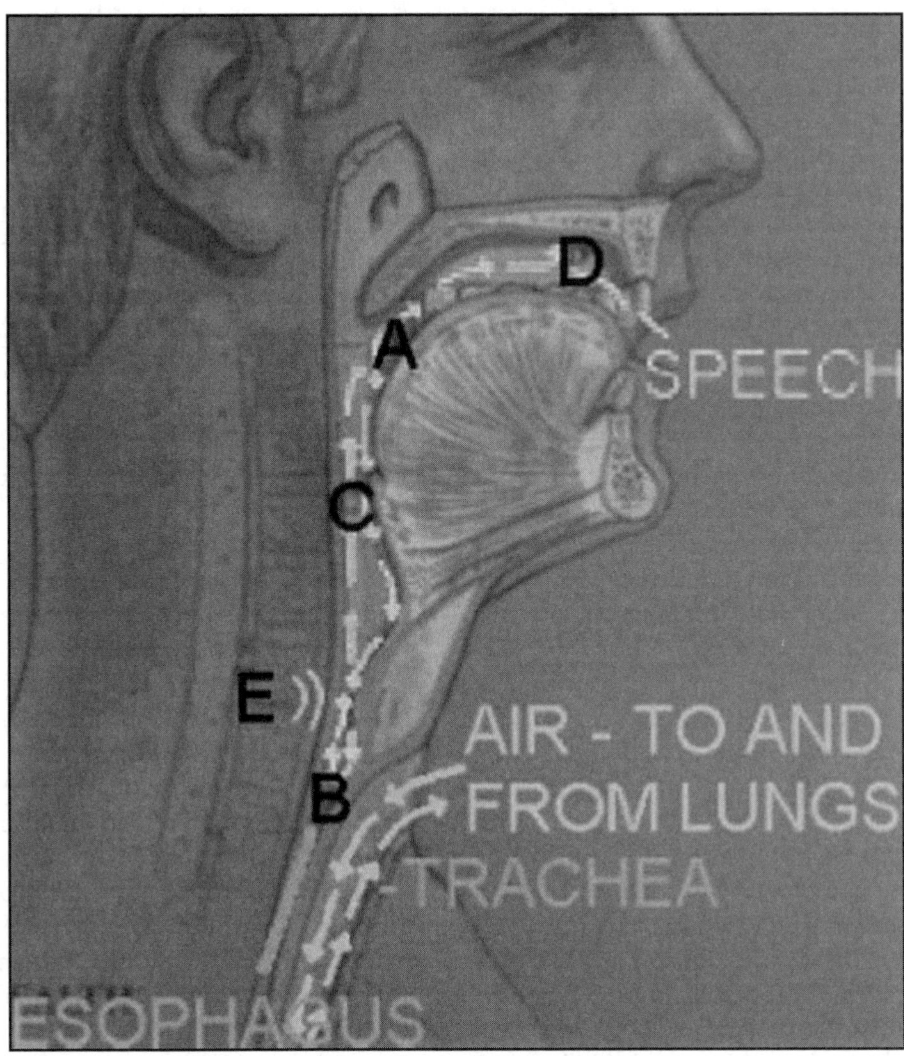

FIGURE 9–18. Representation of speech being produced using esophageal speech. (Photo courtesy of InHealth Technologies, http://www.inhealth.com)

injection (positive pressure approach) and the inhalation (negative pressure approach) methods. The injection method includes glossopharyngeal press and plosive injection. These methods are described by a number of individuals.[8,77,100,105,106] These techniques of esophageal speech production are based on how the PE segment opens to allow for air intake and then expels the air during voicing.

Inhalation Method

The inhalation method involves creating negative pressure in the thoracic cavity, which helps draw ambient air into the esophagus. The esophagus is in a state of negative pressure, and as air is inhaled into the lungs, the intraesophageal pressure drops even further, below atmosphere. Therefore, air from the oral and pharyngeal cavities can be drawn passively into the esophagus. Air pressure in these 2 locations becomes equalized momentarily.[107] This is accomplished when the patient inhales quickly. Upon inhalation, the diaphragm drops, enlarging the thoracic cavity, and thus creating negative thoracic cavity pressure. The inhaled air draws the ambient air into the esophagus. Instructions to the patient may include the following:

- Demonstrate the expansion of the thoracic cavity, using a diagram. This demonstration will make the patient aware of how the normal respiratory system works. As the cavity expands, air is drawn into the lungs; as it contracts, the air is expelled.
- Explain to the patient that as the thoracic cavity expands, so, too, does the diameter of the esophagus. As the esophagus expands, the increased area is filled with ambient air. This air can then be increased to produce vibration of the PE segment.
- The patient is then asked to close his or her mouth and to take air into the stoma through a quick, sharp inhalation. This inhalation may be enhanced by momentarily covering the stoma with the hand. It may be helpful to have the patient imagine that he or she is sniffing through the nose.[66] The patient should then attempt to expel the air by saying "ah." The subsequent decrease in thoracic size will force the air out of the esophagus if esophageal insufflation has occurred. Continue this procedure until sound is produced.

Injection Method

The injection method of air intake is achieved by compressing the intraoral air into the esophagus with assistance from the tongue or lips and sometimes the cheeks. There are 2 types of injection. The first type is air injection by tongue pumping which is also referred to as a glossopharyngeal press or a glossal press.[65] Instructions to the patient for teaching this method may include the following:

- Tell the patient to open his or her mouth and "bite off" a piece of air. This action and imagery helps the patient feel the ambient air from one point to another. It also helps to increase the air pressure in the back of the oral cavity.
- At the end of the "bite" the patient is instructed to close the lips to seal the oral cavity. At the same time, with the tongue tip pushing against the alveolus, the middle section of the tongue should pump the air against both the hard and soft palates. This action will cause the base of the tongue to move backward in a rocking motion, pushing the air into the upper esophagus. In using the glossopharyngeal press, the patient may feel the tongue moving posteriorly and actually making contact with the pharyngeal wall. Once the patient learns this method of air intake, the lips can either be slightly open or closed because the tongue serves to pump the air into the esophagus.
- The patient should feel and perhaps hear the air as it is forced past the PE segment and into the esophagus. When the air passes the segment, an attempt should be made to expel the air by saying "ah."

The consonant injection method of air intake is the second type of injection of air into the esophagus. This method uses the natural intraoral air pressures created by plosive and fricative sounds to inject air into the esophagus. Instructions to the patient for teaching this method may include the following:

- Ask the patient to produce voiceless consonants such as /t/, /k/, /p/, and /sk/ one at a time in quick succession. The consonants should be made firmly with exaggerated oral movement to encourage airflow into the esophagus. This rapid repetition of the consonants, especially a tongue-tip alveolar stop, fricative, or a bilabial, as well as tongue positioning facilitates buildup of air pressure in the esophagus. Production of the consonants forces the air pressure in the esophagus with the result of almost immediate expulsion and sound production. Discourage any stoma noise or sounds made by the tongue and palatal-pharyngeal contact.
- When the esophageal sound is produced consistently utilizing the consonants, add consonant-vowel combinations to the practice regimen. This will force a lengthening of the esophageal sound.
- Constantly add new consonant-vowel combinations, expanding the patient's repertoire of sounds on which injection can take place.
- Finally, attempt to drop the consonant and have the patient inject the air using the tongue for production of the vowel only.

Although the inhalation and injection methods are of primary interest, a swallow method has also been advocated.[108] Using this method, the patient is asked simply to open and close the mouth and to swallow air. The underlying theory of this method is that a normal swallow produces relaxation of the cricopharyngeus, thus allowing air to enter the esophagus. Using this method, the patient is encouraged to swallow air to produce voice. The swallow method of air injection is the least efficient and may be taught as a last resort. One of the problems with this method is that if the swallowed air reaches the stomach, it cannot be readily expelled.

The therapist should encourage practice of the method easiest for the patient to inject air into the esophagus. Often, the most effective approach is a combination of approaches. Isshiki and Snidecor reported that most esophageal speakers actually do use a combination of injection techniques.[109] Perhaps the simplest approach is to ask the patient, "Can you burp on purpose?" It is surprising how many patients can inject air and burp before the therapy program begins. Therefore, before beginning a long explanation of air injection, just ask!

Once the patient can place air consistently into the upper esophagus, by whatever method, much time should be spent practicing single-syllable words. A solid foundation for conversational esophageal speech must be laid at the single-syllable level. All vowel-consonant and consonant-vowel combinations should be practiced and drilled until the percentage of successful intelligible productions is at least at a 90% level. Lengthening the vowels in the single-syllable productions will prepare the patient to move on to 2-syllable words.

From 2-syllable words it is possible to start building phrases. Phrase work may continue from 2-syllable phrases through 8-syllable phrases produced on a single air injection. The average length of a conversational phrase is approximately 7 syllables.

It is important for the patient to inject the air into the esophagus as smoothly as possible and to expel the air producing voicing with minimal effort. Berlin listed 4 training objectives in establishing proficient esophageal speech.[110,111] These objectives may be quantified by the patient and clinician during the training process.

Skill 1: The first skill is the ability to phonate reliably on demand. Proficient esophageal speakers are able to produce phonation 100% of the time.

Skill 2: The second skill is to achieve a short latency period between air injection into the esophagus and phonation. A stopwatch is used to measure the latency period. When the patient signals the clinician that he or she initiated the air injection into the esophagus, the clinician starts the stopwatch and then stops the stopwatch when the clinician hears vocalization. Proficient esophageal speakers are able to maintain a short latency, ranging between 0.2 and 0.6 seconds between air injection and phonation. As the laryngectomee's esophageal air capacity ranges from 40 to 80 cubic centimeters (cc) of air,[112] which is much less than the vital capacity of lungs in healthy adults, frequent reinflation of the esophagus must take place while the patient is talking. Thus, it is important for the patient to quickly inflate the esophagus and expel the air during conversational speech.

Skill 3: The third skill is to maintain an adequate duration of phonation. A stopwatch is also required to record the maximum sustained duration of the vowel /a/ on a single air intake. Good esophageal speakers are able to sustain /a/ for 2.4 to 3.6 seconds.

Skill 4: The fourth skill is the ability to sustain phonation during articulation. This skill refers to the number of times the syllable /da/ can be repeated on a single air intake without consciously reinjecting air into the esophagus. Proficient esophageal speakers are able to phonate 8 to 10 syllables per air intake.

Several factors are monitored and modified throughout the phrase building process. These include stoma noise, air "klunking" noise (caused by forceful air injections), eye blinking, and other unnecessary facial expressions or grimaces. Loudness, inflection, and phrasing exercises are also practiced in treatment, to increase overall speech naturalness.

Proficient esophageal speech is a learned process that requires much work and dedication to be mastered. Motivation, desire, and vigor are essential factors that must be present for successful voice development to occur.[113] Patients who do not make a positive commitment or who are unwilling to devote sufficient time to the process are not likely to do well. Other factors that may have a negative influence on the successful development of esophageal voice include postradiation fibrosis, pharyngeal scarring, esophageal stenosis, recurring suture line fistulas, and defects in neural innervation.[114] Sloane et al[115] found that anatomic differences in the reconstructed PE segment had a profound affect in the acquisition of esophageal speech. They used the Blom-Singer esophageal insufflation test combined with videofluoroscopy to assess the PE segment during esophageal speech and found hypotonicity, hypertonicity, PE spasm, and stricture of the reconstructed pharynx to affect the dynamics of esophageal speech.

Surgical Prosthetics

Another option for speech rehabilitation following a total laryngectomy is the use of a surgical prosthesis. The possible reestablishment of voice through laryngeal reconstruction and prosthetic surgery has long been recognized. Reports dating as far back as 1874 detail the results of voicing achieved either through the spontaneous creation of a tracheoesophageal (TE) fistula or through the creation of planned TE shunts.[116–118] Blom and Singer[119] presented the history of the attempts to restore voicing through various laryngeal reconstruction techniques, shunt surgeries, and surgical prostheses.[119–127]

The primary goal of all the shunt-type surgeries was to effectively channel pulmonary air into the esophagus where the air could set the pharyngoesophageal segment into vibration for the production of voice. Although several of these procedures were very successful in meeting this goal, 2 major problems seemed to persist with these techniques. These problems were aspiration of saliva, liquids, and foods into the trachea through the fistula and breakdown or stenosis of the shunts.[123]

Singer and Blom developed the tracheoesophageal puncture (TEP) voice restoration technique to solve these problems. In this 15- to 20-minute surgical procedure, a fistula is created between the trachea and the esophagus in the superior border of the stoma. The tracheoesophageal puncture can be performed as a primary (at the time of surgery) or secondary surgical voice restoration procedure.[128,129] Following the puncture, a 14-French (Fr) balloon catheter is directed downward through the fistula from the trachea and into the esophagus.[129,130] Approximately 5 cc of water is injected into the catheter balloon to weigh down the distal end, keeping it from dislodging. The proximal end of the catheter is capped and secured to the neck with tape, suture or StatLock. Freeman and Hamaker[128] recommend using a silastic-coated tube due to less tissue reactivity compared to latex rubber catheters. The catheter can serve as a feeding tube following a primary laryngectomy or a myotomy at the time of the tracheoesophageal puncture.

The tracheoesophageal puncture creates a fistula between the posterior wall of the trachea and the anterior wall of the esophagus for the insertion of a voice prosthesis. The voice prosthesis is a one-way valve made of medically high-grade silicone. Once inserted into the tracheoesophageal puncture, the voice prosthesis prevents aspiration during swallowing and fistula stenosis. The one-way valve permits pulmonary air to enter the esophagus when the stoma is occluded while the patient exhales. The valve opens under positive pressure as the air enters the esophagus and closes by elastic recoil. It does not permit a reverse flow of saliva or liquids into the trachea. The voice prosthesis is cylindrical in shape with a neck strap that is taped to the skin of the neck to keep it in place. At the distal end, a slit, hinged, or ball valve is placed in the esophagus. An anterior opening at the proximal end allows pulmonary air to flow through the voice prosthesis and permits internal cleaning. The prosthesis is securely retained in the fistula by a flexible "retention collar" that holds the prosthesis in place by gripping the inside of the esophageal wall preventing dislodgment (Figure 9–19).

The length of the voice prosthesis ranges in size from 4 to 28 mm. The prosthesis diameter is expressed in French—that is, 16-Fr or 20-Fr. There are several manufacturers of voice protheses. InHealth Technologies manufactures 4 styles of Blom-Singer voice prostheses, which include the Duckbill, Low Pressure, Classic Indwelling, and Advantage™ (first and second generation) prostheses (Figures 9–20A and 9–20B).

InHealth Technologies also manufactures special option voice prostheses that are designed to accommodate special anatomical needs, and they

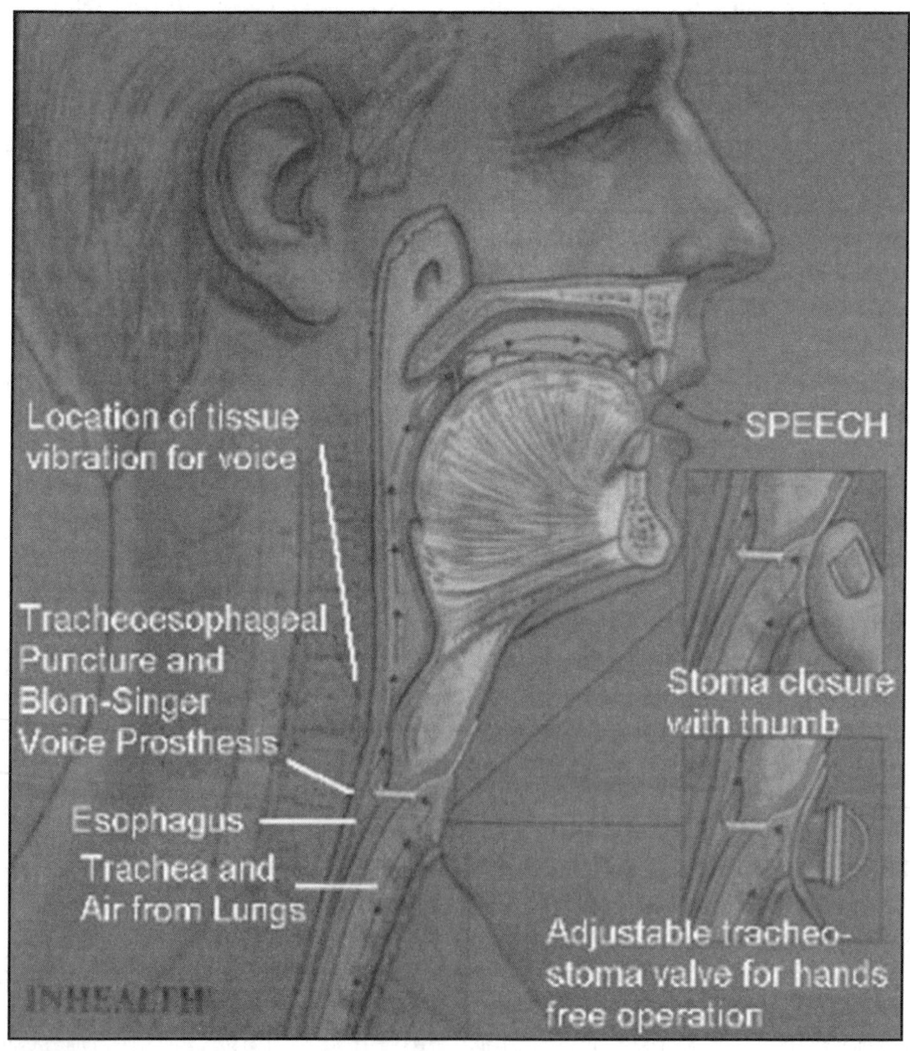

FIGURE 9–19. Representation of speech being produced using a tracheoesophageal voice prosthesis. (Photo courtesy of InHealth Technologies, http://www.inhealth.com)

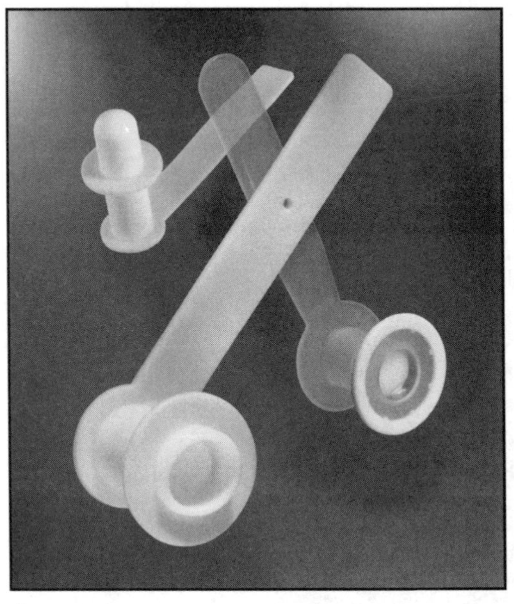

A

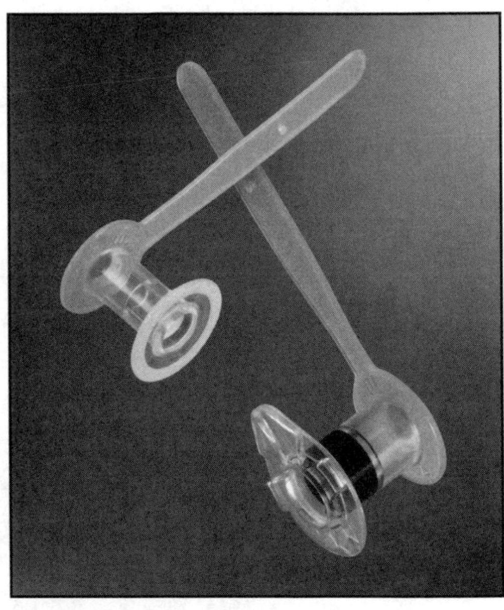

B

FIGURE 9–20. **A.** Blom-Singer Voice Prostheses: Duckbill, Low Pressure, Classic Indwelling. **B.** Blom-Singer voice prostheses: Classic Indwelling and Advantage Indwelling. (Photos courtesy of InHealth Technologies, http://www.inhealth.com)

include the Classic Indwelling with a large esophageal flange (Figure 9–21), large esophageal and tracheal end, Dual Valve, special lengths, or increased resistance.

Atos Medical manufactures 5 voice prostheses which include the Provox 1, Provox 2 (Figure 9–22), Provox Acti-Valve (Figure 9–23) (light, strong, and xtrastrong) Provox NID (Figure 9–24) and Provox Vega.

The Voicemaster Indwelling low-resistance voice prosthesis is manufactured by enterMed from The Netherlands.

When a patient is using a voice prosthesis, the stoma may be occluded manually with a thumb or a finger, or it may be occluded by a tracheostoma valve. The tracheostoma valve has component parts. A housing collar is taped and glued around the stoma. A valve is inserted into the housing collar. When the patient develops sufficient pulmonary air pressure to produce speech, the valve will close, thus occluding the stoma and directing the air into the voice prosthesis.

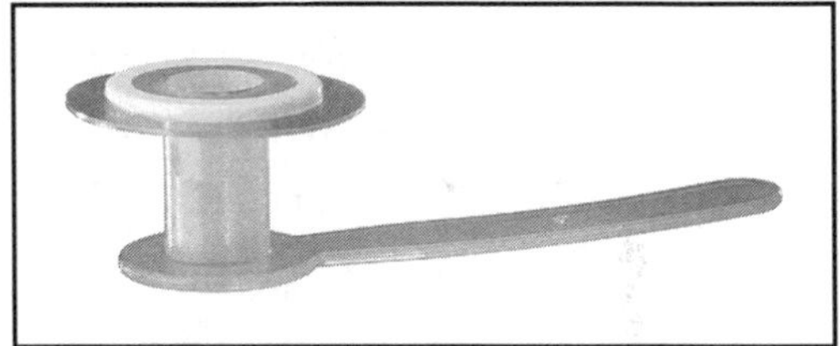

FIGURE 9–21. Modified indwelling with large esophageal flange. (Photo courtesy of InHealth Technologies, http://www.inhealth.com)

The success rate for achieving tracheoesophageal speech is quite high,

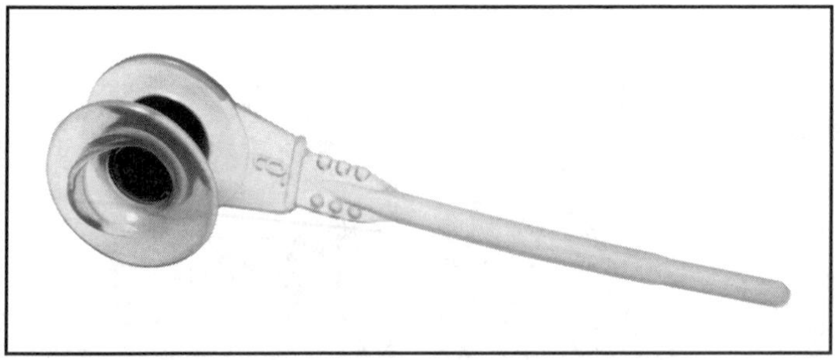

FIGURE 9–22. Provox voice prosthesis. (Photo courtesy of Atos Medical, http://www.atosmedical.com)

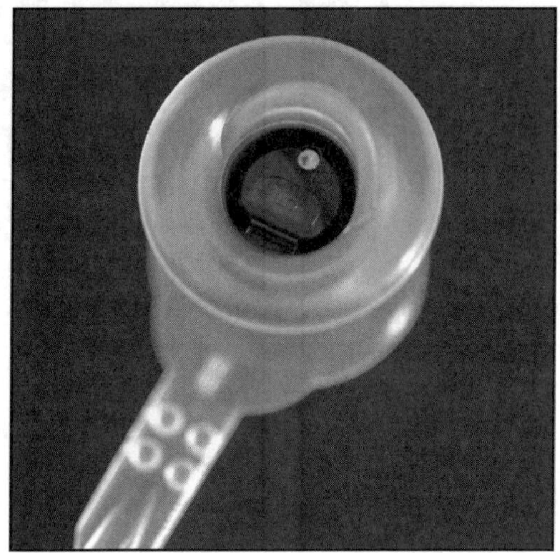

FIGURE 9–23. Provox ActiValve voice prosthesis. (Photo courtesy of Atos Medical, http://www.atosmedical.com)

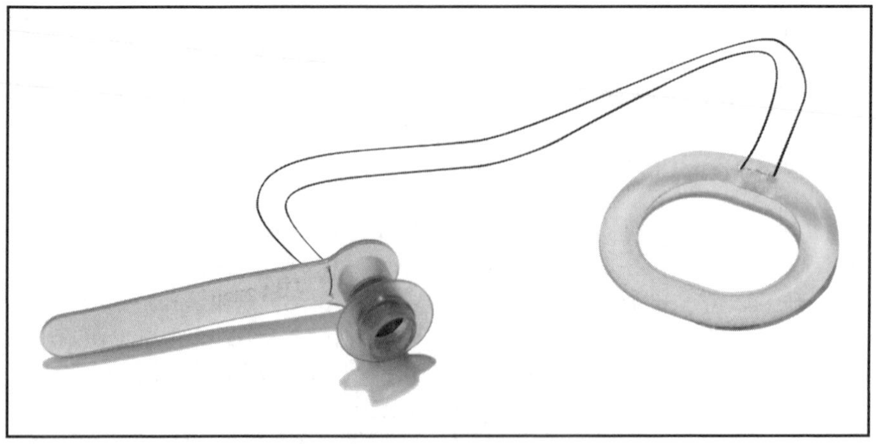

FIGURE 9–24. Provox NID voice prosthesis. (Photo courtesy of Atos Medical, http://www.atosmedical.com)

although some have reported the possibility of long-term problems and complications.[131,132] It has been our experience, however, that if patients are prepared well and properly trained, most total laryngectomy patients can be successful users of this form of communication. We now examine the speech-language pathologist's role with surgical prosthetics.

ROLE OF THE SPEECH-LANGUAGE PATHOLOGIST AND SURGICAL PROSTHETICS

The role of the speech-language pathologist who works with surgical prosthetics is multidimensional and includes the following:

- aiding the surgeon in evaluating the patient's suitability to use the voice prosthesis as a form of communication
- sizing and fitting the prosthesis
- teaching the patient to fit and care for the prosthesis
- maximizing the patient's ability to communicate while using the prosthesis
- fitting and educating the patient on HME system
- fitting and educating the patient on the use of a hands-free speaking valve
- fitting tracheostoma vents/buttons/tubes.

Specialized training is required when working with laryngectomees. The American Speech-Language-Hearing Association has published approved guidelines for "Evaluation and Treatment for Tracheoeosophageal Fistulization/Puncture."[133] A number of workshops and seminars are available for the speech-language pathologist throughout the year for basic training as well as acquiring information on the latest procedures and techniques. The International Center for Post-Laryngectomy Voice Restoration in Indianapolis, Indiana, offers monthly courses, and Atos Medical offers scheduled courses in Voice Restoration and Pulmonary Rehabilitation after Total Laryngectomy. The International Association of Laryngectomees Voice Rehabilitation Institute offers a yearly 5-day training conference. A number of voice institutes also offer courses in laryngectomy rehabilitation. Postings are listed in the *ASHA Leader* or the website.

Patient Evaluation

Although most laryngectomized patients may be candidates for surgical prosthetics, certain social situations and medical and physical conditions may decrease the chances for long-term successful use.

For example, patient motivation is important. At times, the family may be more motivated than the patient to attempt this form of communication. In most cases, however, the patient must be capable of and interested in caring for the prosthesis. Andrews et al listed a number of characteristics necessary for patient selection in using the voice prosthesis.[132] These include the following:

- motivation and mental stability
- adequate understanding of the anatomy and the mechanics of the prosthesis
- adequate manual dexterity and visual acuity to care for the stoma and the prosthesis
- no significant hypopharyngeal stenosis

- speech production with esophageal insufflation via a properly positioned esophageal catheter
- adequate pulmonary reserve
- stoma of adequate depth and diameter to accept the prosthesis without airway compromise.

Singer and Blom reported that chronic pulmonary disease, diabetes, and alcoholism have not presented significant problems.[125] Our experience has not been positive with patients who have chronic drinking problems. Alcohol abuse has also been found to be a major deterrent in the production of efficient voice as well as personal care of the tracheoesophageal puncture.[131,134,135]

Cricopharyngeal spasm[136,137] and pharyngeal constrictor hypertonicity[138] have been implicated as reasons for failure to utilize the voice prosthesis successfully. An esophageal air insufflation test, a procedure described by Blom et al,[139] informs the speech-language pathologist, surgeon, or both of the ability of the PE segment to vibrate. In this procedure a marked 14-Fr catheter is inserted transnasally into the upper esophagus to approximately the 25-cm mark (Figure 9–25).

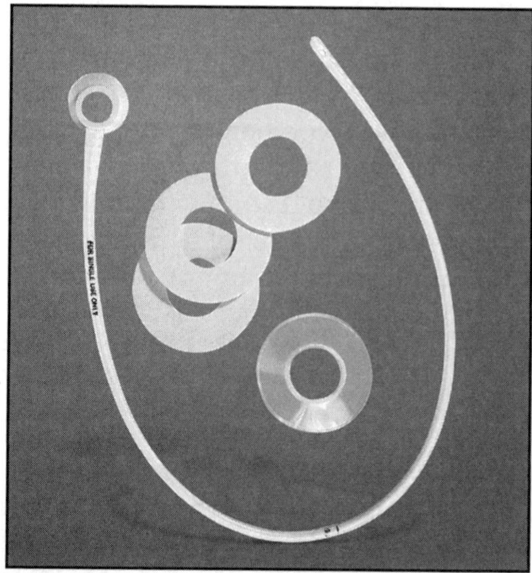

FIGURE 9–25. Blom-Singer Insufflation Test Set. (Photo courtesy of InHealth Technologies, http://www.inhealth.com)

Inserting the catheter to this point ensures the tip of the catheter to be at the approximate level of the cervical esophagus near the proposed tracheoesophageal puncture. Tracheostoma tape housing with an adapter is attached to the peristomal skin. Patients are instructed to open and relax the jaw for the production of the vowel, /a/, inhale deeply, and sustain the vowel for as long as possible while the examiner or patient occludes the stoma adaptor redirecting the air into the esophagus. With this self-insufflation test, the patient should be able to sustain phonation of a vowel without interruption of the sound for 10 to 15 seconds and produce fluent speech when counting or saying sentences. If the patient's sound production is strained or experiences esophageal spasms, the patient may be a candidate for a surgical procedure of botulinum neurotoxin injections to allow the PE segment to vibrate. The air insufflation test is valuable for successful patient selection. This test indicates in advance those patients who are likely to experience esophageal spasms postsurgically. If spasms do occur, the patient is prepared for this possibility. A manometer (Figure 9–26) has also been used to record pressure changes in the esophagus.[139,140]

Yetiser et al[141] found insufflation testing was 43% accurate and manometric measurements 86% accurate in evaluating and predicting patients who would develop esophageal speech or tracheoesophageal speech. Techniques for management of pharyngeal con-

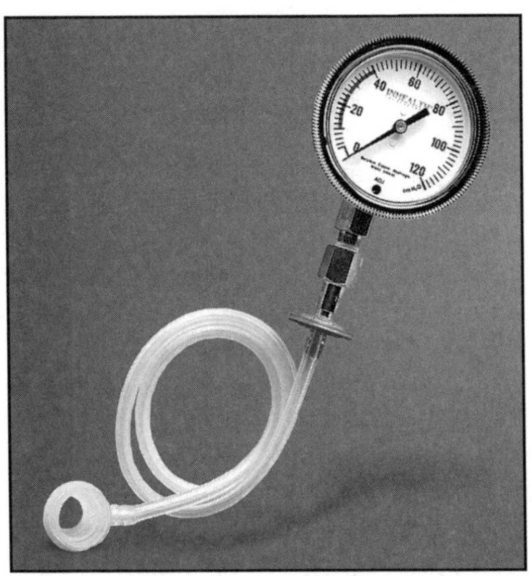

FIGURE 9–26. Manometer with manometer adaptor. (Photo courtesy of InHealth Technologies, http://www.inhealth.com)

strictor hypertonicity included secondary and primary pharyngeal constrictor muscle myotomy, pharyngeal neurectomy, botulinum toxin injections, and Chessman technique.[142] Rather than a surgical approach to treatment of spasms or hypertonicity of the laryngectomized pharynx, unilateral chemical denervation of the pharyngeal constrictor muscles with botulinum neurotoxin type A has proven to be very successful in eliminating muscle spasms.[143,144] A myotomy involves cutting muscle fibers of the pharyngeal constrictors to prevent esophageal spasms when voicing. Pharyngeal neurectomy is a resection of all branches in the nerve plexus to eliminate hypertonicity or spasms. The Chessman technique involves surgical closure of the pharyngeal constrictors to reduce hypertonicity and esophageal spasms.[142]

A trial injection of lidocaine into the pharyngoesophageal segment is a prognostic indicator for successful TEP speech after botulinum neurotoxin injections in an individual with spasms. If the patient has a positive response to the lidocaine block demonstrating decreased phonatory effort and no spasms, percutaneous botulinum neurotoxin type A injections under EMG guidance are administered to the cricopharyngeus at 3 separate sites.[145] Some patients may need repeated injections to help relax the PE segment. Botulinum neurotoxin injections along with voice therapy may facilitate TEP speech and maintain controlled relaxation of the PE segment during speaking. As a result, repeated injections may not be necessary.

Patient Fitting

To prevent the risk of disease transmission from blood-borne pathogens, the speech-language pathologist must follow Universal Precautions when fitting a voice prosthesis. These precautions can be reviewed in the "Centers for Disease Control Morbidity and Mortality Weekly Report"[146] or in ASHA's "Aids/HIV Update."[147] The American Speech-Language Hearing Association also publishes guidelines for "Evaluation and Treatment for Tracheoesophageal Fistulization/Puncture."[132]

Tracheoesophageal punctures can be surgically created primarily, at the time of the total laryngectomy, or as a secondary procedure that can be performed weeks or years after the surgery. If the tracheoesophageal puncture is performed at the time of surgery, the surgeon can place a voice prosthesis into the puncture by retrograde insertion using the Provox voice prosthesis (Provox 1) or an InHealth Classic Indwelling voice prosthesis. Generally, the surgeon places a French balloon catheter through the puncture and directs it into the distal esophagus. Prosthesis sizing and fitting takes place when the patient's surgical incisions show adequate healing, which is usually around 2 weeks following surgery. If the puncture is performed as a secondary procedure, the clinician may need to assess the integrity of the pharyngoesophageal (PE) segment and potential to produce tracheoesophageal speech by performing an insufflation test as described previously. If the insufflation test produces no voice, or poor quality and limited sustained voicing, 4 possible conditions should be considered: (1) hypotonicity, (2) hypertonicity, (3) PE spasm, or (4) stricture.[148] If hypotonicity is suspected, digital pressure to the PE segment or to the external neck may help direct the air for better phonation. When hypertonicity or spasticity is suspected, treatment may include surgical pharyngeal constrictor myotomy, pharyngeal plexus neurectomy, or botulinum toxin (BOTOX) injection with electromyographic or radiographic guidance. Esophageal dilation is the treatment for stricture.

At the time of fitting, the speech-language pathologist will measure the tracheoesophageal lumen for the most appropriate size. For the comfort of the patient, it is important for the clinician to give an overview of the entire fitting process and then explain each step in detail so that no surprises are incurred.[149] The following steps may be taken during the initial voice prosthesis fitting process:

- Clean the stoma area of mucus and any encrusted material using hydrogen peroxide applied with cotton applicators and wipe with 4 × 4 gauze.
- Remove any sutures that are holding the catheter in place.
- Slowly but deliberately remove the catheter from the puncture. In case of an inflated balloon catheter, the residual air or water must be withdrawn using a standard 10-cc syringe before the catheter is removed. Before removing the catheter, instruct the patient to refrain from swallowing to prevent saliva from flowing through the TEP.
- Replace the catheter with a 16-Fr soft red rubber catheter (when using a catheter make sure the larger end is knotted or capped to prevent leaking of fluids through the catheter) or a dilator (Figures 9–27A and 9–27B).

It is strongly recommended to teach the patient to always keep the puncture stented with a catheter, dilator, or voice prosthesis. Teach the patient to insert

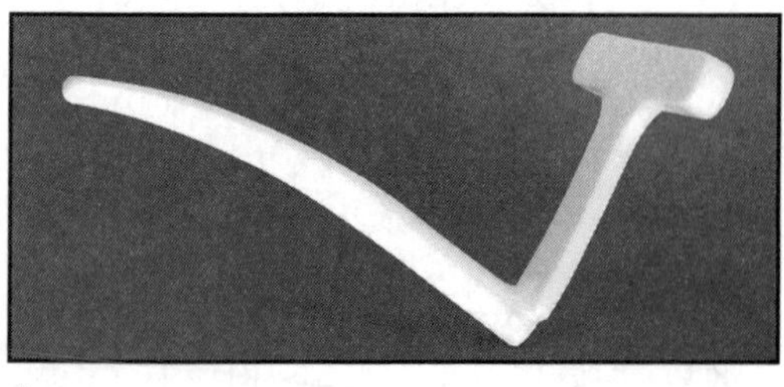
A

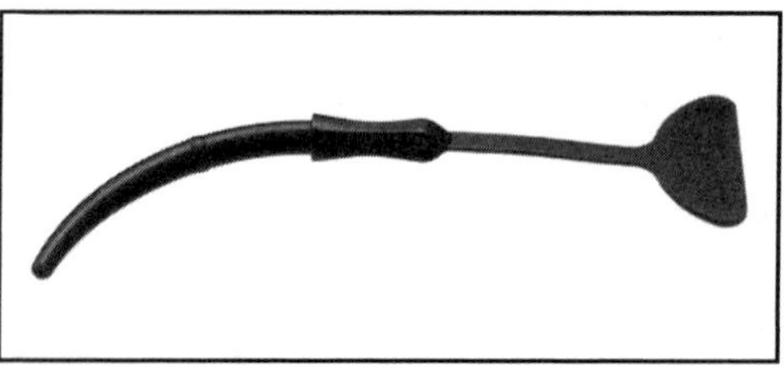
B

FIGURE 9–27. **A.** Blom-Singer tracheoesophageal dilator. **B.** Provox dilator. (Photos courtesy of Atos Medical, http://www.atosmedical.com)

the catheter or dilator in the unlikely event the voice prosthesis would ever come out.

- Control any mucus from the stoma and/or from the oral cavity and nose that was produced when the catheter was removed.
- With the catheter removed and the puncture unstented, the phonatory mechanism can be tested with the least resistance to airflow. Ask the patient to take a breath. Occlude the stoma with your thumb or finger while the patient slowly exhales while saying the vowel /a/. This gives the speech-language pathologist a subjective idea of the ease or difficulty with which the patient can produce voice. If the patient demonstrates much difficulty, then it is possible that internal edema is still present. It may also be an indication of esophageal spasm. If no voicing is produced, one should continue with the sizing and fitting procedure and have the patient return to your office in a week to work on voicing.
- Place a sizing device (Figure 9–28) into the puncture as far as it will go. The sizing device is essentially a dummy voice prosthesis that has incremental markings and numbers that correspond to the various lengths of manufactured prostheses. When the sizing device is completely inserted, you may feel the end of the device touch the posterior pharyngeal wall or go down into the esophagus. The patient can usually indicate when he or she feels the sizer against the posterior pharyngeal wall. Gently pull the sizer out until the retention collar grasps the inside of the anterior wall of the esophagus. Look at the number on the sizer that can be seen on the outside of the puncture. Choose the size prosthesis that corresponds to that number. If the size is between numbers, choose the longer prosthesis. It is best to oversize initially. If the prosthesis is sized too short, the fistula will begin to stenos at the anterior wall of the esophagus, preventing airflow through the prosthesis. The speech-language pathologist should allow for a small amount of "play" (forward/backward movement) when the patient swallows.

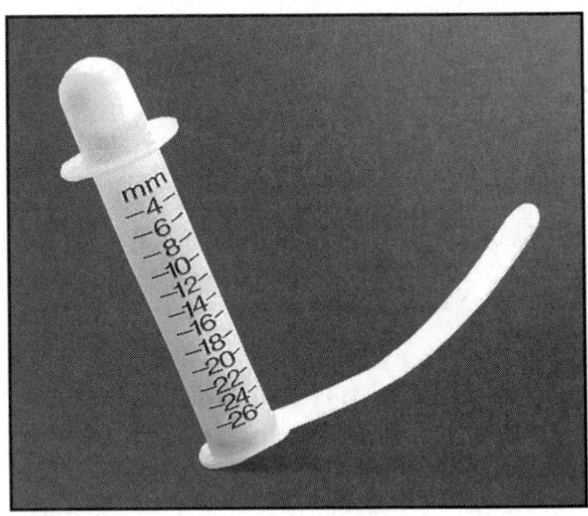

FIGURE 9–28. Blom-Singer voice prosthesis sizer. (Photo courtesy of InHealth Technologies, http://www.inhealth.com)

- Remove the sizing device and insert the correct-sized voice prosthesis into the puncture using the insertion tool. Make sure you follow the angle of the puncture and firmly push the prosthesis until you feel or hear the retention collar "pop" into the esophagus. Hold the outer flange and gently remove the insertion tool by rotating and pulling it forward. When the insertion tool has been removed, check the seating of the prosthesis by tugging gently on the flange. The prosthesis should hold firmly in place. Tape the flange to the neck.

After the prosthesis is fitted, ask the patient to inhale. Occlude the stoma with your thumb or finger while the patient exhales gently sustaining the vowel /a/. If the prosthesis is sized correctly, the diverted air will cause the PE segment to vibrate. The patient must increase effort and air pressure to speak. This air pressure is greater with the prosthesis in place than when attempting voice with an open tract.

- Check to make sure there is no leaking of fluids either around or through the voice prosthesis by having the patient drink water. If leaking is noted around the prosthesis, allow more time for the fistula to seal around the prosthesis. A new or different prosthesis should be inserted if leaking is noted through the prosthesis.
- The patient should be taught to occlude the stoma with his or her own thumb or finger and to produce voice independently. Start with sustained vowels then words such as counting. Speech material should be provided and the patient encouraged to practice frequently throughout the day.
- Teach the patient or significant other to clean the voice prosthesis without removing it. Mucus and crusts can be softened by using cotton applicators dipped in hydrogen peroxide applied to the anterior opening of the prosthesis. Using a long forceps, these crusts can then be removed.
- Schedule the patient to be seen back in the office a few days after the initial voice prosthesis fitting to learn independent care.

Independent Care

If a patient will be using a voice prosthesis that will be maintained by the patient such as the Blom-Singer Duckbill or low-pressure voice prosthesis or the Provox NID, the clinician needs to teach the patient and/or significant other to remove, clean, and reinsert the prosthesis. The prosthesis should be removed for cleaning as needed. Some patients may choose to do so weekly, and others may choose to leave the prosthesis in place for several weeks or replace when needed. It is preferred that cleaning the prosthesis as well as the stoma be performed simultaneously with adequate lighting and use of a mirror. To remove the prosthesis, the patient is instructed to firmly grasp the flange and pull forward. When the prosthesis is removed, a size 16-Fr catheter or a tracheoesophageal puncture dilator is immediately inserted into the fistula to prevent aspiration and stenosis. The prosthesis is cleaned according to the instructions given by the manufacturer. Care should be taken not to violate the valve end of the prosthesis. Solvents or petroleum-based cleaning products should not be used as they might damage the silicone.

Patients may also clean the voice prosthesis without removing the device (Figure 9–29) from the tracheoesophageal puncture by using a flushing device and/or brush (Figure 9–30).

These devices, similar to a pipette, have a plastic tapered tube with a bulb

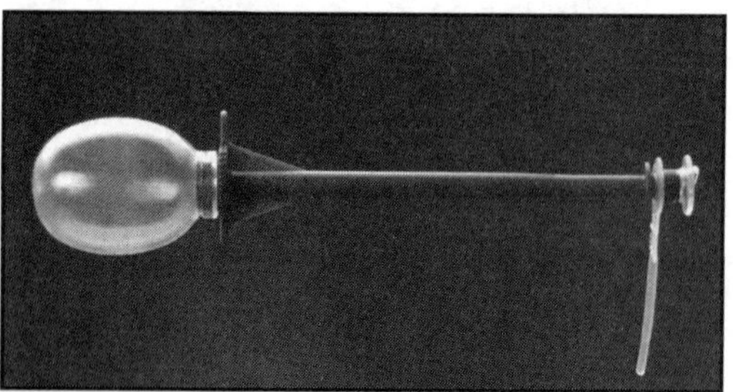

FIGURE 9–29. Provox Flush use with Provox 2 voice prosthesis. (Photo courtesy of Atos Medical, http://www.atosmedical.com)

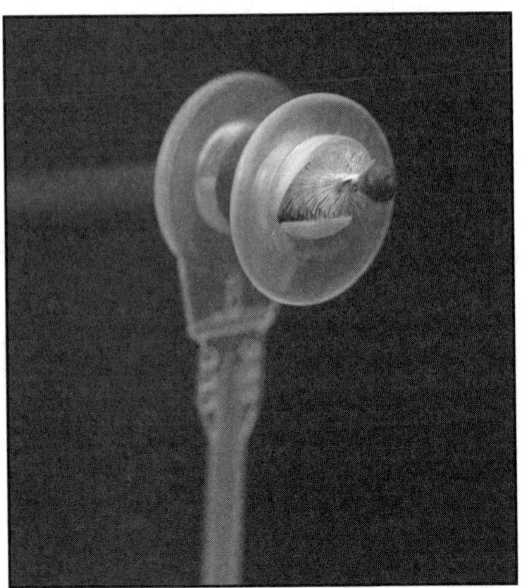

FIGURE 9–30. Provox brush in use with Provox 2 prosthesis. (Photo courtesy of Atos Medical, http://www.atosmedical.com)

on one end. The patient is instructed to fill the device with water and position the device into the voice prosthesis until it abuts against the stopper on the stem of the pipette. Once properly positioned, the patient quickly squeezes the bulb on the pipette to inject the water through the prosthesis, flushing out any debris that may have accumulated inside the prosthesis. The debris is then flushed into the esophagus. Removing the prosthesis for cleaning is recommended if a large mucous plug is contained within the prosthesis.

Instructions for self-fitting the voice prosthesis include:

- Check the slit valve or flapper valve to make sure the edges are not stuck together. Place the tip of the insertion tool into the open end of the voice prosthesis. Avoid squeezing or damaging the slit valve at the tip of the prosthesis.
- Place a small amount of oil-free, water-soluble lubricant such as Surgi-Lube on the tip of the prosthesis. Place the tip of the voice prosthesis in the fistula with the neck strap pointed upward. Firmly insert until the circular retention collar "snaps" open within the esophagus. (Insertion or removal of the prosthesis occasionally causes slight bleeding at the fistula. Persistent bleeding should be brought to the attention of the physician.)
- Place a finger against the flange and gently withdraw the insertion tool from the fully inserted prosthesis.
- Apply a small strip of hypoallergenic adhesive tape over the flange to secure it to the neck to prevent movement or accidental dislodgment.

The low-pressure voice prosthesis has a recessed valve and a low-profile tip making insertion more difficult into the fistula. An easier method of insertion for the Blom-Singer Low Pressure Voice Prosthesis is using the Blom-Singer Gel Cap Insertion System (Figure 9–31).

The gel cap provides a smooth, rounded shape to the tip by folding the retention collar in a forward position inside the cap making insertion of the prosthesis less traumatic to the surrounding tissue. The gel cap is designed to dissolve inside the esophagus within minutes after insertion. After the voice prosthesis is correctly placed in the tracheoesophageal puncture, it is important for the patient to hold the prosthesis in place with the inserter tool for at least 3 minutes, allowing time for the gel cap to dissolve and the retention collar to unfold. Explicit instructions in applying the gel cap are provided by the manufacturer.

In 1995, the Blom-Singer Indwelling Low Pressure Voice Prosthesis (Figure 9–32) was designed for patients who are unable or resist changing the Low Pressure Voice Prosthesis every 2 to 3 days as recommended.[150]

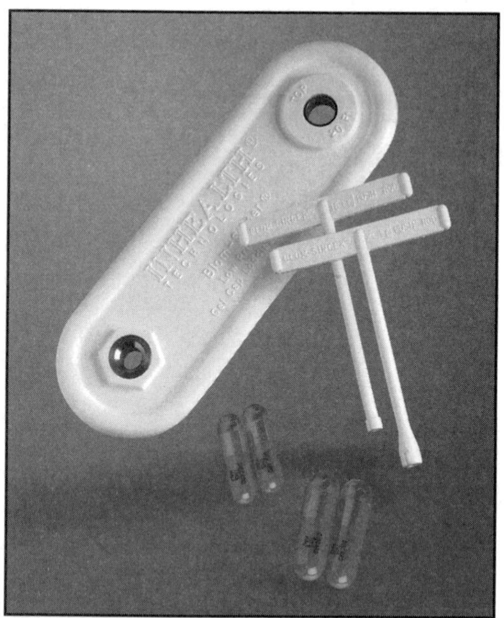

FIGURE 9–31. Blom-Singer gel cap insertion system. (Photo courtesy of InHealth Technologies, http://www.inhealth.com)

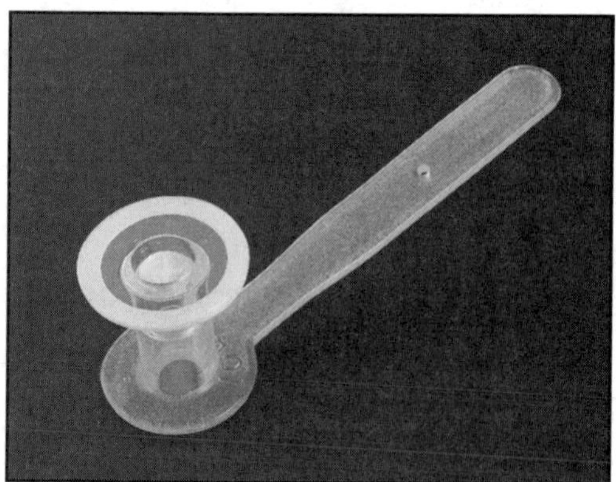

FIGURE 9–32. Blom-Singer indwelling classic voice prosthesis. (Photo courtesy of InHealth Technologies, http://www.inhealth.com)

The Blom-Singer Indwelling Low Pressure Voice Prosthesis (now referred to as the Classic Indwelling Voice Prosthesis) is a 16- or 20-Fr prosthesis inserted and removed by a physician or a trained speech-language pathologist. Inserting the prosthesis requires using the gel cap (as previously described). The Provox 2 Voice Prosthesis uses a single-use insertion tool to place the prosthesis into the tracheoesophageal puncture, and the Provox Vega uses a SmartInserter. These devices must be inserted by a trained professional.

A 22-Fr tracheoesophageal puncture dilator is inserted into the fistula to slightly dilate the opening. The dilator is removed and the voice prosthesis is inserted with the neck strap pointed upward. After insertion, the voice prosthesis is held into position for at least 3 minutes, allowing the gel cap to dissolve and the retention collar to unfold within the esophagus. Check to make sure the prosthesis is secured by rotating the prosthesis 360°. Once the prosthesis is correctly placed, the voice prosthesis strap is detached from the safety peg on the inserter. If the prosthesis does not rotate freely, an A-P radiographic examination of the tracheostoma is recommended to confirm the retention collar is positioned within the esophagus.[149]

The indwelling prosthesis may be worn until it ceases to function correctly or begins to leak. A hemostat is used to remove the prosthesis by grasping the outer rim of the device, and pulling gently and firmly until the prosthesis is completely removed. Once removed, a 22-Fr tracheostoma dilator is inserted into the puncture. Keep the dilator in the tracheoesophageal lumen for at least 5 minutes before inserting a new prosthesis. The Blom-Singer voice prosthesis is available from InHealth Technologies, and the Provox voice prosthesis is available from Atos Medical Inc.

Maximizing Communication

Once fit with the prosthesis, some patients readily occlude the stoma and speak with excellent phrasing and inflection, similar to their prelaryngectomy speech patterns. Other patients may need instruction in occluding the stoma and to coordinate proper breath control for phrasing and articulation. Patients who have used esophageal voice prior to surgical prosthetics may have to work on eliminating the habit of injecting air into the esophagus. The result of the use of a surgical prosthesis is a superior esophageal voice.

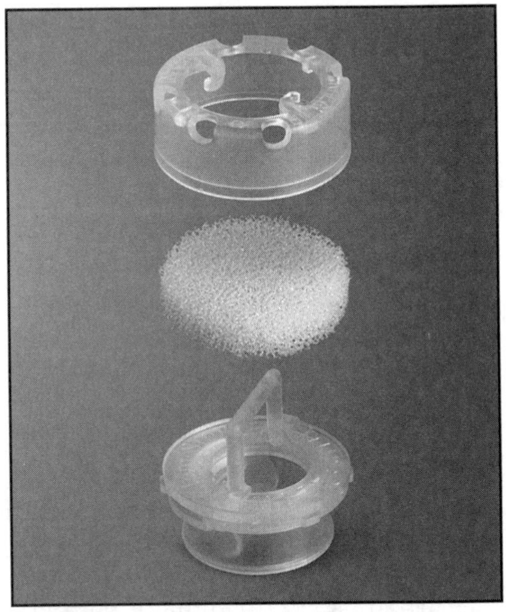

FIGURE 9–33. Blom-Singer adjustable tracheostoma Valve II with cap + foam + valve. (Photo courtesy of InHealth Technologies, http://www.inhealth.com)

Hands-Free Speaking Valve

The hands-free speaking valve is a device designed for laryngectomees who have undergone a tracheoesophageal puncture and communicate with various types of voice prosthesis. The use of this valve negates the need to manually occlude the stoma for speech production, thus freeing both hands. The Blom-Singer Adjustable Tracheostoma Valve II (Figure 9–33) is available from InHealth Technologies, and the Provox FreeHands HME (Figure 9–34) is available from Atos Medical.

In evaluating patient use of the valve, the speech-language pathologist focuses on the size, shape, and contour of the stoma and surrounding tissue. Each device comes with its own heat moisture exchange filter to moisten, warm, and filter inspired air.

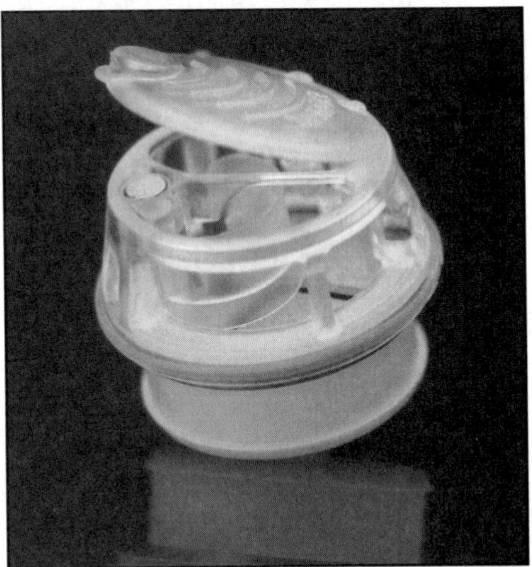

FIGURE 9–34. Provox FreeHands HME. (Photo courtesy of Atos Medical, http://www.atosmedical.com)

Successful use of the speaking valve depends on the ability to tape and glue the valve collar to a sufficient amount of tissue surrounding the stoma to prevent it from being dislodged by the pulmonary air pressure. Patients with sunken stomas or uneven skin tissue surrounding the stoma may not have an adequate skin surface for collar adhesion. Other factors that may influence wearing a speaking valve include phlegm production, back-pressure, age, and motivation.[73]

The first step in evaluating patient use is to attach the peristomal housing. Once the adhesive base plate is in place, the tracheostoma valve is fitted. The Blom-Singer Tracheostoma Valve has an internal adjustment sensitivity that allows the patient to adjust the valve from ultralight to medium sensitivity by rotating the faceplate. There are three membranes, each with different closing resistance that comes with the Provox FreeHands HME speaking valve. The proper membrane weight (light, medium, or strong) is the weight that does not close during heavy respiratory effort but will close when sufficient air pressure is exhaled to produce speech. The speech-language pathologist should help the laryngectomee select a speaking valve that requires a lower resistance during resting breathing and not too much effort to close the valve for speaking.[151]

A simple way to determine the degree of valve closure or proper valve weight (depending on the type of valve) is to have the patient walk up and down steps. Begin with the ultralight setting or valve in place. If the valve closes when the patient is breathing heavily, turn the valve slightly, or if using a valve or spring move up to the next weight. Continue this process until a valve that does not close during heavy breathing is found. The device will allow for the patient to breathe without closure of the membrane/valve during heavy demands on breathing when the device is turned to an open position.

Excessive intratracheal pressure can contribute to an adhesive seal breakdown of the housing when using the tracheostoma valve. Manometric measurements can assess intratracheal back-pressure. This measurement is performed by placing the adapter from a disposable Blom-Singer Insufflation test kit into the tracheostoma valve housing and attaching a manometer to the adapter. For normal conversational intensity levels, manometric readings should range between 30 and 35 cm H_2O. Measurements greater than 35 cm H_2O indicate higher intratracheal airflow pressure and less time the patient may be able to wear the valve. The manometer may be used as a visual feedback tool to monitor the degree of pressure and serve to control intensity levels.[152] Contributing causes for increased intratracheal pressure may be the voice prosthesis diameter (16-Fr versus 20-Fr) and/or pharyngeal constrictor muscle hypertonicity.

Coughing can present a problem for all tracheostoma valve users. The valve may need to be completely removed when coughing as a result of increased air pressure produced when coughing. Sometimes repeated coughing causes strain on the adhesive discs that hold the housing collar in place, causing premature leaking of air around the housing. Increased mucus may also work the adhesive free from the skin. Still, another complication is skin irritation from the adhesive. At times even when a commercial skin preparation is brushed on the skin prior to the adherent, some patients still experience skin irritation.

SUMMARY

Although significant advancements have been made in the treatment of head and neck cancer, total rehabilitation of the laryngectomized patient continues to present challenges for the patient, the patient's family, and for all professionals involved in this process. Rehabilitation involves a multidisciplinary approach in addressing the patient's physical and psychosocial needs in a comprehensive and timely manner. The speech-language pathologist's role in working with the cancer patient and family involves both counseling and management of all communication and swallowing needs. Our interactions with the patient and family may, at times, be challenging and personally stressful, but most often the results of our efforts are both satisfying and rewarding. No other group of communicatively impaired patients has the potential to progress from very limited communication to functional oral communication as rapidly as the laryngectomized patient.

The total laryngectomy has several communication options from which to choose. The speech-language pathologist is encouraged to become familiar with all options and for the sake of the patient, to show no biases against any. As research continues to expand and improve these options, so too will the role of the speech-language pathologist.

HELPFUL WEBSITES ON HEAD AND NECK CANCERS

American Academy of Otolaryngology-Head and Neck Surgery (AAO-HNS)
http://www.entnet.org

American Association for Cancer Research (AACR)
http://aacr.org

American Cancer Society
http://www.cancer.org

American Cancer Society
http://cancer.org/clinical trials/

American Cancer Society has a section called "Caregivers"
http://www.cancer.org/treatment/caregivers/index

American Head and Neck Society (AHNS)
http://ahns.info

American Head and Neck Society
http://www.headandneckcancer.org

American Institute for Cancer Research (AICR)
http://aicr.org

American Society of Clinical Oncology (ASCO)
http://asco.org

American Society of Clinical Oncology's People with Cancer
http://www.plwc.org

American Society for Therapeutic Radiology & Oncology (ASTRO)
http://astro.org

Association of Cancer Online Resources (ACOR)
http://www.acor.org

Australia "Cancer Council Australia"
http://www.cancer.org.au

Canadian Cancer Society
http://www.cancer.ca

CancerCare
http://www.cancercare.org

Cancer Council New South Wales
http://www.cancercouncil.com.au

Cancer.net
http://www.cancer.net

Cancer Survivors Network
http://csn.cancer.org

CarePages
http://www.carepages.com

Chemocare.com
http://www.chemocare.com

Chemotherapy and You National Cancer Institute
http://www.cancer.gov/cancertopics/covers-chemotherapy-and-you.pdf

Eating Hints—National Cancer Institute
http://www.cancer.gov/cancertopics/eatinghints.pdf

Head and Neck Cancer Alliance
http://www.headandneck.org

International Association of Laryngectomees (IAL)
http://www.theial.com

Irish Cancer Society
http://www.cancer.ie

Medlineplus
http://www.medlineplus.gov

Medlineplus (cancers)
http://www.nlm.nih.gov/medlineplus/cancers.html

Medlineplus (head and neck cancer)
http://www.nlm.nih.gov/medlineplus/headandneckcancer.html

Mouth Cancer Foundation
http://www.mouthcancerfoundation.org

National Cancer Institute
http://www.cancer.gov

National Cancer Institute
http://www.cancer.gov/clinicaltrials

National Cancer Institute (head and neck cancers)
http://www.cancer.gov/cancertopics/factsheet/Sites-Types/head-and-neck

National Cancer Institute's Cancer Information Service (CIS) http://www.cancer.gov/aboutnci/cis

National Coalition for Cancer Survivorship
http://www.canceradvocacy.org

National Comprehensive Cancer Network (NCCN)
http://nccn.org

National Institute of Dental and Craniofacial Research
http://www.nidcr.nih.gov

National Library of Medicine (NLM)
http://nlm.nih.gov

Oral Cancer Foundation
http://www.oralcancerfoundation.org

Patient Advocate Foundation
http://www.patientadvocate.org

RadiologyInfo
http://www.radiologyinfo.org

Radiation Therapy: the USA's National Cancer Institute has an online book, *Radiation Therapy and You: Support for People with Cancer*
http://www.cancer.gov/cancertopics/coping/radiation-therapy-and-you

Society of Otorhinolaryngology and Head-Neck Nurses (SOHN)
http://sohnnurse.com

Support for People with Oral and Head and Neck Cancer (SPOHNC)
http://www.spohnc.org

Surveillance Epidemiology and End Results (SEER)
http://seer.cancer.gov

The Centers for Disease Control and Prevention
http://www.cdc.gov/hpv/cancer.html

United Kingdom's big Macmillan Cancer Support
http://www.macmillan.org.uk

USA Government Clinical Trials
http://www.clinicaltrials.gov

US Department of Veteran Affairs (VA)
http://va.gov

WebWhispers–Internet Support Group for Laryngectomees
http://www.webwhispers.org

REFERENCES

1. Parkin DM, Bray F, Ferlay J, Pisani P. Global cancer statistics, 2002. *CA Cancer J Clin*. 2005;55(2):74–108.
2. Carew JF, Shah JP. Advances in multimodality therapy for laryngeal cancer. *CA Cancer J Clin*. 1998;48:211–228.
3. Siegel R, Naishadham D, Jemal A. Cancer statistics, 2013. *CA Cancer J Clin*. 2013;63:11–30.
4. Jaworowska E, Serrano-Fernández P, Tarnowska C, et al. Clinical and epidemiological features of familial laryngeal cancer in Poland. *Cancer Detect Prev*. 2007;31:270–275.
5. Shah JP, Karnell LH, Hoffman HT, et al. Patterns of care for cancer of the larynx in the United States. *Arch Otolaryngol Head Neck Surg*. 1997;123:475–483.
6. Seiwert TY, Cohen EEW. State-of-the-art management of locally advanced head and neck cancer. *Br J Cancer*. 2005;92:1341–1348.
7. Rothman KJ, Cann CI, Flanders D, Fried MP. Epidemiology of laryngeal cancer. *Epidemiol Rev*. 1980;2:195–209.
8. Casper J, Colton R. *Clinical Manual for Laryngectomy and Head/Neck Cancer Rehabilitation*. 2nd ed. San Diego, CA: Singular Publishing Group; 1998.
9. Goldenberg D, Lee J, Koch WM, et al. Habitual risk factors for head and neck cancer. *Otolaryngol Head Neck Surg*. 2004;131:986–993.
10. Dahlstrom BS, Little JA, Zafereo ME, Lung M, Wei Q, Sturgis EM. Squamous cell carcinoma of the head and neck in never smoker-never drinkers: a descriptive epidemiologic study. *Head Neck*. 2008;30:75–84.
11. D'Souza G, Kreimer AR, Viscidi R, et al. Case-control study of human papillomavirus and oropharyngeal cancer. *N Engl J Med*. 2007;356:1944–1956.
12. deVilliers EM, Fauquet C, Broker TR, Bernard HU, zurHausen H. Classification of papillomaviruses. *Virology*. 2004;324:17–27.
13. Kroupis C, Vourlidis N. Human papilloma virus (HPV) molecular diagnostics. *Clin Chem Lab Med*. 2011;49:1783–1799.
14. Tran N, Rose BR, O'Brien, CJ. Role of Human Papillomavirus in the etiology of head and neck cancer. *Head Neck*. 2007;29:64–70.
15. Parkin DM, Bray F. The burden of HPV-related cancers. *Vaccine*. 2006;24(suppl 3):S11–S25.
16. Tachezy R, Klozar J, Rubenstein L, et al. Demographic and risk factors in patients with head and neck tumors. *J Med Virol*. 2009;81:878–887.
17. El-Serag HB, Hepworth EJ, Lee P, Sonnenberg A. Gastroesophageal reflux disease is a risk factor for laryngeal and pharyngeal cancer. *Am J Gastroenterol*. 2001;96:2013–2018.
18. Koufman JA. The otolaryngologic manifestations of gastroesophageal reflux disease (GERD): a clinical investigation of 225 patients using ambulatory 24-hour pH monitoring and an experimental investigation of the role of acid and pepsin in the development of laryngeal

injury. *Laryngoscope*. 1991;101(4, pt 2, suppl 53):1–78.
19. Qadeer MA, Colabianchi N, Vaezi MF. Is GERD a risk factor for laryngeal cancer? *Laryngoscope*. 2005;115:486–491.
20. Bacciu A, Mercante G, Igegnoli A, et al. Effects of gastroesophageal reflux disease in laryngeal carcinoma. *Clin Otolaryngol*. 2004;29:545–548.
21. Pressman J, Dowdy A, Libby R, Fields M. Studies upon the submucosal compartments and lymphatics of the larynx by the injection of dyes and radioisotopes. *Ann Otol Rhinol Laryngol*. 1956;65:766–980.
22. American Cancer Society. *Cancer Statistics*. 2008. Atlanta, GA: American Cancer Society.
23. Stenson KM, MacCracken E, List M, et al. Swallowing function in patients with head and neck cancer prior to treatment. *Arch Otolaryngol Head Neck Surg*. 2000;126:371–377.
24. Raber-Durlacher JE, Brennan MT, Rouleau TS, et al. Swallowing dysfunction in cancer patients. *Support Care Cancer*. 2012;20:433–443.
25. Schuller DE, Schleuning AJ, Schleuning II J. *Deweese and Saunders' Otolaryngology-Head and Neck Surgery*. 8th ed. St. Louis, MO: CV Mosby; 1994.
26. Raitiola H, Pukander J. Symptoms of laryngeal carcinoma and their prognostic significance. *Acta Oncolog*. 2000; 39:213–216.
27. Dammann F, Horger M, Mueller-Berg M, et al. Rational diagnosis of squamous cell carcinoma of the head and neck region: comparative evaluation of CT, MRI, and 18F-FDG PET. *Am J Roentgenol*. 2005;184:1326–1331.
28. Ha PK, Hdeib A, Goldenberg D, et al. The role of positron emission tomography and computed tomography fusion in the management of early-stage and advanced-stage primary head and neck squamous cell carcinoma. *Arch Otolaryngol Head Neck Surg*. 2006;1:12–16.
29. Adams S, Baum RP, Stuckensen T, Bitter K, Hor G. Prospective comparison of 18F-FDG PET with conventional imaging modalities (CT, MRI, US) in lymph node staging of head and neck cancer. *Eur J Nucl Med*. 1998;25:1255–1260.
30. Compton CC, Byrd DR, Garcia-Aguilar J, Kurtzman SH, Olawaiye A, Washington MK. *AJCC Cancer Staging Atlas: A Companion to the Seventh Editions of the AJCC Cancer Staging Manual and Handbook*. 7th ed. New York, NY: Springer; 2012.
31. Harrison JA, Wilson KM. Current trends in head and neck cancer. ASHA: *Perspectives on Voice Voice Dis*. 2006;16:3–9.
32. Patel SG, Shah JP. TMN staging of cancers of the head and neck: striving for uniformity among diversity. *CA Cancer J Clin*. 2005;55:242–258.
33. Robbins KT, Clayman G, Levine PA, et al. Neck dissection classification update: revisions proposed by the American Head and Neck Society and the American Academy of Otolaryngology-Head and Neck Surgery. *Arch Otolaryngol Head Neck Surg*. 2002;128: 751–758.
34. Kumar P. Radiation therapy of the larynx and hypopharynx. In: Cummings C Jr, Haughey BH, Thomas JR, et al, eds. *Cummings Otolaryngology: Head and Neck Surgery*. 4th ed. Philadelphia, PA: Elsevier Mosby; 2005:2401–2419.
35. Department of Veterans Affairs Laryngeal Cancer Study Group. Induction chemotherapy plus radiation compared with surgery plus radiation in patients with advanced laryngeal cancer. *N Engl J Med*. 1991;324:1685–1690.
36. Al-Sarraf M, LeBlanc M, Giri PG, et al. Chemoradiotherapy versus radiotherapy in patients with advanced nasopharyngeal cancer: phase III randomized intergroup study 0099. *J Clin Oncol*. 1998;16(4):1310–1317.
37. Forastiere A, Maor M, Weber RS, et al. Long-term results of intergroup RTOG 91-11: a phase III trial to preserve the larynx-induction cisplatin/5FU and radiation therapy versus concurrent cisplatin and radiation therapy ver-

sus radiation therapy. *J Clin Oncol.* 2006;24:18s.
38. Bourhis J, Pignon J-P. Update on MACH-NC (meta-analysis of chemotherapy in head neck cancer) database focused on concomitant chemoradiotherapy. *J Clin Oncol.* 2004;22(14S):Abstr 5505.
39. Lefebvre JL. Laryngeal preservation in head and neck cancer: multidisciplinary approach. *Lancet Oncol.* 2006;7:747–755.
40. Forastiere AA, Goepfert H, Maor M, et al. Concurrent chemotherapy and radiotherapy for organ preservation in advanced laryngeal cancer. *N Engl J Med.* 2003;349:2091–2098.
41. Fung K, Lyden TH, Lee J, et al. Voice and swallowing outcomes of an organ-preservation trial for advanced laryngeal cancer. *Int J Radiat Oncol Biol Phys.* 2005;63:1395–1399.
42. Kuppersmith RB, Greco SC, Teh BS, et al. Intensity-modulated radiotherapy: first results with this new technology on neoplasms of the head and neck. *Ear Nose Throat J.* 1999;78:238–251.
43. Lee N, Puri DR, Blanco AI, Chao KSC. Intensity-modulated radiation therapy in head and neck cancers: an update. *Head Neck.* 2007;10:387–400.
44. Kian Ang K, Trotti A, Garden AS, Foote RL. Importance of overall time factor in postoperative radiotherapy. In: *Proceedings of the Fourth International Conference on Head and Neck Cancer,* July 28–August 1; Toronto, Canada. Arlington, VA: Society of Head and Neck Surgeons; 1996:231–235.
45. Parsons JT, Mendenhall WM, Stringer SP, Cassisi NJ, Million RR. An analysis of factors influencing the outcome of postoperative irradiation for squamous cell carcinoma of the oral cavity. *Int J Radiat Oncol Biol Phys.* 1997;39:137–148.
46. Seiwert TY, Salama JK, Vokes EE. The concurrent chemoradiation paradigm-general principles. *Nat Clin Pract Oncol.* 2007;4:86–100.
47. Clayman C. *The American Medical Association Home Medical Library: Fighting Cancer.* Pleasantville, NY: American Medical Association; 1991.
48. Chan ATC, Ma BBY, Lo YMD, et al. Phase II study of neoadjuvant carboplatin and paclitaxel followed by radiotherapy and concurrent cisplatin in patients with locoregionally advanced nasopharyngeal carcinoma: therapeutic monitoring with plasma Epstein-Barr virus DNA. *J Clin Oncol.* 2004;22: 3053–3060.
49. Garden AS, Harris J, Vokes EE, et al. Preliminary results of Radiation Therapy Oncology Group 97-03: a randomized phase II trial of concurrent radiation and chemotherapy for advanced squamous cell carcinomas of the head and neck. *J Clin Oncol.* 2004;22:2856–2864.
50. Seiwert TY, Salama JK, Vokes EE. The chemoradiation paradigm-head and neck cancer. *Nat Clin Pract Oncol.* 2007;41:56–171.
51. Adelstein DJ, Saxton JP, Lavertu P, et al. Maximizing local control and organ preservation in stage IV squamous cell head and neck cancer with hyperfactionated radiation and concurrent chemotherapy. *J Clin Oncol.* 2002;20:1405–1410.
52. Haraf DJ, Rosen FR, Stenson K, et al. Induction chemotherapy followed by concomitant TFHX chemoradiotherapy with reduced dose radiation in advanced head and neck cancer. *Clin Cancer Res.* 2003;9:5936–5943.
53. Vokes EE, Stenson K, Rosen FR, et al. Weekly carboplatin and paclitaxel followed by concomitant paclitaxel, fluorouracil, and hydroxyurea chemoradiotherapy: curative and organ-preserving therapy for advanced head and neck cancer. *J Clin Oncol.* 2003;21:320–326.
54. Pfister DG, Su YB, Kraus DH, et al. Concurrent cetuximab, Cisplatin, and concomitant boost radiotherapy for locoregionally advanced, squamous cell head and neck cancer: a pilot phase II study of a new combined-modality paradigm. *J Clin Oncol.* 2006;24: 1072–1078.

55. Suntharalingam M. The use of carboplatin and paclitaxel with daily radiotherapy in patients with locally advanced squamous cell carcinomas of the head and neck. *Int J Radiat Oncol Biol Phys*. 2000;47:49–56.
56. Bourhis J. Update of MACH-NC (meta-analysis of chemotherapy in head and neck cancer) database focused on concomitant chemoradiotherapy. *J Clin Oncol*. 2004;22:5505.
57. Forastiere AA, Goepfert H, Maor M, et al. Concurrent chemotherapy and radiotherapy for organ preservation in advanced laryngeal cancer. *N Engl J Med*. 2003;349:2091–2098.
58. Huntley TC, Borrowdale RW. Tracheoesophageal voice restoration following laryngopharyngectomy and laryngopharyngoesophagectomy. In: Blom ED, Singer MI, Hamaker RC, eds. *Tracheoesophageal Voice Restoration Following Total Laryngectomy*. San Diego, CA: Singular Publishing Group; 1998:41–49.
59. Ariyan S. The pectoralis major myocutaneous flap. A versatile flap for reconstruction in the head and neck. *Plast Reconstr Surg*. 1979;63:73–81.
60. Murakami Y, Saito S, Ikari T, Haraguehi S, Okada D, Maruyama T. Esophageal reconstruction with a skin grafted pectoralis major muscle flap. *Arch Otolaryngol Head Neck Surg*. 1982;108:719.
61. Anthony JP, Singer MI, Mathes SJ. Pharyngoesophageal reconstruction using the tubed radial forearm flap. *Clin Plast Surg*. 1994;21:137–147.
62. Shangold LM, Urken ML, Lawson W. Jejunal transplantation for pharyngoesophageal reconstruction. *Otolaryngol Clin North Am*. 1991;24:1321.
63. Smith BG, Lewin JS. Lymphedema management in head and neck cancer. *Curr Opin Otolaryngol Head Neck Surg*. 2010;18:153–158.
64. Humphris GM. The missing member of the head and neck multidisciplinary team: the psychologist. Why we need them. *Curr Opin Otolaryngol Head Neck Surg*. 2008;16:108–112.
65. Campinelli PA. Audiological considerations in achieving esophageal voice. *Eye Ear Nose Throat Monthly*. 1964;43:76–80.
66. Diedrich WM, Youngstrom KA. *Alaryngeal Speech*. Springfield, IL: Charles C. Thomas; 1966.
67. LaBorwit L. Speech rehabilitation for laryngectomized patients. *Ear Nose Throat J*. 1980;59:82–89.
68. Clark J, Stemple J. Assessment of three modes of alaryngeal speech with a synthetic sentence identification (SSI) task in varying message-to-competition ratios. *J Speech Hear Res*. 1982;25:333–338.
69. Hilgers FJ, Aaronson NK, Ackerstaff AH, Schouwenburg PF, van Zandwikj N. The influence of a heat and moisture exchanger (HME) on the respiratory symptoms after total laryngectomy. *Clin Otolaryngol*. 1991;16:152–156.
70. Ackerstaff AH, Hilgers FJ, Aaronson HK, Balm AJ, van Zandwikj N. Improvements in respiratory and psychosocial functioning following total laryngectomy by the use of a heat and moisture exchanger. *Ann Otol Rhinol Laryngol*. 1993;102:878–883.
71. Grolman W, Schouwenburg PF. Postlaryngectomy airway humidification and air filtration. In: Blom ED, Singer MI, Hamaker RC, eds. *Tracheoesophageal Voice Restoration Following Total Laryngectomy*. San Diego, CA: Singular Publishing Group; 1998:109–121.
72. Grolman W, Blom ED, Branson RD, Schouwenburg PF, Hamaker RC. An efficiency comparison of four heat and moisture exchangers used in the laryngectomized patient. *Laryngoscope*. 1997;107:814–820.
73. Grolman W, Schouwenburg PF, deBoer MF, Knegt PP, Spoelstra HA, Meeuwis CA. First results with the Blom-Singer adjustable tracheostoma valve. *ORL J Otorhinolaryngol Relat Spec*. 1995;57:165–170.
74. Keith R. *Looking Forward: A Guidebook for the Laryngectomy*. 2nd ed. New York, NY: Thieme Medical Publishers; 1991.

75. Bohnenkamp TA. The effects of a total laryngectomy on speech breathing. *Curr Opin Otolaryngol Head Neck Surg.* 2008;16:200–204.
76. Ward EC, Hartwig P, Scott J, Trickey M, Cahill L, Hancock K. Speech breathing patterns during tracheoesophageal speech. *Asia Pacific J Speech Lang Hear.* 2006;10:33–42.
77. Gardner W. *Laryngectomee Speech Rehabilitation.* Springfield, IL: Charles D. Thomas; 1971.
78. Logemann JA, Veis S, Colangelo L. A screening procedure for oropharyngeal dysphagia. *Dysphagia.* 1999;14: 44–51.
79. McConnel FM, Mendelsohn MS, Logemann JA. Examination of swallowing after total laryngectomy using manofluorography. *Head Neck.* 1998;9:3–12.
80. Manikantan K, Khode S, Sayed SI, et al. Dysphagia in head and neck cancer. *Cancer Treat Rev.* 2009;35(8):724–732.
81. Sullivan PA, Hartig GK. Dysphagia after total laryngectomy. *Curr Opin Otolaryngol Head Neck Surg.* 2001;9:139–146.
82. Smit CF, Tan J, Mathus-Vilegen LMH, et al. High incidence of gastropharyngeal and gastroesophageal reflux after total laryngectomy. *Head Neck.* 1998;20:619–622.
83. Herranz J, Sarandeses A, Fernandez MF, Barro, CV, Vidal JM, Gavilan J. Complications after total laryngectomy in nonradiated laryngeal and hypopharyngeal carcinomas. *Otolaryngol Head Neck Surg.* 2000;122:892–898.
84. Cady J. Laryngectomy: beyond loss of voice-caring for the patient as a whole. *Clin J Oncol Nurs.* 2002;6:1–5.
85. Van As-Brooks C, Finizia C, Ward EC. Rehabilitation of olfaction and taste following total laryngectomy. In: Ward EC, van As-Brooks CJ, eds. *Head and Neck Cancer: Treatment, Rehabilitation, and Outcomes.* San Diego, CA: Plural Publishing; 2007:325–346.
86. Doty RL, Cometto-Muniz JE. Trigeminal chemosensation. In: Doty RL, ed. *Handbook of Olfaction and Gestation.* 2nd ed. New York, NY: Marcel Dekker; 2003:981–1000.
87. Van Dam FS, Hilgers FJ, Emsbroek G, Touw FI, Van As CJ, de Jong N. Deterioration of olfaction and gestation as a consequence of total laryngectomy. *Laryngoscope.* 1999;109:1150–1155.
88. Welge-Lussen A, Kobal G, Wolfensberger M. Assessing olfactory function in laryngectomees using the Sniffin´ Sticks test battery and chemosensory evoked potentials. *Laryngoscope.* 2000;110:303–307.
89. Hilgers FJM, Van Dam FS, Keyzers S, Koster MN, Van As CJ, Muller MJ. Rehabilitation of olfaction after laryngectomy by means of a nasal airflow-inducing maneuver: The "polite yawning" technique. *Arch Otolaryngol Head Neck Surg.* 2000;126:726–732.
90. Hilgers FJM, Jansen HA, van As CJ, Polak MF, Muller MJ, vanDam S. Long-term results of olfaction rehabilitation using the nasal airflow—inducing ("polite yawning") maneuver after total laryngectomy. *Arch Otolaryngol Head Neck Surg.* 2002;128:648–654.
91. Risberg-Berlin B, Moller RY, Finizia C. Effectiveness of olfactory rehabilitation with the nasal airflow-inducing maneuver after total laryngectomy. *Arch Otolarhyngol Head Neck Surg.* 2007; 133:650–654.
92. Pressman J, Bailey B. The survey of cancer of the larynx with special reference to subtotal laryngectomy. In: Snidecor J. ed. *Speech Rehabilitation of the Laryngectomized.* Springfield, IL: Charles C. Thomas; 1968.
93. International Association of Laryngectomees. *First Aid for (Neck Breathers) Laryngectomees [No. 4521].* New York, NY: National Office of the American Cancer Society.
94. Levin, SK. Emotional aspects of laryngectomees. In: Lauder E, ed. *Self-Help for the Laryngectomee.* Unpublished manuscript; 2009:59–63.
95. Sindecor J. *Speech Rehabilitation of the Laryngectomized.* 2nd ed. Springfield, IL: Charles C. Thomas; 1968.

96. International Association of Laryngectomees, Laryngectomees Speaker's Source Book [No. 4522]. New York, NY: National Office of the American Cancer Society.
97. Blood G, Blood I. A tactic for facilitating social interaction with laryngectomees. *J Speech Hear Dis*. 1982;47:416–418.
98. Watterson TL, McFarlane SC. The artificial larynx. *Semin Speech Lang Laryngectomee Rehab*. 1995;16:205–214.
99. Keith RL, Shanks JC. Historical highlights: laryngectomy rehabilitation. In: Keith RL, Darley FL, eds. *Laryngectomee Rehabilitation*. 3rd ed. Austin, TX: Pro-Ed; 1994;1–48.
100. Shanks JC. Essentials for alaryngeal speech: psychology and physiology. In: Keith RL, Darley FL, eds. *Laryngectomee Rehabilitation*. 3nd ed. Austin, TX: Pro-Ed; 1994:191–203.
101. Xu JJ, Chen X, Lu MP, Qiao MZ. Per-ceptual evaluation and acoustic analysis of pneumatic artificial larynx. *Otolaryngol Head Neck Surg*. 2009;141:776–780.
102. Meltzner G, Hillman RE. Impact of aberrant acoustic properties on the perception of sound quality in electrolarynx speech. *J Speech Lang Hear Res*. 2005;48:766–777.
103. Graham MS. Strategies for excelling with alaryngeal speech methods. *Persp Voice Voice Dis*. 2006;16:25–32.
104. Lundstrom E, Hammarberg B, Munck-Wikland E, Edsborg N. The pharyngoesophageal segment in laryngectomees-videoradiographic, acoustic, and voice quality perceptual data. *Logopedics Phoniatrics Vocol*. 2008;33:115–125.
105. Doyle PC. *Foundations of Voice and Speech Rehabilitation Following Laryngeal Cancer*. San Diego, CA: Singular Publishing Group; 1994.
106. Duguay MJ. Esophageal speech training: the initial phase. In: Solmon SJ, Mount KH, eds. *Alaryngeal Speech Rehabilitation, for Clinicians by Clinicians*. Austin, TX: Pro-Ed; 1991:47–78.
107. Salmon S. Methods of air intake for esophageal speech and their associated problems. In: Keith RL, Darley FL, eds. *Laryngectomee Rehabilitation*. 3rd ed. Austin, TX: Pro-Ed; 1994;219–234.
108. Morrison W. The production of voice following total laryngectomy. *Arch Otolaryngol*. 1981;14:413–431.
109. Isshiki N, Snidecor J. Air intake and usage in esophageal speech. *Acta Otolaryngol*. 1965;59:559–574.
110. Berlin CI. Clinical measurement of esophageal speech. I. Methodology and curves of skill acquisition. *J Speech Hear Dis*. 1963;28:42–51.
111. Berlin CI. Clinical measurement of esophageal speech: III. Performance of nonbiases groups. *J Speech Hear Dis*. 1964;30:174–183.
112. Van den Berg J, Moolenaar-Bijl AJ. Cricopharyngeal sphincter, pitch, intensity, and fluency in oesophageal speech. *Practica Otorhinolaryngol*. 1959; 21:298–315.
113. Gates G, Ryan W, Cantu E, Hearne, E. Current status of laryngectomy rehabilitation: causes of failure. *Am J Otolaryngol*. 1982;3:8–14.
114. Aronson A. *Clinical Voice Disorders: An Interdisciplinary Approach*. New York, NY: Brian C. Decker; 1980.
115. Sloane P, Griffin J, O'Dwyer T. Esophageal insufflation and videofluoroscopy for evaluation of esophageal speech in laryngectomy patients: clinical implications. *Radiology*. 1991;181:433–438.
116. Gussenbauer C. Ueber die erste durch Th Billroth am Menschen ausgefuhrte Kehlkopf-Ecstirpation und die Anwendung eines kunstlichen Kokokopfes. *Arch. F Klin. Chir.* 1874;17: 343–356.
117. Guttman MR. Rehabilitation of the voice in laryngectomized patients. *Arch Otolaryngol*. 1932;15:478–479.
118. Kolson H, Glasgold A. Tracheo-esophageal speech following laryngectomy. *Trans Am Acad Ophthalmol Otolaryngol*. 1967;71:421–425.

119. Blom E, Singer M. Surgical-prosthetic approaches for post-laryngectomy voice restoration. In: Keith RL, Darley FL, eds. *Laryngectomy Rehabi*litation. Austin, TX: Pro-Ed; 1979.
120. Amatsu M, Matsui T, Maki T, Kanagawa K. Vocal reconstruction after total laryngectomy: a new on-stage surgical technique. *J Otolaryngol, Japan.* 1977;80:779–785.
121. Arslan M, Serafini I. Reconstructive laryngectomy: report of the first 35 cases. *Ann Otol Rhinol Laryngol.* 1972; 81:479–486.
122. Asai R. Laryngoplasty after total laryngectomy. *Arch Otolaryngol.* 1972;95: 114–119.
123. Conley J, DeAmesti F, Pierce M. A new surgical technique for the vocal rehabilitation of the laryngectomized patient. *Ann Otol Rhinol Laryngol.* 1958; 67:655–664.
124. Shedd D, Schaaf N, Weinberg B. Technical aspects of reed-fistula speech following pharyngolaryngectomy. *J Surg Oncol.* 1976;8:305–310.
125. Singer MI, Blom E. An endoscopic technique for restoration of voice after laryngectomy. *Ann Otol Rhinol Laryngol.* 1980;89:529–533.
126. Staffieri M. Laryngectomie totale avec reconstitution de la glotte phonatoire. *Rev Laryngol Otol Rhinol.* 1973;95:63–68.
127. Taub D. Air bypass voice prosthesis for vocal rehabilitation of laryngectomees. *Ann Otol Rhinol Laryngol.* 1975; 84:45–48.
128. Freeman SB, Hamaker RC. Tracheoesophageal voice restoration at time of laryngectomy. In: Blom ED, Singer MI, Hamaker RC, eds. *Tracheoesophageal Voice Restoration Following Total Laryngectomy*. San Diego, CA: Singular Publishing Group; 1998:19–25.
129. Singer MI. DeLassus Gress C. Secondary tracheoesophageal voice restoration. In: Blom ED, Singer MI, Hamaker RC, eds. *Tracheoesophageal Voice Restoration Following Total Laryngectomy*. San Diego, CA: Singular Publishing Group; 1998:27–32.
130. Hamaker RC, Singer MI, Blom ED, Daniels HA. Primary voice restoration at laryngectomy. *Arch Otolaryngol.* 1985;111:182–186.
131. Donegan J, Gluckman J, Singh J. Limitations of the Blom-Singer technique for voice restoration. *Ann Otol Rhinol Laryngol.* 1981;90:495–497.
132. Andrews JC, Mickel RA, Hanson DG, Monahan GP, Ward PH. Major complications following tracheo-esophageal puncture for voice rehabilitation. *Laryngoscope.* 1987;97:562–567.
133. American Speech-Language Hearing Association. Position statement and guidelines: evaluation and treatment for traceoesophageal fistulization/ puncture. *ASHA.* 1992;34(suppl 7): 17–21.
134. Johns ME, Cantrell RW. Voice restoration of the total laryngectomy patient: The Singer-Blom technique. *Otolaryngol Head Neck Surg.* 1981;89:82–86.
135. Schuller DE, Jarrow JE, Kelly DR, Miglets AW. Prognostic factors affecting the success of duckbill vocal restoration. *Otolaryngol Head Neck Surg.* 1983; 91:396–398.
136. Isdebski K, Reed CG, Ross JC, Hilsinger RL. Problems with tracheoesophageal fistula voice restoration in totally laryngectomized patients. *ArchOtolaryngol Head Neck Surg.* 1994;120:840–845.
137. Simpson CB, Postma GN, Stone RE, Ossoff RH. Speech outcomes after laryngeal cancer management. *Otolaryngol Clin North Am.* 1997;30:189–205.
138. Singer MI, Blom E. Selective myotomy for voice restoration after total laryngectomy. *Arch Otolaryngol.* 1981;107: 670–673.
139. Blom ED, Singer MI, Hamaker RC. An improved esophageal insufflation test. *Arch Otolaryngol.* 1985;111:211–212.
140. Martinkosky SJ. Tracheoesophageal puncture: general considerations. In: Solmon SJ, Mount KH, eds. *Alaryngeal*

Speech Rehabilitation, for Clinicians by Clinicians. Austin, TX: Pro-Ed; 1991: 107–138.

141. Yetiser S, Serce G, Mus N. Evaluation of esophageal speech in patients with total laryngectomy: a comparison of esophageal insufflation and intra-esophageal manometric tests. *Phonoscope*. 1998;4:255–264.
142. Hamaker RC, Cheesman AD. Surgical management of pharyngeal constrictor muscle hypertonicity. In: Blom ED, Singer MI, Hamaker RC, eds. *Tracheoesophageal Voice Restoration Following Total Laryngectomy*. San Diego, CA: Singular Publishing Group; 1998:83–87.
143. Crary MA, Glowasky AL. Using Botulinum toxin A to improve speech and swallowing function following total laryngectomy. *Arch Otolaryngol Head Neck Surg*. 1996;122:760–763.
144. Hoffman HT, Fisher H, VanDemark D, et al. Botulinum neurotoxin injection after total laryngectomy. *Head Neck*. 1997;19:92–97.
145. Hoffman HT, McCulloch TM. Botulinum neurotoxin for tracheoesophageal voice failure. In: Blom ED, Singer MI, Hamaker RC, eds. *Tracheoesophageal Voice Restoration Following Total Laryngectomy*. San Diego, CA: Singular Publishing Group; 1998:83–87.
146. Centers for Disease Control. Perspectives in disease prevention and health promotion update: universal precautions for prevention of transmission of human immunodeficiency virus, hepatitis B virus, and other bloodborne pathogens in health-care settings. *Morbidity and Mortality Weekly Report*. 1988; 37:377–388.
147. American Speech-Language-Hearing Association. AIDS/HIV: implications for speech-language pathologists and audiologists. *ASHA*. 1990;32:46–48.
148. Sloan PM, Griffin JM, O'Dwyer TP. Esophageal insufflation and videofluoroscopy for evaluation of esophageal speech in laryngectomy patients: clinical implications. *Radiology*. 1991:181: 433–437.
149. Leder SB, Blom ED. Tracheoesophageal voice prosthesis fitting and training. In: Blom ED, Singer MI, Hamaker RC, eds. *Tracheoesophageal Voice Restoration Following Total Laryngectomy*. San Diego, CA: Singular Publishing Group; 1998:57–65.
150. Blom ED, Hamaker RC. Tracheoesophageal voice restoration following total laryngectomy. In: Myers EN, Suen J, eds. *Cancer of the Head and Neck*. Philadelphia, PA: WB Saunders; 1996: 839–852.
151. Grolman W, VanSteenwijk RP, Grolman E, Schouwenburg PF. Airflow and pressure characteristics of three different tracheostoma valves. *Ann Otol Rhinol Laryngol*. 1998:107:312–318.
152. Blom ED. Tracheostoma valve fitting and instruction. In: Blom ED, Singer MI, Hamaker RC, eds. *Tracheoesophageal Voice Restoration Following Total Laryngectomy*. San Diego: Singular Publishing Group. 1998:103–108.

Index

Note: Color Plates are numbered consecutively, with the Color Plate page numbers preceded by CP. Page numbers in **bold** reference non-text material.

D

E

F

G

H

I

J

K

M

N

O

P

Q

R

T

U

V

W

Y

Z